BEST 162 MEDICAL SCHOOLS

AF874475

The Princeton Review

BEST 162 MEDICAL SCHOOLS

2005 EDITION

Random House, Inc.
New York
www.PrincetonReview.com

Malaika Stoll

Princeton Review Publishing, L.L.C.
2315 Broadway
New York, NY 10024
E-mail: bookeditor@review.com

© 2004 by Princeton Review Publishing, L. L. C.

All rights reserved under International and Pan-American Copyright Conventions. Published in the United States by Random House, Inc., New York, and simultaneously in Canada by Random House of Canada Limited, Toronto.

ISBN: 0-375-76420-8

Manufactured in the United States of America.

Editor: Erica Magrey
Account Manager: David Soto
Designer: Scott Harris
Production Coordinator: Greta Blau
Production Editor: Vivian Gomez

9 8 7 6 5 4 3 2 1

2005 Edition

Acknowledgments

Malaika Stoll would like to thank Steven for his support and assistance.

Special thanks must go to the hundreds of med students and scores of admissions officers who have supplied information for this book over the years. This year's edition owes a great debt to the efforts of many: to Erica Magrey for her editorial talents; to David Soto for heading the data collection efforts, and to Steven Aglione and Michelle Arnove for assisting him; to Ben Zelevansky for his data pouring wizardry and sense of humor; to Robert Franek, Editorial Director, for his enthusiasm; and to Vivian Gomez and Greta Blau for their patience and understanding.

Contents

Preface

For the past twenty-three years, The Princeton Review has offered preparatory courses and tutoring for standardized tests such as the SAT, MCAT, LSAT, GRE, GMAT, and USMLE. More than 100,000 students took our courses last year, and hundreds of thousands have bought our "Cracking" series test-prep books. At the center of our approach is the desire to help students tear away the anxiety and sense of helplessness that have surrounded these entrance exams for so many years. The Princeton Review has long been an advocate of students' right to be informed consumers.

Besides being consumers of entrance exams, students are also consumers of education. Before investing in a graduate degree, they have the right and the need to gather as much information as possible. We hope that this publication will provide students with a viable means of achieving this goal. The *Best 162 Medical Schools* contains the essentials students will need to answer both basic and advanced questions regarding their list of prospective medical schools. The 2005 edition is our most complete medical school handbook to date; it contains 128 accredited allopathic schools in the United States, including 3 in Puerto Rico, 15 accredited allopathic schools in Canada, and 19 accredited osteopathic schools.

When viewing individual schools listed in this year's guide, you will find the union of painstakingly researched school profiles coupled with school-specific statistical data. Each profile has been sent to the medical school itself for review prior to publication so that we may provide our readers with the most accurate and current information about the programs. We hope this book will serve as an important guide as you research, gather, and consider information before embarking on your medical career.

We wish you good luck as you pursue your career in medicine. If you have questions, comments or suggestions, we welcome them. Please give us your insights:

The Princeton Review
Best 162 Medical Schools
2315 Broadway
New York, NY 10024
medicaleditor@review.com

We appreciate your input and want to make our books as useful to you as they can be.

Sincerely,
Erica Magrey
Senior Editor
Admissions Services
The Princeton Review

1 How to Use This Book

Although some people describe medical school education as somewhat canned—and downplay the differences between schools—real, concrete differences do exist. Some differences, like the fact that a family medicine clerkship is two weeks at one school and eight at another, might not seem like a big deal, but such details may help convey a school's priorities. The school profile section of this guide will help you to discern such differences, and in doing so match your interests with the school that can best fulfill them. But don't just use this book to decide where to apply; also use it as a resource to help you decide when to apply or if you really want to go to medical school after all. The detailed information about course offerings and facilities will be helpful in preparing for interviews. Look at the descriptions of such pertinent information as each program's fundamental academic approach and resources, the student body, and the school's emphasis as evident in the path its graduates take—all good points to bring up in an interview and to aid in your decision of where to attend.

As you review the school profiles, keep the following in mind:

- *Just as admissions offices rely too heavily on quantitative measures to evaluate candidates (MCAT and GPAs), applicants probably rely too much on school ranking in deciding where to apply and where to go to school. Often, the criteria for ranking have little to do with how well a school will train you or how enjoyable your experience will be (NIH research dollars for example). Thus, you will find no quantitative rankings in this book.*
- *Our goal is to present accurate and complete descriptions of medical schools. Note that the admissions offices of each medical school had the opportunity to read and edit our write-ups. In deciding where to apply or where to go, you should use this book as part of your research. Take every opportunity to meet with medical students at the schools in which you are interested. Speak with more than just one student at each school, and with students in different years at each school.*
- *In response to managed care and other trends, many medical schools that traditionally focused on research or specialty medicine claim now to focus on primary care. Whether a school really has changed its focus may be partially gleaned*

from the percentage of graduates who enter primary care fields. Note, however, that definitions of primary care vary (some include Ob/Gyn for example).

- *In the Graduates section (under Students) a statistic on what percent of students match within their top one, two, or three may appear. It is interesting that the less prestigious schools often have impressive rates. This is in part because students only rank schools that they have a good chance of getting into (and at which they were successful in obtaining an invite to interview). In addition, students at less prestigious schools are less likely to enter highly specialized residency positions that are typically the most competitive. Please make note that this stat is often misleading.*
- *For most schools, we list website addresses—they are often helpful and some include candid student opinions, so try to visit them before you make a commitment to apply, interview, or attend.*

HOW THIS BOOK IS ORGANIZED

The 2005 edition of *Complete Book of Medical Schools* includes 143 U.S. and Canadian accredited medical schools. You may notice that we no longer list Puerto Rican schools separate from U.S. schools. The AAMC lists them under one umbrella, and now, so do we. The profile of each school is broken down into five text sections—Overview, Academics, Students, Admission, and Costs. The general data in the allopathic profiles is supplemented by three categories of hard stats—Student Body, Admissions, and Cost and Aid—listed in the shaded sidebar column. We also created a supplementary chapter of a complete list—including a general overview and admissions requirements—of the 19 accredited osteopathic schools.

Here's what you will find in the various text and statistic sections for each allopathic school profile:

PROFILE

ACADEMICS

First we give you a basic look at the academic program—quarter system or semester, pass/fail or honor, and USMLE requirements. Then we break it down in accordance with how your own studies will be broken down—Basic Sciences and Clinical Training—outlining the academic requirements and path of each. Here you will find out how much time you have to spend hunched over a book vs. the fun part—hunched over, say, a cadaver. We will often use the term "selective" to describe certain clinical requirements. It means that students have some choice within a specified area. Selective courses are less "free" than an "elective" (which might also have some restrictions).

Students

Discover where your potential classmates call home and who they are—percentage-wise. In the Student Life section we describe what kind of recreation facilities are available, where you might live, where you might go out. We also include information about the graduates. Who are the grads of this school—primary care physicians, surgeons, public health administrators—and in what type of community do they choose to practice?

Admissions

Pretty straightforward: The Requirements section details what the school is looking for in its prospective students. Pay special attention to Suggestions for some hints about how to impress the school. Then whip out your date book—the Process section will tell you the dates you need to know and key stats about who gets interviews and then who the lucky recipients of the fat envelopes are.

SIDEBAR

The shaded column next to each school listing contains the following information:

Student Body

Type: Is the school private or public? This is important information that is closely tied to the cost of tuition. In addition, public schools are often open to only state residents.

Enrollment: Total number of students enrolled in the medical school.

% male/female: Gender breakdown based on total enrollment.

% underrepresented minorities: Percentage of African Americans, Native Americans, Mexican Americans, and mainland Puerto Ricans in the total enrollment.

 # applied: The number of people who applied to the school in the most recently reported year, presented as the total number and the number of out-of-state/province residents who applied.

% interviewed: The percentage of applicants who interviewed at the school in the most recently reported year. Also broken down in terms of total interviewed versus out-of-state/province applicants interviewed.

% accepted: The percentage of applicants who were accepted at the school in the most recently reported year. Also broken down in terms of total and out-of-state/province.

% enrolled: The percentage of people who were accepted who actually entered the school as first-year medical students in the most recently reported entering class, in terms of total and out-of-state/province.

Average age: The average age of entering class.

ADMISSIONS

Average GPA

Overall undergraduate grade point average of the students who matriculated in the most recently reported entering class.

Average MCAT

Average MCAT scores of the students who matriculated in the most recently reported entering class, broken down into the following areas: Biology, Verbal, Physics, and Essay.

Application Information

Outlines all the dates and facts you need to know:

Regular application: The latest date by which the school must receive all application materials for regular admission.

Regular notification: The latest date by which the school will notify prospective students its decisions concerning regular admission.

Early application: The latest date by which the school must receive all application materials for the early decision plan.

Early notification: The latest date by which the school will notify prospective students of its decisions concerning admission to the early decision plan.

Transfers accepted? Yes or No.

Admissions may be deferred? Yes or No.

Interview required? Yes or No.

Application fee: How much to apply?

COSTS AND AID

Tuition & Fees

Most recent yearly tuition figures available for both state residents and nonresidents. The amount of money students can expect to spend on books and fees is listed here as well.

Financial Aid

% students receiving aid: Percentage of medical students at the school receiving some sort of financial aid.

Average grant: The amount of money in grants students receive on average.

Average loan: The amount of money lent to students on average.

Average debt: How much do students owe when they get out?

2 So You Want to Be a Doctor . . .

A GLIMPSE AT MEDICINE IN THE TWENTY-FIRST CENTURY

Do you want to be a doctor? If your answer is yes, use this chapter to prepare you for what lies ahead. (That includes medical school interviews—you can impress interviewers with your knowledge of current trends in health care!) If you're not yet sure whether medicine is the career for you, this chapter will help you decide. Learn about current issues as well as potential future trends in health care, medicine, and physician practice. The purpose of this chapter is to provide a glimpse of what life will be like for you as a doctor. Although it is impossible to predict the future, research and analysis allow us to identify some of the issues that will shape medicine in the coming years.

DECISIONS, DECISIONS . . .

Becoming a doctor requires a real commitment, so the decision to pursue this career path should be an informed one. You should consider information from discussions with medical professionals as well as from books such as this one. Talk to as many doctors as you can. Find out how they spend their days, and what they love and don't love about their profession. Think about whether you could fill their shoes, and whether you would thrive in doing so. Always consider your source when gathering information. For example, TV shows with exciting plots and attractive actors glamorize medicine, whereas newspapers sometimes do the opposite by highlighting negative trends and emphasizing scandal.

While you are fortunate to have hundreds of career options to choose from, this amount of choice can be confusing and overwhelming. Don't let indecision paralyze you. Consider taking time off after college to work in medical or nonmedical fields, to travel, or to volunteer before applying to medical school. This type of experience serves the dual purpose of allowing you to assess your interest in medicine and giving you something to write about in your medical school application essays (not to mention that it can be fun and meaningful, depending on what you do). The chapter in this book on nontraditional medical school applicants discusses several alternative paths to medical school. In deciding whether medicine is the career for you, you should also reflect on the paths that you won't be taking. Are you deciding between being a teacher or a doctor? Why not teach for a year or two and then reconsider medical school? The skills you learn teaching will help you explain medical issues to patients if you decide to become a physician.

Perhaps you feel that there are too few rather than too many career possibilities from which to choose. Some people consider medicine, law, and other obvious professions because they just don't know what else is out there. In this situation, there is nothing like spending a couple years in the "real" world. This will expose you to various professions and career options. Even working for a temp agency can be beneficial, in that it can provide exposure to a number of fields and organizations. Learning about other options might confirm your interest in medicine, or could lead you in another direction. Either way, it will be valuable use of time.

WHAT IT TAKES TO BE A DOCTOR

In some ways, being a doctor in the United States in the twenty-first century is similar to being a doctor in any number of cultures during just about any time period. There are a few traits that are essential, no matter what century it is. Consider the following questions:

Do you want to spend your life helping others?

Doctors heal people, save lives, and help others—often through direct, face-to-face interactions. According to a recent survey of medical school students, "helping others" is the primary motivation for pursuing an MD.[1] If this is your motivation, you're in good company. However, there are other altruistic careers out there, all of which involve less schooling and less debt than medical school. The desire to help others should be one, but not your only, reason for becoming a doctor.

Do you enjoy working hard?

Medicine is an incredibly challenging field. This was the case a hundred years ago when doctors worked to fight yellow fever, polio, and influenza, and it is the case today as health professionals try to prevent and treat heart disease, cancer, AIDS/HIV, and influenza, while dealing with the constraints of managed care. Consider medicine only if you love challenges, and if you know you want tremendous challenge in your professional life. As you read through this chapter, think about whether the challenges involved in practicing medicine are the ones that appeal to you. For example, a physician who is twenty years out of medical school is still expected to be familiar with the latest medical developments. One of the challenges of practicing medicine is a commitment to lifelong learning.

[1] Princeton Review survey of medical students

Are you interested in science and health issues?
If you enjoyed some aspects of your science courses (few people enjoy all aspects of premedical course work) and you find yourself drawn to health issues, there is a good chance that you will enjoy studying and practicing medicine. Although medicine has changed significantly over the years, its roots remain in basic science.

Do you like working with different people?
With the exception of a few fields, medicine involves working with people, many of whom may be very different from you. If science interests you but working with people does not, you may wish to consider a PhD rather than an MD (this choice also involves less debt). You might also look into an MD that allows you to do only research.

WHAT IT'S LIKE TO BE A DOCTOR

What is life like as a doctor in the twenty-first century? Although it varies a great deal depending on specialty, geographic region, employment situation, and so on, we get a general idea by examining recent data.[2,3]

PATIENT CARE

Most doctors—90 percent—spend their time seeing patients, in fact, seeing twenty to twenty-five patients per day on average. Doctors generally work in one of three situations: solo, as part of a group practice, or as an employee of a hospital or organization. The most common reason people go to the doctor is for some sort of check-up or test. Other common reasons for doctor visits are respiratory (allergies, the flu), gastrointestinal (heart burn, nausea), and psychological (e.g., depression) complaints. An important responsibility of the primary care physician is to identify potentially serious issues during routine examinations. On the other side of the spectrum, a major challenge for doctors with highly specialized training (e.g., oncologists, cardiologists, and surgeons) is to work intensely to save and improve lives. The most common causes of mortality (death) in the United States are listed below.

***Top Ten Causes of Mortality in the United States*[4]**

1. *Diseases of heart (heart disease)*
2. *Malignant neoplasms (cancer)*
3. *Cerebrovascular diseases (stroke)*
4. *Chronic lower respiratory diseases (e.g., emphysema, asthma, bronchitis)*

[2] Association of American Medical Colleges. AAMC Data Book. Statistical Information Related to Medical Schools and Teaching Hospitals. January 2003.
[3] The Future of American Medicine. American Medical Association, Council on Long Range Planning and Development, 1994
[4] National Center for Health Statistics, Deaths: Leading Causes for 2000.

5. *Accidents*
6. *Diabetes mellitus (diabetes type 2)*
7. *Influenza and pneumonia*
8. *Alzheimer's disease*
9. *Nephritis, nephrotic syndrome, and nephrosis (kidney disease)*
10. *Septicemia (blood poisoning)*

Please note that all of the above except Alzheimer's are preventable. Preventive medicine and the interdisciplinary approach are important elements of practicing medicine.

Workload and Compensation

On average, doctors work fifty-eight hours per week. Obstetricians work longer hours, sixty-two per week, while the typical psychiatrist works shorter hours, forty-nine per week. Although their annual incomes have decreased over the past few years, physicians are still the highest paid professionals in the country. The following table presents median annual income for nine areas of practice. Incomes listed are after expenses (such as staff and malpractice insurance) but before taxes.

Medical Field	Annual Income
Anesthesiology	$210,000
General/Family Practice	$130,000
Internal Medicine	$150,000
Ob/Gyn	$200,000
Pathology	$184,000
Pediatrics	$126,000
Psychiatry	$130,000
Radiology	$230,000
Surgery	$240,000
ALL PHYSICIANS	$160,000

The figures listed above do not account for residents, who are notoriously underpaid. The national median salary for a resident is about $35,000. In the interest of patient safety there have been some efforts—at the state and hospital level, and among residents themselves—to limit the number of hours that residents work each week. These efforts have been successful. However, despite the rules limiting the work week to 80 hours, many residents continue to work more than 100 hours per week. Why are residents required to work so hard? In part because hospitals depend on residents as a cheap source of labor, as they are paid much less than other physicians and somewhat less than nurses and other health professionals.

PRESTIGE

Almost universally, being a doctor carries prestige. Doctors are generally thought to be smart, well educated, hard working, caring, and dedicated. Even in this era of managed care and malpractice lawsuits, doctors are well respected. In a recent Harris poll, Americans ranked "doctor" as the most prestigious profession/occupation.[5] In another poll, 65 percent of respondents viewed doctors positively, compared with 22 percent who viewed teachers positively, and only 4 percent who viewed lawyers positively.[6] You should consider the degree to which having a prestigious career is important to you. Other health professions, although perhaps less glamorous, also involve healing and helping others.

TRENDS IN MEDICINE IN THE TWENTY-FIRST CENTURY

Several trends that began during the past few decades are likely to continue well into the twenty-first century. These trends have implications for you, the aspiring doctor. They will impact the nature of your work, the structure of the organization in which you work, your salary, the relationship you have with patients, and above all the quality of the health care you deliver.

In the sections that follow, we consider some important trends (we call them the Top Ten, with a disclaimer that predicting the future is difficult) affecting medicine in the twenty-first century.

Top Ten List: Trends in Medicine in the Twenty-First Century

1. *Development of new technology*
2. *Increased health care costs*
3. *Evolution of health care delivery and payment systems*
4. *Greater reliance on primary and preventive care*

[5] Doctors reign, teachers gain, lawyers wane in public esteem. *New York Times*. 11/1/2000.

[6] An Honorable Profession. *Industry Week*. April 20, 1998. 247 (8).

5. *More guidelines for patient care*
6. *A possible surplus of physicians, at least in certain specialty areas*
7. *Better gender and ethnic diversity among physicians*
8. *An aging patient population*
9. *The emergence of new ethical issues*
10. *Changes in academic medicine and medical education*

Note that above list is by no means complete. Also, trends listed are inter-related and are not necessarily in order of importance.

New Technology

Medicine and health care has improved during the past few decades largely because of technological advancement. And there are probably even more exciting developments on the horizon. The term *technology* is often used broadly. In the health care arena, it means the development of new drugs, procedures, techniques, and means of communication that, if used correctly, have the potential to improve diagnosis, care, and patient outcomes.

- ***Medications and Procedures.*** *The increase in life expectancy over the past few decades is partially due to improvements in medications and procedures. For example, the death rate due to heart disease is declining because of better drugs (hypertension, heart, and cholesterol medications) and surgical techniques.*
- ***Laboratory Techniques.*** *Often, improvements in laboratory tools or techniques lead to important discoveries. For example, better tools allowed the human genome to be mapped.*
- ***The Internet.*** *Patients who are Internet users arrive at their doctor's office well-informed about their illness. On the other hand, the Internet houses a great deal of misinformation. The physician who is Web savvy can guide patients to informative websites and Web-based support groups. The Internet is invaluable for research.*
- ***Telemedicine.*** *Telemedicine is defined by the American Telemedicine Association as "the use of medical information exchanged from one site to another via electronic communication for the health and education of the patient or healthcare provider and for the purpose of improving care." Sharing of radiographic images and patient information (X-rays, MRIs) via computer between physicians is an important current application. In the future, we may see telemedicine bringing the expertise of specialists to rural or other remote areas.*
- ***Other Computer Applications.*** *Computerized database systems are used for billing and patient records. Some physicians take advantage of software programs made for*

hand-held devices. These can be used for note-taking, reference, or even patient management. Not surprisingly, it is often the younger doctors (and medical students) who are the most comfortable with computer technology. Interest and understanding of relevant computer applications can give you an advantage when it comes to working with older, more experienced doctors; instead of just learning from them, you will have something to contribute. The key is being able to explain, teach, and pass on your knowledge effectively.

Health Care Costs

The United States spends more money per capita on health care than any other country in the world. Some believe that the U.S. offers the best medical care in the world, thereby justifying the cost. Others note that according to indicators such as life expectancy and infant mortality, the U.S. lags behind other industrialized countries. In 1960, 6 percent of the U.S. Gross Domestic Product (the sum total of all expenditures, by all people, in a given country) went to health care. In 2000, that figure climbed to 20 percent, meaning that nearly a fifth of the GDP went to health-related goods and services. There are many theories as to what has caused this escalation, two of which are discussed below.

Technology

As discussed above, technological advances usually serve to improve health care and health outcomes. However, technology is often cited as a major cause of rising health care costs. When new tools are developed and advertised, hospitals and physicians may feel pressure to purchase and use them, sometimes even if the benefit of the new device is questionable. Someone ultimately pays for such purchases, and thus we see rising health care costs. The MRI—an imaging device that, for about $2,000, provides pictures of a patient's organs—is often thought to be over-used in this country. For example, there are more MRI machines in Orange County, California, than in all of Canada.[7] It is important to remember, however, that technological advances can also serve to reduce costs. By preventing illness and reducing spread of disease, new vaccines (anti-influenza for example) lower the cost of treatment for society overall. New surgical instruments and the development of medication in pill form facilitate the use of outpatient procedures instead of expensive hospital stays.

Incentives

Patients are generally far removed from the cost of their care, and therefore have little incentive to keep costs down. Employers and the government—not patients themselves—foot most of the bill for health care, creating a system of "third-party payers."[8]

[7] By the Numbers: Health Care Costs. *Scientific American*. April 1999.

[8] The United States relies largely upon an employer-based, health care financing system which means that most people (60%) receive health benefits through their work. In other words, employers pay for employees' health care—typically by taking responsibility for paying monthly premiums. Twenty percent of the population receives government health care benefits, in the form of Medicare (everyone over 65 is eligible) or Medicaid (eligibility based on financial need).

Some believe that since patients don't pay much for their own health care, they "over-use" it, thereby driving government and employer health care expenditures up.

As a physician, you will undoubtedly feel pressure to keep health care costs down. In many practice settings, doctors are scrutinized on the basis of the cost of the tests and treatments they prescribe. For example, primary care doctors are sometimes encouraged to limit referrals to specialists. All doctors may be monitored for "over-use" of expensive tests and equipment. Physicians face difficult decisions as they attempt to provide excellent care at a lower cost: if a patient has a slim chance of benefiting from an expensive treatment, should that treatment be employed? The physician must balance the cost of treating with the risk of not treating.

HEALTH CARE DELIVERY SYSTEMS

The push for management of health care costs has led to the growth of managed care. One of the most important trends of the past few decades has been the replacement of simple fee-for-service plans by the growth of the managed care industry.

Fee-for-Service

Before managed care, health care was delivered on a "fee-for-service" basis. Medicare (federally funded health insurance for those over 65 years of age) remains a fee-for-service program. Under a fee-for-service system, doctors and hospitals perform a service (a check-up, an operation, etc.) and charge a fee for the service. Typically, the patient's health insurance company pays the fee for whatever medical service the patient wants or needs. The patient pays the health insurance company a monthly premium or, if the patient has health benefits from his employer, the employer pays the monthly premiums. The insurance company calculates monthly premiums based on how much it pays out to hospitals and doctors each year for all people enrolled in the insurance plan.

Managed Care

Managed care was introduced as a response to rising health care costs, and has succeeded in slowing the rate at which health care costs rise. Thus, the trend towards managed care will probably continue. Although managed care is often thought to be synonymous with Health Maintenance Organizations (HMO), an HMO is, in fact, just one of many systems for managing care.[9]

Managed care usually involves set monthly premiums that are lower than those in fee-for-service plans, and this makes those paying the premiums (usually the employers) happy. How do managed care organizations keep their premiums down? By keeping their financial outlays down. Under managed care, expenditures are typically controlled through several mechanisms:

[9] HMOs specify the doctors and hospitals that participants must use. Another example of a managed care organization is a Preferred Provider Organization (PPO). PPOs encourage the use of certain providers ("preferred providers") but will also cover part of the cost of doctors and hospitals outside of the preferred provider network.

- *Participants in a managed care plan agree to use doctors and hospitals that are part of the plan, and these providers are either paid yearly salaries or charge reduced fees for services rendered.*
- *Primary care physicians serve as "gatekeepers" in limiting the use of expensive medical specialists.*
- *Guidelines/regulations are implemented that attempt to limit the use of expensive tests and equipment in unnecessary situations.*
- *Inpatient care is reduced and there is more emphasis on outpatient services (care that does not involve an overnight hospital stay). Associated with the movement towards outpatient care, hospitals are filling fewer of their beds and are seeing a decline in length of stay (LOS) for hospital patients.*

Managed care has generated discontent among some patients and providers. In a recent study,[10] over half of those surveyed said that managed care lessens quality of care. Patients are often frustrated by red tape, the inability to choose one's own doctor, short visits, long waits, obstacles to seeing specialists, and limitations on coverage. Many doctors object to managed care because the cost-cutting mechanisms may compromise patient care, and because physician salaries and autonomy are reduced under managed care arrangements.

However, there can be advantages in working for a managed care organization. For one, doctors are often salaried, which means that they earn a specified amount each year, and their income does not depend on finding clients. Doctors also tend to work fewer hours per week, which is probably good both for doctors and for patients. For better or for worse, being a doctor in the twenty-first century is likely to involve practicing in a managed care environment of some form.

The Uninsured

This section on health care delivery and payment would be incomplete without a discussion of the uninsured. At least 15 percent of people in the United States have no health insurance. The U.S. is unique among industrialized nations in that respect, and it is not exactly something to be proud of. Individuals without health insurance tend to seek medical care—typically through an emergency room—only after a health problem has become really serious. This is obviously bad for the patient, who with early treatment might have avoided serious complications. It is also costly to society, because prevention and early treatment are less expensive than late intervention. Most people—physicians and nonphysicians alike—believe that everyone should have access to health care. However, there is less agreement on how universal access should be achieved and funded. Doctors will need to speak out to assure that this issue is addressed as soon, and as equitably, as possible.

[10] Harvard/Harris Poll, analyzing 25 public opinion surveys. 1997.

Primary and Preventive Care

Most observers predict that as managed care grows, primary care physicians will continue to play a very important role, and the demand for primary care doctors will remain relatively high. Primary care physicians may be either MDs or DOs (see page 17 for a description of both degrees).

Gatekeepers

Before the days of managed care, if a person discovered an odd-looking spot on his skin, he could go directly to a dermatologist and be reimbursed by his insurance company for the visit. An important tenet of managed care has been the requirement that enrollees see a primary care physician prior to visiting a specialist. Family practice, pediatrics, internal medicine, and Ob/Gyn are typically considered primary care fields. The primary care physician serves as a "gatekeeper," presumably reducing unnecessary visits to expensive specialists.

Without the training of a specialist (a dermatologist in our example above), the primary care physician may not be equipped to judge the seriousness of some conditions. Missing a pre-cancerous skin lesion, for example, may cause hardship for the patient later on. On the other hand, if a primary care doctor refers *all* patients with skin lesions to the dermatologist, the system has failed because each patient required two doctor visits rather than one.

Integrated Approach

A benefit of this emphasis on primary care is that, in theory, patients develop a long-term relationship with their primary care doctor who is better able to understand the social, economic, and community-related issues associated with their health. The primary care doctor presumably has an understanding of all physiologic systems. This comprehensive knowledge facilitates diagnosis or at least allows the physician to make the initial decision about what next steps will lead to diagnosis. Primary care physicians are well-positioned to address behavioral changes, such as exercise programs, that aid in the prevention of disease.

Prevention

Several of the major causes of morbidity (illness) and mortality (death) in the U.S. are preventable. Emphysema, for example, is often the result of heavy smoking. The most common type of diabetes is linked with obesity. We have learned that the spread of HIV can be reduced through educational programs and behavioral interventions. The high death rate in this country due to violent crime is often attributed to the prevalence of hand guns, a situation that could be addressed through legislation. Advances in genetics could potentially revolutionize preventative medicine by allowing physicians to identify people who are going to get sick before they show any symptoms of disease.

Prevention is preferable to treatment for the obvious reason that, with prevention, illness is reduced or even eliminated altogether. Whether prevention efforts are cost-effective depends upon the disease, its prevalence, and the technology employed. For example, mammography is helpful in detecting breast cancer at a treatable stage and can potentially prevent mortality and reduce the high costs associated with treating end-stage cancer. It is sensible and cost-effective to offer mammograms to women above a certain age. However, it is probably unreasonable to encourage women in their twenties to have annual mammograms because breast cancer at this age is rare and, furthermore, can be difficult to spot on mammogram.

Guidelines for Patient Care

Fundamental to medicine are the doctor-patient relationship, the belief that each patient must be considered individually, and the principle that doctors should be allowed to use their best judgment when providing care. Do these ideals conflict with the recent trend of using guidelines in clinical medicine?

Evidenced-Based Medicine or Cookbook Medicine?

Doctors vary tremendously in their approach to medicine and disease treatment. This is why, in serious illness, a second opinion is usually recommended. In recent years, there has been increased use of Evidenced-Based Medicine (EBM) in clinical practice. EBM employs *scientific evidence* for the purpose of standardizing and improving patient care. Quantitative indicators such as rate of reduction of disease are typically used to evaluate procedures and treatments. The goal of EBM is to establish guidelines for clinical decision-making based on the results of studies, particularly randomized clinical trials (these are generally considered the most accurate type of study).

Some doctors worry that the trend towards EBM de-emphasizes physician judgment, results in strict guidelines for treatment, and amounts to "cookbook medicine." In fact, this has not been the case. EBM, with its population-based approach, actually complements the one-on-one tradition of medicine by allowing doctors to defend their decisions with data. However, there are many diseases and clinical situations for which the literature fails to provide clear evidence. In some cases, the risks and benefits of a particular therapy may differ depending on the study examined.

Cost Consciousness

Occasionally, guidelines that dictate clinical care are based on cost-cutting objectives rather than on sound medical evidence. Such "guidelines" may compromise patient care. Going back to our mammogram example, an HMO might encourage physicians to recommend mammograms to all women over fifty, when research suggests that mammograms are highly beneficial for women in their forties as well. It is the physician's ethical responsibility to give his patient honest and up-to-date medical advice (in this case, to recommend mammograms after age forty). At the same time, the physician may want to support the cost-cutting goals of his employer. This is the type of conflict that doctors face in the current era of cost-consciousness. There are no easy answers. However, familiarity with medical evidence and the rules of the organization will at least allow you make informed decisions.

Physician Surplus or Physician Shortage?

From 1970 to 1990 there was a sharp increase in the number of residency positions in the U.S., largely as a result of government policy encouraging such growth. During the same period, there was a much less dramatic increase in the patient population. Some said that we were training too many doctors and that we would see a surplus. Since 1990, however, the number of residency programs has remained relatively stable, while the patient population has grown (partially as a result of an aging population). The surplus never occured; now some experts predict a shortage.

Whether we have a physician surplus, shortage, or neither, there will always be rural and inner-city areas that are in need of doctors. To combat this problem, federal and state-funded programs offer financial incentives to doctors who agree to work in underserved areas. There is also a shortage of physicians from certain ethnic backgrounds. It is important to have a physician population that represents the population that it serves. Most medical schools attempt to recruit students of ethnic backgrounds that are underrepresented in medicine.

Diversity Among Physicians

Increased diversity among physicians is a very positive trend and may result in better patient care.

Women

Approximately 49 percent of entering medical students are women. This is remarkable considering that just twenty years ago women accounted for about 30 percent of medical students, and in 1960 less than 7 percent of medical students were women. Today, about 25 percent of practicing physicians are women, and this percentage will continue to rise. There are outstanding women physicians in every imaginable medical field. However, women are especially well represented in fields like pediatrics and Ob/Gyn, and less well represented in other fields like surgical subspecialties. Several theories and generalizations have been put forth to help explain why women are attracted to some fields more than others. First, once there is a critical mass of women within a field, it becomes a more welcoming environment for other women. Also, people tend to be interested in fields that have personal relevance. Finally, many women tend to avoid fields with the very longest residencies (only 10 percent of neurosurgery residents, for example, are women).

Minorities

The medical profession is slowly becoming more ethnically diverse, as increased numbers of nonwhite medical school graduates enter the work force. This increase in diversity reflects the changing demographics of the U.S. population, better and more widely available educational opportunities, and active minority recruitment on the part of medical schools. If this trend continues, we will someday have a physician work force that is representative of the population at large, including African Americans, Mexican Americans, Puerto Ricans, other Hispanics, Native Americans, and other underrepresented minorities. In 2003, underrepresented minorities made up 11 percent of entering medical school classes.

Aging Population

In 2020, the median age in the U.S. will be 40 years, up from 36 in 2000 and 30 in 1960. As the population ages, the demand for medical care increases: the average number of doctor visits per year is three for the population at large, but is six for those over 74 years old. The aging of the American population contributes to rising health care costs. Because 99 percent of individuals over 65 are covered by Medicare, government expenditures on health care are expected to rise. The paperwork involved in treating a patient with Medicare is notoriously time-consuming.

An older population will cause growth within certain fields, such as geriatrics, internal medicine, orthopedics, and cardiovascular medicine. The incidence of chronic disease, meaning disease that is long-lasting and often incurable, will increase. Thus, physicians will often be called upon to provide palliative care that addresses symptoms when the underlying disease cannot be cured. Physician-researchers will be encouraged to find treatments for conditions that afflict the elderly, such as Alzheimer's Disease.

Ethical Issues

Physicians have always dealt with important ethical issues related to life and death. As a physician in the twenty-first century, some of your ethical dilemmas are likely to involve the conflict between saving money and saving lives. Consider the following scenario:

> *You are a pediatrician, seeing a patient you have never seen before. The patient is a very ill 6 year old without health insurance. Do you treat her, knowing that you will hear about it later? Or, do you send her to the Free Clinic across town even though it will entail a long bus ride for the sick girl?*

Ethical issues about end-of-life care will become increasingly relevant because of an older patient population. For example:

> *Your patient is 80 years old and suffers from terminal lung cancer, which has spread to his brain. There are no cures for this man at this stage, so your care has been focused on keeping him comfortable. He can't breath on his own, is incoherent, and has been more or less motionless in the hospital for one week. His daughter does not want you to remove life support. What do you do?*

The rule of doctor-patient confidentiality can be the basis for ethical issues. Consider this situation:

> *You have been treating a young man in the hospital for a lung infection. During his hospital stay, he was tested for HIV and the test results were positive. He is unwilling to discuss the matter, does not want medications that will help his HIV symptoms, and appears to be in denial. Do you have a responsibility to alert the man's wife?*

Unfortunately, some medical schools barely address ethics, leaving you on your own to learn about and think through important ethical issues. A mentor, someone whose opinion you respect, can serve as a resource for sorting out ethical questions. If you feel strongly about a particular issue, you should consider getting involved—through writing, attending conferences, or engaging in dialogue.

Changes in Academic Medicine and Medical Education

Most medical schools are directly affiliated with teaching hospitals. Three advantages to this arrangement are

- *Medical students have the opportunity for hands-on learning*
- *Patients are treated by expert physicians and benefit from the latest technology*
- *The academic environment coupled with the clinical facilities provide an ideal setting for research that ultimately pushes medicine forward and improves care*

Academic medical centers throughout the country are having a tough time financially, leading some experts to question their future viability. Although medical school tuition seems incredibly high, it does not cover the actual cost of medical education; academic medical centers have historically depended on income from clinical activities to subsidize medical education, research activities, and management of a teaching hospital. As discussed, the shift toward outpatient medicine has resulted in reduced earnings for hospitals. For academic medical centers, this means less revenue to cover their high costs. As more and more academic medical centers face financial crisis, there will be pressure to cut costs and/or raise revenue significantly. We might see academic medical centers restrict their patients to those who can pay higher fees, or perhaps we'll see an increase in government funding and/or medical school tuition.[11]

In response to these changes in medicine and health care, most medical schools are attempting to revise their curriculum. Some of the revisions we see are

- *Less time spent in lecture. Educators recognize that in this age of technology and information there are simply too many facts to learn. Rather than inundate students with a massive amount of information, some medical schools hope to teach students general concepts that will prepare them for a lifetime of learning.*

[11] Keynotes on Health Care. AAMC. 34 (1) Winter, 2000

- *More clinical problem-solving during the first two years. With all that we know, and all the treatment options available today, physicians must be thinkers and problem-solvers.*
- *Greater emphasis on health economics, health care management, and public health. Doctors should understand the interdisciplinary nature of health care, and the forces that affect medicine.*
- *Better training in outpatient medicine, with the use of outpatient clinics and doctors' offices for clinical rotations of outpatient facilities.*

With the requirement of at least eleven years of post–high school training, becoming a physician takes longer in the U.S. than anywhere else in the world. This is costly to society. Some people predict that, as a result of financial pressures, the amount of schooling required to become a doctor will be reduced. For the time being, however, you have a long (but exciting) road ahead of you.

CONCLUSION: IS MEDICINE YOUR CALLING?

This chapter describes some of the major issues and trends that characterize medicine in the twenty-first century. Whether you will be able to work effectively amidst all these changes depends in part on your flexibility. According to the American Medical Association, ". . . the next ten to fifteen years will be a period of substantial change for physicians. Physicians who are flexible, adaptable, and responsive to changing circumstances are likely to prosper during such a period."[12]

Apart from flexibility, what other traits will help you succeed and find job satisfaction as a physician in the twenty-first century?

What It Takes to Be a Doctor in the Twenty-First Century

C*ompassion—a critical part of healing*

A*dvocacy—for your patients and for those without health care*

L*eadership—in improving health care at the team, hospital, and policy level*

L*ifelong learning—there will always be more to know*

I*nterpersonal skills—communication with patients and among providers is key*

N*egotiation—to work around bureaucratic constraints*

G*rasp—of increasing amounts of medical knowledge and of a health care system in flux*

Ask yourself: Is medicine your CALLING?

[12] ibid

3 So You Still Want to Be a Doctor . . .

Congratulations! You are on your way to entering one of the most rewarding and respected fields, one of the few altruistic careers that pays a livable wage. The bad news is that even armed with all the information we can give you and the help of a pre-med advisor, the application process is still tough. The painful reality is that there are about 33,000 applicants for approximately 18,000 spots. The good news, however, is that if you are persistent and have worked hard for the past several years to make yourself a competitive candidate, you have a good chance at a certified letter and a career that will keep you challenged and fulfilled for the rest of your life.

WHAT MAKES A COMPETITIVE APPLICANT?

Well, that's the $103,855 question (average debt of current medical school graduates). In 2001 the average matriculated (accepted) medical student had an undergraduate science GPA of 3.53, a nonscience GPA of 3.69, and an overall GPA of 3.61; the average matriculated (accepted) medical student had average MCAT scores of 9.5 Verbal Reasoning, 10.0 Physical Science, 10.2 Biological Sciences, and a P on the Writing Sample. But, while GPA and MCAT scores will play a large role in the admissions decision, they aren't everything. Solid numbers are a good start, but medical schools are also quite interested in who you are, why you want to be a physician, and whether or not you have a clue about what being doctor is like. Therefore, in addition to strong grades and scores, your application will be strengthened by volunteer time, some experience in scientific academic research, demonstrated leadership roles, interesting extracurricular activities, a well-written personal statement, excellent communication skills, and solid recommendation letters. All these application pieces will provide the admissions committee with a fuller picture of who you are than mere numbers can convey.

Also, keep in mind that, despite the odds, there are always large numbers of normal, sane people who actually didn't get straight A's or perfect MCATs who still manage to get into medical school. You can be one of them, and this book can help you to package yourself and target schools that are likely to appreciate your unique strengths. If you have a hunch that your set of qualifications is not what traditional medical school admissions committees are looking for, consider a few alternate career paths. This book covers allopathic (MD) programs in the U.S., Puerto Rico, and Canada (many Canadian schools accept only Canadians), as well as osteopathic (DO) programs. Don't rule out programs or schools in other health fields, such as dental school, nursing school, and physician assistant programs.

Allopathic Medicine

Allopathic schools confer the MD on their graduates, and allopathic training is by far the most widely available and recognized type of medical training. Both the Canadian and Puerto Rican medical schools in this book are fully accredited allopathic institutions and are part of the American Association of Medical Colleges (AAMC). Teaching methodology varies among schools. The "traditional" model consists of two years of basic science followed by clinical rotations. The "systems-based" program is organized around physiologic systems, such as the lung or kidney. The "case-based" model teaches through clinical vignettes. There are also schools offering hybrids of these approaches. Most schools have made a concerted effort to get students together with patients at a much earlier stage in their education—it used to be that medical students might not come in contact with any patients until they'd already been through two years of school. At most schools, the last two years are spent doing clinical rotations. Even if you're sure that your calling in life is plastic surgery, you're going to have to do a pediatrics rotation. Most medical students really enjoy having a chance to delve into the various specialties, and this structure provides an excellent opportunity to learn about the areas you hope to pursue.

Allopathic training will give you the option to practice in any of the medical specialties and the MD is universally recognized worldwide as a medical degree. For an abundance of information on all aspects of allopathic training and practice, visit the AAMC website (www.aamc.org).

Osteopathic Medicine

Osteopathic medicine in the United States got its start in the late 1800s. Its founding father was Dr. Andrew Taylor Still, who established the American School of Osteopathy in Kirksville, Missouri, in 1892. The various regulatory bodies (osteopathic versions of AAMC and the AMA) were well under way by the early 1900s, and are now the American Osteopathic Association (AOA) and the American Association of Colleges of Osteopathic Medicine (AACOM). There are currently nineteen colleges of osteopathic medicine throughout the United States, and the DO is only issued in the United States. Visit the AOA's website at www.aoa-net.org and the AACOM's website at www.aacom.org to find out more information about these organizations.

Osteopathic medicine has an interesting history; until fairly recently, its insistence on preventive care, communication with the patient, and a holistic approach to health was considered to be somewhat radical. Now, of course, much of what osteopathic medicine has always espoused is rapidly becoming part of all medical training. In addition to a philosophical difference in approach, an important distinction between osteopathic and allopathic training is that osteopaths are taught an additional modality of treatment called manipulation (not to be confused with chiropractic manipulation, which has an entirely different system of education and is not recognized as a fully licensed medical degree). The osteopathic philosophy posits that there is a unity between a living organism's anatomy and physiology. Osteopathic science includes "the behavioral, chemical, physical, spiritual, and biological knowledge related to the establishment and maintenance of health as well as the prevention and alleviation of disease." Osteopathic concepts emphasize the following principles:

1. *The human being is a dynamic unit of function.*
2. *The body possesses self-regulatory mechanisms that are self-healing in nature.*
3. *Structure and function are interrelated at all levels.*
4. *Rational treatment is based on these principles.*

(AOA Yearbook of Osteopathic Physicians 1996, Chicago: AOA, p. 732.)

What this means to the average osteopathic student is that he or she has to learn all of the same science as his or her allopathic counterpart, plus osteopathic diagnosis and treatment, in the same amount of time. Practicing osteopaths have another way of helping their patients that allopaths do not. Osteopaths achieved full-practice rights in 1973, although some states certified osteopaths to practice in all public hospitals as complete physicians and surgeons much earlier.

As you might guess from their philosophy and training, many osteopathic doctors choose to become primary care physicians. Most work in Family Practice, Internal Medicine, Pediatrics, Ob/Gyn, and General Surgery. In the words of one osteopathic dean, they tend to be generalists first and specialists second. However, there are DOs in just about every area of modern medical practice, from Neurological Surgery to Psychiatry, Oncology, and Emergency Medicine. Although DO was not traditionally considered a research degree, the DO/PhD combination is becoming more common, and the AOA is becoming much more active in encouraging research activities, particularly in primary care.

At most osteopathic schools, matriculates have undergrad GPAs of about a 3.4 and combined MCAT scores of just under 25. Last year, there were 55,000 applications from 9,500 applicants for 2,500 seats. However, osteopathic schools do have a reputation for "looking past the numbers" and put a very strong emphasis on the whole picture of the candidate. This often makes osteopathic school an attractive choice for nontraditional, older students whose GPAs from their first trek through undergraduate school prove prohibitive in most allopathic programs. If you have a few blemishes on your academic record but a life that suggests you'll make a dedicated physician, you should consider applying to osteopathic schools.

Most pre-meds trying to decide whether or not to apply to osteopathic schools worry about what will happen to them after they graduate and apply for a residency. Osteopathic graduates participate along with allopaths and foreign medical graduates (both American and nonresident) in the National Resident Matching Program (NRMP)—the Match. DOs can apply for either osteopathic or allopathic residencies, and for that reason many take both the USMLE (United State Medical Licensing Examination) and the COMLEX (Comprehensive Osteopathic Medical Licensing Examination, which is a series of exams administered by the National Board of Osteopathic Medical Examiners). Louisiana is the only state that does not recognize the COMLEX and requires DOs to pass the USMLE to be licenced. The best way to decide which path is right for you is to spend time with both MDs and DOs, and talk to them at length about their practices.

Foreign Medical Schools

If you are seriously considering attending a foreign school but want to practice in the U.S., make sure you take a hard look at the prospective school's USMLE pass rate and residency placement rate. Although foreign schools are much easier to get into, they will put you in just as much debt as U.S. schools, without the same assurance of a career that will render you capable of paying it off.

THE NUMBERS GAME

Because of the sheer volume of applications they have to wade through, admissions officers have to make some initial screening decisions based largely on GPA and MCAT scores—deceptively simple acronyms for the arcane processes they represent.

Your GPA, for the purposes of applying to medical school, consists of your science GPA (biology, chemistry, physics, and math), your nonscience GPA (every other class you ever suffered through), and your cumulative GPA. These are calculated for your undergraduate career, any nondegree-seeking post-secondary work, and any degree-seeking post-secondary programs. In other words, you could conceivably have nine GPAs. Each medical school has its own policies for deciding which GPA means the most to them when they're choosing which applicants to interview and/or matriculate. The average GPA of all applicants (not necessarily accepted) in 2002 was a 3.36 science, a 3.59 nonscience, and a 3.46 overall.

Although community college classes may count as part of your GPA, they may not always be acceptable as prerequisite, pre-medical course work. If you are planning to take some of your core pre-med courses (biology, chemistry, physics, etc.) at a community college, it's an extremely good idea to do some advance planning and call some of the schools that you're interested in to make sure that they have no qualms about community college credit. Similarly, if you took an AP class in high school and then tested out of a core class, such as physics, you may run into trouble when you apply unless you've taken upper-division course work in that subject. Again, it is very much to your advantage to check with a few medical schools and your pre-health advisor to make sure that your academic record doesn't have any holes in it.

Your MCAT score is made up of four separate marks: verbal reasoning, physical sciences, biological sciences, and the writing sample. Verbal reasoning and the science sections are scored from 1 to 15, although in recent years the top verbal score has been designated as 13 to 15. The writing portion of the MCAT requires that you write two essays, which generate a single score. This score is reported as a letter J–T, where J is low and T is high, presumably to emphasize that the writing sample is totally useless as a means of judging skills. The average score for all applicants on each section in 2002 was 8.7 verbal, 9.1 physical sciences, 9.3 biological sciences, and an O on the writing sample.

The writing sample, added to the MCAT a few years ago in an attempt to ensure the applicant's ability to communicate, is largely ignored by admissions committees. Virtually the only time the writing sample is looked at very carefully is in the case of a disconnected application—a beautifully written personal statement with low verbal scores and/or a low writing sample score. Some schools will also consider the writing score if they are evaluating the English ability of English as a Second Language applicants. This does not mean that you can take a nap during the writing sample. You should make every effort to answer the questions in a coherent and focused way on the off-chance that the committee decides to look at your score.

THE SUM OF YOUR EXPERIENCE

Although your GPA and MCAT score play a large role in your application, admissions committees are also looking for several other attributes. They are quite interested in who you are, why you want to be a physician, and whether or not you have a clue about what being a doctor is really like.

Exposure to the Health Care Field

Although students with no discernible exposure to health care still matriculate, the vast majority of successful pre-meds have some experience, usually volunteer work, in a hospital, clinic, hospice, or other health care setting. Some pre-meds are qualified enough to find part-time paying positions as emergency medical technicians (EMTs), nurse's aids, or organ and blood bank workers, while other "nontraditional" applicants had full-time careers in health care. Your goal should be to hold a volunteer or paid position for at least six months. Many pre-medical programs have specific classes you can take that include organized volunteer time as part of their course work—even if you are a returning adult student and not officially registered as pre-med. You can often get college credit for community service work in the medical field. Although it may seem difficult to find the time to volunteer, it will make a huge difference as you work on your personal statement and get through your interviews. You will have stories to tell, and will be able to speak far more effectively about the reasons that you want to become a physician.

Leadership Experience and Community Service

Leadership can mean many things, and being a leader, say, within your family, can be as important as being class president. One of the simpler ways to prove your abilities is to join a club or campus organization and get elected to office. You can also lead youth- or religious-affiliated organizations, or participate in a variety of community service organizations such as food banks, literacy programs, and mentoring. The key is to demonstrate sincere commitment and have some longevity with whatever cause you decide to embrace, so that you can achieve a measure of responsibility. If you are serious about practicing primary care medicine, for example, this is your chance to build your resume and to start proving yourself. Find a clinic that needs a dedicated volunteer, and get your feet wet.

Research

Academic research is quite a bit easier to get involved with than you might think. Research labs are always looking for drones—read "undergrads"—to help with the unlovely business of test-tube cleaning and organism counting. With any luck, however, you should be able to find a program in which you will actually be able to conduct experiments and write about the results. If you are considering a career in academic medicine, you should try to get involved in research projects as early in your undergraduate career as you can convince someone to take you. One way to find out about cool research projects is to bribe a teaching and research assistant with a cup of coffee and ask about the various projects in their departments. Alternatively, check out the science department websites at your university for information on current research.

Humanity

Medical schools are interested in training bright, empathic, communicative people who have a strong interest in science and a wide-ranging intellect. They are not interested in students with perfect grades who have clearly never done anything else with their lives than try to break the curve in chemistry class. The schools want to graduate physicians who will listen to their patients and be able to effectively use the myriad tools available to heal them. What this means is that there is no magic system that will create an unbroken path into medical school. You can major in art history, modern dance, or biochemistry—it doesn't matter, as long as you take the classes you need to fulfill medical school requirements. You can take a few years off and join the Peace Corps or go straight to med school upon college graduation. Admissions committees will be trying to discern what you have learned from your experiences, and how the things you have seen and done have nurtured the values that have led you to pursue a medical career.

THE APPLICATION PROCESS

There are many factors to consider when applying to medical schools. The first rule of thumb is to apply broadly and include "safety" schools where you will most likely be accepted. Besides the obvious clinical and scholastic goals, it is important to look for a school in a location that suits you. Although you may think that you won't see the light of day for four years, you should apply to schools that are in geographic areas that appeal to you and will provide outlets for your hobbies and interests.

Applying to Allopathic Medical Schools

Most allopathic medical schools use AMCAS®, the American Medical Colleges Application Service, which is a centralized and standardized application that is handled by the AAMC, the Association of American Medical Colleges. In the spring of 2001, the AAMC switched to an entirely Web-based AMCAS application. The Web-based application is available directly from www.aamc.org. The AMCAS application costs $150 for the first school; for each additional school the fee is $30. If you have significant financial hardship, you can apply directly to AMCAS for a fee waiver on their services. You will also need to prepare transcript requests for every post-secondary school you ever attended, even if you only took one class there or the credits transferred elsewhere. Undergraduate colleges will send transcripts to AMCAS, who then forwards them to all medical schools to which you are applying. AMCAS begins accepting transcripts on March 15 each year and completed applications on June 1. It will take a couple of weeks for AAMC to process everything, at which point you'll receive a "transmittal notification." You can call and use AAMC's voicemail to check your status. You can reach AAMC on the Web at www.aamc.org or by phone at 202-828-0600. At most universities and colleges, your pre-health advisor will help you navigate the AMCAS application, which can be fairly baffling. One of the toughest parts of the application is the "Personal Comments" page, where you have exactly one typewritten, single-spaced page to explain your life and convince them that you should be one of the chosen few. Needless to say, this part of the application takes time and patience—be sure to read through the suggestions and advice for working on it that are included later in this chapter.

When you are choosing which schools to apply to, make sure that you check their in-state residency requirements. Although many allopathic schools are private, there are quite a few public schools that receive free money every year from out-of-state applicants they are prohibited from accepting into their programs; it doesn't matter how qualified you are, if you aren't a state resident, you can't get in.

Applying to Osteopathic Schools

Osteopathic schools use their own internal system, called AACOMAS®, which in many respects works exactly the same way as AMCAS. They have both paper and electronic applications. You can request an application from their website at www.aacom.org, or call 301-968-4100. Like the AMCAS application, AACOMAS takes some time to fill out, so make sure you get started early. It also includes a personal statement, but it's even shorter than AMCAS's—you only have half of a page to explain why you want to be an osteopathic physician. You will also need to get a recommendation from a DO, a fact that takes some applicants by surprise. If you are serious about osteopathic school, search for a mentor DO as early as possible. One of the nice things about AACOMAS is that all osteopathic schools use it—you don't have to worry about tracking down additional applications. Because osteopathic schools are private institutions, they don't have residency requirements (although some may have tuition breaks for residents of particular states). If you are interested in going to osteopathic school, investigate all of the colleges and choose based on your interest in the program and living conditions in the area.

When to Apply to Medical School

Whether you're applying to osteopathic or allopathic medical schools, you need to apply as early as you can in the process. In general, pre-medical students begin the application process in the spring semester of their junior year, or approximately a year and a half before they want to enter medical school. The vast majority of medical schools engage in some type of rolling admissions, which means that they read and evaluate applications as the folders arrive. Admissions officers are only human. Even though they make every effort to give the same consideration to applicant number 6,005 as they give to applicant number 1, the sheer volume of applications takes its toll on their patience and enthusiasm. In practical terms, this means that if you take the April MCAT (Medical College Admission Test) and get your applications in by late June, you will have a distinct advantage over someone taking the August test. Even if you turn in your AMCAS or AACOMAS application early, many medical schools will not look closely at your application until they have a copy of your MCAT scores. Each year, students are accepted with August test scores and applications that arrived late in the process. Unfortunately, there are also large numbers of students who are not accepted but would have had a decent chance had they applied earlier. Basically, you should try to for every possible advantage. Turning in your application early can certainly help to give you an edge. Also, procrastinators take note: AMCAS is serious about its deadlines. If an application or transcript is late, you'll get it back.

When to Take the MCAT

Virtually all U.S. and Canadian osteopathic and allopathic medical schools require the MCAT, which is given in April and August of each year. According to the "AMCAS Survival Guide" (an official publication of the AAMC) you should, "if possible, take the Medical College Admissions Test (MCAT) on the April test date." As evidence, they cite the admissions cycle—earlier is better. Of course, not all applicants' academic schedules realistically allow them to take the April test.

There are three ways to get the forms you need to register for the MCAT. You can request them at the AAMC website, pick them up from a pre-med advisor, or contact the MCAT program office at the following address:

MCAT Program Office
PO Box 4056
Iowa City, IA 52243

If you have not finished most of the prerequisites for the test—two semesters each of biology, physics, general chemistry, and organic chemistry—you probably should not sit for the exam. If you are determined to try the test without being fully prepared, take advantage of the fact that you can take a practice test at any Princeton Review office. It is much, much better to find out precisely what your current scoring levels are on a practice exam than to have to explain a woefully low score on a later medical school application.

It is possible, although it's certainly not the best idea, to take the last semester of one of the required science courses concurrently with studying for the MCAT. If you find yourself in this situation, it is vitally important to lighten your course load so that you will be able to adequately study for the exam while maintaining good grades in your courses. Thoroughly studying for the MCAT is not a small task.

How to Study for the MCAT

You are correct in assuming that since you're reading a book published by The Princeton Review, we're a little biased as to how we think you should study for the MCAT. The short answer here is that for most people, taking a course to prepare for the MCAT is worth the investment in both time and money. This is simply because MCAT scores are as important as your GPA in terms of admissions criteria. The MCAT is a tedious and wretched business, and having a class full of fellow sufferers at least makes you feel less alone in your pain. A class also forces you to study in a reasonable way, cover the material effectively, get plenty of practice, and gives you the resources to shore up any gaps in your academic preparation.

There are some people who do not need much preparation for the MCAT, and you'll meet them in medical school. They'll be getting honors designations in all of their classes while maintaining their world rankings as premier ice climbers/Sanskrit poets/master chefs. Unless you're pretty sure you're one of them (you might qualify if you're reading this while skydiving) you'll need some help with the test.

First, assume that you will be spending about twenty hours a week for several months studying for the MCAT. Although it doesn't test everything you've learned in school, it will feel that way. And, if you're rusty or haven't studied one of the subjects in awhile—physics, general chemistry, organic chemistry, and biology—you're going to have to do some in-depth review. At the same time, you have to keep in mind that this is a standardized test, and even though it's one of the better ones available, it still suffers from the same flaws as all other standardized tests—a fact that you can use to your advantage.

The key to doing well on the exam is to know the material, and then to know the test. The MCAT consists of four timed sections administered over a period of more than seven hours.

As you can see from the grid below, the MCAT tests basic sciences—but don't assume that the exam is a science test similar to the kind you have learned to take as an undergraduate. Fundamentally, the MCAT is a verbal test, which is why on average, humanities majors tend to get slightly better scores in all of the sections than any other major. They are seeing a test format that they are used to: passages and questions. Science majors, on the other hand, are generally used to manipulating formulas and answering questions that may have a setup, but are not embedded in a long series of paragraphs.

In practice, it is much easier to raise your score if you start with low science numbers but a high verbal score. Unfortunately, most examinees are in exactly the opposite position. This is of real concern because more and more medical schools have come to regard scores that are out of balance as undesirable. They will often look more favorably on a candidate with three tens than someone with an eight verbal and two twelves. In order to change your verbal score you will have to practice the type of causal, linear logic that it tests. AAMC releases five previous MCATs, including one that is free, and a couple of books of practice items (any formal test preparation course should give you reams of additional practice material). If you don't have access to test preparation courses, you will probably find yourself rapidly running out of verbal practice material, although most college bookstores are reasonably well stocked with practice materials relating to the science portions of the MCAT. You can use reading comprehension sections from other graduate-level standardized tests such as the GRE or LSAT to supplement your verbal study, but keep in mind that the passages in these tests were not written to be read under the same time constraints as were the MCAT passages. In addition, you may want to consider using online training materials.

The MCAT

Section	Questions	Time	Score
Physical Sciences	77	100 minutes	1–15
Verbal Reasoning	60	85 minutes	1–15
Writing Sample	2	60 minutes	J–T
Biological Sciences	77	100 minutes	1–15

MCAT Score Reporting—Full Disclosure

Gone are the days when prospective med students could choose whether or not to release their MCAT scores to schools before seeing them. The MCAT is, in fact, moving toward a "full disclosure" policy, whereby scores from any MCAT taken in 2003 or later will automatically be reported as part of the examinee's test history. AMCAS and the medical schools you're applying to will always receive your MCAT Testing History Report, or THx Report (previously known as the Additional Score Report). If you took the MCAT between 1991 and 2002, those scores won't be released unless you request it. Still, the dates of those tests will appear on the THx Report.

Although you'll no longer have the option to withhold MCAT scores except in the case of older test dates, this isn't necessarily a bad thing. In the past, schools knew when you withheld your scores, and as you might imagine, they could interpret this in many different ways. Although some schools told us that they did not hold it against you if you withheld your scores, other said they were inclined to look negatively on withheld scores and would rather see your entire test history. Problem solved! Seriously though, these issues may still come into play if you choose to withhold test scores from 2002 or earlier.

There are a few perks to the new THx Report online system, too: the reports are free, and you can check out your score online much earlier—as soon as it's available to the AAMC.

Check out www.PrincetonReview.com for more information on the MCAT, including some changes to the April 2003 test.

Your Budding Career as a Novelist

If you've ever harbored any fantasies of becoming a writer, now is your chance. If you've ever harbored fantasies of wiping the art of composition from human memory in retaliation for the suffering you endured in your Freshman English class, you're going to have to find a way to cope. The personal comments section of the ACOMAS and AMCAS application is your chance to convince the committee that you are more than the sum of your numbers and that you deserve a chance at an interview.

Idea Generators

It is extremely difficult to write about anything important in a page or less, so assume that you will be spending some quality time with your computer. To get started, you can try a couple of different approaches to get your fingers moving:

Clustering

You may remember this from Freshman Comp. You probably thought it was silly back then, but it just might save you now. Get a large blank piece of paper and write down a few words to describe some of the experiences that have led you to pursue medical school. Or, jot down some interesting, sad, or memorable experiences and later link them to your interest in medicine. You don't have to write them down in any particular order, just scatter your thoughts across the page. After you have several topics to work with, see if you can spot any patterns. Some of them will probably be interrelated. Next, generate longer descriptions of the words you wrote. For example, try to explain what you mean by "intellectual challenge." Was there a particular class you took? A paper you wrote? After you have some ideas on paper, try pulling them together based on the patterns of relationships you see between the topics. For example, telling a story about helping to clean a wound while volunteering in the ER might be a good way of letting them know that compassion is one of your qualities. It is often more effective to let the reader draw conclusions rather than spelling them out. For example, relate how you felt while treating a patient and let the reader see that you are compassionate. Don't write, "That experience demonstrates my compassion."

Free Writing

This is particularly helpful if you find that you are having trouble figuring out where to start. All you have to do is sit down and force yourself to write about anything that comes into your mind. Don't worry about punctuation or grammar—just write for several pages. Take a break and look back at what you wrote. Most of the time, you'll be surprised to discover the beginnings of an idea. Keep a notepad with you and by your bed. Jot down ideas as they come to you.

Talk, Talk, Talk

One way to avoid writer's block and get started is to talk into a tape recorder, or bribe a friend to write as you speak. Sometimes, an empty screen or page can be intimidating in and of itself. You can get started on your essay by telling your story to a tape recorder, or by having a friend write down what he or she thinks is interesting or important as you explain why you want to go to medical school. Don't expect to have suddenly generated your essay in this way. However, you can generate some material with which to start writing.

Three Basic Approaches

There are many different ways to structure the personal essay, but there are three basic approaches that can be used alone or in combination.

"My History in School"

This essay focuses on college experiences. It works well for people whose grades are fairly high and who want to emphasize their growth during the college years. The essay should be about your development, specialties, and strengths. The best essays usually have specific examples. It helps to have a specific class, professor, paper, or experience that crystallizes your experiences and ties into your goals. One of the benefits of this essay is a built-in chronology and organizational structure.

"My Life History"

In this essay, focus on a few events or main ideas that illustrate the qualities you can bring to medicine. If your whole life clearly leads up to being a physician (even if it might not have seemed that way at the time) this can be a good choice. One of the pitfalls of this structure is that it can let you ramble and lose coherency. Although you need to give a brief overview of your life, you also need to concentrate your paragraphs around individual ideas.

"The Story"

This is often the most effective essay if it's done correctly. Focus on one or two stories that illustrate some of the points listed above. The story essay is the most fun for admissions officers to read, and is the most likely to be coherent and cohesive. You don't have to go overboard with adjectives and turns of phrase to write effective narrative. Just pick a few moments that most clearly define why you want to be a physician.

Key Bragging Points

No matter the subject you plan to focus on, the following are points that you should consider incorporating into the finished essay:

Academic Strength

You can discuss this generally, or with a specific example of a class, an assignment, or a moment in which you enjoyed an intellectual challenge. Medical school will require a lot of hard work. What demonstrates your love of hard work?

Commitment to Ideals

No one expects you to be Mother Teresa, but most good physicians have a streak of empathy and altruism.

Balance

What makes you whole? What balances the hardworking academic powerhouse that you are?

Careful, Complex Thinking

It is very difficult to explain something as complicated as your motivation to be a physician. Most people, when writing about a defining moment in their lives, assume that the audience is right there with them. This is not the case. You have to explain what you think and feel after you describe the event. Don't assume that the admissions committee is going to fill in the blanks for you.

Why You Want to Be a Doctor

The question you should ask yourself is why—when many other people who've had similar life/career/academic experiences take one look at the horrendous hours involved in medical training and decide that teaching or counseling are perfectly good alternatives—you want to be a doctor. For instance, although many physicians decide to be doctors because of an early experience with the illness of a family member, there are far greater numbers of people with the same background who never consider medicine—but would still describe themselves as compassionate and moved to help people. You have to force yourself to ascertain what odd mixture of qualities—intellectual and emotional—have convinced you that going more than $100,000 in debt in the era of HMOs is a good idea.

Reasons, Not Excuses, for Weakness

Do not attempt to cover up or gloss over any deficiency, academic or otherwise. You will earn yourself points by honestly and openly dealing with your less than sterling qualities. If you have a couple of low grades or if you had a bad semester, briefly explain what happened, discuss what the experience taught you, and move on.

Good, Clever, Interesting Writing

Translation: Lots and lots and lots of drafts. Everybody has a distinct voice, and you're not going to survive medical school without a sense of humor. Find a way to get both qualities across without resorting to clichés. Prohibited phrases include: Lifelong learning, challenge of a lifetime, healing the mind as well as the body, childlike wonder, frail hands, quiet desperation, and any variations on these themes.

Overall Conservative Tone

Shock value doesn't work, despite the tales you might have heard about cartoons and poems. Admissions committees expect you to take the exercise seriously, and to treat the process with respect. Humor is fine, but it needs to be subtle.

Show, Don't Tell

One of the traps of the personal statement is to rewrite your resume in prose. Instead of listing your accomplishments, explain what they mean to you and show how they have affected your life. For example, if you really want to practice primary care, it is far more effective for you to explain in detail what motivates you than to simply state your goal.

The Evolution of the Essay

Good essays tend to evolve, and often bear very little resemblance to rough drafts. Don't be afraid to start over, or to let the essay build on itself. If you write something that doesn't use any of the forms described above but that you feel gets across the points you want to make, then that is the essay you should stick with. Don't force yourself into a mold.

No matter what your eventual essay looks like, however, there are a few general issues that you should think about.

Focus

Your essay must communicate specific points clearly and effectively. This means that every time you write a sentence that could be used in any other essay, you need to cross it out and start over. For example, "I truly enjoy working with people" could be the opening line in an application for Fry Guy at McDonald's just as easily as it could be a statement about the profound impact you want to have on your patients' health.

Editing

No mistakes. If you are not one of those people who go around making a pest of themselves by correcting everyone else's grammatical errors, you need to find one. Most colleges and universities have writing centers with free editorial assistance, or you can check the local college paper for teaching assistants who are willing to edit for food. No matter what, make sure someone else reads your essay.

Interest

Everyone has an interesting style, and you need to write until you find it. You are who you are for a reason; you have to write until that reason becomes apparent to anyone reading the essay.

Relevance

At some point, the reader will have to have a very clear sense of just why they should let you into their medical school. Don't get so caught up in explaining your inner child that you forget to mention your desire to become a doctor.

Coherence

Make sure your essay fits together. You shouldn't be able to move a paragraph or a sentence when you're finished.

Remember that your entire personality is not going to be reflected in this essay, nor can you entirely offset an otherwise weak application. But this is your big chance to talk to the committee, so make the most of it. Spend the necessary time to draft and rework your essay until it is the best measure of your writing ability and candidacy for medical school.

Secondaries and Letters of Recommendation

After medical schools receive your application, they will send you what's called a "secondary." Some schools send all of their applicants a secondary, while others go through an initial cut (usually based totally on GPA and MCAT score). One of the reasons that schools like to send out secondaries is that they usually charge you about fifty dollars for the privilege of filling them out. Secondaries usually include a variety of essays that are slightly more directed than the "personal comments" in either the ACOMAS or AMCAS. Some typical secondary questions are:

- *What is your favorite novel?*
- *What are your hobbies?*
- *Where do you see yourself in ten years?*
- *Name a leadership role that you've taken and what it taught you about yourself.*
- *What has been your greatest academic achievement? What has been your greatest academic failure?*
- *What type of medicine do you think you might want to practice?*

As you can see, most of these essays seem fairly simple, but that doesn't mean you shouldn't spend time thoughtfully filling them out. Many secondaries are quite lengthy, so it's a good idea to fill them out as you get them, unless you've decided for some reason not to continue with your application to the school. If you find that the cost of sending back secondaries rapidly becomes prohibitive, you can call the individual schools and request a fee waiver. If you were eligible for a waiver from AMCAS, for example, you will probably be able to have most of your secondary fees waived.

You should also take care of your letters of recommendation at the secondary stage. If you are a student who is still in school and you have access to pre-health advising, your letters will probably be handled by that office, and at least one of your letters will probably be from the pre-health advisor. Usually, your recommenders will write one letter that the advising office will copy and send to your list of schools. If you are a returning adult, you may have to take care of all the requests and letters yourself.

Letters of recommendation for medical school work in much the same way as any other such letters; you will have much better luck if you approach your potential recommender with a copy of your resume, transcript, and personal statement. Try to make an appointment to speak to the person to explain to them about the various schools to which you are applying, and to make your case. Even if you have been out of school for awhile, you should try to get at least one letter from a former professor. Medical schools are interested in your character, your desire to be a physician, your academic preparedness, and your intellectual ability. Although most employers could attest to some of those qualities, you will probably need a letter from a professor that discusses your academic abilities. As an undergrad or in your post-bacc program, try to build relationships with faculty members so they can write something meaningful about you. Don't ask for a letter from someone famous unless they know you pretty well. Name dropping is not considered to be particularly attractive in a prospective medical student.

Although many returning adults feel awkward approaching professors they might not have spoken with in several years, most are pleasantly surprised to discover that for the most part, professors do tend to remember their students, and most are happy to write them letters of recommendation. Both current and former students should also consider asking for letters from doctors with whom they have worked or volunteered—and remember that if you're applying to osteopathic school, you have to have a letter from a DO.

Once you discover how painless it really is to get a letter of recommendation, you may be tempted to go into overdrive on the theory that inundating the committee with reams of stationary will force them to recognize your worthiness. Resist this! Do not send more letters than the school asks for. The committee will not read them, and you will not have done yourself any favors. The only time you might consider sending extra letters is if you are placed on hold after an interview, and have in the meantime been working with someone who you feel would be able to contribute some additional information about your abilities.

Minority Recruitment

Minority status refers to ethnicities that are *underrepresented* in medicine, such as Native Americans, African Americans, Latinos, Native Hawaiians, and some other specific groups. If you are not sure whether you are a minority in this sense, you should contact AMCAS. Many public and private medical schools recognize the value of educating physicians who will work in underserved areas and communities. Some committees look favorably on a candidate with a background that suggests he or she will fill this need. In some cases, this amounts to a preference for candidates with specific ethnic backgrounds—but it is a preference that occurs after a field of equally qualified applicants is generated from the initial pool. Medical schools are simply too competitive to accept candidates who are not up to the intellectual challenge of medicine. This selectivity advantage often extends to people of any ethnicity who come from under-served rural areas and seem inclined to return there to practice medicine.

There is also a type of minority status that AMCAS recognizes that deals only with economic factors, and does not take into account ethnicity or country of origin. To be considered a "financially disadvantaged" minority, you need to have been under financial strain for a long period of time, and to have been the recipient of federal aid in the form of AFDC, welfare, food stamps, or other such programs. Your financial situation needs to have had an ongoing and persistent negative effect on your ability to procure education, housing, food, etc. In other words, the average two-job-struggling-to-make-ends-meet college student does not qualify. This minority status is reserved for those who have struggled uphill their entire lives, and have somehow managed to make it through undergraduate school. The basic rule of thumb here is: If you are a financially disadvantaged minority, you probably know it. If you're in doubt, you probably aren't.

Medical schools are faced with a problem that is actually a boon for the quality of health care in the U.S.: they literally have more good applicants that they can take. This means that medical schools can easily fill their classes with students who are academically qualified. Medical schools have the opportunity to select from this pool those students who are most likely to improve under-served communities and help those with the most need. The AAMC has sought to increase enrollment of underrepresented minorities in recent years. AOA has recently instituted a minority scholarship, the Sherry R. Arnstein Minority Student Award, to boost minority recruitment at osteopathic schools.

WHAT HAPPENS AFTER YOU'VE BEEN ACCEPTED

So you've achieved the impossible, the best-case scenario: multiple acceptances. First, congratulations. Second, it's probably not a good idea to share your good fortune with too many of your pre-med friends, unless you don't particularly want to keep them and you've first removed all the sharp objects from the room.

Back to Reality

After the giddiness wears off, you will have to deal with the best problem you will ever have: choosing which school to attend. Remember that you have lots of time to choose the medical school that best fits your goals and lifestyle. You can hang on to your acceptances until May 15, at which point schools will begin dropping your name off of their acceptance lists if you have not committed. Remember, however, that most of your fellow pre-meds do not share your enviable position. If you are accepted by a school that you know you will not attend, notify them before the deadline so that they can offer the seat to someone else. If you are on the waitlist for a school you really want, don't heisitate to write a short note letting the committee know the school is your first choice.

Factors to Consider

So, while you are basking in your acceptance, think seriously about the following factors, but don't selfishly hold onto too many acceptances while you are deliberating.

How much does the school emphasize and reward teaching?

This is a huge concern and often overlooked. Look into how much the school values teaching vs. how much they emphasize research. This can be the difference between being taught and being forced to teach yourself. The best way to determine teaching quality is to ask current students for their opinions.

What are community, social life, and support systems like?

Talk to current students to determine the overall community of the school. You'll be there for four years, and you certainly won't be studying all—OK, most, but not all—of the time. Do the students seem to be accepting the rigors of med school with a positive view or do they waste all extra energy complaining? What is the quality of life in general like at this school? Do students study together? Is it a community or commuter lifestyle?

What's the quality of the residents?

The residents are the ones who will be teaching you when you're a med student, so of course you want them to be good. You should presumably be able to approximate the quality of residents based on the quality of post-graduate training programs (residency programs) at the hospitals affiliated with the school.

How family-friendly are the school and its surroundings?

If you're a returning adult student with a family, check into the spouse/partner support available at the schools you're considering. Getting through medical school will be hard on you and your family, and many places have begun programs that allow spouses/partners to attend special seminars and support groups that acclimate you to the pressures of your chosen educational and career path. Will your partner be able to find work/activities he or she enjoys?

Where will you be living?

Believe it or not, you will occasionally escape to the outside world. Make sure that the activities and hobbies you enjoy are available somewhere in the general vicinity. If you come from one climate and are moving to another, consider how that will affect you. Also, find out how close the clinical facilities are to the school and housing. The closer the better.

What kind of research opportunities are available?

Some schools are much better equipped than others, and it's not always the "name" schools that are doing the most cutting-edge research. Different schools have different specialties, and some benefit from affiliated schools of public health, business, or law. Other schools offer paid research opportunities.

Traditional or systems-based?

Teaching methodologies include traditional (two years of science plus two years of rotations), organ-based (learn everything about the liver), case-based (learn science by delving into patient histories), and everything in between. Which method will be best for you? It is difficult to know. It is also likely that other issues are more important for you to consider, such as regard for education, commitment to teaching, and responsiveness to student input and overall academic climate. These issues may prove more important than the curricular grid (i.e., when you take Anatomy), in terms of how much you learn and how much you enjoy learning.

What kind of financial aid offer are they making?

Is the offer good for all four years? In comparing offers between schools, consider cost of living differences and variation in the terms of loans.

How much will you owe?

This is the most important financial aid statistic a school can offer because it encompasses tuition, expenses, and financial aid. No matter what kind of financial package you get, you will most likely owe a staggering sum when you graduate, and it all eventually has to be paid back. As an intern and resident, you won't be making much in the way of a salary ($38,000 in 2002). Although most physicians eventually achieve a comfortable living (average of $160,000 annual salary in 2002), the practice of medicine is in such a state of flux that it is impossible to predict what kinds of jobs and compensation will be available ten years from now. A public university education, while perhaps not carrying quite the cachet as a private school, may save you tens of thousands of dollars and relieve some of the stress associated with gargantuan debt.

BEHIND DOOR NUMBER 1 . . . MORE STANDARDIZED TESTS!

Most medical students take the USMLE Step 1 (and/or the first COMLEX—the COMLEX exams go in the same order as the USMLEs) at the end of the second year of medical school. Osteopathic students must pass the USMLE to obtain allopathic residency spots. Step 1 is often used to determine whether or not a student has "passed" their pre-clinical course work and can continue into their third and fourth years of training. Step 2 is usually taken during the third or fourth year of school during clerkships. At this point, the vast majority of senior U.S. medical students go through the Match in order to obtain residency positions. Very few contract privately for their first year of graduate medical training. Most programs in the Match now use ERAS

(Electronic Residency Application Service), which is administered by AAMC, rather than a traditional paper application. Step 3 is usually taken after at least one year of residency (most physicians do at least three years of residency, but still take the test after the first year). The USMLE is written and scored by the National Board of Medical Examiners, which administers Steps 1 and 2. Step 3 is administered by the state. The state confers the license; the USMLE is a prerequisite.

International Medical Graduates

International medical graduates (IMG) go through a special process to be granted licensure in the U.S. Before you can start a residency program, you need to be certified by the Education Commission for Foreign Medical Graduates (ECFMG). To be certified, an IMG must complete the following five steps:

- *Take USMLE Steps 1 and 2.*
- *Send medical credentials and fill out the paperwork necessary to show proof of medical education.*
- *Take the English test administered by the ECFMG.*
- *If you don't pass the English test, you can take the Test of English as a Foreign Language instead.*
- *Take the Clinical Skills Assessment, which is a live "standardized patient" exam.*

After this, contact the board of the state in which you want to practice for the Step 3 requirements (each state determines its own passing score). You can get a residency either through the NRMP Match or through a private contract. After passing Step 3 and following any other state guidelines, you are granted a temporary license to practice in that state.

If you are currently in a medical program abroad and thinking about transferring to a U.S. medical school, you need to contact the school and ask about its transfer policies. In general, it is extremely difficult to transfer into a U.S. medical school.

ANOTHER PRINCETON REVIEW RESOURCE FOR PROSPECTIVE MED STUDENTS

For more in-depth information about putting together a winning application, look out for our new medical school admissions guide, available in the spring in our online bookstore: www.princetonreview.com/medical/bookstore.asp.

HIGH SCHOOL STUDENTS

If you've picked up this book and you're still in high school, you're very much ahead of the game. You can get started on the road to medical school by participating in volunteer activities and researching potential college choices to learn about their pre-medical training. Remember, you can major in any subject that interests you as long as you complete your pre-medical courses. Choose a subject you enjoy, and you are more likely to earn good grades and get into medical school. A few schools have special programs that funnel students through their undergraduate education directly into medical school. If you are interested in these programs, you should contact the following schools directly for more information:

Boston University

Brown University

Case Western University

East Tennessee State University

George Washington University

Howard University

Louisiana State University—New Orleans

Louisiana State University—Shreveport

Michigan State University

New York University

Northwestern University

University of Alabama

University of Miami

University of Michigan

University of Missouri, Kansas City

University of Rochester

University of South Alabama

University of Southern California

University of Wisconsin

IMPORTANT CONTACT ORGANIZATIONS

American Osteopathic Association (AOA)

142 E. Ontario Street
Chicago, IL 60611-2864
800-621-1773
www.aoa-net.org

American Association of Colleges of Osteopathic Medicine (AACOM)

5550 Friendship Boulevard
Suite 310
Chevy Chase, MD 20815-7231
301-968-4100
301-968-4101 (fax)
www.aacom.org

AMERICAN ASSOCIATION OF MEDICAL COLLEGES (AAMC)
2450 N. Street, NW
Washington, DC 20037-1126
202-828-0400
202-828-1125 (fax)
www.aamc.org

EDUCATIONAL COMMISSION FOR FOREIGN MEDICAL GRADUATES
3624 Market Street
Fourth Floor
Philadelphia, PA 19104-2685
215-386-5900
www.ecfmg.org

FEDERATION OF STATE MEDICAL BOARDS
400 Fuller Wiser Road
Suite 300
Euless, TX 76039-3855
817-868-4000
817-868-4099 (fax)
www.fsmb.org

NATIONAL BOARD OF MEDICAL EXAMINERS
3750 Market Street
Philadelphia, PA 19104
215-590-9500
215-590-9555 (fax)
www.nbme.org

THE TEXAS MEDICAL AND DENTAL SCHOOLS APPLICATION SERVICE
702 Colorado, Suite 6400
Austin, TX 78701
512-499-4785
www.utsystem.edu/tmdsas
(Texas public schools do not use AMCAS)

4 Advice for the "Nontraditional" Applicant

Forty years ago, most medical school applicants shared certain traits. The "traditional" medical school applicant was white, male, and just older than twenty. Most likely, he majored in biology or chemistry while in college. Although he knew that medical school would be difficult and that his career would be challenging, he looked forward to choosing from a wide range of medical specialties and being financially secure. As a trained professional, he would possess real skills and expertise and, as a result, could expect to enjoy authority and autonomy.

The past few decades have seen substantial changes both in the composition of the medical school applicant pool, and in the professional opportunities available to medical school graduates. Based on the previous idea of the "traditional" medical student, women and minority applicants could be considered "nontraditional," but the term is currently used to describe applicants who are older than most med students. The average age of applicants is between 23 and 26, but a significant and increasing proportion of applicants are several years older.

Some of these older applicants, always intending to apply to medical school, completed pre-medical requirements during their years as undergraduates, and simply postponed medical school to work, travel, or start a family. Others were unsuccessful at gaining admission directly out of college and are attempting a second or third time. Another group considered medical school in college, but did not complete requirements or the application process. Some older applicants never seriously considered medicine until after they graduated college and were involved in another occupation. Whatever the reason for postponing, older applicants now represent a significant proportion of the medical school candidate pool.

Aspiring doctors who did not take the prerequisite science courses in college or did not excel in them face a formidable challenge. These individuals have a minimum of seven years of medical school and residency on the horizon and, in addition, must complete (and do well in) one to two years of basic science courses before even applying to medical school. Nonetheless, thousands of adults, despite the arduous path ahead of them, decide to tackle this challenge. This chapter is intended as a source of information and support for nontraditional applicants in all stages of the application process. It is written by a nontraditional applicant with the input of others who are or were in the same category. Follow eight nontraditional applicants through the entire process—from decision-making, to post-bacc training, to MCAT preparation, and acceptance. The group is composed of real individuals[1] coming from a wide range of backgrounds, some elements of which will hopefully resemble aspects of your own situation. When these people decided that medical school was their goal, this is who they were and what they were doing:

- *Becky, a 28-year-old who completed two years of college and had worked as a medical assistant for ten years.*
- *Pete, a 28-year-old with a law degree who was unhappy in his field.*
- *Tina, a 27-year-old art history major who was working in a gallery and dating a medical student.*
- *Bob, a 35-year-old chemistry professor at a small college.*
- *Mitch, a 30-year-old former Peace Corps volunteer, who was working in international development.*
- *Jacob, a 24-year-old volunteer firefighter. A car accident and subsequent hospitalization kept him from completing organic chemistry while in college. Discouraged, he dropped out of the pre-medical track.*
- *Eve, a 42-year-old wife and mother of three who graduated college twenty years ago, and had little experience working outside of the home.*
- *Donald, an engineering graduate student who decided that he needed more human contact in his work.*

DECIDING THAT MEDICINE—AND MEDICAL SCHOOL—IS WHAT YOU WANT

Some of these people were absolutely sure about going to medical school. Jacob, for example, had always known. Tina, who was fascinated by what her boyfriend studied in medical school, had a strong hunch. Donald imagined that being a physician would give him what he felt was missing from his career, but he had limited contact with the medical field and had not fully considered other options that would give him more personal interaction.

[1] Names have been changed.

Being reasonably sure about medicine is important because you will invest time, money, and energy into the medical school preparation and application process. It is also important because admissions officers will look for indications of your commitment. If you are sure of it, your commitment is more likely to come through in your personal statement and your interview.

If you have never worked or volunteered in a medical setting, you should explore your opportunities. You might arrange to informally shadow a physician or to volunteer in a hospital that has a formal program. Some volunteers find that they are given more responsibility at a small clinic than they are in a large hospital, so look into clinic programs as well. Explore opportunities to volunteer in overseas medical projects. Of our eight subjects, those who had more than one medically related experience felt that it was beneficial because they were exposed to the variation that exists within the field. Not only are volunteer activities helpful in your decision-making process, but they will become significant resume builders should you decide to apply to medical school. In addition, they are likely to be valuable and, hopefully, enjoyable experiences.

One way to help determine if medicine is the right career for you is to talk to others who have made the choice. Interview as many people as you can. Talk to practicing physicians, residents, medical students, and those involved in academic medicine such as researchers. Find out what they love and hate about their work. Ask questions that will help you put their comments about medicine in perspective. For example, if you come across someone who positively hated medical school and dislikes being a physician, ask him what part of medical school he hated the least. If his favorite part of the experience was the relaxing cruise-ship vacation he took after his first year, he probably could have made a better career choice for himself. His views of medical school may not be an indication of what the experience will be like for you.

If possible, talk to medical students, practicing physicians, and resident physicians who are or were nontraditional. Find out whether they feel that they made the right decision. What were the biggest sacrifices they had to make? Visit the pre-medical and medical student discussion pages on the Internet where many nontraditional applicants and students share their thoughts. Although we are unaware of books documenting the experiences of nontraditional medical students, at least one book does give accounts of nontraditional applicants.[2] A commonly held view is that nontraditional medical students have more difficulty with the pre-clinical medical curriculum, but excel during the clinical years.[3] Based on our own discussions, however, nontraditional medical

[2] Goss, Bryan. *Applying to Medical School for the Nontraditional Student.* 1997: Lakeshore-Pearson Publications. Contact Mountain Books, Albuquerque, NM.

[3] Some studies indicate that nontraditional students do less well in basic science courses. See Blacklow HM et al. *Postbaccalaureate Preparation and Performance in Medical School.* Academic Medicine 1990 June; 65 (6). Other studies refute the claim. See Hall ML, Stocks MD. *Relationship Between Quantity of Undergraduate Science Preparation and Preclinical Performance in Medical School.* Academic Medicine 1995 March; 70:3.

students express fewer doubts about their decision to go to medical school than those who went directly from college. Perhaps this is because they appreciate having a second "chance" at a career, or perhaps it is because they gave the decision more thought.

Bob's decision to apply to medical school was influenced by his sister-in-law. She works in medical equipment sales and is five years older than Bob. She encouraged him to follow his dream, saying that she, too, had entertained the idea of becoming a physician when she was thirty. She decided against it and at forty still dreams about doing it today. But with two young children, she feels that it would be too difficult. Bob decided that it would be more painful to spend his life wondering if he should have gone to medical school than to go and—in the worst-case scenario—drop out and return to teaching.

Mitch also found it helpful to talk to people working in totally unrelated fields. He had worked for two years in a clinic in rural Africa, and thought that he wanted to become a pediatrician. However, he became discouraged while talking to his friends who were medical students, residents, or newly graduated practicing physicians because it seemed that few people loved everything about what they were doing. Many of his friends warned him of the burden of debt and the prospect of having little free time. One friend told him that in comparison to Mitch's current job, which involved traveling around the world, he would be *bored* in medicine. Mitch then took an informal poll of all his friends who included teachers, writers, business owners, software designers, lawyers, and full-time parents. He found that people in all occupations both love *and* hate certain things about their work.

Although medical students and physicians complain about debt, teachers complain about low salaries, and business owners complain about financial insecurity. All of Mitch's friends in their early thirties complain about working too hard, and about the difficulty of balancing their personal and family lives with their careers. Mitch concluded that, despite the initial discouragement he got from friends in the medical profession, people in medicine are among the *most* professionally fulfilled. Although medical students and physicians had complaints, they were engaged in their work and most couldn't imagine a better career. He also noticed that a significant number of nonphysicians he spoke to, although unhappy with their own jobs, still discouraged him from going into medicine. He realized that some of these people had, at one point in their lives, entertained the idea of becoming a doctor. They had successfully talked themselves out of medical school and were sold on all the reasons why *not* to go into medicine. As far as his friend's comment about being bored, Mitch realized that others tended to glamorize his current work because it involved travel. He knew that being a pediatrician would, on a day-to-day basis, be more interesting than the paperwork he dealt with in his current job. Furthermore, he could probably work overseas as a physician if he found himself yearning for travel.

After you follow Mitch's example and grill everyone you know, ask yourself some serious questions. What jobs and experiences have you loved most in your life? Do you foresee medicine providing similar satisfaction? Have you enjoyed some aspects of your medically related work? Do you have the skills it takes to become a physician? To be fulfilled as one? Whether or not to pursue a career in medicine is an important decision that will affect many years of your life. Give yourself time, both for information gathering and personal reflection. Write down your thoughts on what is influencing your decision. Whether or not you decide to go for it, if you carefully weigh the decision now, you will be less likely to doubt it later on.

Resist feeling that, because you are "older," you should make your decision to enter medical school as quickly as possible. Medical school, internship, and residency require at least seven years to complete. Moreover, medicine is a career of lifelong learning. Start finding things to enjoy about the process of becoming a doctor now. Deciding to go to medical school is part of the process. Try not to stress too much about the decision, and find some satisfaction in your information gathering and self-reflection.

GETTING INTO MEDICAL SCHOOL AS A NONTRADITIONAL APPLICANT

If you are reading this, you have probably decided to move forward with your plan to become an MD or a DO Hopefully, your level of maturity and your life experience have allowed you to make a well-informed decision that a student just out of college may not be in a position to make. Between 20 percent and 30 percent of applicants in the 24- to 37-year-old age range are admitted to medical school, while approximately 45 percent of 21 to 23 year olds are admitted. Although these statistics suggest that the odds are against older applicants, age itself is not regarded as a disadvantage, and may in some cases be a plus. The smaller percentage of older applicants admitted may be partially due to lower GPAs[4] and test scores. Even the most exciting and unique older applicant must have a competitive GPA and MCAT score.

The timing of the admissions process is often an issue for nontraditional applicants. Donald started thinking about medical school mid-way through his first year of graduate school. We will call this January of Year 1. He realized that he had prerequisites to fulfill and that he wouldn't be eligible to enter medical school the following fall, but thought he would be able to matriculate in the fall of Year 3. Donald quit his graduate program and entered an intensive pre-medical curriculum, completing his requirements by January, Year 2. He took the MCAT in April, Year 2. If Donald had taken pre-medical courses part-time rather than full-time, he could not have adhered to this schedule. Had he done poorly on the MCAT the first time, he could have been delayed

[4] Smith, SR. *A Two-Year Experience with Premedical Postbaccalaureate Students Admitted to Medical School.* Academic Medicine; 1991: 66:1.

an entire year and postponed entrance until Year 4. As a result of the timing of the admissions process, it takes two to four years to matriculate after deciding to pursue medical school. The following are the important dates to remember as you think about timeframe and requirements:

- *April: MCAT is given. You should have completed all prerequisite science courses by this date.*
- *June: AMCAS (preliminary) applications are accepted. Filling out the AMCAS application requires all undergraduate, graduate, and post-bacc transcripts (they accept transcripts beginning on March 15, but the completed application isn't accepted until June 1). You will need your own copies, and you will need to have copies sent directly to AMCAS. It is important to submit AMCAS applications as soon as possible because most schools offer rolling admissions.*
- *August: MCAT is given. Use this test date only if you need to improve your scores from the April test. You will indicate on your AMCAS application whether you intend to take (or retake) the test on this date. If so, many schools will not look at your application until August scores are available (some time in October). The penalty for this delay may very well outweigh your score improvement. Thus, unless you anticipate significant score improvement, the August MCAT is not advised.*
- *August: Medical schools to which AMCAS applications have been submitted begin sending secondary applications. Some schools will review AMCAS applications closely, and send secondary ones to a limited number of applicants. Others send them to everyone who applies through AMCAS. There is almost always an additional fee. In some cases, secondary applications require essays or short-answer questions that focus on motivation, personal characteristics, values, and experiences. In other cases, the application is very simple and similar to the AMCAS application. Thus, receiving a secondary application may be an indication that a school is interested in you. When you return the application and fee, you demonstrate your interest in the school. Schools often want these back within two to four weeks. You will also need to submit recommendations at this time. Some schools ask for a photo.*
- *August–May: Based on AMCAS and secondary applications and recommendations, applicants are invited to interview during this period. Some schools conduct all their interviews during one or two months, while others spread them out. Most schools accept 25–50+ percent of interviewed candidates. Thus, getting an interview is an excellent sign. Most admissions decisions are also made during this period, with the exception of applicants who fall into a "hold" or "wait list" category.*
- *June–August: Wait-listed candidates may be accepted.*

ACADEMIC REQUIREMENTS

Most medical schools require or strongly prefer that applicants have a BA or BS degree from a four-year accredited college or university. All medical schools require a minimum level of science preparation that includes approximately one year each of biology, chemistry, organic chemistry, and physics. Some nontraditional candidates meet these requirements by taking night courses while simultaneously working part- or full-time. Others enroll full-time at private or public undergraduate institutions. Some choose to enroll in special "post-baccalaureate pre-medical" programs (we call them post-bacc programs) offered by a surprisingly large number of colleges and universities (see chapter 8 for a comprehensive listing of post-bacc programs). Post-bacc programs vary widely in terms of cost, rigor of course work, grading system, percentage of graduates admitted to medical school, structure and flexibility of curriculum, duration, size, and class composition. Unlike medical schools, post-bacc programs are neither accredited as such, nor ranked.

Becky needed to complete her BA in addition to fulfilling science prerequisites. When she decided it was time to take a shot at fulfilling her long-time dream of becoming a physician, she lived and worked in California, which has some of the most selective state-affiliated medical schools in the country. Becky decided to move to another state and complete her BA there so that she would be qualified for admission to the state's medical school. Becky enrolled full-time for three years to complete her BA—not all of her previous college credits transferred—and fulfill all her science requirements.

Becky's strategy is interesting and may be advisable for others in similar situations who are prepared to relocate. Before moving across the country, be sure that you understand your new state's criteria for determining residency. In some states, being a full-time student does not ensure resident status. Becky might have saved herself a year of schooling had she looked at more colleges and possibly uncovered schools willing to award her credit for all her previous college work.

Tina graduated from a prestigious college, but had taken neither science nor math classes while in school. She was also concerned about her undergraduate GPA, which was 2.9. To make herself a more competitive applicant, she wanted to demonstrate both competence in the sciences and overall improved study skills. Some post-baccalaureate pre-medical programs are quite structured and involve only the minimum science prerequisites; Tina felt that she needed more than this to make up for her undergrad GPA. One of Tina's options was to apply to a post-bacc program that allows participants to take additional courses beyond those in the required scientific disciplines. This type of program tends to be somewhat flexible, allowing students to spend as much time as needed to fulfill requirements and take any additional courses. Students get the opportunity to learn foreign languages, improve writing or math skills, or take courses often recommended—but not required—by medical schools such as biochemistry or statistics. Other post-bacc programs apply students' course work toward a master's degree.

Tina decided not to enter an organized post-bacc program. Instead, she enrolled full-time as a non-degree candidate at a local, private university. This gave her access to larger course offerings. One of the advantages of post-bacc programs is that they are compact, scheduling courses and labs so students may complete all requirements within a year. Tina was less worried about speed, and more interested in earning excellent grades. Another important consideration for Tina was letters of recommendation. Medical schools usually prefer that applicants submit a composite letter from their pre-medical advisor who is typically an administrator or dean, a department head, a specified faculty member, or some type of counselor. The letter discusses the student's qualifications and incorporates comments from his or her pre-medical professors. Because Tina chose a small school, she had the opportunity to get to know her professors and, presumably, to secure meaningful comments from them. At some colleges, only degree-earning students have full access to pre-medical and other advisors, but Tina was able to identify one who agreed to write a letter for her. One advantage to true post-bacc programs is that the pre-medical advisors are able to write appropriate letters of recommendation for nontraditional applicants.

Some pre-medical candidates are highly concerned with getting through the application process quickly and have no interest in prolonging pre-medical course work. Pete had a 3.7 GPA in college and an excellent record in law school. He had no need to prove himself scholastically, but just wanted to "get the sciences out of the way." He was a good candidate for a highly selective post-bacc program. To be admitted to one of these programs, applicants must submit detailed information including personal statements, prior standardized test scores, and several recommendations. Interviews are often required. These programs seek to admit students who will not only complete the course work, but who are likely to be accepted to medical school. Often, the brochures for these programs boast the percentage of graduates who have been admitted into medical school. Although a high acceptance rate is partially a reflection of the quality and resources of the program itself, it also indicates that they accept well-qualified students. In one year, Pete was able to complete all his sciences and study for and take the MCAT.

Pete took advantage of an arrangement between his post-bacc program and a medical school, allowing him to enter medical school in the fall following completion of pre-medical course work. Thus, he avoided an "in between" year generally devoted to the medical school application process. Several selective post-bacc programs offer this type of arrangement, affiliation, or linkage with a number of medical schools. In some cases, the medical school and the post-bacc program are part of the same university. Many nontraditional candidates are disappointed to discover that top medical schools such as Harvard, University of Pennsylvania, and Columbia do not offer these arrangements with their own university's post-bacc program.

Pete took the shortest path possible to medical school. In the fall of 1996 he left the law firm where he was working, and in the fall of 1997, he was beginning medical school. He was happy to skip the long and stressful medical school application process, having been through a similar experience with law school. While ideal for some, Pete's path is neither available nor advisable for everyone. The short, intensive post-bacc programs are grueling and may be too fast-paced for some people. Graduates of these programs often claim their post-bacc work was more demanding than medical school itself. Although these programs can serve as excellent preparation for medical school, they may discourage people who could have succeeded had they enrolled in a more relaxed program.

Earning acceptance to a post-bacc program with affiliated medical schools does not assure your acceptance to medical schools. Post-bacc students in these programs usually apply to the affiliated schools, but acceptances are only provisional, and based on securing a minimum GPA and MCAT score. Only a handful of medical schools participate in these linkages, and each school limits the number of positions available through the direct admissions route. Pete chose his post-bacc program in part because one of the linked medical schools interested him. If none of the medical schools that allow admission through this route appeal to you, saving one year now is probably not worth spending four years someplace you don't want to be. Generally, medical schools agree to these arrangements as a means of enrolling students who they would otherwise not attract. Thus, if you are accepted as a post-bacc student to one of these schools, you are not likely to be accepted to other schools if you apply through the regular admissions process. Another disadvantage to these arrangements is that they are usually binding: if you get in, you must go. If you earn a perfect score on the MCAT, you cannot withdraw and apply to your dream school for the following year. Additionally, you have no opportunity to compare financial aid packages.

While Donald, Tina, Pete, and Becky quit their jobs to enter pre-medical studies full time, Mitch, Jacob, and Eve opted for part-time schooling. Eve wanted to ease into school, and decided to take one course at a time. She enrolled in a general chemistry class through the extension office of a local public university. Her children spent summers at camp and with relatives, allowing her to take a compact organic chemistry course during the summer. The following school year, she enrolled in a two-semester biology course, and she took an intensive physics course the next summer. Eve was concerned that her age would hurt her chances of being accepted to medical school. Some pre-medical advisors believe that being older than forty may be a slight disadvantage.[5] However, had she crammed all of the required science courses into just one year, she would have only been one year younger when she applied to med school, but a whole lot more frustrated and perhaps not as appealing a candidate because her grades could have suffered. In retrospect, Eve's only regret about taking courses "on her own" is that she missed the camaraderie and support that she might have had in a post-bacc

[5] See the article, "Is It Too Late For Me To Go To Medical School?" by Leon C. Dorosz, Professor and Chair, Department of Biological Sciences, San Jose State University.

program. An advantage to post-bacc programs is that you will meet people facing challenges similar to your own.

Most medical schools advise nontraditional applicants to demonstrate success in *recent* course work. Bob had fulfilled all the prerequisites in college about fifteen years earlier. Since Bob had a graduate degree in science, and remained active in an academic environment, the fact that he completed his prerequisite courses years earlier did not hurt him. His hurdle was the MCAT, for which he reviewed intensely.

The grading systems vary tremendously among undergraduate institutions and post-bacc programs. Some material that you learn as a pre-med, such as the basic biochemical processes, will serve you in medical school. Other topics, like whether your rowboat sinks or rises if you fall into the water, might not. As a pre-medical student, your goals should be to figure out whether you enjoy studying science, to learn the material for the MCAT, and to get good grades.

Some colleges and universities with post-bacc programs assign nontraditional students to regular, undergraduate science courses. You attend lectures, labs, and exams alongside undergraduates, and may or may not be graded on the same curve as your younger classmates. Most likely, the mean score of post-bacc students is somewhat higher than that of the rest of the class. Undergraduates shouldn't be penalized by your presence since, after all, you already have your BA Thus, schools with significant numbers of post-bacc students are likely to separate them from the undergraduates for grading purposes. Unfortunately, this practice could hurt you because you may be competing with your undergraduate classmates for positions in medical schools. Your cumulative test score of 90 percent put you in the middle of the post-bacc curve and earned you a C, while your classmate's 90 percent put him at the front end of the undergraduate curve and earned him an A. Although a letter of recommendation could explain that you did in fact maintain a 90 percent average, a C is still a C.

Some post-bacc programs address this issue by setting the post-bacc curve higher. The mean score will represent a B grade rather than a C grade. Highly selective post-bacc programs usually recognize that all their students were strong in college, and will set the mean somewhere in the A– or B+ range. If a college that does not have a formal post-bacc program allows you to enroll in science courses, your GPA might be slightly higher because you will be graded with your classmates, many of whom are probably less focused and less serious than you about maintaining excellent grades. Note, however, that many medical schools consider the caliber of undergraduate institutions when evaluating GPAs. This applies to traditional and nontraditional applicants alike.

THE MCAT

The MCAT is a day-long exam that is offered twice yearly at locations throughout the country. It is composed of four sections. An individual's raw score (number wrong out of number possible) on each section is compared with those of test-takers nationwide and is converted to a scaled score. Because most MCAT takers have never sat through an all-day exam, many find the experience a test of endurance and concentration as much as a test of knowledge (see page 23 for more information on the MCAT).

Virtually all medical schools require the MCAT. Schools evaluate MCAT scores in different ways. Some have devised formulas that incorporate MCAT results and GPAs and produce numerical scores. In some cases, if an applicant's score falls above a cutoff, he will receive a secondary application or perhaps be invited to interview. Although certain sections of the MCAT may be weighted more heavily than others by some admissions offices, most schools regard all sections except the essay as equally important. In some formulas, the MCAT and GPA carry roughly equal weight, while in others one is weighted more heavily. A number of schools claim that GPA is more important than MCAT. Although this may be true, consider such statements in light of the recent outcry against standardized tests. A school that admits to using test scores as its primary means of weeding out applicants could be regarded as lazy and discriminatory.

Most schools claim not to use specified formulas or cut-off points and indicate that they might consider an applicant with a very low MCAT score if other aspects of his application are extraordinary. But generally, admissions committees rely heavily on MCAT scores because they are considered a strong indicator of success in the first two years of medical school, and because they are the easiest part of an application to judge. Examining the average MCAT scores of accepted students at a school gives you a rough idea of what you will need to gain admission there.

The MCAT is important for all applicants, but may be especially so for nontraditional applicants. Eve's college grades were twenty years old. Over the years, colleges and universities have made changes and adjustments to grading scales and curricular requirements. Thus, her GPA might not be comparable to that of someone who graduated from the same school in 2004. Furthermore, how she performed in college twenty years ago is probably not a great indicator of how she will fare in medical school today. Grades in post-bacc courses are important, but as mentioned earlier, there is wide variation in grading policies among post-bacc programs and between regular undergraduate courses and the same courses within post-bacc programs. The benefit of the MCAT is that it is standardized, supposedly allowing admissions committees to compare the aptitude of people with different backgrounds.

When preparing for the MCAT, consider that the results of that one day of work are nearly as important as all your other academic achievements. Beyond striving for a sound academic background, most medical school applicants—both traditional and nontraditional—take some sort of MCAT preparation course like the ones offered by The Princeton Review. For some, a test-prep course teaches material never learned, or never absorbed, in class. For others, it relieves some anxiety associated with standardized tests, and thereby allows for an improved performance. For those lacking self-motivation, taking a course is a good way to encourage studying.

Some post-bacc programs offer an MCAT review along with pre-medical courses.

Usually, such a review will be much less intensive than a course offered by an outside organization. In Pete's post-bacc program, most students enrolled in a private course that met twice weekly for three months prior to the April MCAT. Since the post-bacc program itself was so intensive and required many hours per day of studying, the students needed to be pushed to devote time to MCAT preparation. Pete did not take the course because he felt confident that he would enter medical school the following fall through the arrangement he had made with an affiliated medical school. The medical school required Pete to take the MCAT and to score at least a nine in all subjects. By January of his post-bacc year, Pete was scoring eights or higher in all sections, and reasoned that, by finishing his pre-medical courses and studying for the MCAT on his own, he could score nines.

Formal MCAT courses typically include three or four practice, full-length MCATs. The exams are scored, giving students an idea of their strengths, weaknesses, and overall progress throughout the course. Pete obtained practice MCATs through the Association of American Medical Colleges (AAMC), and set aside three Saturdays prior to the April exam to take them. For those who do not take a course, it is important to order these practice exams and to be disciplined about taking them.[6] The exams come with tables that allow you to convert your raw score to the scaled score that gives you an accurate idea of how you'll score on an actual MCAT. There are a number of books available that review important MCAT topics and offer tips for taking the exam.

Review books and courses are a good idea for both nontraditional and traditional students, although nontraditional students who have been out of the standardized test scene for many years may particularly need the help. For example, when Becky took her first practice exam, she was discouraged because she was barely able to complete half of the questions in the science sections. MCAT questions are not arranged in order of difficulty, and Becky was spending too much time on really tough passages that appeared early in the sections. She improved her score significantly on the science sections just by training herself to skip and go back to difficult passages.

Some nontraditional applicants have an advantage on the verbal section. Just being older, you may have had more time than a college student to read a wide variety of books. Eve loves reading, and found the verbal section to be a confidence builder. Becky, who did not read extensively for work or pleasure, found the verbal section very difficult. Donald, who learned English as his second language, studied more for the verbal section than for both science sections combined. Becky improved her verbal score by focusing on concentration skills. One way to do this is to read slightly complicated or technical magazine and journal articles every day for several months before the MCAT. Force yourself to concentrate for an extended period of time each day.

[6] Practice exams are real MCATs from years past. Visit www.aamc.org/students/mcat/start.htm.

THE PERSONAL STATEMENT AND INTERVIEW

Health care has changed dramatically in the United States, and some argue that physicians in the twenty-first century (see chapter 2) will have to possess a wider range of skills than was previously considered adequate. Not only must physicians be experts in their respective fields, but it is advantageous to understand the financial, legal, ethical, and political issues surrounding health care provision. Medical schools recognize the need for well-rounded physicians. The schools now offer revised curriculums that include nonscience courses, and they admit more and more nonscience majors.

As a nontraditional applicant, you have unique experiences and skills. These will differentiate you from other applicants and can be an important strength. The AMCAS personal statement, essays for secondary applications, and the interview are opportunities for you to shine. Although you are probably tired of being asked why you want to become a doctor, you will have to figure out how to answer the question with sincerity and enthusiasm. As a nontraditional applicant, your motivation is an extremely important consideration for admissions committees.

Despite recognizing the value of nontraditional students, admissions committees may be skeptical of applicants who are embarking on their second or third career. Essays and interviews also allow you to address their concerns and doubts about your motivation. In interviews, Donald was often asked what made him so sure he wouldn't drop out of medical school as he had engineering school. The concern is partially that poor judgment with respect to your first career choice suggests the possibility of poor judgment in your decision to apply to medical school. Or, perhaps the worry is that some people are eternally unfulfilled, and will therefore be unfulfilled by a career in medicine. Many people believe that if you are good at something, you enjoy it. Thus, not liking your previous job suggests to some that you were bad at it and that you may possess some hidden faults.

All medical school applicants—both traditional and nontraditional—must figure out how to package themselves. Like wrapping a present that is oddly sized, some nontraditional applicants have to be creative in their packaging. Donald's strategy was to maintain a positive attitude. He told interviewers that some of what attracted him to engineering, such as the analytic thinking required, also applies to medicine. He asked interviewers whether some of the principles in engineering would translate to physiological issues. He emphasized his excellent academic record, his success in science courses, and his demonstrated willingness to work hard in school. He also stressed how much he enjoyed volunteering at a clinic. He did his best to be personable and talkative, thereby showing off his "people skills" rather than restating what was written in his essay—that he was switching fields because he wanted to work directly with people.

Tina's story—that she was bored working in an art gallery and envious of her boyfriend's career—would not get her into medical school without clarification. Tina enjoyed certain aspects of her job, such as interacting with artists and clients. She loved much of the art with which she worked, particularly the pieces that were highly expressive and revealed human emotion. On the other hand, she missed a sense of social purpose in her gallery work, and she felt that she wasn't being intellectually challenged. Tina packaged herself as passionate, people-oriented, and interested in helping others. She was good at her job, but knew that it would not engage her for life. Through her work, she came to know what she liked and disliked, what fulfilled her and what did not. Unlike children of physicians who are likely to consider medicine as a potential career from an early age, Tina never thought about it as a realistic pursuit until her twenties when her boyfriend entered medical school. Now that she had an idea of what medical school and medicine were like, and now that she knew herself better, she was ready to commit to the career. Because she enjoyed working with people, she envisioned a career in primary care. She believed that as a result of her studies and work in the art world, she had good insight into the mental capacity and emotions of people. She wondered if psychiatry was the field for her.

Packaging Jacob was relatively straightforward. He had a reasonably consistent interest in medicine, demonstrated by earlier pre-medical courses and more recent firefighting work that involved some emergency medical skills. In Jacob's personal statement, he needed to address the reasons he dropped out of the pre-medical track in college. Jacob had been hospitalized, and this experience was emotionally difficult for him. Being in a hospital and being around sick and dying people was enough to make him question whether he really could be a physician. When he returned to school, he was less committed to going to medical school and decided to focus on completing his major and general requirements with good grades. After graduation, he fully recovered and had regained his interest in medicine. He took several first aid courses, volunteered in an emergency room, trained to become a fireman, and looked around for post-bacc programs. In his essay, Jacob brought up the doubts that he had about becoming a physician, and discussed how he overcame them. Had he glossed over his hospital experience and the fact that he only took one semester of organic chemistry in college, admissions committees may have concluded that he "just couldn't cut it" as a pre-med. By addressing the situation, he presented himself as someone who matured and grew from a difficult experience.

Some medical schools read the essays and personal statements of all applicants and use them, along with grades and scores, for initial screening. Others only read essays after some applications have been weeded out. If you are filling out applications, you are at the point where you can't do much about your grades or scores. However, you can write an excellent personal statement. Enlist a friend, relative, advisor, or coworker who is well read and writes well to review your statement and make suggestions. Have someone who really knows you read it to be sure that you have conveyed your strengths. On the AMCAS application, exactly one page is provided for an applicant's personal statement. The resume of a nontraditional applicant is probably longer than that of a college senior, and limiting your statement to one page may seem difficult. However, you need not mention all of your accomplishments, experiences, or reasons for pursuing medicine. Choose your most impressive accomplishments, your most meaningful experiences, and your most compelling reasons for pursuing medicine (see page 25 for more advice on how to compose a good essay).

There are countless approaches to writing a personal statement. Becky wrote about learning. By focusing on a concept, she subtly brought up her relevant accomplishments and experiences, and explained her motivation for wanting to go to medical school. During her career as a nurse, she learned a tremendous amount from doctors, other nurses, patients, and families. She loved applying her knowledge to her daily work, and seeing her work pay off in the people she helped. However, she felt that her formal education did not enable her to really understand disease, treatments, and the healing process. Having worked closely with physicians, she understood that they didn't always know everything. She felt, however, that they had the tools to ask the right questions. Asking and answering questions, addressing problems and solving them, observing others, and analyzing their techniques are among the activities Becky looked forward to in medical school.

Eve concentrated on the doctor-patient relationship, discussing vivid memories of her own pediatrician and comparing the relationship she had with him to that of her children and their current pediatrician. She was able to elaborate on her accomplishment of raising three well-adjusted children, a feat that involved serving as caretaker, healer, friend, manager, teacher, advisor, and so on. Mitch described a few of his work experiences in Africa and Latin America, focusing on the ones that were most directly related to health care issues. He wrote that although he enjoyed working overseas, he felt that he would be able to contribute more as a physician than as a project manager. Jacob's prose included personal accounts of saving peoples' lives as a firefighter, and how fulfilling he found that aspect of his work.

The secondary application may have general questions that allow you to elaborate on topics mentioned in the AMCAS essay. Some secondaries contain questions about particular experiences that you may have had, such as research, community service, or employment. Some questions focus on your values and personal experiences. Chapter 7 of this book includes a profile of each medical school. In the "Application Process" section of each description, we give the percentage of AMCAS applicants who generally receive secondaries. Some schools send secondary applications to a very limited number of applicants, and receiving a secondary from these schools means that you made it through a significant screening.

All schools limit the number of applicants that they interview. If you have been invited to interview, it is a sign that you are a "competitive" applicant and you should be pleased. If you receive several interview invitations, the odds are that you will get into medical school. Nontraditional applicants who have interesting life experiences have an advantage in interviews because there is more to talk about than college courses or summer jobs. In addition, you may have had more experience interviewing for jobs and other educational programs than a college student. Hopefully, this will allow you to be more relaxed during the interview process.

In writing a personal statement, you are able to edit, rewrite, rethink, and start over. In an interview, you don't have this luxury. Being relaxed is important, but so is being prepared. Interviewers may ask about courses you have taken. Before going into an interview, review your academic transcripts. Which courses were your favorites? Your least favorite? Why? How do your preferences relate to your desire to go to medical school? If there are any particularly low or high grades, be prepared to discuss what went on in those classes. Review your AMCAS and secondary applications. Be sure that you can discuss every experience you have listed or discussed. Think of some sort of interesting, impressive, (tastefully) funny, or meaningful comment for each experience. Be prepared to answer questions about your childhood. What aspect of yourself do you really hate talking about? Be ready to talk about it, or figure out a good way to divert the conversation from it. What (of relevance) do you know about and enjoy talking about? Think about ways to introduce this subject into an interview.

Although most interviews are one-on-one, some schools use panels of more than one interviewer. Some schools offer group interviews where you interview alongside other applicants. Interviewers may be faculty members, administrators, medical students, or members of the community. Older applicants may find that interviewing with current students, who could be somewhat younger, challenging. An important part of being a physician is the ability to communicate and to get along with all types of people in all types of positions. The interview is an opportunity to demonstrate your skills in this area.

There are predictable interview questions, such as, "Why do you want to go to medical school?" Others are much less predictable, and may even be surprising or shocking. You may be asked about your strategy for balancing personal/family life and medical school, or whether you intend to have children. These questions might seem to be inappropriate, particularly to women. However you choose to answer such questions, it is probably best *not* to get defensive. It is reasonable to have concerns about these issues. Tina found that she got a good response when she turned the questions around and asked the interviewer whether *he* felt being a medical student/resident/physician was stressful on a marriage and what *he* felt about having children while in medical school. For more advice on interviewing techniques, turn to chapter 6.

CHOOSING YOUR MEDICAL SCHOOL

Due to the intense competition in medical school admissions, most pre-medical advisors recommend that applicants apply to at least ten schools. Some applicants, particularly those from states with competitive state-affiliated medical schools and whose grades and test scores are below average, should apply to thirty or more schools. In deciding which and how many schools to apply to, it is valuable to talk to a pre-medical advisor. They will help you determine how strong your application is.

The average MCAT scores of students at a particular school are an indicator of how difficult it is to get in. Be sure to apply to a few "safety" schools to which you have a better chance of being admitted. Medical school admission and rejection decisions don't always make sense. Donald was accepted to some of the most prestigious schools in the country, but not to his own state school. This element of chance is a reason to apply to a number of schools, and not to set your hopes on a single school.

For legal reasons, most schools claim that "age is not a factor in admissions." One way to evaluate a school's attitude toward nontraditional students is to look at its student body. Are there a significant number of nontraditional students? What is the average age of incoming students, and what is the age range? Typically, a school's student body reflects its applicant pool, and some schools with fewer nontraditional students simply have fewer nontraditional applicants. If a school that interests you has few nontraditional students, you may want to ask why. It is possible that the school is looking to diversify its students, and will be particularly interested in your application. Medical schools that have arrangements with post-bacc programs are clearly interested in nontraditional students. You should explore them carefully.

Some people argue that all the medical schools in the United States are very good and that there is no particular reason to aspire towards a "top" school. An important difference between medical school and many other graduate or professional degree programs is that medical training does not end at graduation. Rather, a physician's formal education continues during internship, residency, and possibly into fellowship experiences. In terms of job opportunities, where you do your residency could be more important than where you go to school. While attending a well-reputed school will help in residency placement, doing very well at a lesser-known school will also allow you to secure a desirable residency. On the other hand, an advantage to attending a well-reputed school is the comfort of knowing that you don't necessarily have to graduate at the top of the class.

For those who want to practice strictly clinical medicine, there are factors to consider that may be equally as important as, if not more important than, a school's general reputation, which is often based largely on the research associated with the institution. In evaluating the training you will receive, some of the issues to consider are the school's location, the patient population to which students are exposed, the extent to which first and second year students learn clinical medicine, the format of the basic science curriculum,[7] interdisciplinary aspects of the curriculum,[8] the learning resources available to students, the school's role in the community and as a health care provider, the emphasis on primary care, the grading system, and the accessibility of faculty. Even if you are uninterested in a career in medical research, there are educational benefits to becoming involved in research efforts while in medical school, and you may be interested in schools that facilitate faculty/student collaboration and encourage student participation in research.

Rather than focusing on prestige or a published ranking,[9] concentrate on what you want from a school. Among other features, Mitch wanted access to a school of public health so that he could continue working in public and international health issues. Eve looked for schools that devoted significant resources to primary care. Donald looked for more structured programs, while Becky was interested in programs that allowed flexibility. Jacob applied primarily to schools with strong reputations for emergency medicine. Bob hoped to continue teaching part-time or during summers while in school. He looked for schools that would allow this.

Beyond academic features, there are lifestyle issues to consider that may be quite different from those faced by recent college graduates. In college, Mitch enjoyed being part of a cohesive student body at a small, remote, private school. As a thirty-year-old who had spent significant time overseas, he wanted to live in a more multicultural environment. He hoped to have a social life that, to some degree, involved people other than his medical school classmates. Most of the schools he applied to were either in urban areas or were closely associated with a larger university. Tina wanted to remain near her boyfriend, and decided to limit her applications to schools in the region of the country where he was studying. Because of her family, Eve had location issues as well. As a nontraditional student, you are likely to have more responsibilities and complexities in your life than a recent college graduate. As a result, you may find that lifestyle issues play a more important role in determining where you apply and where you go to school.

Interview day is a rare opportunity to hear first-hand what it is like to be a student at a particular medical school. During the course of the day, you will probably speak with current students, either formally or informally. Ask the students you meet for the names of nontraditional students within the class. If you have a spouse and/or children, ask for the names of students in similar situations. While interviewing, you will be focused on making a good impression and getting in. Later, however, you might have

[7] Some schools use lectures and labs while others have an entirely case-based approach. A number of schools fall somewhere in the middle, incorporating some of each educational methodology. There is no evidence that a particular curriculum is "best." You need to consider your own learning style.

[8] Presumably, nontraditional students bring an interdisciplinary perspective and benefit from this approach.

[9] There is no definitive ranking. *U.S. News & World Report* publishes a yearly report ranking graduate schools. Be sure to understand the methodology used when reading their findings.

some choices to make and you may be desperately trying to differentiate one school from the next. Input from current students, particularly those with backgrounds similar to your own, will be invaluable (for more advice on how to choose a school, turn to page 17).

Financial Issues

The cost of a medical education is daunting for traditional and nontraditional students alike. With the exception of those who have accrued savings in former careers, financing medical school as a nontraditional student involves challenges. Nontraditional students often have higher living expenses associated with off-campus living, dependents, debt, and other financial responsibilities. With few exceptions, financial aid offices will look at your parents' income and assets in determining assistance packages. This applies to all students, regardless of their age and whether they themselves are parents. If you are married, medical schools will expect your spouse to contribute to the extent that he or she can. If your parents and/or spouse are less than thrilled about supporting you in this endeavor, financial questions can translate to personal/emotional issues. Older medical students will have less time in the workforce to pay off educational debt, and it is unclear whether financial aid offices consider this in making awards (for more information on financial issues, turn to Chapter 5).

Consider the financial implications of going to medical school, and try to come up with a strategy for dealing with them. If your heart is set on going, financial issues alone should probably not stop you. When deciding where to apply, add to your list of considerations the average debt of graduating students. Even if this figure is not published, financial aid offices will probably provide it. Look very closely at your state-affiliated medical school because in-state tuition is typically much less than private school costs. Ask financial aid offices about loan repayment programs. Think about ways to trim your budget, such as living with relatives or giving up your car. The material possessions you forego now, and the loan payments you make in the future, should be weighed against the value of having a truly fulfilling career.

5 Financing Medical School

HOW MUCH IS ALL OF THIS GOING TO COST?

There's no doubt that med school is expensive. The average first-year tuition for a U.S. private medical school is upwards of $32,000, and the average at public schools is upwards of $13,000 for in-state residents. When planning for the cost of attending medical school, however, tuition is only part of the picture. You must also pay for books, equipment, housing, utilities, food, insurance, transportation, and miscellaneous costs. All of these expenses add up quickly; depending on where you attend school, they may equal or exceed the price of tuition. Note that tuition is 30 percent higher during second and third years to cover the cost of year-round education.

The cost of a medical education is daunting, but once in practice, physicians are among the most highly paid professionals. Currently, the average physician earns $160,000 annually. Although it will be years before today's first-year students make that kind of money, they can assume the financial burden of their education with the confidence that they will one day make enough money to justify the investment.

AND HOW CAN I PAY FOR IT?

Since the medical student of today will be the well-paid physician of tomorrow, medical schools expect the students and their families to be responsible for the cost of their education. Except in cases in which a student has exceptional financial resources, it is essential to rely on outside sources of financial assistance to pay the bill.

Financial Aid Programs

There are two general types of financial assistance: loans and scholarships/grants. Loans must be repaid, and have varying interest rates, deferment options, and repayment periods. Many subsidized loans will be available to you only if you have documented need, while other funds are available regardless of your financial situation. Most medical students borrow heavily, relying on the potential of a generous salary once they begin practice. For 2002 med school graduates, the average debt was $123,780 for students from private schools and $91,389 for students from public schools, and by all indications, these amounts will continue to increase. Scholarships and grants are gifts that need not be repayed. They can be awarded on the basis of several factors—financial need, outstanding academic merit, specific criteria such as gender, or a promise of future service—or a combination of those factors. Note that the financial aid offices of the schools you are accepted to should provide you with a package that covers all costs somehow. The question is how much of the package comes from you or your parents or from high interest loans.

Loans

Anyone with good credit can borrow enough money to finance a medical education. Borrowing is simplified if you take advantage of federal lending programs. Qualifications are:

- *American citizenship or permanent U.S. resident status*
- *If you are a male 18 years of age or older, you are registered for Selective Service or you have documentation proving that you are not required to register.*
- *You have a good credit history, including good standing on prior student loans.*
- *You are an active, enrolled student in good academic standing.*

If you have financial resources that disqualify you for some types of need-based aid, but you meet the above requirements, you are still eligible for federal loans (unsubsidized and private loans). The loans for which you qualify may have higher interest rates and offer less favorable repayment schedules than the subsidized loans that are aimed at those with financial need.

Following is a description of five basic types of loans: federal, state, private, charitable, and institutional.

Federal

Federal loan programs are funded by the federal government or are funded by banks and guaranteed by the federal government. Federal loans, particularly the Stafford Loan, are usually the "first resort" for medical student borrowers. Some federal loans such as Perkins or Stafford subsidized loans are need-based, but some higher-interest loans are available to students or their families regardless of financial circumstance.

State

Students who are residents of the state in which they attend medical school may be eligible for state loan programs. Eligibility is often based on need and may be further tied to specific segments of the population (e.g., minority or disadvantaged students, or students who are interested in practicing family medicine in underserved areas of the state). Individual schools can provide you with information about state loan programs.

Private

Privately funded, commercial loans are available from banks and other financial institutions. Interest rates are high! The banks benefit as much from the loan as you do.

Charitable

Charity loans are funded by contributions from foundations, corporations, and associations. A number of private loans are targeted to aid particular segments of the population (e.g., minority or disadvantaged students, women, or students who are interested in practicing family medicine in under-served areas of the state). You may have to investigate to identify all of the charitable loans for which you qualify. The best place to begin your search is in public, undergraduate, and med school libraries. There are also a number of commercial financial aid search services available, but beware—financial aid officers warn that search services sometimes charge hefty fees for information that, in the majority of cases, students can obtain themselves. Private financial aid resources are also available on the Internet. Visit the Financial Center at www.PrincetonReview.com to find many of them.

Institutional

The amount of loan money available, and the method by which it is disbursed, varies greatly from one school to another. As part of the shift toward emphasizing primary care, some schools offer assistance to students who are committed to providing primary care after graduation. To find out about the resources available at a particular school, refer to its catalog or contact its financial aid office.

In the chart on pages 66 and 67 we have compiled a table of the most commonly used loan programs. Included in this table is information about the characteristics of each loan. The following defines each category.

Name: The full name of the loan and the acronym, if applicable, by which it is most commonly known.

Source: Information about who funds and who administers each loan.

Note that regardless of your age or how long you have been independent of your parents, their income is considered in calculating your need in almost all cases.

Eligibility: Some loans are need-based. Others are open to people regardless of their financial situation. A few federal and private schools require that a student fit a specific demographic profile. Note that regardless of your age or how long you have been independent of your parents, their income is considered in calculating your need in almost all cases.

TABLE OF LOANS

NAME OF LOAN	SOURCE	ELIGIBILITY	MAXIMUM ALLOCATION
Federal Stafford (Subsidized) Student Loan (SSL, formerly GSL) www.ed.gov/prog_info/SFA/StudentGuide/2002-3/	Federal, administered by participating lender	Demonstrated financial need	$8,500/year. The maximum aggregate total for subsidized loans is $65,000. The maximum aggregate total includes any Stafford loans received for undergraduate study.
Unsubsidized Stafford Student Loan www.ed.gov/prog_info/SFA/StudentGuide/2002-3/	Federal, administered by participating lender	Not need-based	The total Stafford loan limit is $38,000, including Unsubsidized loans and Subsidized loans not to exceed $8,500. The maximum aggregate total of Stafford loans is $189,125, including Unsubsidized loans and Subsidized loans not to exceed $65,000.*
Health Professions Student Loan/Primary Care Loan (HPSL) Contact school for more information	Federal, administered by school	Exceptional financial need; commitment to primary care	Tuition plus $2,500 stipend.
Perkins Loan (formerly NDSL) Contact school for more information	Federal, administered by school	Demonstrated financial need	$6,000/year, with aggregate of $40,000. Aggregate amount includes undergraduate loans.
Alternative Loan Program (ALP) www.aamc.org/students/medloans/start.htm	AAMC, administered under MEDLOANS division of AAMC	Not need-based	Cost of attendance minus other aid received. Aggregate: original principal of debt may not exceed $200,000.

*Students pursuing certain health professions and enrolled in programs accredited by the appropriate approved accreditation agency are eligible to receive increased amounts of Unsubsidized Stafford loans. If a student is granted the maximum additional allocation, the maximum aggregate total will be $189,125. This number includes all undergraduate and graduate Subsidized and Unsubsidized Stafford loans. See "Increased Eligibility for Health Professions Students" in the Federal Student Aid Handbook for details and updates.

TABLE OF LOANS (continued)

REPAYMENT AND DEFERRAL OPTIONS	INTEREST RATE	PROS	CONS
10–30 years to repay. Begin repayment 6 months after graduation. Forbearance possible for up to 3 years of residency training.	Variable, 91-day T-Bill plus 2.3%. Capped at *8.25%.	Most common medical school loan. Interest is paid by the government during school. Once you get a loan, later loans are at the same rate.	None
10–30 years to repay. Interest begins to accrue from day loan is disbursed; you can pay the interest or have it capitalized (added to principal). Begin repayment 6 months after graduation. Forbearance possible for up to 3 years of residency training.	Variable, 91-day T-Bill plus 2.3%. Capped at *8.25%. (While in school, the rate is variable, 91-day T-bill plus 1.7%. Capped at *8.25%.)	Not need-based.	Interest is not paid by the government while you're in school.
10 years to repay, beginning 1 year after graduation. Deferrable during residency and under special circumstances.	Fixed, 5%.	Fixed, relatively low interest rate	Very limited availability.
10 years to repay. Begin repayment 9 months after graduation. Can be deferred for 2 years during residency.	Fixed, 5%.	Fixed, relatively low interest rate	Low maximum allocation.
Standard: 20 years of interest and principal payments. Alternative: 3 years of interest only and 17 years of interest and principal. Repayment generally begins 3–4 years after graduation, depending on length of residency.	Based on prime rate, about 10%.	High maximum allocation; not need-based.	"Loan of last resort." High interest rate.

*Check www.ed.gov/prog_info/SFA/StudentGuide/2002-3/ to confirm most recent rates. Rates are variable, and the T-bill is reset on July 1 each year

Maximum Allocation: There is a maximum amount of money you can borrow from any one program, so many medical students find it necessary to borrow from more than one source. Most loans have both maximum yearly and aggregate loan amounts. Amounts you borrowed from the same loan program for your college education are deducted, in some cases, from the aggregate amount you can borrow in medical school.

Repayment and Deferral Options: Important considerations in structuring your educational debt are how long you have to pay back loans and whether principal and/or interest may be deferred until you have completed your education. This column provides information about the repayment period and deferral options for each loan. It is important to remember that, no matter what the source of a loan, the responsibility for keeping track of loan activity is yours.

Interest Rate: This column provides information about the current interest rate of the loan. Fixed-rate loans use the same interest rate throughout the life of the loan. Variable-rate loans base their interest rate on established financial values, usually ninety-one-day Treasury Bills (T-Bills) or the prime lending rate. Since these rates fluctuate greatly, you should check with a bank to find out the exact interest rate.

Pros: Listed in this category are factors that make this an attractive loan source. Attractive features include long repayment terms, deferral policies that waive both interest and principal throughout medical school and all or part of residency training, and low, fixed-rate interest.

Cons: Listed in this category are factors that make a particular loan unattractive. Such features include short repayment times, limited deferral options, or variable, high-interest rates.

Scholarships/Grants

Some grant, or gift money, comes with no strings attached; these are nonobligatory scholarships. Although such scholarships may be available on the basis of outstanding academic merit alone, others are based on a combination of merit and need. In fact, all federal, nonobligatory scholarships are based on need and may also require that you fit a particular demographic profile. Scholarship amounts vary, and they are administered by the same groups as loans: federal and state governments, private foundations, and institutions. For more information about private, state, and institutional scholarships, contact the financial aid offices at some of the schools to which you are going to apply, or visit the Financial Center at www.PrincetonReview.com.

Obligatory Scholarships

Some federal scholarships are available to students who agree to serve at the Public Health Service, at the Veterans Administration, or in the Armed Forces. These scholarships provide full tuition, some or all expenses, and a monthly stipend. Service-based scholarships, which are not based on need, all carry an obligation to serve at least one

TABLE OF GRANTS

NAME OF GRANT	SOURCE	ELIGIBILITY	SERVICE OF OBLIGATION	AMOUNT OF GRANT
National Health Service Corps (NHSC)	Federal	Need-based; former EFN recipients and students with interest in primary care are preferred.	Two to four year contract. Years spent in residency do not count toward fulfilling obligation.	Maximum amount is full tuition and fees plus stipend
Financial Assistance for Disadvantaged Health Professions Students (FADHPS)	Federal, administered through school	Exceptional financial need and disadvantaged background; family contribution not to exceed the lesser of $5,000 or one-half the cost of education.	None	Varies
National Medical Fellowship Scholarship (NMF)	Private	First- or second-year underrepresented minority, female, rural, or disadvantaged background with documented financial need.	None	Varies
Scholarship Program for Students of Exceptional Financial Need (EFN)	Federal, administered through school	Exceptional financial need and disadvantaged background; family contribution not to exceed the lesser of $5,000 or one-half the cost of education.	None	Varies; tuition and other educational expenses
Armed Forces Health Professions Scholarship Program (HPSP)	U.S. Army, U.S. Navy, and U.S. Air Force	Able to serve in military; age restrictions; U.S. citizens only.	One year for every year of support. Years spent in residency do not count toward fulfilling obligation.	Full tuition, "reasonable" fees, and stipend. Student becomes officer in service branch upon matriculation and receives all benefits of rank.

year for every year of support. The advantage—a "free" medical education—is obvious, but this is not an option to take lightly. Time spent in residency—which is often restricted to only military residencies—does not count toward your service debt, so you may be out of medical school for seven to twelve years before you're free of your obligation. Some states and counties also offer service-based scholarship programs or tuition remission programs. Despite their lengthy obligations, service-based scholarships are in high demand. To increase your chances of obtaining one, apply as early as possible. Ask the financial aid offices of schools in which you are interested who to contact locally for more information. There are also loan repayment programs available to which you apply after you have accrued debt and when you are ready to start working in an underserved area.

THE FINANCIAL AID PROCESS

PREPARING TO APPLY

Many students miss out on potential assistance by making some basic, avoidable mistakes. Top financial aid officers supplied the following common errors and their remedies.

Missing Deadlines and Keeping Poor Records

Like your applications for admission, your financial aid applications should be submitted as early as possible. File your income tax forms early and encourage your parents (all med students are considered dependent by med schools, even if they have been independent for years) to do the same. Photocopy all forms that you submit and note the date you send them. File these forms along with any material related to the decisions of the financial aid committees of the schools to which you apply. Keep careful track of deadlines, which are strongly enforced.

Submitting Information to the Wrong Needs Analysis Service

There are several third-party organizations that assist medical schools in determining the financial need of entering and continuing students. Many applicants assume that because they have submitted information to one of the services for one school, they have done everything they need to do for all the schools they are considering. Making this assumption can have serious repercussions. Until the proper service completes the needs analysis, the financial aid office cannot package your financial aid. To avoid making this mistake, check with the financial aid offices of all the schools you are applying to, to see which service they use. Submit the proper materials to the appropriate service. More detailed information on the needs analysis services and their function can be found under "Calculating Your Contribution."

Having a Poor Credit History

People are often unpleasantly surprised when they see their credit histories. Even relatively minor financial problems, like making a couple of late payments on loans or credit cards, can lower your credit rating. Also, credit bureaus sometimes make mistakes, causing negative, but false, information to show up on your record. Since a bad credit history will make you ineligible for many, if not all, loan programs, it is a good idea to check your credit history before you apply for financial aid. Because it usually takes several weeks to obtain a copy of your history, you should order one well in advance of the time you will begin to submit your applications. There is usually a fee for this, but it's worth the few dollars to check to make sure it is accurate. You can obtain your credit history on-line at www.equifax.com, www.experian.com, or www.transunion.com.

Defaulting on Undergraduate Student Loans

If you have not kept up with your student loan payments, you will have a very hard time qualifying for loans, especially those funded by the federal government. Clear up any problems with prior student loans well before applying for additional assistance. If you are still in school and have not yet begun repaying your loans, talk to your undergraduate financial aid officer to clarify repayment and deferral options on your loans. Remember that the burden of keeping track of your loan activity is on you, and that once you start medical school, you must keep the lenders apprised of your whereabouts.

Applying for Aid

Schools' policies may vary somewhat, but they all follow the same general lines. To determine whether you qualify and for how much, schools must first determine how much it will cost for you to attend, and then how much of that cost you and your family can bear.

How Schools Determine Their Cost

Each medical school prepares a student budget that reflects the expenses associated with being a first-year medical student. Included in this budget are items such as tuition and fees, books, equipment, housing, utilities, food, insurance, transportation, and personal expenses. To some degree, schools customize expenses if a student has particular needs. For example, costs may be considered higher if you live off campus.

Calculating Your Contribution

To determine how much you and your family can contribute, medical schools use a needs analysis service. Refer to the financial aid guidelines of the schools you are considering attending. Some schools use more than one service to calculate need, and many ultimately use their own formulas to determine institutional assistance. To make sure you have all the information required to fill out the forms completely, file your previous year's income tax returns early. Because some federal loan programs and some institutions require parental information even from independent or married students, your parents should also file their income tax forms as early as possible.

On the basis of the information you give them, the needs analysis calculates your financial need by subtracting your expected personal and family contribution from the total student budget furnished by the school. If expenses are higher than the estimated contribution, you show financial need.

Your Tentative Financial Aid Package

Most schools will only prepare a financial aid package for accepted students. Once you have been accepted to a school, be on the lookout for a financial aid package. The package can include loans, scholarships, grants, or a combination of these elements. If financial aid is an important consideration in deciding between schools, be sure that you have estimates from all schools by the applicant decision deadline.

Accepting Your Financial Aid Package

Once you matriculate at a school, the financial aid office will put together your actual financial aid package. In most cases, loans will make up a portion of the package. Remember, loans must be repaid—with interest—and the amount of this debt will affect your lifestyle far beyond medical school and residency. For instance, if you borrow a large sum of money for medical school, you may have trouble later obtaining a loan for a large purchase like a car or a house. You are not required to accept all the aid you are offered, so it is in your best interest to borrow only what you need to meet your expenses.

CUTTING COSTS

Medical schools formulate their student budgets by using average expenses for everything except tuition. By making some adjustments to your lifestyle, it is usually possible to undercut this budget, and therefore decrease the amount of money you borrow. Following are some strategies recommended by financial aid professionals to reduce debt.

Books and Equipment

Buy good-quality used textbooks and equipment whenever possible. Use the Internet (eBay!). Selling books and equipment you no longer need is a good way to earn extra cash.

Transportation

Automobile loan payments, insurance premiums, licensing fees, fuel, and maintenance really add up. Evaluate your need for a car before taking one to medical school. If you attend school in a place where public transportation is available or where you can bike or walk to school, leave the car behind. If you must have a car, you can save by raising insurance deductibles and carpooling with fellow students.

Insurance

Most medical schools require you to carry medical and, in some cases, disability insurance. Before you buy into the school's plan, check your existing coverage. If your parents still claim you as a dependent, or if you have a spouse whose medical benefits extend to you, you may already have adequate coverage.

Other Expenses

Millions of Americans find themselves in financial straits each year because of revolving credit. Medical students are no exception. If you find that you have trouble avoiding the temptation of pulling out the plastic for purchases you can't afford, cut up your cards. Remember, if you can't afford to pay for something with cash or a check, you probably can't afford to charge it, either. To keep discretionary expenses from getting out of hand, set up a detailed budget and stick to it. If you've never used a budget before and need help, there are many computer software programs that help you set up a budget, track expenses, and give you reports on how you're doing.

A FINAL WORD

Your Financial Aid Rights

- *You have the right to expect that the financial aid office will assist you in obtaining financial aid and information about financial aid opportunities.*
- *Financial aid officers who you give information to about your/your family's financial profile can not publicize this information.*
- *You have the right to accept or decline all or part of the aid offered.*
- *You have the right to appeal your financial aid package if your financial aid picture changes for the worse. (This does not necessarily mean, however, that the amount of aid will increase.)*
- *You have the right to examine your financial aid file at any time.*
- *You are entitled to treatment that does not discriminate on the basis of race, creed, age, handicap, gender, or national origin.*

YOUR FINANCIAL AID RESPONSIBILITIES

- *You are responsible for meeting the expenses related to attending medical school.*
- *You are responsible for reading and understanding the conditions and terms of all of the elements in your financial aid package.*
- *You are responsible for submitting financial aid applications on time.*
- *You are responsible for obtaining and filling out financial aid forms and supplying accurate and complete information on these forms.*
- *You are responsible for reporting to your financial aid office any outside scholarships or loans that may affect your amount of need.*
- *You are responsible for using loan funds to pay tuition.*
- *You are responsible for repaying all loans.*
- *You are responsible for notifying all lenders of all changes of address during and after medical school.*
- *You are responsible for keeping accurate and complete records of all financial aid applications and transactions.*

6 The Interview:
Separating the Merely Qualified from the Truly Worthy

Be proud if you're invited to an interview. You've made it through two initial screenings, one before and one after the supplemental application. Usually, this means that the Admissions Committee thinks you're qualified to attend their school. Unfortunately, they also invite a lot of other qualified people, and they don't have space to admit all of you. The object is to convince everyone who interviews you that the school would be a better place with you in it. Easy to say, a little harder to do. It is important to realize that the weight of the interview varies from school to school. At some schools it is the key, while at others it is mainly a formality—more for you than for them.

Because almost everyone has heard horror stories about someone else's interview, most people start to worry about the interview before they even submit their applications. Try to relax. A good interview begins with good preparation. You can start by becoming familiar with the interview process.

WHO CONDUCTS INTERVIEWS?

Different schools have different policies about who conducts the actual interview. In general, schools have a Medical Selection Committee made up of professional admissions or student affairs people and faculty members. Often, especially in more progressive schools, upper-level med students also participate. At some schools, you'll have a couple of separate, one-on-one interviews; at others, you'll be interviewed by a panel. You may be the only applicant in front of a panel (this really seems like an inquisition), or you may be joined by other candidates.

At many schools, the person or people you speak with become your advocates in the final selection process. When all the interviews in a certain time period are finished and the Selection Committee meets, these people share their observations about you and sometimes recommend a particular action. The final decision, of course, is up to the entire committee.

WHAT CAN I EXPECT?

Expect some interviews to go well and others to go poorly. In the vast majority of cases, the interviewers are trying to build an honest picture of you beyond the numbers, and most try to reduce stress during the interviews. Despite this, you will probably experience one or two "bad" interviews with interviewers who have not read your file and therefore seem disinterested, are insecure or awkward themselves, or are simply having a bad day. Keep this in mind as your interviews approach.

HOW SHOULD I ACT?

The golden rule for interviews is "Be Yourself." Interviewers have been through all of this before, and they're pretty good at spotting people who are putting on an act or reading from a mental script. What they're trying to find out from this interview is what kind of person you are and how you relate to others. Up until now, you've been only a few sheets of paper, a bunch of numbers, and (probably horrible) photograph. Now's the time to show them your stuff. But, remember: no lying and no b.s.

BE PREPARED

You should be ready to answer questions about your motivation to become a physician, your academic background, your extracurricular and leisure activities, your job or research experience, and your views on medical problems and ethical issues. Later in this chapter is a sample of questions that current medical students were asked in their interviews. Some of them are typical; others are truly strange. As you get ready to interview, try to answer some of these questions to yourself, and then to a friend, parent, or professor. In addition, you may want to audiotape or videotape mock interviews to see how you sound and look. When you choose a guinea pig to be your surrogate interviewer, select someone who will be honest with you about the strengths and weaknesses of your responses. Don't try to memorize answers word for word; canned responses, no matter how valid, are stiff and unconvincing (just look at a tape of a presidential debate). It is a good idea, however, to enter an interview with several "stories" or points in mind. Questions are often open-ended, giving you the chance to direct the conversation toward your strengths and away from your weaknesses.

APPROACH WITH CONFIDENCE

Like dogs, interviewers seem to smell fear. The tone of your interview is often set in the first few seconds, so approach with confidence. Greet your interviewer with a firm handshake and look him in the eye. During the interview, be positive. Think of it as a pleasant conversation with someone you'd like to get to know better. A good interview is a dialogue, where there is considerable "give and take." Unless your interviewer brings them up, avoid controversial or emotionally charged subjects like abortion. If you're asked your views, state them and move on.

Take Your Time

In the course of your interviews, you may be asked scores of questions, some on issues to which you haven't given a great deal of thought. Your interviewers don't expect you have a ready answer for every one of these questions, but they do expect you to come up with a coherent, well-thought-out response. Many applicants are afraid that if they hesitate, it will seem that they are unprepared. Not so. Good physicians don't rush to a conclusion without considering the facts; rather, they think through a problem before they decide how to act. If a question catches you off guard, take a second to think it through. If it seems ambiguous, don't be afraid to ask for clarification. If you don't know, admit it and ask the interviewer to share the answer. By taking the time to make sure that your response is well conceived and well spoken, you will impress the interviewers as thoughtful and articulate—two characteristics essential in a good doctor.

Ask Questions

Although the interview is the time for medical schools to find out about you, it is also an excellent opportunity for you to find out more about the school. Before you go to an interview, make sure you've studied the school's information packet and are ready to ask intelligent questions about the program. Do a search at your undergraduate or public library to see if the school has been in the news and, if so, for what. Remember that most people love to talk about themselves. Ask the interviewer about his work or impressions of the curriculum.

Be on Time

Make sure that you get detailed directions before you make the trip, and arrive with enough time to park and find the office. If you are invited to interview at several schools in the same geographic region, you might save on travel costs and time by making an interview "circuit," visiting several schools on the same trip. This can mean that you have several interviews in the same week or even the same day. Give yourself as much time as possible at each, so that you have time to make the transition, both physically and mentally, from one school to the next. If you can, try to get to each campus early enough to walk around, talk to students, and formulate questions that are specific to the school.

Dress for Success

Like it or not, looks count. No matter what your usual mode of dress, you should dress conservatively and professionally for your interviews. For men, this means a suit, or a blazer and nice slacks (and, of course, a tie); for women, a suit, blazer and skirt or dress slacks, or a business-style dress is appropriate. Regardless of your gender, keep an eye to detail; even the most beautiful suit looks shabby if your shoes are scuffed and worn, and the effect of a great-looking blazer is ruined by a ragged backpack. Polish your shoes, invest in a nice portfolio or case for your papers, and by all means, iron your clothes. If you are generally somewhat less than conservative in your dress, you may want to tone it down: men, replace the big hoop earring with a stud; women, take off the gold glitter polish and paint on clear. After all, you don't want to be asked, as one of the respondents to our survey was, "Why are you dressed the way you are? Why did you come here looking the way you do?"

Conduct Yourself Professionally

Admissions committees can see from your application that you are smart, accomplished, and highly regarded by your professors. The interview is an opportunity for them to gauge things that are not so easily conveyed on paper. Medical schools are looking for students with maturity, empathy, and superior interpersonal skills. All of these things come through in the interview. In a group setting, where the committee talks with more than one candidate at a time, you will be observed not only when you answer a question, but also when your fellow applicants are speaking. Keep alert, and show interest. After all, you never know what you may learn that you can use in your next interview.

HOW AND WHEN TO FOLLOW UP ON YOUR INTERVIEWS

First, don't forget to send a thank you note after each set of interviews. You can write several different notes to each of your interviewers, or send just one addressed generally to the interview committee. Don't write a novella in your thank you note. It's fine to mention a particular question or topic you found interesting during your interview, but you should confine yourself to only a few lines. As you might have guessed, it's a good idea to take a few brief notes, such as the interviewer's names and some of the topics they covered, right after you leave the interview. For the thank you notes themselves, you can use any nice stationary paper.

If the school is not entirely certain of the strength of your application relative to other candidates after your interviews, you may be placed on a "hold" list. Don't despair. You made it as far as the interview process, which (except in the case of some public schools who interview every candidate) means that you have survived some of the initial cuts. Sometimes being put on hold simply means that the school has already accepted enough students that month. You can, however, send supplementary information to further support your application. For example, if you have been doing research, volunteer work, or taking classes that didn't appear on your initial application, and if you didn't get a chance to talk about your new activities during the interview, you can write a short—less than one page—letter outlining your recent accomplishments and send it to the school. This shows that you are still working hard to better your chances of acceptance into medical school.

WHAT ARE THEY GOING TO ASK?

Over the past several years, The Princeton Review has surveyed current medical students about their schools and the medical school application process. The sample interview questions in this section come from those surveys. Although the following list of questions is by no means exhaustive, it is a good sampling of questions that were asked in real interviews in the recent past. When we first decided to ask current med students what they were asked in their interviews, we had no idea how strange—and it some cases disturbing—some of their responses were going to be. Get ready, because, while some of the questions are pretty standard, others are truly bizarre.

So You Want to Be a Doctor?

Some of the students we surveyed were unprepared for questions like those that follow, thinking them so mundane that they wouldn't be asked. From our research, however, we can say with confidence that if you're granted even one interview, you're almost sure to be asked several questions about your motivation and suitability for medical school.

- *Why do you want to be a doctor?*
- *The future of medicine looks bleak. Why do you want to go into it?*
- *What articles have you read recently that relate to the reasons you want to become a doctor?*
- *What do you see yourself doing with a medical degree?*
- *Were you influenced by relatives to pursue a career in medicine?*
- *Why do you want to attend [name of school]?*
- *Why should we accept you?*
- *How are your accomplishments better than those of the other candidates in this interview?*
- *Evaluate yourself based on the required evaluation of the interviewer.*
- *Do you think you are motivated enough for medical school?*
- *When you don't get into medical school, what will you do?*
- *What would you do if Saddam Hussein took over our country and wouldn't allow women in medical school?*
- *What career path would you follow if all the medical schools closed today?*
- *You've taken an odd, nontraditional path to get here. Why are you interested in medicine?*

- *What disadvantages do you see in being an older student?*
- *Can you afford to come here?*
- *How will you finance your medical education?*
- *Describe what you believe to be the financial rewards of medicine.*
- *If doctors were paid as much as teachers, would you still want to be a doctor?*
- *Doctors have the power to give or take life. How do you feel about "playing God"?*

Tell Me a Little Bit About Yourself . . .

Selection committees use the interview as an opportunity to find out what makes you tick. Prepare yourself for personal questions about your character traits, your coping mechanisms, and your life experiences. You may also be asked to comment on your interpersonal relationships. Always be honest.

- *What is your worst quality?*
- *If you could change anything about yourself, what would it be?*
- *Are you aggressive?*
- *What makes you a fun person?*
- *What makes you angry?*
- *What makes you sad?*
- *What scares you?*
- *Do you like sick people?*
- *Are you afraid of death?*
- *What are you the most proud of?*
- *One of the people who wrote a letter of recommendation for you described you as [adjective]. Do you agree with that description?*
- *Was there a time in your life when you had tremendous responsibility?*
- *What is the wackiest thing you've ever done?*
- *What was the biggest mistake you ever made?*
- *What is the worst thing that has happened to you in the past four years?*
- *Tell me something you wanted to achieve but did not, or something you've failed at. How did you cope with failure?*
- *What role has stress played in your life?*
- *How could you prove to me that you can perform well under stress?*

- *What do you do to alleviate stress?*
- *Tell me about your family.*
- *What role do you play in your family dynamic?*
- *How is your relationship with your parents?*
- *What is the physical health of your parents, and how would you handle an illness of theirs while attending school?*
- *Who is the person in the world to whom you are closest?*
- *Describe your best friend.*
- *What does your closest friend think about your relationship with him or her?*
- *Give one word that a friend would use to describe you.*

It's All Academic

Grades, MCAT scores, and courses are fair game for the inquisitive interviewer. You may be asked to explain your performance in a course or to tell what you learned. A hint: To be better prepared for questions of this type, get a copy of your transcript and take a look at it. Look for things that might cause an interviewer to ask a question. Lower than normal grades stick out, as do courses with funny names (like Rocks for Jocks). Then, again, only be honest.

- *What do you think of the GPA as a valid method of categorizing students?*
- *Why were your first-year grades so bad?*
- *Why do you have so many C grades on your transcript?*
- *Explain your low math grade.*
- *Why are your grades high compared to your MCAT scores?*
- *Do you realize that your MCAT scores aren't anything special?*
- *Tell me about your research.*
- *Have you taken any humanities classes, and what papers did you write in them?*
- *What did you learn in [name of course]? (It's worth noting that some people were asked about normal courses like "Philosophy 101" and others were asked about bizarre courses like "The Art of Murder," "Fairy Tales," and "Play, Games, Toys, and Sports.")*
- *Who was the author of your biochemistry textbook?*

Extra, Extra, Read All About It!

Whatever your extracurricular activities and work experiences, you will most likely be asked how they relate to your commitment to and preparedness for studying medicine. Think about your extracurricular experiences and what you learned about yourself, the medical field, and/or working with people as a result of participating in these activities. If you've been out of school for a while and have worked extensively in another field, be ready for questions about why you decided to change fields. Scientific or medical research experience is a plus, but can be a real liability if you're not able to discuss it in detail.

- *What are your hobbies?*
- *How does your hobby relate to being a doctor?*
- *Have you taught yourself to do anything, and if so, what?*
- *How has working as a [name of job] made you a better candidate for medical school?*
- *What volunteer work contributed to your commitment to become a doctor?*
- *What did you do with your job earnings?*

Medical Issues and Ethics: Where Do You Stand?

Interviewers love to ask students about a medical issue or about an ethical dilemma related to medicine. In general, there is no wrong answer to these questions. You should know the terminology (for example, what is the difference between euthanasia and euthenics?), and be aware of some pros and cons for each of these issues. Since the health care crisis and attendant problems in reforming the health care delivery system have been grabbing headlines, you should be prepared to discuss the issues intelligently. No one expects you to be an expert on this or any other issue, but you should do some research before your interviews (read the chapter on medicine in the twenty-first century in this book for a review). Don't be surprised if an interviewer challenges your view on an issue; usually, he is trying to see how well you support your argument.

- *What is the greatest problem facing medicine today?*
- *What do you consider the most important thing medicine has done for mankind?*
- *What do you think will be the most significant scientific breakthrough in the next ten years?*
- *If you could find a cure for AIDS or for cancer, which would you choose and why?*
- *If you were Surgeon General, what is the first thing you would do?*
- *If you were the Health Commissioner of [a large city], what would you do?*
- *What is preventive medicine?*
- *What is the biggest problem family practitioners face?*

- *What are your views on euthanasia?*
- *What do you think about euthenics (not euthanasia)?*
- *What would you do about the alcoholism problem in this country?*
- *What do you think about condoms being distributed in high schools?*
- *What are your views on mandatory HIV testing for doctors and patients?*
- *Current AIDS education programs aren't working; what should we do?*
- *Why will organ rationing be the problem of the future in medicine?*
- *Should people have the right to sell their own organs?*
- *Do you think it's ethical to take the life of a fetus for a cell line to save the life of a sibling with cancer?*
- *Should we spend so much time and effort trying to keep premature infants alive?*
- *If a cure were invented for aging, what repercussions would it have on society in general and the medical profession in particular?*
- *How do you feel about animal research?*
- *What role should politics play in medicine?*
- *Is health care a right or a privilege?*
- *What is your opinion of socialized medicine?*
- *How would you organize health care in an ideal world?*
- *Discuss the health care system of Australia.*
- *What do you think should be done about patients who can't pay for treatment?*
- *What is the difference between Medicare and Medicaid?*
- *What is your opinion of HMOs and PPOs?*
- *How will you react to the death of your first patient?*
- *Who would you go to if your mom needed surgery: a surgeon with good hands and a bland personality or a surgeon with not as good hands with a great personality?*
- *How would you tell your best friend's wife (who is your patient) that she has cancer? What would you do if she then refused to tell her family?*
- *You have to amputate one of the legs of an eight-year-old child. How would you tell him?*
- *Would you give a transfusion to a child whose parents were Jehovah's Witnesses?*

- *If a Hindu, for example, comes in and refuses surgery on the basis of religion, and the surgery is his only hope, what would you do? Also, what if the patient is this man's child?*
- *If you diagnosed a patient with a terminal illness as having only two months to live and the family and the patient wanted to end the turmoil ("pull the plug"), would you allow it or strongly disagree?*
- *What would you do if you saw a bleeding child on the side of the road?*
- *What would you do if you had a female patient who was trying to conceive, and your colleague had that patient's husband, and the husband was HIV positive?*
- *If one of your colleagues refused to treat a patient with AIDS, how would you address that colleague?*
- *How would you react if a fellow medical student had AIDS and entered surgery with you?*
- *Would you let a surgeon with AIDS operate on you?*
- *Would you treat a white supremacist, and should physicians be forced to treat such a patient?*
- *If you made a mistake as a physician, how would you handle it?*

To Choose, or Not to Choose

Abortion is not only a hot political topic, it also seems to be a hot topic for interviews. Some schools are affiliated with hospitals where abortions are performed; some are not. Don't try to guess if the interviewer is hoping you will espouse a particular position; honesty seems the best policy on this issue. If you are asked about your willingness to perform an abortion (as a large number of those we surveyed were), you may want to mention that it is not only your conscience but also the rules of the hospital or laws of the land that you must consider.

- *What should a physician's role be in the politics of abortion?*
- *What would you do as a physician if you were asked to do something contrary to your stand on abortion?*
- *Would you perform an abortion for a teenager, and would you tell her parents?*
- *How do you justify being a Catholic and going to an institution that allows abortion?*
- *If you wouldn't perform an abortion because of your religious beliefs, but you would refer a patient to another physician who would perform an abortion, are you not just as guilty in God's eyes?*

Have You Heard the News?

Good doctors are aware of, and involved in, the world around them. You may be asked about current events, even things completely unrelated to medicine. The questions that follow are only examples; in most cases, these events are no longer current. To prepare for questions like these, keep up with what's happening. If you get most of your news from the TV or radio, start reading newspapers and news magazines for more in-depth coverage.

- *Who is the U.S. Secretary of State?*
- *What do you think about the current situation in Bosnia?*
- *What do you think about the current social climate in Mozambique?*
- *What do you think about the political situation in Iraq and surrounding countries?*
- *What is your opinion on the confirmation hearings of Clarence Thomas?*
- *Why did Margaret Thatcher resign?*
- *Do you think the Israelis beat up on the Palestinians?*

Philosophy 101

From the serious to the silly, questions interviewers ask can make you stop and think. (And, for some of these questions, one of the things you might think is, "What does this have to do with med school?")

- *What are the top five priorities of society?*
- *Do you see any parallels between medicine and the priesthood?*
- *What is Zen Buddhism?*
- *Explain Hinduism.*
- *Are you a racist?*
- *Do you believe that racism still exists?*
- *How do you feel about affirmative action?*
- *Would you move to Canada to avoid serving active duty during a military conflict abroad?*
- *What is your view on censorship in the arts?*
- *What would you do if you saw a classmate cheating on a test?*
- *Do you believe in drug legalization?*
- *Do you believe that volunteerism could help eliminate greed from society's social structure?*
- *Is altruism ever pure, without some kind of motive?*

- *Do you believe in life after death?*
- *What is your opinion about natural law ethics?*
- *Explain the mind-body problem.*
- *Are you a vertical or horizontal thinker?*
- *If you could be any cell in the human body, what would you be?*
- *If you were to build a human being, what would you include and exclude?*
- *Define hope.*

TRIED AND TRUE

Some questions sound more like pickup lines than med school interview questions. Although none of those surveyed was asked, "What's your sign?" there were plenty of old favorites that you may as well be prepared for.

- *Are you a person who thinks a glass is half empty or half full?*
- *If you could go back in history and meet anyone, who would it be and why?*
- *If you could talk to someone from the future, what would you ask him?*
- *If a genie were able to grant you three wishes, what would they be?*
- *If you were stranded on a desert island, what five books would you want?*
- *If your house was burning down, and you could save only one thing, what would it be?*
- *If you could be any vegetable, what would you be?*
- *If you could be any kind of fruit, what would you be?*
- *If you could be any kind of animal, what would you be?*
- *What is your favorite color?*
- *What was the last book you read, and how did it influence your life?*
- *What was the last good movie you saw?*
- *Tell me what you see when you look in the mirror.*
- *What was the most embarrassing moment in your life?*
- *Who is your hero?*
- *If you could invite three role models to dinner, who would they be and why, and what would you serve them?*
- *When you die, what would you like your tombstone to read?*

I'll Take Potpourri for $500, Alex

The students we surveyed were asked some trivia worthy of "Final Jeopardy." The bad news is that, because of the very nature of these questions, you can't prepare for them. The good news is that a simple "I don't know" seemed to satisfy the interviewers. For bonus points, ask for the answer, or, as one student did, tell them you'll check and get back to them. He did and, subsequently, he got in.

- *What is the largest lobbyist group in the U.S.?*
- *Which state first had women's suffrage?*
- *What language did Abraham (of the Bible) speak?*
- *When did Iraq become an independent nation?*
- *How many numbers that contain 9 are there between 1 and 100?*
- *What is the capital of Vietnam?*
- *When and how was Pakistan formed?*
- *Who won the 1969 World Series?*
- *What is the difference between European and American eighteenth-century poetry?*
- *Why was the Civil War fought?*
- *What is the origin of the name "Cincinnati"?*
- *What do the e's in e.e. cummings' name stand for?*
- *When and why was the March of Dimes founded?*
- *When did Istanbul become Istanbul?*
- *Name the four non-Arabic-speaking countries in the Middle East.*
- *What was Thomas Aquinas famous for?*
- *Who was the architect who built the Great Wall of China?*
- *Where was Millard Filmore born?*
- *Give a brief history of the Jesuit order.*
- *Define the Apollonian and the Dionysian as they figure in the philosophy of Nietzsche.*
- *Who was the head of NATO during World War II?*
- *What size tippets do you use on your fly lines with a 14X fly?*

A Corollary: I'll Take Science & Medicine for $1,000, Alex

A few interviewees were asked trivia questions that actually related to science and medicine. For the most part, they knew the answers. When they didn't, and the question was obscure, it didn't seem to hurt their chances of getting in. Your undergraduate coursework and MCAT review should be preparation enough for a lot of these questions.

- *What was the first industrialized country to practice socialized medicine? The second?*
- *How much does the U.S. spend each year on medical care?*
- *How does a lightbulb work?*
- *Why don't fish die in winter?*
- *Why does ice float on the top of water?*
- *How do you make a protein?*
- *So, what is Alzheimer's disease anyway?*
- *Where is your hamstring region?*
- *Tell me what you know about DNA.*
- *What is the Grignard Reaction?*
- *What is Poisson's equation?*
- *Describe protein structure.*
- *What is PKU?*

Anita Who?

Despite the media attention focused on the issues of gender discrimination and sexual harassment, medical school interviewers are still asking questions that, if they were asked in a job interview, would be deemed inappropriate or illegal. These kinds of questions are more common than you would expect. The students who told us they'd been asked these questions (and there were lots of them, mostly female) expressed emotions from confusion to outrage. Still, most admitted to being intimidated that they would be rejected if they did anything but reply calmly, and therefore they answered honestly and without additional comment. How you handle a question like this is up to you. At this point, you too might feel that there is too much at stake to make waves, but, on the other hand, it is certainly within your rights to ask how the question is relevant or even to politely decline to answer.

- *How did you get such a high score in math? I've never seen such a high score from a woman!*

- *Do you know that you have extraordinarily good looks?*
- *Why do you want to be a doctor rather than a nurse?*
- *Will you faint if I take you into surgery?*
- *Would you feel uncomfortable being alone with a male patient?*
- *How did taking a nude art class make you feel?*
- *What would your ideal date be?*
- *Do you find it hard to find educated black men to date?*
- *Why don't you like men?*
- *How does your boyfriend feel about your going to medical school?*
- *Would having a boyfriend affect your decision in choosing a medical school and career?*
- *Are you prepared to handle possibly losing your boyfriend/girlfriend over the stress and distance?*
- *Are you married?*
- *What kind of person would you like to marry?*
- *Do you plan to marry while in medical school?*
- *Why aren't you married?*
- *How will you deal with being married while in medical school?*
- *What does your husband do?*
- *Why did you get divorced?*
- *Do you plan to remarry?*
- *Do you expect to have a family? If so, why are you applying to medical school?*
- *If you become pregnant, what will you do?*
- *How do you plan to manage a family and a career? After all, you are a woman.*
- *How would you raise your children if you were a doctor?*
- *What would you do if you were sexually harassed at any time during school, residency, or your career?*
- *Are you prepared for the sexual discrimination you are most likely to face as a student, resident, intern, and so on?*

EXPECT THE UNEXPECTED

Although most of the questions fall into one of the previous categories, some of the questions are just plain off the wall. Some of the following questions were logical from the perspective of the candidates' background, so be prepared to answer questions about the leisure activities you listed on your application or the experiences you related in your essays. Other questions came straight out of left field. These are unlikely to be repeated, but they give you an idea of the kind of things interviewers ask to catch you off balance. If you're asked a question like this, take your time and think it through. If all else fails, remember, it's better to say "I don't know" than to try to "baffle 'em with bull." As one of those surveyed said after an unsuccessful attempt at bluffing, "It doesn't work—they've heard it all before."

- *What would you do if I dropped unconscious right now?*
- *What would you say if you smashed your finger with a hammer?*
- *How tall are you?*
- *How did you get your hair to do that?*
- *Is that your natural hair color?*
- *Why are you dressed the way you are? Why did you come here looking the way you do?*
- *Do you think that anyone can become a singer?*
- *Do you know how to play an instrument?*
- *Who is your favorite classical music composer?*
- *What's your favorite Beatles album?*
- *What is your favorite college football team?*
- *What do you think the chances are that the [team name] will make the playoffs?*
- *Why are the majority of NBA players black?*
- *How much can you bench press?*
- *If you're accepted, will you play on our softball team?*
- *What was your opinion of the rich, yuppie Greek students on your undergraduate campus?*
- *How much do you drink?*
- *Have you ever cheated?*
- *Have you ever tried an illegal substance?*

- *Have you ever stolen a car?*
- *What kind of car do you drive?*
- *What is your opinion of Charlie Brown?*
- *Do you prefer the old* Star Trek *or the new one?*
- *Why didn't you take Latin?*
- *Do you dream in Chinese or English?*
- *Do you know how to surf?*
- *Are you most like Madonna, Margaret Thatcher, or Mother Theresa, and why?*
- *What is your favorite card game?*
- *Do you play bingo?*
- *Does your mother know where you are?*

7 Allopathic Profiles

ALBANY MEDICAL COLLEGE

47 NEW SCOTLAND AVENUE, MAIL CODE 3, ALBANY, NY 12208 • ADMISSION: 518-262-5521 • FAX: 518-262-5887 • E-MAIL: ADMISSIONS@MAIL.AMC.EDU • WEBSITE: WWW.AMC.EDU

STUDENT BODY

Type	Private
Enrollment	514
% male/female	49/51
% underrepresented minorities	6
# applied (total/out)	6,103/4,778
# accepted (total/out)	375/269
# enrolled (total/out)	89/88
Average age	24

FACULTY

Total faculty (number)	1,534
% female	22
% minority	6
% part-time	65
# student/faculty ratio	3:1

ADMISSIONS

Average GPA and MCAT Scores

Overall GPA	3.5
MCAT Bio	9.78
MCAT Phys	9.34
MCAT Verbal	9.27
MCAT Essay	P

Application Information

Regular application	11/15
Regular notification	10/15
Are transfers accepted?	No
Admissions may be deferred?	Yes
Interview required?	Yes
Application fee	$100

Academics

Albany Medical College administrators responded to the changing health care needs in the United States by restructuring the curriculum in 1993 to better address contemporary issues in health care, while simultaneously providing a solid clinical and scientific education. The curriculum specifically focuses on the principles and practices of comprehensive care—health care that addresses the full spectrum of patient needs from medical and preventive to palliative and psychosocial. Grades of honors, excellent, good, marginal, and unsatisfactory are used to evaluate student performance. In the clinical years narrative assessments of performance are also used as an important evaluation tool. Graduation requirements include passing Step 1 of the USMLE and taking Step 2, including the clinical skills exam.

BASIC SCIENCES: Basic science education is coordinated and integrated in a manner that spans all four years of medical school and systematically increases within the context of clinical medicine. By teaching within a clinical context, professors offer a learning environment where students develop problem solving skills. Basic science concepts are divided into themes or modules that are most often organ based. Taught in conjunction with clinical case experience, these modules come together to form the foundation of clinical education. In the first year students combine basic science instruction with clinical cases to focus on normal function. In the second year students further expand their knowledge and focus primarily on abnormal function and the disease state. Students learn clinical skills beginning in their first year by working within small groups and interacting with patients (standardized patients who are trained to simulate evaluation purposes. Students explore legal, ethical, and humanistic concerns in a four-year module called health care and society. Systems of health care, epidemiology, biostatistics, and evidence-based medicine are concurrently studied in a four-year module called comprehensive care case study. Fundamental knowledge of nutrition also begins in year one and is integrated in all four years of the curriculum. Managing information is a key component throughout all thematic modules. The Schaffer Library of Health Sciences houses more than 144,000 volumes and 974 journals in print, and it contains 8,500 journals (available online) and 3,900 multimedia programs; there are forty computer stations in the independent learning center. Throughout their medical education, students rely on these resources as well as the support of the library faculty.

CLINICAL TRAINING

An innovative experience called the Orientation Clerkship transitions students from the first two years of the curriculum to the clinical and rotation requirements of the final two years. This two-week clerkship occurs during the summer prior to year three. These learning opportunities on standardized patients enable medical students to develop, practice, and enhance their clinical skills and abilities. Students participate in mock preceptor rounds, assess their own clinical skills, and perform basic medical procedures. The third year required clinical clerkships are in the process of changing from hospital-based experiences to hospital- and ambulatory-based experiences. The third-year required clerkships are medicine (includes radiology, twelve weeks), surgery (eight weeks), obstetrics/gynecology (six weeks), pediatrics (eight weeks), family practice (six weeks), and psychiatry (six weeks). Fourth-year rotation requirements are surgery (four weeks), emergency medicine (four weeks), neuro/opthomology (four weeks), critical care (four weeks), and an elective in either family practice, medicine, surgery, or pediatrics (four weeks). Required rotations take place primarily at Albany Medical Center Hospital, other regional and local community hospitals, community health centers, psychiatric inpatient units, nursing homes, adult homes, and patients' homes. The remainder of the fourth year includes electives that students choose.

Students

Of students in the 2003 entering class, 8 percent were underrepresented minorities. Geographic representation was as follows: Northeast (60 percent), South (8 percent), Midwest (7 percent), West (23 percent), foreign countries (2 percent). There is usually a wide variety of ages within the student body. Average class size is 130.

STUDENT LIFE

The student community is very active both on and off campus. There are about thirty campus clubs and organizations, including a student newspaper, outdoor and athletic clubs, support groups for students with similar backgrounds or situations, and groups focused on community activities. For example, one student organization arranges activities for the medical center's pediatric cancer patients, while another brings AIDS education programs to local schools. Residence halls in the vicinity of the school are available for single students. Off-campus housing is generally comfortable and affordable.

GRADUATES

Graduates gain acceptance into some of the top institutions in the nation. Forty-six percent of the 2003 graduates entered residency programs in primary care.

Admissions

REQUIREMENTS

Requirements are six semester hours each or nine quarter hours of biology, general chemistry, organic chemistry, and physics—all of which must include associated labs. When assessing GPAs, the Admissions Committee considers the intensity of all students' course loads as well as their undergraduate institutions. The MCAT is required of all applicants. The school considers the best set of scores the most important when making their decision; however, candidates should submit all their scores.

SUGGESTIONS

Community service and medically related activities are valued. College courses should be varied and demonstrate breadth and depth. There is no preference for New York State residents.

PROCESS

All AMCAS applicants are sent secondary applications. About 25 percent of cadidates who complete secondaries are interviewed. Interviews take place from September through April and are conducted by faculty, students, administrators, and local physicians. The interview day also features a group orientation and the opportunity to meet with deans, faculty, and students. Candidates are notified on a rolling basis and are either accepted, rejected, or wait-listed. About 50 percent of interviewees are accepted. Albany Medical College offers combined degree programs with Siena College, Union College, and Rensselaer Polytechnic Institute with a special focus on community service, business management, or research, respectively. Interested students should apply during their senior year in high school. The MCAT is waived for students admitted through these joint programs. Students admitted to the programs earn both degrees in seven or eight years depending on the undergraduate institution.

Admissions Requirements (Required)

MCAT scores, science GPA, non-science GPA, letters of recommendation, interview, essays/personal statement.

Admissions Requirements (Optional)

state residency, extracurricular activities, exposure to medical profession.

COSTS AND AID

Tuition & Fees

Tuition	$38,860
Cost of books	$1,200

Financial Aid

% students receiving aid	85
Average grant	$2,913
Average loan	$41,111
Average debt	$147,337

BAYLOR COLLEGE OF MEDICINE

OFFICE OF ADMISSIONS INFORMATION, ONE BAYLOR PLAZA, HOUSTON, TX 77030 • ADMISSION: 713-798-4842 • FAX: 713-798-5563 • E-MAIL: MELODYM@BCM.TMC.EDU • WEBSITE: WWW.BCM.TMC.EDU

STUDENT BODY

Type	Private
Enrollment	682
% male/female	58/42
% underrepresented minorities	18
# applied (total/out)	2,734/1,336
# accepted (total)	8
# enrolled (total/out)	168/74
Average age	23

FACULTY

Total faculty (number)	1,574
% female	33
% minority	21
% part-time	6
# student/faculty ratio	1:1

ADMISSIONS

Average GPA and MCAT Scores

Overall GPA	3.8

Application Information

Regular application	11/1
Regular notification	rolling
Early application	8/1
Early notification	10/1
Are transfers accepted?	Yes
Admissions may be deferred?	Yes
Interview required?	Yes
Application fee	$35

Academics

Students enjoy a flexible curriculum with various opportunities for individualized experiences. Grades of honors, pass, marginal pass, and fail are used to evaluate all students in basic science courses. During clinical training, students are evaluated with honors, high pass, pass, marginal pass, and fail. The USMLE is not a specified academic requirement. About 12 students each year enter a combined MS/PhD program and earn the doctoral degree in biochemistry and molecular biology, cardiovascular sciences, molecular and cellular biology, developmental biology, immunology, molecular and human genetics, molecular physiology and biophysics, molecular virology and microbiology, neuroscience, or pharmacology. Interdisciplinary programs at Baylor and the University of Houston and an engineering program with Rice University are also options. Nineteen MS/PhD students are funded annually by the NIH MSTP training grant. Other students are supported by private or institutional sources.

BASIC SCIENCES: Complementing basic science courses are clinical experiences, behavioral sciences, and social/ethical perspectives. Throughout the first year and a half, students take integrated problem solving (IPS) and patient, physician, and society (PPS). The IPS course develops lifelong learning skills by focusing on problem solving and the use of modern informational systems. The PPS course introduces basic clinical skills such as the physical diagnosis and examination along with principles of patient care. Other first-year subjects are organized into blocks. Courses include gross anatomy and embryology, cell biology and histology, biochemistry, physiology, immunology, general pharmacology, bioethics, nervous system, behavioral sciences, infectious disease, and general pathology. The first semester of the second year is organized around body/organ systems: immunology/rheumatology, cardiology, genetics, respiratory, gastroenterology, dermatology, renal, genitourinary/gynecology, endocrinology, age-related topics, and hematology/oncology. Both faculty and student tutors are available for additional instruction outside of the classroom. Basic sciences are taught primarily at the DeBakey Biomedical Research Building. The Learning Resources Center provides study areas and educational aids such as computers with medical software and Internet access, videotapes, and interactive learning programs. The Houston Academy of Medicine—Texas Medical Center Library contains more than 260,000 volumes, making it one of the largest medical libraries in the country.

CLINICAL TRAINING

Clinical rotations begin in January of year two. Required clerkships are pediatrics (eight weeks), obstetrics/gynecology (eight weeks), psychiatry (eight weeks), family and community medicine (four weeks), medicine (twelve weeks), surgery (twelve weeks), surgical subspecialties (four weeks), and neurology (four weeks). Throughout year three, students participate in longitudinal ambulatory care experience (LACE) that requires one half-day each week. Other requirements include four weeks of selectives and twenty weeks of electives in addition to a yearlong course on the mechanisms and management of disease (MMD). The MMD course is made up of modules that correlate basic science principles with clinical concepts. At the end of the fourth year, students may elect a two-week course in integrated clinical experiences (ICE), which serves as a transition to postgraduate training. Students train in the Baylor Affiliated Teaching Hospitals in the Texas Medical Center complex and at other sites around the city. In total, Baylor's teaching facilities hold approximately 5,000 beds. Elective credits may be earned at institutions throughout the United States and overseas.

Students

Approximately 70 to 75 percent of all students are Texas residents. Students in the class that entered in 1999 came from sixty-four undergraduate institutions. About 16 to 20 percent of all students are underrepresented minorities, and a wide age range is seen within the student body. Entering class size is 168.

STUDENT LIFE

A two-day orientation introduces entering students to the school's academic and nonacademic resources and promotes a supportive atmosphere from the beginning. First-year students also benefit from peer counseling groups and professional advising. Numerous organizations promote extracurricular, professional, community service, and religious interests or offer support for minority or other groups of medical students. Some examples include the Family Practice Club, the Texas Medical Association Medical Student Section, and the Baylor Association of Minority Medical Students. An athletic center with exercise equipment and weights; basketball, racquetball, and volleyball courts; and aerobics studio is available to medical students. Houston is home to almost two million people and is a center for commerce, industry, arts, and recreation. A dormitory operated by the Texas Medical Center is located near Baylor, although most medical students opt to live off campus in nearby residential areas.

GRADUATES

Graduates are successful in securing residencies in all generalist and specialty areas. Baylor also administers post-graduate programs.

Admissions

REQUIREMENTS

Prerequisites are one year each of biology, chemistry, organic chemistry, and English. Science courses must include associated labs. The MCAT is required and must be from within the past five years. For applicants who have taken the exam on more than one occasion, the most recent set of scores is weighted most heavily.

SUGGESTIONS

Approximately 70 to 75 percent of the positions in each class are reserved for Texas residents, making nonresident positions highly competitive. The April MCAT is recommended over the August MCAT. Beyond intellectual ability, Baylor is interested in personal integrity and demonstrated interest in medicine.

PROCESS

Baylor does not participate in AMCAS. Institutional applications are available in June preceding the year of anticipated entrance. Approximately 15 percent of all applicants are interviewed between September and February. Interviews usually consist of three thirty-minute sessions each with a faculty member or medical student. The interview weekend features a group orientation session, a campus tour, and the opportunity to informally meet with students and faculty members. Of interviewed candidates, about 40 percent are accepted on a rolling basis.

Admissions Requirements (Required)

MCAT scores, science GPA, non-science GPA, letters of recommendation, interview, essays/personal statement.

Admissions Requirements (Optional)

state residency, extracurricular activities, exposure to medical profession.

COSTS AND AID

Tuition	$6,550
Room and board	$12,595
Cost of books	$6,298
Fees	$3,008

Financial Aid

% students receiving aid	68
Average grant	$9,048
Average loan	$10,732
Average debt	$55,555

BOSTON UNIVERSITY
SCHOOL OF MEDICINE

715 ALBANY STREET, BOSTON, MA 02118 • ADMISSION: 617-638-4630 • FAX: 617-638-4718 •
E-MAIL: MEDADMS@BU.EDU • WEBSITE: WWW.BUMC.BU.EDU

STUDENT BODY

Type	Private
Enrollment	612
% male/female	54/46
% underrepresented minorities	15
# applied (total/out)	8,698/8,142
# accepted (total/out)	367/217
# enrolled (total/out)	155/132
Average age	22

FACULTY

Total faculty (number)	1,040
% female	34
% minority	8
% part-time	10
# student/faculty ratio	1:1

ADMISSIONS

Average GPA and MCAT Scores

Overall GPA	3.5
MCAT Bio	10
MCAT Phys	10
MCAT Verbal	9
MCAT Essay	Q

Application Information

Regular application	11/1
Regular notification	rolling
Early application	8/1
Early notification	10/1
Are transfers accepted?	No
Admissions may be deferred?	No
Interview required?	Yes
Application fee	$100

Academics

Several combined degree programs are offered, including the MD/MPH, to which all students accepted into the medical school may apply. Qualified students may pursue a joint MS/PhD program and earn the doctoral degree in anatomy, biochemistry, biomedical engineering, biophysics, behavioral neuroscience, cell biology, genetics, immunology, microbiology, molecular biology, pathology, pharmacology, or physiology. Most students take part in a four-year curriculum of basic and clinical science that leads to the MD. However, up to ten students each year enter an alternative curriculum that spreads out the first year of study into two years, thereby freeing up time for academic or personal interests. Grades of honors, pass, and fail, in addition to narrative reports whenever possible, are used to evaluate students. Passing the USMLE Step 1 is a requirement for promotion to year three.

BASIC SCIENCES: An integrated problems course supplements the traditional lecture/lab format of first- and second-year courses. In the integrated problems course, students meet in small groups; the course's interdisciplinary approach allows students to tackle case studies that relate to subjects discussed in other courses. First-year courses are gross anatomy, histology, biochemistry, physiology, endocrinology, neuroscience, principles of psychiatry in medicine, essentials of public health, immunology, genetics, and introduction to clinical medicine I (ICM I). In ICM I, students develop an understanding of the doctor/patient relationship and discuss sociocultural issues related to it. Second-year courses are pathology, pharmacology, microbiology and infectious diseases, biology of disease I, biology of disease II, ICM III, psychiatry, and integrated problems. In ICM II, students learn to conduct patient interviews and physical examinations. A benefit of the ICM continuum is that instruction involves mentorships with practicing physicians, often in primary care settings. Most basic science instruction takes place in the instructional building, which has classrooms, administrative offices, and a library with 117,000 volumes and 1,300 periodicals. This building connects to the Housman Research Building, which has a learning center and a computer room.

CLINICAL TRAINING

Required third-year clerkships are family medicine (six weeks), medicine (eleven weeks), surgery (eleven weeks), obstetrics/gynecology (six weeks), pediatrics (six weeks), and psychiatry (six weeks). More than half of the fourth year is reserved for electives. Required fourth-year clerkships are home medicine/geriatrics (four weeks), neurology (four weeks), radiology (four weeks), primary care (four weeks), and a subinternship (four weeks). Clinical training takes place at the Boston Medical Center (633 beds), the Veterans' Affairs Administration Medical Center (535 beds; located in Jamaica Plain), and at least eighteen other affiliated hospitals and health care facilities. Several research centers are part of the Medical Center and also serve as educational facilities for medical students.

Students

Underrepresented minorities account for about 15 percent of the student body. The average age of entering students is twenty-two, with a very broad range. Although a large number of states and colleges are represented, a significant proportion of students have completed their undergraduate education on either the East or West coasts.

STUDENT LIFE

Students are involved in a large number of student organizations, both professional and nonprofessional. These activities include The Creative Arts Society; volunteer efforts such as the Outreach Van, which provides medical care to the poor and homeless, and the Domestic Violence Awareness Project; and interest groups in the various specialties. Housing is conveniently located by instructional facilities and promotes cohesion among students. Medical students have access to the academic and athletic facilities of the medical campus as well as those on the Charles River campus, including the student union and several athletic facilities that offer swimming pools, an ice skating rink, dance, and sailing or rowing on the Charles River.

GRADUATES

In the 2003 graduating class, the most prevalent specialties were internal medicine (17 percent), pediatrics (16 percent), emergency medicine (8 percent), general surgery (8 percent), family practice (7 percent), anesthesiology (5 percent), diagnostic radiology (5 percent), obstetrics/gynecology (4 percent), and urology (4 percent). In recent years 85 to 92 percent of all graduating students have placed in one of their top three choices in the intern match.

Admissions

REQUIREMENTS

Prerequisites include one year each of English, humanities, general chemistry with lab, organic chemistry with lab, biology with lab and physics with lab. In evaluating GPAs, professors consider factors such as in the intensity of the undergraduate workload. The MCAT is required and must be taken within three years of the date of matriculation. For applicants who have taken the exam more than once, the committee looks at the best set of scores. The Committee on Admissions prefers that advanced placement courses and community or junior college courses not be utilized to fulfill prerequisites.

SUGGESTIONS

In addition to requirements, calculus is recommended, as is a broad background in the humanities and social sciences. Applicants are encouraged to take the April MCAT. For applicants who have been out of college for a period of time, some recent course work in the biological or physical sciences is advised.

PROCESS

BUSM uses a very limited secondary application, but applicants are invited to provide any additional materials that they believe might be helpful to the Committee on Admissions. About 10 percent of the approximately 9,000 AMCAS applicants are invited to interview; the school holds interviews between October and February. The interview day consists of an introductory session with the Associate Dean for Admissions, a session with staff from the Offices of Student Affairs and Financial Services, lunch with first- and second-year students, and a tour of the facilities with third- and fourth-year students. The interview consists of a one-hour session with a faculty member who is on the Admissions Committee. With only one hundred positions available for applicants to the four-year program, admission is very competitive. There are several alternate paths to gaining admission. A seven-year program, leading to a BA/MD degree is offered in conjunction with BU's undergraduate college. The MMEDIC program at BU offers an integrated curriculum made up of liberal arts and medical school courses, enabling preselected students to fulfill portions of the requirements of the medical school curriculum. The ENGMEDIC program at BU offers a joint, early selection program for the training of biomedical engineers interested in becoming physicians. The EMSSP program was developed with a consortium of historically Black undergraduate institutions and colleges with large Hispanic populations to provide an early and more gradual transition into the medical school curriculum beginning with the summer after the second year of undergraduate study.

Admissions Requirements (Required)

MCAT scores, science GPA, non-science GPA, letters of recommendation, interview, essays/personal statement, extracurricular activities, exposure to medical profession.

Admissions Requirements (Optional)

state residency.

COSTS AND AID

Tuition	$36,530
Room and board	$10,887
Cost of books	$2,118
Fees	$450

Financial Aid

% students receiving aid	79
Average grant	$2,500
Average loan	$41,669
Average debt	$138,909

BROWN UNIVERSITY
BROWN MEDICAL SCHOOL

97 WATERMAN STREET, BOX G-A212, PROVIDENCE, RI 02912 • ADMISSION: 401-863-2149 • FAX: 401-863-3801 •
E-MAIL: MEDSCHOOL_ADMISSIONS@BROWN.EDU • WEBSITE: HTTP://BMS.BROWN.EDU/MED/

STUDENT BODY

Type	Private
Enrollment	330
% male/female	42/58
% underrepresented minorities	55
# applied (total/out)	1,711/1,655
# accepted (total/out)	133/118
# enrolled (total/out)	69/57

FACULTY

Total faculty (number)	2,209
% female	34
% minority	13
# student/faculty ratio	7:1

ADMISSIONS

Average GPA and MCAT Scores

Overall GPA	3.6
MCAT Bio	10.2
MCAT Phys	10
MCAT Verbal	9.9
MCAT Essay	Q

Application Information

Regular application	12/15
Regular notification	12/15
Are transfers accepted?	Yes
Admissions may be deferred?	Yes
Interview required?	Yes
Application fee	$85

Academics

Most students enter the medical school after the fourth year in an eight-year BA/MD program at Brown to which they were admitted out of high school. Although curricula of this type are offered at other schools, Brown is unique in that it admits the majority of its medical students through this program, called the Program In Liberal Medical Education (PLME). Brown-Dartmouth program participants study basic sciences at Dartmouth and join Brown students for clinical training. They receive their MD degrees from Brown. Applicants may be considered for MS/PhD programs in conjunction with Brown graduate departments in the following fields: artificial organs, biomaterials, cellular technology, ecology, epidemiology, gerontology, molecular biology, biochemistry, molecular pharmacology, physiology, neuroscience, and pathobiology.

BASIC SCIENCES: Principles of patient care and of the social and behavioral aspects of medicine are integrated into the basic science curriculum. The first two years are organized into semesters. During the fall semester of year one, students take physiology, anatomy, histology, and medical interviewing. During the spring semester of year one, students take biochemistry, microbiology, pathology, brain and behavior, and neurobiology. The basic science courses are taught primarily through lectures and labs and also utilize small group teaching and clinical correlations. Pathophysiology provides a structure for year two, which is organized around organ systems or concepts such as cardiovascular, renal, hematology, pulmonary, human reproduction, gastroenterology, infectious diseases, supporting structures, endocrine, pharmacology, pathology, introduction to clinical medicine, neurologic pathophysiology, and epidemiology. Preclinical instruction takes place in the Biomedical Building, which is central to the Brown campus. The Science Library is fully computerized and has online database systems. Medical students have access to all of Brown's academic facilities, including the main library, which houses two million volumes. Grades of honors, pass, and fail are used to evaluate students. Passing Step 1 of the USMLE is not a requirement for promotion.

CLINICAL TRAINING

Patient contact begins in the first year (fall semester) with medical interviewing. Formal clinical training, made up of required core rotations and electives, occupies years three and four. In total, fifty weeks are devoted to core clerkships and thirty-two weeks to electives. Requirements are medicine (twelve weeks), surgery (eight weeks), pediatrics (six weeks), obstetrics/gynecology (six weeks), family medicine (six weeks), psychiatry (six weeks), community health (six weeks), medicine or pediatrics subinternship (four weeks), and longitudinal ambulatory (one half-day per week for 2six weeks). Clinical training takes place at seven affiliated teaching hospitals in the Providence area: Bradley Hospital, Butler Hospital, The Miriam Hospital, Memorial Hospital of Rhode Island, Rhode Island Hospital, Hasbro Children's Hospital, VA Medical Center, and Women and Infants Hospital. The hospitals attract an ethnically and socioeconomically diverse urban population. Noteworthy areas of clinical care and research include child/adolescent medicine, psychiatric care, international health, cancer, AIDS, artificial organs, and diabetes. Grades of honors, pass, and fail are used to evaluate clinical performance, as are narratives. Students are required to take the USMLE Steps 1, 2, and 2B prior to graduation.

Students

PLME students make up about 63 percent of the student body. Students who studied basic sciences at Dartmouth account for 9 percent. Rhode Island residents who entered through the EIP make up 8 percent of students, and those who attended post-baccalaureate programs make up about 9 percent of each class. The remaining 11 percent of students are post-baccalaureate students, MS/PhD candidates, former Brown students, or advanced standing/transfer students. Fifty percent of the students majored in the natural or physical sciences as undergraduates. Women make up 58 percent of the student population, while men make up 42 percent. About 18 percent of students are underrepresented minorities, and about 24 percent of entering students are twenty-five years old or older upon matriculation.

STUDENT LIFE

Medical students have full access to the school's recreational activities and facilities. Brown has over 200 student clubs and organizations that unite students. Although most students choose to live off campus, residence halls and housing co-ops are available.

GRADUATES

In recent years, approximately 15 percent of graduates entered residency programs at hospitals affiliated with Brown. About half of each class enters primary care residencies.

Admissions

REQUIREMENTS

Students admitted to Brown Medical School must attain competence in the sciences basic to medicine and sufficient to provide adequate preparation for medical school. Applicants are expected to demonstrate competence by successfully completing courses in quantitative reasoning (one course dealing with the elements of probability and statistics, preferably biostatistics and epidemiology); biology (at least one introductory course and one course in introductory biochemistry for which a laboratory experience in one of the courses is recommended); chemistry (two courses in general inorganic chemistry and one course in organic chemistry); physics (a two-course sequence is necessary for coverage of topics in mechanics, heat, electricity, optics, and radiation physics); and social and behavioral sciences (at least two courses of the applicant's choice, preferably in anthropology, sociology, psychology, economics, or political science). The MCAT is required for students applying to the Brown-Dartmouth Program and through the new standard route of admissions.

SUGGESTIONS

The only way for a typical medical school applicant to gain admission to Brown is through the Brown-Dartmouth program or as an MS/PhD candidate. About 15 students enter the Brown-Dartmouth program each year.

PROCESS

For the first time in more than fifteen years, Brown Medical School will accept applications from qualified graduates of any college or university for the fall 2005 entering class. As a result, the medical student body—which currently comprises PLME, post-baccalaureate, Brown Avenue, EIP, Brown-Dartmouth students, and advanced standing/transfer students—will also include eight to ten matriculants from a standard route of admissions, starting with the class entering in September 2005.

The first step in applying through both the standard route of admissions and the Brown-Dartmouth Program is filing an application with the American Medical College Application Service (AMCAS). Interviews are required of most applicant groups.

Admissions Requirements (Required)

MCAT scores, science GPA, non-science GPA, letters of recommendation, interview, state residency, essays/personal statement, exposure to medical profession.

Admissions Requirements (Optional)

extracurricular activities.

COSTS AND AID

Tuition	$31,872
Room and board	$11,792
Cost of books	$1,690
Fees	$2,138
Financial Aid	
% students receiving aid	63
Average grant	$17,810
Average loan	$27,800
Average debt	$100,407

Case Western Reserve University
School of Medicine

Associate Dean of Admissions, 10900 Euclid Avenue, Cleveland, OH 44106 • Admission: 216-368-3450 • Fax: 216-368-4621 • E-mail: emr3@po.cwru.edu • Website: http://mediswww.cwru.edu

STUDENT BODY

Type	Private
Enrollment	587
% male/female	57/43
% underrepresented minorities	14
# applied (total/out)	7,308/6,217
# accepted (total/out)	35/7
# enrolled (total)	12

ADMISSIONS

Application Information

Early application	11/15
Early notification	1/15
Are transfers accepted?	Yes
Interview required?	Yes
Application fee	$60

Academics

The curriculum is decidedly nontraditional, combining several approaches to learning and two distinct and flexible paths. All students participate in the Core Academic Program (CAP), which incorporates the Core Physician Development Program (CPDP), a case-based system. Patient Based Learning (PBL) is introduced in year one and required clerkships in year three; the Flexible Program allows students to participate in preclinical and clinical electives throughout the four years. Students who elect the Primary Care Tract (PCT) have enhanced clinical opportunities early in the program and have direct contact with primary care providers throughout medical school. Joint MS/PhD programs are offered in physiology, engineering, and biophysics and in thirteen divisions of biomedical sciences, including nutritional sciences and environmental health. Approximately ten students in each class are admitted as MS/PhD candidates. A BA/MD is offered in conjunction with the undergraduate college, and approximately ten students matriculate yearly as part of this program.

BASIC SCIENCES: During the first year, students are presented cellular and developmental biology, integrated human physiology, and the cellular basis of disease by faculty teaching teams representing both basic science and clinical departments. Each course lasts two months and is followed by an exam. For the remainder of the first year and for the duration of the second year, students cover basic sciences through study of the individual organ systems, and students retain the information with the help the case study approach. With this integrated approach to learning, students attend class, and student note-taking collectives are not emphasized. Afternoons are generally free from scheduled courses, which allows students time for elective study or research. Computer facilities support classroom learning, and computers loaded with first- and second-year course material are available in the MicroComputer Lab. The Health Center Library houses 150,000 volumes. Grading is pass and fail. Students choose their own academic advisers and have a great deal of control over their own courses of study. The USMLE Steps 1 and 2 are required for graduation.

CLINICAL TRAINING

Students have ample opportunity for clinical training outside of traditional clerkships. Most students begin their clinical responsibilities during the first year when they are assigned to either a pregnant woman in the family clinic or a patient in the geriatric care program. For two years students follow their patients and their development. Second-year students learn physical diagnosis and history-taking under the supervision of physician preceptors. In the third year, required rotations include medicine, obstetrics/gynecology, pediatrics, psychiatry, surgery, neuroscience, and family medicine. Fourth year is devoted to clinical electives. Training takes place at affiliated teaching hospitals, including the University Hospitals of Cleveland, Metro-Health Medical Center, Saint Luke's, VA Cleveland, Mount Sinai Medical Center, and the Henry Ford Health System. Some training takes place in clinics rather than in traditional hospital settings. The patient population represents urban Cleveland and rural Ohio. The Primary Care Tract is a relatively new mechanism for encouraging and training primary care physicians; it promotes ongoing student-physician mentorships and intensive primary-care clinical training. Grades of pass, fail, and honors are used to evaluate students during years three and four.

Students

Case Western is partially supported by the State of Ohio and gives preference to in-state residents, which is reflected in its matriculates: 60 percent of its students are Ohio residents. The student body is slightly more mature than average and is particularly diverse in terms of experience and background. Class size is about 135.

STUDENT LIFE

Although campus residence halls are available, most students choose to live off campus and most of them rely on cars for transportation to and from school. University-sponsored married student housing is unavailable. Student groups are involved in both community and social activities. The structure of the academic program allows time for extracurricular activities, and students participate in both university and community events.

GRADUATES

Of the 140 graduates of a recent class, fifty-two people went on to residency programs in Cleveland; another five people remained in Ohio. The rest of them went to different places as follows: California (seven), Georgia (four), Illinois (five), Maryland (five), Michigan (six), New York (seven), Pennsylvania (eight), Texas (four), Washington (eight), and other states. Graduates specialized in family medicine (twenty-two), surgery (seventeen), pediatrics (thirteen), radiology (seven), obstetrics/gynecology (nine), orthopedic surgery (five), psychiatry (five), emergency medicine (four), anesthesiology (three), neurology (three), ophthalmology (three), pathology (three), urology (two), transitional (two), neurosurgery (two), physical medicine (one), and plastic surgery (one).

Admissions

REQUIREMENTS

Students are required to take one year of biology, one of physics, and two of chemistry, which should include cover both organic and inorganic. In addition, students should demonstrate writing ability through course work. Recent academic performance is more heavily weighted, and although many older students are admitted, most of them have taken some relevant courses within the past two years. The MCAT is required, and the most recent set of scores is considered. Due to the rolling admissions process, applicants are encouraged to submit materials as soon as possible.

SUGGESTIONS

Case Western offers no further recommendations for college courses and accepts students from all undergraduate majors.

PROCESS

About half of all candidates who submit AMCAS applications receive a secondary. Secondaries should be promptly completed and are due no later than December 15. Less than one-third of all candidates who complete secondaries are interviewed, and interviews are held from September to March. Students have a one-on-one interview with a faculty member that generally lasts one hour. Those interviewed are notified shortly afterward of their status: accept, reject, or wait-list. The wait-list is not ranked. About half of the students who are accepted decline the offer, freeing up spaces for wait-listed applicants. Wait-listed candidates may submit additional material and should indicate if Case Western is their top choice. All Case Western undergraduates are invited to interview at the Medical School.

Admissions Requirements (Required)

MCAT scores, science GPA, non-science GPA, letters of recommendation, interview, state residency, extracurricular activities, exposure to medical profession.

Admissions Requirements (Optional)

essays/personal statement.

COSTS AND AID

Tuition	$36,500
Room and board	$7,260
Fees	$866

Columbia University
College of Physicians and Surgeons

Admissions Office, Room 1-416, 630 West 168th Street, Box 41, New York, NY 10032 • Admission: 212-305-3595 • Fax: 212-305-3601 • E-mail: psadmissions@columbia.edu • Website: http://cumc.columbia.edu/dept/ps/

STUDENT BODY

Type	Private
Enrollment	633
% male/female	54/46
% underrepresented minorities	12
# applied (total/out)	2,544/2,069
# accepted (total/out)	280/213
# enrolled (total/out)	150/101
Average age	24

ADMISSIONS

Average GPA and MCAT Scores

Overall GPA	3.7
MCAT Bio	12
MCAT Phys	12.2
MCAT Verbal	11.2
MCAT Essay	Q

Application Information

Regular application	10/15
Regular notification	2/15
Are transfers accepted?	Yes
Admissions may be deferred?	Yes
Interview required?	Yes
Application fee	$75

Academics

The Columbia curriculum is multidisciplinary and integrated; it focuses not only on understanding the science, skills, and techniques of medicine but also appreciating the art and ethics involved in it. Several joint degree programs such as the MD/MPH and MD/MBA are offered in conjunction with other schools and departments at Columbia. Qualified students who are interested in scientific research careers may pursue a combined MS/PhD and earn the doctorate in fields such as anatomy, biochemistry, biophysics, cell biology, genetics, immunology, microbiology, molecular biology, neuroscience, pathology, pharmacology, and physiology. Grades of honors, pass, and fail are used to evaluate medical students. Successful completion of Steps 1 and 2 of the USMLE are required for graduation.

BASIC SCIENCES: The first two years provide students with essential information and experience. The majority of instruction is conducted in lectures and labs, but small group teaching is increasingly emphasized. Students spend approximately twenty-five hours per week in scheduled activity. The first year (forty-two weeks) includes gross anatomy, neural science, clinical practice, and an integrated course that covers biochemistry, cell biology, genetics, human development, and physiology. The majority of the second year (forty weeks) is devoted to a multidisciplinary course that examines the basic concepts of immunology, pathology, microbiology, and pharmacology. Physical diagnosis, basic psychiatry, and clinical practice are also taught. Columbia has extensive laboratory, informational, and computer facilities that enhance classroom learning. The Augustus C. Long Health Sciences Library houses nearly 450,000 volumes and is one of the largest medical center libraries in the nation.

CLINICAL TRAINING

In the third year, students complete required rotations in the following: medicine (ten weeks), surgery (five weeks), pediatrics (five weeks), obstetrics/gynecology (five weeks), primary care (five weeks), psychiatry (five weeks), neurology (five weeks), anesthesiology/dermatology (two weeks), orthopedics (two weeks), urology (two weeks), otolaryngology (one week), and ophthalmology (one week). The fourth year consists of one- and two-monthlong electives drawn from a large number of offerings and student-designed experiences. There are extensive opportunities for clinical electives abroad. Each student is also required to complete one back-to-basic science elective. Science electives include one month seminars in advanced pathophysiology, clinical pharmacology, or clinical pathology. Rotations are conducted at various medical centers and hospitals throughout the metropolitan area, including Columbia-Presbyterian Medical Center, Harlem Hospital Center, Roosevelt Hospital, St. Luke's Hospital, and other institutions.

Students

Columbia attracts an extremely diverse, nationally represented student body. About 10 percent of all students are underrepresented minorities. There is a wide age range among incoming students, with significant numbers of students in their late twenties and thirties.

STUDENT LIFE

Although the schedule is rigorous, student life abounds at Columbia. Medical students have access to the recreational and athletic facilities of Columbia University and to university-sponsored cultural events. The P & S Club, the oldest student organization of its kind at any medical school in the United States, provides a variety of extracurricular activities. Students have opportunities in the fine arts, athletics, and service-oriented projects. In addition, Manhattan offers unparalleled access to museums, concerts, and every imaginable type of dining. Most students live in on-campus housing. Both residential halls and apartments buildings are available. Newly accepted married students are guaranteed married-student housing.

GRADUATES

Graduates gain acceptance to the most competitive residency programs in the nation. A Columbia education allows students to emphasize academic medicine, research, or primary care.

Admissions

REQUIREMENTS

One year each of English, biology, physics, chemistry, and organic chemistry are required for admission along with the MCAT. For students who have taken the MCAT more than once, the most recent scores are weighed most heavily. Thus, there is no advantage in withholding scores. Columbia does not admit students on a rolling basis. Therefore, submitting MCAT scores from the fall of the admission year does not place applicants at a disadvantage.

SUGGESTIONS

The Admissions Committee is interested in the depth and breadth of an applicant's extracurricular experiences. Community service, artistic activities, athletics, and medically related experiences are all valuable. It is valuable for applicants to denote that Columbia is their first choice for medical school, particularly for those who have been placed on the wait list.

PROCESS

Columbia does not participate in AMCAS. Rather, applications should be requested from the address above early in the summer. Between Labor Day and early March, approximately 25 percent of all applicants are invited for an interview. The interview day consists of one session with a faculty member who is a member of the Admissions Committee. Applicants also have lunch and tour the facilities with a current medical student. About 15 percent of interviewed applicants are accepted and are notified in February and March. A wait list is also created at this time. Wait-listed applicants may send additional information to update their files.

Admissions Requirements (Required)

MCAT scores, science GPA, non-science GPA, letters of recommendation, interview, essays/personal statement, extracurricular activities, exposure to medical profession.

Admissions Requirements (Optional)

state residency.

Overlap Schools

Harvard University

COSTS AND AID

Tuition	$35,036
Room and board	$14,550
Cost of books	$1,750
Fees	$2,700

Cornell University

Weill Medical College of Cornell University

Office of Admissions, 445 East 69th Street, New York, NY 10021 • Admission: 212-746-1067 • Fax: 212-746-8052 • E-mail: cumc-admissions@med.cornell.edu • Website: www.med.cornell.edu

Student Body

Type	Private
Enrollment	416
% male/female	48/52
% underrepresented minorities	18
# applied (total)	4,915
# accepted (total)	259
# enrolled (total)	101

Faculty

Total faculty (number)	938
% female	36

Admissions

Average GPA and MCAT Scores

Overall GPA	3.7
MCAT Bio	11.7
MCAT Phys	11.7
MCAT Verbal	10.6
MCAT Essay	Q

Application Information

Regular application	10/15
Regular notification	3/10
Early application	8/1
Early notification	10/1
Are transfers accepted?	Yes
Admissions may be deferred?	Yes
Interview required?	Yes
Application fee	$75

Academics

A curriculum revised to limit the time students spend in lectures promotes independent and interactive learning and research. The curriculum integrates basic and clinical sciences, utilizes problem-based learning, includes principles of public health, and encourages student research efforts. Students can pursue joint MS/PhD programs in conjunction with the Weill Graduate School of Medical Sciences, Rockefeller University, and the Sloan-Kettering Institute in the following fields: biochemistry, cell biology, immunology, molecular biology, and genetics; molecular pharmacology, neuroscience, and physiology; and microbiology. Fifteen students per year may enter joint programs.

BASIC SCIENCES: The curriculum was completely revised in 1996 and has been both highly successful and widely emulated. The first and second years of study consist of six basic science courses and medicine, patients, and society. In the first year, basic science courses are molecules to cells, fundamentals of genetic medicine, human structure and function, and host defenses. In the second year, basic science are brain and mind and basis of disease. The core basic science courses are sequential, integrated, interdisciplinary block courses that employ problem-based learning (PBL) in small groups. PBL emphasizes active learning and requires the student first to identify the issues needed to solve a medical problem, next to seek out the information needed to solve the problem, and last to reconvene in small groups with the faculty to apply the information learned. Lectures are few and emphasize the conceptual framework of a field. Anatomic dissection and experimental laboratories complete the learning experience. The course medicine, patients, and society approaches the doctor-patient relationship from both the conceptual and practical perspectives. For one day each week throughout each year, students spend the morning in seminar and the afternoon in physicians' offices. Areas treated include medical interviewing, physical diagnosis, human behavior in illness, medical ethics, public health, biostatistics, clinical epidemiology, and others. Thus, students learn these vital topics in a patient-centered context. Grades of honors, pass, and fail are used to evaluate students.

CLINICAL TRAINING

Upon completion of the second year and after taking the USMLE Step 1, students take three introductory clinical courses: clinical pharmacology, anesthesia, and the introductory clerkship. The third year is dedicated to clinical learning and emphasizes the core clerkships, including medicine, surgery, pediatrics, obstetrics-gynecology, psychiatry, neurology, and primary care. In these courses, students are assigned to clinical inpatient and outpatient services at New York-Presbyterian Medical Center and throughout the network of clinical affiliates. Clinical affiliates include the Hospital for Special Surgery, a leader in the fields of orthopedics, rheumatology, and sports medicine; Memorial Sloan-Kettering Cancer Center, one the premier facilities in the world devoted to the study and treatment of cancer; The New York Methodist Hospital; and others throughout the city. Students are integral members of the health care team and actively care for patients, under the supervision of the faculty. The fourth year centers on completion of clinical requirements, a subinternship, and electives. While students can take electives at any time in the third or fourth years, most of them focus on three major types of electives in the fourth year: clinical electives, often in subspecialty areas; research; and international electives. Each year up to half of the fourth-year class spends time abroad, typically in

Cornell-funded programs that combine clinical care and research in South America, the Caribbean, Africa, and Asia. In the month before graduation, eight weeks of advanced basic science allow students to study in-depth leading-edge biomedical science.

Students

In a typical class, students graduated from over forty-five different undergraduate institutions and came from over twenty-five different states. Class size is 101.

STUDENT LIFE

Although the school is located in an urban environment, students are cohesive and student life is apparent around the medical college. Ninety-five percent of all students live within three blocks of campus, generally in college-owned dorms or apartments. The rent is subsidized and competitive for New York. Students have access to athletic facilities in the residence halls. Student organizations, including organizations that support women and minority students, are active. Parks, including Central Park, are accessible, as are countless museums, theaters, shops, and restaurants. Students do not own cars.

GRADUATES

Graduates gain acceptance to the nation's top residency programs. Many graduates stay in New York City for post-graduate training.

Admissions

REQUIREMENTS

Weill/Cornell requires twenty-four semester credit hours in science courses, including two semesters each of biology, general chemistry, organic chemistry, and physics. In addition, six semester hours of English are required. The science GPA is given considerable weight. The MCAT is required and is used to assist the Admissions Committee in assessing the GPAs of applicants who typically come from a wide variety of undergraduate backgrounds. If an applicant has repeated the MCAT, the best score is considered.

SUGGESTIONS

Beyond required courses, Weill/Cornell recommends one to two additional upper division biology courses for nonscience majors. For students who graduated college several years ago, recent science course work is suggested. The medical college is interested in the extracurricular activities of applicants, particularly if they demonstrate commitment and dedication. Some exposure to the field of medicine is also desirable. Biomedical research is recommended.

PROCESS

All AMCAS applicants receive secondary applications. About 13 percent of applicants who complete secondaries are invited to interview, and about 20 percent of those who interview are offered a place in the first-year class. Interviews are held from October through February and consist of two thirty-minute sessions, each with a member of the Admissions Committee. Decisions are announced by March 15. Wait-listed candidates are encouraged to submit supplemental material as it can strengthen their applications and demonstrates their interest to attending Weill/Cornell.

Admissions Requirements (Required)

MCAT scores, science GPA, non-science GPA, letters of recommendation, interview, essays/personal statement, extracurricular activities, exposure to medical profession, secondary application.

Admissions Requirements (Optional)

state residency.

COSTS AND AID

Tuition	$31,085
Room and board	$9,224
Cost of books	$1,800
Fees	$910

Financial Aid

% students receiving aid	80
Average grant	$25,160
Average loan	$23,870
Average debt	$86,850

Creighton University
School of Medicine

Office of Admissions, 2500 California Plaza, Omaha, NE 68178 • Admission: 402-280-2799 • Fax: 402-280-1241 • E-mail: medschadm@creighton.edu • Website: http://medicine.creighton.edu/

STUDENT BODY

Type	Private
Enrollment	460
% male/female	54/46
% underrepresented minorities	8
# applied (total/out)	3,948/3,759
# accepted (total/out)	315/285
# enrolled (total/out)	120/106
Average age	23

FACULTY

Total faculty (number)	295
% female	23
% part-time	7
# student/faculty ratio	1:1

ADMISSIONS

Average GPA and MCAT Scores

Overall GPA	3.7
MCAT Bio	10
MCAT Phys	9.9
MCAT Verbal	9.5
MCAT Essay	P

Application Information

Regular application	12/1
Regular notification	Rolling
Early application	6/1-8/1
Early notification	10/1
Are transfers accepted?	Yes
Admissions may be deferred?	Yes
Interview required?	Yes
Application fee	$75

Academics

The educational program is divided into four years based on biomedical fundamentals, organ- and disease-based concepts, clinical clerkships, and elective clinical experiences. Students may apply to PhD programs in several areas of biomedical science, medical microbiology, or pharmacology and pursue the degree jointly with the MD. Grades of honors, pass, and fail are used to evaluate students; grades are supplemented with written evaluations. Students are not ranked against their peers.

BASIC SCIENCES: Professors use both the traditional lecture/lab format and small group/case-based learning approches to teach the basic sciences. First- and second-year students are in scheduled sessions of some sort for about twenty-five hours per week. First-year courses, which make up the first unit, are molecular and cell biology, anatomy, pharmacology, microbiology, host defense, neuroscience, interviewing and physical exam, ethics in medicine, evidence-based medicine, and human development in medicine. Many students participate in funded research projects during the summers between years one and two. The second component, organized by organ-and disease-based concepts, occurs during year two. Concepts or systems include cardiovascular, respiratory, renal-urinary hematology/oncology, gastrointestinal, muscular/skeletal, endocrinology reproductive, psychiatry, infectious disease, and multisystems courses. Throughout year two, students take psychological and social dimensions of medical practice, in which they are exposed to health policy, public health, medical ethics, and behavioral science issues. During years one and two, students also participate in clinical activities related to the patient physical and examination. Tutoring and review sessions for the USMLE Step 1 are provided. Creighton's Bio-Information Center houses 200,000 books and maintains extensive multimedia resources, computer teaching laboratories, and computerized literature search facilities. Passing the USMLE Step 1 is a requirement for progression to year three. Students at Creighton benefit from the new on-site computer testing facility, which is one of eight in the nation, for administration of their exams.

CLINICAL TRAINING

Second-year students take part in a longitudinal care clerkship, which demands one half-day per week. This allows students to develop longer-term relationships with mentors and patients. Third-year, core clerkships are primary care (eight weeks, encompassing internal medicine and family medicine); inpatient general medicine (eight weeks); psychiatry (eight weeks); surgery (eight weeks); pediatrics (eight weeks); and obstetrics/gynecology (eight weeks). Fourth-year guidelines require that students select one surgery elective, one critical care elective, one primary care subinternship, and one neurology clerkship; they must also participate in senior colloquium. The remaining twenty-eight weeks are reserved for residency interviewing and electives. CUMC (404 beds) is the primary teaching hospital. Other sites for clinical training include Omaha Children's Hospital, Omaha Veterans Medical Center, and Bergen Mercy Medical Center. During the summer, Creighton students have the opportunity to gain clinical experience through volunteer efforts in medical settings in the Dominican Republic or in communities closer to home.

Students

Among the 115 students in a recent class, 37 percent of them were from California, Minnesota, and Nebraska. The remaining students come from twenty-eight states and three foreign countries. Furthermore, students represented sixty-four colleges, and about 30 percent of the class graduated from Creighton with either an undergraduate or a graduate degree. About 84 percent of the students were science majors. The age range was twenty-one to thirty-seven, with an average age of twenty-three. Of the entire class, 50 percent were women, 6 percent were members of underrepresented minority groups (mostly Hispanic and African American), 10 percent were married, and 6 percent had at least one parent who is an MD alumnus/alumna of Creighton.

STUDENT LIFE

The student body is cohesive and supportive, as evidenced by the student-published Wellness Chronicle that offers tips and shares experiences on issues such as exercise, nutrition, mental health, relationships, and spirituality. Through clubs, organizations, and extensive volunteer opportunities, students associate with each other outside of an academic setting. The School of Medicine is part of the main campus of Creighton, allowing medical students to take advantage of programs and facilities of the greater university and to integrate with students from other programs. The Physical Fitness Center, the Student Center, and graduate student housing are all conveniently located by the School of Medicine. Omaha is a comfortable, friendly, and inexpensive city that allows students to meet their own lifestyle needs. Affordable off-campus housing is widely available.

GRADUATES

Our students have gained entrance into virtually all available specialty areas and prestigious programs throughout the United States. Over the last three years an average of 52 percent of the graduates enter primary care specialties, defined as internal medicine, family practice, or pediatrics. This is well above the national average of 48 percent. Creighton alumni are found in every state but are more numerous in the Midwest and Western regions.

Admissions

REQUIREMENTS

Requirements are biology (eight semester hours), chemistry (eight hours), organic chemistry (eight hours), physics (eight hours), and English (six hours). The MCAT is required, and scores must be from within the past three years. The school considers the best set of scores for applicants who have retaken the exam.

SUGGESTIONS

No particular courses or majors are recommended beyond requirements, but advanced courses including biochemistry and/or molecular biology are a plus. Studying overseas is encouraged, as are volunteer and community activities that demonstrate motivation and character.

PROCESS

All AMCAS applicants receive a secondary application, and about 15 percent of returning secondaries are invited to interview. Interviews are held from September through the spring and consist of one thirty-minute session with a faculty or alumnus member of the admissions committee and one session with a medical student who is usually a committee member. A tour of the campus and lunch with current medical students are also provided. About half of the interviewed candidates are initially offered a place in the class and are notified on a rolling basis. Wait-listed candidates may send supplementary information such as grades and updates on extracurricular activities.

Admissions Requirements (Required)

MCAT scores, science GPA, non-science GPA, letters of recommendation, interview, essays/personal statement, extracurricular activities, exposure to medical profession, volunteer service.

Admissions Requirements (Optional)

state residency.

Overlap Schools

Georgetown University, Loyola University Chicago, Medical College of Wisconsin, Saint Louis University, University of Iowa, University of Minnesota, University of Nebraska at Omaha.

COSTS AND AID

Tuition	$35,364
Room and board	$12,250
Cost of books	$2,665
Fees	$72,000

Financial Aid

% students receiving aid	94
Average grant	$20,000
Average loan	$53,599
Average debt	$142,000

DALHOUSIE UNIVERSITY

DALHOUSIE MEDICAL SCHOOL

5849 UNIVERSITY AVENUE, HALIFAX, NS B3H 4H7 • ADMISSION: 902-494-1874 • FAX: 902-494-6369 •
E-MAIL: MEDICINE.ADMISSIONS@DAL.CA • WEBSITE: WWW.MEDICINE.DAL.CA/

STUDENT BODY

Type	Public
Enrollment	90
% male/female	37/63
% underrepresented minorities	37
# applied (total)	479
# accepted (total)	90
# enrolled (total)	90

FACULTY

Total faculty (number)	1,311
% female	30
% part-time	32

ADMISSIONS

Average GPA and MCAT Scores

Overall GPA	3.5
MCAT Bio	10
MCAT Phys	10
MCAT Verbal	9
MCAT Essay	0

Application Information

Regular application	10/31
Regular notification	3/1
Are transfers accepted?	No
Admissions may be deferred?	No
Interview required?	Yes
Application fee	$70

Academics

The progressive case-oriented problem-stimulated (COPS) curriculum, which was introduced in 1992, prepares students for the pressures and problems facing physicians today. The COPS curriculum uses real life patient cases and is based on a tutorial system that emphasizes group learning, contextual learning, communication skills, and clinical interaction with patients. In addition to the MD curriculum, programs leading to MA and PhD degrees are offered. Some students opt for a combined degree program, earning both an MD and a graduate degree in a biomedical or related field.

BASIC SCIENCES: During their first two years, students are organized into small groups and build their basic science knowledge by examining matter relevant to patient cases. Faculty/staff tutors guide the group's learning process. Students also choose specific areas of medicine for an elective period and begin to acquire clinical skills in the first month of school. The first academic period lasts forty weeks and covers the following subjects: human body; metabolism and function; pathology, immunology, and microbiology; genetics, embryology, and reproduction; pharmacology; and clinical epidemiology and critical thinking. During the second academic period, students learn brain and behavior; skin, glands, and blood; respiratory and cardiovascular; genitourinary, gastrointestinal, and musculoskeletal; and population health, community service, and critical thinking. Throughout the first and second years, students have ongoing patient contact through the patient-doctor unit and have the opportunity to take elective courses. Teaching, research, and administration take place within two buildings: the Sir Charles Tupper Medical Building and the Clinical Research Center. The patient-doctor sessions are organized within the hospitals and pair the students with a clinical preceptor each week. Additionally, students attend the Learning Resource Centre weekly, where they participate in small groups in hands on skills and procedures such as casting, blood gases, and tubes and wires. Each student also completes case practice sessions that support each unit and use simulated patients. The students gain exposure to pediatrics, psychiatry, and various disciplines of medicine. The Kellogg Health Sciences Library houses more than 150,000 books and journals. The library is fully computerized and provides links to other libraries on campus.

CLINICAL TRAINING

The clerkship is organized into two phases, each of which has a central theme. All clerks will begin in a one-month introduction to clerkship unit in which clinical skills, procedures, history-taking, and physical-taking skills will be reviewed for all students. Phase 1 includes medicine, surgery, obstetrics and gynecology, pediatrics, family medicine, emergency medicine, and psychiatry. Each unit will be accountable for integrating objectives from other disciplines, and ambulatory and community experiences will be expected. Phase 2 begins with elective rotations offering the clerks maximum choice or remediation depending on their performance. In the final unit, continuing and preventive care, clerks are required to complete three-week rotations in long term care and care of the elderly and again have an opportunity for a choice of rotations. Clerks will be frequently evaluated so they can receive feedback on their progress to guide self directed learning. The major teaching hospitals are within walking distance of the school. They include a 202-bed pediatric hospital, a 254-bed obstetrics hospital, a psychiatric hospital, a rehabilitation center, and two large tertiary care adult hospitals. Other affiliated hospitals, clinics, and outpatient facilities also provide important training sites for medical students.

Students

Each entering class has ninety students. In a recent class, eighty-one students were from the Maritime Provinces and nine were from nonmaritime regions. At least 50 percent of students are women.

STUDENT LIFE

Although the academic workload is heavy, students are encouraged to pursue nonacademic interests. All students belong to the Dalhousie Medical School Society (DMSS), which promotes the interests of medical undergraduates. The DMSS organizes social and sporting events and raises money to support various nonprofit organizations. Through the Student Advisory, students have access to informal counseling, activities, and organized discussions that are coordinated and sponsored by other students. Dalhousie offers a variety of housing options on campus including residencies, singles rooms, and shared apartments. Outside of the campus, the city of Halifax offers a wide variety of entertainment, leisure, and shopping activities.

GRADUATES

Many graduates choose to enter post-graduate training at Dalhousie. Areas of training include family practice, numerous surgical and medical specialties, and laboratory medicine.

Admissions

REQUIREMENTS

The MCAT is required, and scores cannot be more than five years old. A baccalaureate degree is required for entrance to Dalhousie Medical School. There are no absolute prerequisite courses, although a minimal science background is advisable for success on the MCAT. Maritime applicants (candidates from Nova Scotia, New Brunswick, and Prince Edward Island) should have a minimum academic average of a B+, while nonmaritime applicants should have at least an A average.

SUGGESTIONS

Applicants from nonmaritime provinces and countries other than Canada should be exceptionally qualified. In addition to place of residence and academic credentials, the Admissions Committee reviews recommendations, results of personal interviews, and the applicant's extracurricular interests and activities.

PROCESS

For applications and details on the admissions cycle, view the website at www.medicine.dal.ca or contact the Admissions Office at the phone number and/or address above. Applications are available online only beginning September 1 of each year.

Admissions Requirements (Required)

MCAT scores, nonscience GPA, letters of recommendation, interview, essays/personal statement, extracurricular activities, exposure to medical profession, official school transcripts.

Admissions Requirements (Optional)

science GPA, state residency.

Overlap Schools

Memorial University Newfoundland

COSTS AND AID

In-state tuition	$10,460
Out-of-state tuition	$14,960
Cost of books	$2,000
Fees	$519

Financial Aid

Average grant	$4,000
Average loan	$12,000

DARTMOUTH COLLEGE
DARTMOUTH MEDICAL SCHOOL

3 ROPE FERRY ROAD, HANOVER, NH 03755-1404 • ADMISSION: 603-650-1505 • FAX: 603-650-1560 •
E-MAIL: DMSADMISSIONS@DARTMOUTH.EDU • WEBSITE: WWW.DARTMOUTH.EDU/DMS

STUDENT BODY

Type	Private
Enrollment	294
% male/female	52/48
% underrepresented minorities	22
# applied (total/out)	5,010/4,942
# accepted (total)	260
# enrolled (total)	78
Average age	24

FACULTY

Total faculty (number)	2,249

ADMISSIONS

Overall GPA	3.7
MCAT Bio	10.6
MCAT Phys	10.6
MCAT Verbal	9.8
Regular application	11/1
Regular notification	rolling
Are transfers accepted?	Yes
Admissions may be deferred?	Yes
Interview required?	Yes
Application fee	$75

Academics

Dartmouth Medical School (DMS), founded in 1797, is the fourth oldest medical school in the United States. Well-known for its commitment to teaching, excellence in clinical care, and strong sense of collegiality, DMS is also an important research institution. In the past decade, annual research grants and contracts awarded to DMS increased by more than 100 percent. Annual grant support today totals over $112 million. The innovative new directions curriculum integrates study of the basic and clinical sciences throughout the four years of medical school. Dartmouth's new directions combines small group discussions, problem-based learning, independent study, and traditional classroom presentations in the right mix to supply focus and support without hindering individual learning and creativity. DMS is a small school with a national student body, where opportunities for collaboration with the faculty abound. The medical school is located on the campus of Dartmouth College in Hanover, New Hampshire, one of the United States' classic college towns. DMS students are well traveled and enjoy opportunities to participate in clinical clerkships and electives around the U.S. and throughout the world.

BASIC SCIENCES: Structured class time in the first two years totals approximately twenty hours per week. During the three thirteen-week terms of the first year, students focus on the human organism's physical and psychosocial functioning. Students gain strong basic science grounding through course work in human gross anatomy and embryology, microscopic anatomy, microbiology, immunology, neuroscience, pathology, and physiology. The year also includes an integrated biochemical and genetic basis of medicine course. Topics in biostatistics and epidemiology are introduced, as well as biochemistry and metabolism. The major component of the second year is an interdisciplinary pathophysiology course called scientific basis of medicine. Another important second-year course is principles of medical pharmacology.

CLINICAL TRAINING

Clinical training begins at the start of the first year when students are paired with a faculty preceptor in the on doctoring course. On doctoring continues through the second year. The Dartmouth-Hitchcock Medical Center was recently identified by Solucient, a leading health care data company, as one of top sixteen major teaching hospitals in the U.S. A second major training facility, the White River Junction VA hospital, was awarded the Robert W. Carey Quality Achievement Award (the highest quality award of the Department of Veterans' Affairs) two years in a row. System-wide the Dartmouth-Hitchcock Clinic conducted almost 1.5 million patient visits last year. In addition to other teaching sites in New England, students can complete clinical clerkships in Dartmouth-affiliated teaching hospitals in Alaska, Arizona, California, Connecticut, Florida, New Mexico, and New Zealand. Fellowships from the Dartmouth International Health Group have made it possible for DMS students to explore health care opportunities throughout the world.

Students

DMS is located on the campus of Dartmouth College, an Ivy-League institution with an international student body and reputation. DMS students fully participate in the life of the institution and have access to the facilities, events, activities, and society that are part of the academic community. Students may enjoy national performing arts groups, professional theater, and high quality films at Dartmouth's Hopkins Center. The Hood Museum of Art, the Berry Sports Center, Thompson Arena, and Alumni Gymnasium are other focal points of interest. Dartmouth's athletic facilities include a ski area, golf course, horse farm, boathouses, and approximately 5,000 acres on Mt. Moosilauke. Many medical students volunteer in the community through such organizations as Planned Parenthood, the Good Neighbor Health Clinic, HEART (Health Education and Rescue Training), and the DMS Dermatones, a singing ensemble. There are several medical interest groups at the medical school. On-campus housing is available; however, the majority of students live off-campus.

STUDENT LIFE

Student life at DMS is marked by a strong sense of community and collaborative spirit. In an entering class of approximately eighty-five individuals, approximately sixty different undergraduate institutions are represented along with every region of the country and several foreign countries. Students of color and international students make up approximately one-quarter of the student body. Although medical education is demanding, DMS students do not typically view medical school as four years that are set aside. The environment is rich in opportunities for intellectual and personal growth.

GRADUATES

Graduates are successful in securing residencies in all fields at locations across the country. The Dartmouth-Hitchcock Medical Center sponsors thirty-four ACGME accredited residency and fellowship training programs.

Admissions

REQUIREMENTS

One year (eight semester hours) each of general biology, general chemistry, organic chemistry, physics, and one-half year of calculus are required. Facility in written and spoken English is also required. MCAT results are strongly recommended and must be no more than three years old.

SUGGESTIONS

Biochemistry is a recommended course, although it is not required. In addition to scientific acumen, applicants should demonstrate motivation and interest in their chosen major, which need not be science. Relevant research, medical experience, social service, and other cocurricular activities are important evidence of commitment.

PROCESS

All AMCAS applicants to DMS receive a secondary application, which must be completed by December 31. Approximately 700 applicants are invited to interview from a pool of roughly 5,000 candidates. Interviews occur from October to April and take place on the Dartmouth campus. Dual degree applicants (MD/PhD, MD/MBA) also interview at Dartmouth. After the interview, students are asked to indicate their program of preference: either the four-year MD program at DMS or the Brown/Dartmouth program in medical education, a unique affiliation between DMS and Brown Medical School. Students in the Brown/Dartmouth program spend the first two years of medical school at Dartmouth, years three and four at Brown. About 30 percent of those interviewed are admitted. A small number are placed on the waiting list.

Admissions Requirements (Required)

science GPA, non-science GPA, letters of recommendation, interview, essays/personal statement.

Admissions Requirements (Optional)

MCAT scores, extracurricular activities, state residency, exposure to medical profession.

COSTS AND AID

Tuition & Fees

Out-of-state tuition	$31,600
Cost of books	$2,800
Fees	$1,950

Financial Aid

% students receiving aid	88
Average grant	$17,655
Average loan	$27,055
Average debt	$93,000

DREXEL UNIVERSITY
COLLEGE OF MEDICINE

2900 QUEEN LANE, PHILADELPHIA, PA 19129 • ADMISSION: 215-991-8202 • FAX: 215-843-1766 •
E-MAIL: MEDADMIS@DREXEL.EDU • WEBSITE: WWW.DREXEL.EDU/MED

STUDENT BODY

Type	Private
Enrollment	1,019
% male/female	51/49
% underrepresented minorities	51
# applied (total/out)	4,453/3,930
# accepted (total/out)	974/717
# enrolled (total/out)	250/179
Average age	24

FACULTY

Total faculty (number)	2,599
% female	23
% minority	8
% part-time	82
# student/faculty ratio	1:1

ADMISSIONS

Average GPA and MCAT Scores

Overall GPA	3.5
MCAT Bio	10.2
MCAT Phys	10.2
MCAT Verbal	9.1
MCAT Essay	0

Application Information

Regular application	1/5
Regular notification	Rolling
Early application	8/1
Early notification	10/4
Are transfers accepted?	Yes
Admissions may be deferred?	Yes
Interview required?	Yes
Application fee	$75

Academics

Most students follow a four-year curriculum that leads to the MD. Students gain research experience through the Summer Research Fellowship Program, which provides a stipend in exchange for full-time research in the laboratory of a participating mentor. The combined MD/MHP program is available, as are MD/MS and MS/PhD programs, through which students may earn graduate degrees in bioengineering, cardiovascular biology, clinical microbiology, interdepartmental medical science, laboratory animal science, medical science preparatory, microbiology and immunology, molecular and cell biology, molecular and human genetics, molecular pathobiology, neuroscience, pharmacology, and physiology and radiation sciences. The medical humanities scholars program allows students who are particularly interested in the humanistic elements of medicine to graduate with the designation of humanities scholar. Several programs aimed at encouraging primary care, including a six-year combined medical school-residency option, are offered. Grades of honors, pass, and fail are used to evaluate students, and Step 1 of the USMLE is required for promotion to year three.

BASIC SCIENCES: As an alternative to the traditional preclinical curriculum, the program for integrated learning (PIL) offers a problem-based learning track to selected entering students. Students in PIL work in small groups and on their own, learning principles of basic sciences and applying them to clinical cases. Although the learning modality differs, students in both tracks cover similar topics and are in class or other scheduled sessions for about twenty hours per week. During the first year, topics are biochemistry, gross anatomy and embryology, microscopic anatomy and cell biology, human and molecular genetics, neuroscience and medical physiology, bioethics, nutrition, human sexuality, behavioral science, principles of medical research, and clinical skills. Second-year topics are medical microbiology, community and preventive medicine, psychopathology, pathology and laboratory medicine, medical pharmacology, and introduction to clinical medicine (a continuation of the first-year Clinical Skills course). The clinical continuum teaches interviewing techniques, the physical examination, and problem solving skills that are relevant to the practice of medicine. Standardized patients and model examination rooms are some of the facilities used to enhance clinical instruction in the course. Students also spend time in the offices of primary care physicians, thereby gaining firsthand experience with patient care. All students are involved in the school's computer-based learning program, which takes advantage of extensive educational and informational software programs.

CLINICAL TRAINING

Required rotations, most of which are completed in the third year, are medicine (twelve weeks), surgery (twelve weeks), pediatrics (six weeks), obstetrics/gynecology (six weeks), psychiatry (six weeks), neurology (four weeks), a subinternship (four weeks), and family medicine (six weeks). Among the clinical training sites in the Philadelphia area are Allegheny University Hospitals in Hahnemann (618 beds), Allegheny University Hospitals MCP (465 beds), Allegheny University Hospitals City Avenue (228 beds), Allegheny University Hospitals Elkins Park (280 beds), Allegheny University Hospitals Mt. Sinai (235 beds), Allegheny University Hospitals Parkview (200 beds), Allegheny University Hospitals Rancocoas (318 beds), and St. Christopher's Hospital for Children (183 beds). In the Pittsburgh area, teaching sites include Allegheny General Hospital (728 beds) and Allegheny University Medical Center Forbes-Metropolitan (172 beds). There are numerous other affiliated hospitals throughout Pennsylvania and New Jersey, in addition to community-based clinical facilities.

Students

About 17 percent of all students are underrepresented minorities, and at least one-quarter of all students are older, having pursued other interests or careers in between college and medical school.

STUDENT LIFE

Although the class size is relatively large, students are cohesive and supportive. The School of Medicine offers a variety of clubs and activities that are both academically and nonacademically oriented. Many students are involved in community outreach activities in local public schools, health clinics, and rehabilitation centers. Students have access to a new on-site fitness center and to the local YMCA. Philadelphia is a diverse and interesting city with a large student population. Students can find additional attractions in New York and other urban areas, which they can easily reach by train. There is no campus-owned housing in Philadelphia.

GRADUATES

Graduates are successful in securing residency positions. As one of sixteen schools nationwide to receive an implementation grant from the Robert Wood Johnson Foundation's Generalist Physician Initiative, MCP Hahnemann is focused on training primary care physicians.

Admissions

REQUIREMENTS

Requirements are two semesters each of biology, general chemistry, organic chemistry, physics, and English. Science courses should include associated labs. The MCAT is required, and scores should be from within the past two years. The most recent set of scores is weighed most heavily for applicants who have retaken the exam.

SUGGESTIONS

Beyond prerequisites, recommended courses include philosophy, ethics, history, psychology, and other social science and humanities courses. An advanced course in molecular biology or genetics is strongly encouraged. The Admissions Committee regards an applicant's background and experience as important. Women, older students, minorities, and students from rural areas are encouraged to apply. Pennsylvania residents are given slight preference.

PROCESS

All AMCAS applicants receive secondary applications of which about 10 percent are interviewed between September and March. The interview typically consists of two sessions, each with a faculty member or administrator. About one-third of interviewed candidates are accepted on a rolling basis. Wait-listed candidates may send transcripts or other material to update their files. An alternate route to admissions is through BA/MD and BS/MD programs organized in conjunction with Leigh University and Villanova University. A provisional acceptance to the School of Medicine may be granted to highly qualified post-baccalaureate students at participating institutions, contingent on their successful completion of the pre-medical curriculum. Post-baccalaureate programs where this type of arrangement is possible are Bryn Mawr, Bennington, Columbia, Duquesne, Goucher, University of Pennsylvania, and West Chester University.

Admissions Requirements (Required)

MCAT scores, science GPA, non-science GPA, letters of recommendation, interview, essays/personal statement, extracurricular activities, exposure to medical profession.

Admissions Requirements (Optional)

state residency.

COSTS AND AID

Tuition	$31,670
Cost of books	$2,500
Fees	$952

Financial Aid

Average grant	$8,430
Average loan	$39,067

DUKE UNIVERSITY
SCHOOL OF MEDICINE

COMMITTEE ON ADMISSIONS, PO BOX 3710, DUMC, DURHAM, NC 27710 • ADMISSION: 919-684-2985 • FAX: 919-684-8893 • E-MAIL: MEDADM@MC.DUKE.EDU • WEBSITE: WWW.DUKEMED.DUKE.EDU/

STUDENT BODY

Type	Private
Enrollment	401
% male/female	51/49
% underrepresented minorities	22
# applied (total/out)	2,525/2,322
# accepted (total)	240
# enrolled (total/out)	99/11

ADMISSIONS

Average GPA and MCAT Scores

Overall GPA	3.7
MCAT Bio	12
MCAT Phys	12
MCAT Verbal	11
MCAT Essay	Q

Application Information

Regular application	11/15
Regular notification	2/26
Are transfers accepted?	No
Admissions may be deferred?	Yes
Interview required?	Yes
Application fee	$75

Academics

By condensing the basic sciences into the first year and scheduling required clinical clerkships for the second year, Duke allows medical students additional opportunities for research, clinical, or other enriching experiences during their third year. Those who are particularly interested in research may apply for joint MS/PhD programs in fields such as anatomy, biochemistry, biomedical engineering, cell biology, genetics, immunology, microbiology, molecular biology, neuroscience, pathology, pharmacology, and physiology. Other joint degree programs are the MD/JD, MD/MBA, MD/MPH, MD/MPP, and the medical historian program, which leads to an MD and either an MA or PhD in history. In most courses, grades of pass with honors, pass, incomplete, or fail are used to evaluate medical students. The USMLE is not required for graduation, although most students opt to take it; virtually all of them pass each section with scores in the 90th percentile or higher.

BASIC SCIENCES: A new introduction to critical care course meets weekly during the first and second years and integrates clinical and basic science concepts. Each week during the first year, practice alternates between the classroom, where students meet in small groups, and the clinics, so that students can apply lessons shortly after they learn them. Computers are issued to all students to be used in the practice course for informational and instructional purposes. Also, part of the course is an intensive three-week preparation for year II segment, which prepares students for clinical rotations. Other first-year courses, taught primarily in a lecture/lab format, are organized into five blocks, so that no more than three subjects are tackled at a time. Courses are biochemistry, cell biology, genetics, gross anatomy, microanatomy, physiology, neurobiology, microbiology, immunology, pathology I, pharmacology, and pathology II. In total, first-year students are in class or at scheduled sessions for approximately thirty hours per week. Classes are held in buildings central to the medical complex. The Medical Center Library houses 276,000 books, including a renowned medical history collection. The Medical Library Education Center has electronic classroom and multimedia areas. Basic science concepts are reinforced during clinical rotations in year two.

CLINICAL TRAINING

Preparation for and exposure to clinical medicine begins during the first year, as part of the introduction to critical care course. The yearlong preparation for clinical clerkships provides students with significant experience in clinical settings before the beginning of their formal clerkships in year two. Clerkship requirements are fulfilled in the second year and include medicine (eight weeks), obstetrics/gynecology (eight weeks), pediatrics (eight weeks), psychiatry (six weeks), cost-effective care (two weeks), surgery (eight weeks), and family medicine (eight weeks, or neurology and family medicine, four weeks each). Clinical training takes place at Duke Hospital (1,124 beds), Durham Veterans' Affairs Medical Center (455 beds), Lenox Baker Children's Hospital, Durham Regional Hospital (451 beds), and at multiple affiliated hospitals and clinics. Students spend their third year conducting research as part of an independent scholarship project, which may be in behavioral neuroscience, biomedical engineering, biometry, biophysics, cancer biology, cardiovascular studies, cell and regulatory biology, epidemiology health services and health policy, immunology, infectious diseases, neurobiology, ophthalmology and visual studies, and pathology. Third-year students may design a year of mentored research at Duke or at approved extramural sites such as NIH; students may also begin the dual-degree curricula. During their fourth year, students complete clinical training through elective clerkships. There are more than 150 electives offered at Duke. In addition, students may spend up to two months in rotations at other institutions.

Students

In the most recent class, 22 percent of the students are underrepresented minorities, most of whom are African American. Women account for 49 percent of the class. The average age is twenty-two, with an age range of nineteen to forty-two. Forty-three undergraduate institutions are represented, the top six being Duke, Harvard, North Carolina State, Johns Hopkins, UNC at Chapel Hill, and Yale. Twenty-eight states are represented, and the top five are North Carolina, California, New York, Ohio, and Virginia. Class size is 100.

STUDENT LIFE

Students, faculty, and administrators come together for events that promote a sense of community, congeniality, and friendship within the medical school. For example, the dean hosts five Dean's Desserts so that medical students can interact with teaching, research, and clinical faculty during the year. Organizations based on volunteer work, professional goals, or extracurricular interests are numerous. Medical students have access to all of Duke's athletic and recreational facilities. Durham is popular with students since they can enjoy themselves at parks, shopping districts, restaurants, and museums. Mountains and beaches are just a few hours away. Convenient campus-owned apartments, some of which have athletic facilities, are available on a limited basis. Social events sponsored by various medical school-based organizations provide opportunities for students to interact together. A fitness facility located with the major hospital complex for medial students and house staff has only recently opened.

GRADUATES

Graduates enter top residency programs in primary and specialty fields. Most students get their top choice for residency appointment.

Admissions

REQUIREMENTS

Prerequisites are one year each of English, inorganic chemistry, organic chemistry, physics, biology, and calculus. The MCAT is required, and scores must be from within the past four years. The most recent set of scores is generally considered for students who have taken the exam on multiple occasions. Students who have taken time off after college, must complete science work no more than seven years before matriculation.

SUGGESTIONS

An introductory course in biochemistry is recommended. The character, motivation, and dedication of applicants is considered along with academic merits. Extracurricular activities (particularly activities that are medically related), community service, volunteer experience, research exposure, and work experience are all considered in admission.

PROCESS

About 60 percent of AMCAS applicants receive secondary applications, ofwhich approximately 30 percent are interviewed. Interviews are conducted from September through February and consist of two thirty-minute sessions with members of the Admissions Committee. On interview day, students also receive a campus tour and have the opportunity to eat lunch and speak with students. About one-third of interviewees will be considered for admission.

Admissions Requirements (Required)

MCAT scores, science GPA, non-science GPA, letters of recommendation, interview, essays/personal statement, extracurricular activities, exposure to medical profession.

Admissions Requirements (Optional)

state residency.

Overlap Schools

Harvard University, Johns Hopkins University, University of Pennsylvania, Washington University.

COSTS AND AID

Tuition	$28,566
Cost of books	$2,420
Fees	$2,563

Financial Aid

% students receiving aid	80
Average grant	$17,514
Average loan	$19,569
Average debt	$68,981

East Carolina University

Brody School of Medicine

Office of Admissions, Brody School of Medicine at ECU, Greenville, NC 27858 • Admission: 252-744-2202 • Fax: 252-744-1926 • E-mail: somadmissions@mail.ecu.edu • Website: www.ecu.edu/bsomadmissions

STUDENT BODY

Type	Public
Enrollment	288
% male/female	50/50
% underrepresented minorities	34
# applied (total/out)	1,092/464
# accepted (total)	72
# enrolled (total)	72
Average age	25

ADMISSIONS

Average GPA and MCAT Scores

Overall GPA	3.5
MCAT Bio	9
MCAT Phys	9
MCAT Verbal	9
MCAT Essay	P

Application Information

Regular application	11/15
Regular notification	rolling
Early application	6/1-8/1
Early notification	10/1
Are transfers accepted?	Yes
Admissions may be deferred?	No
Interview required?	Yes
Application fee	$50

Academics

All first- and second-year students are paired with community physician mentors, and have the opportunity for ongoing patient contact and exposure to primary health care settings. Grades of A, B, C, and F are used to evaluate students. In addition, honors may be awarded in some instances. Passing the USMLE Step 1 is a requirement for promotion to year three, and passing the USMLE Step 2 is a requirement for graduation. Joint PhD/MD programs can be arranged on a case-by-case basis.

BASIC SCIENCES: During the first two years, students spend about twenty-eight hours per week in classes, most of which are taught in a lecture/lab format. Small group discussions, problem-based learning, and an introduction to clinical medicine are also part of the basic science curriculum. First-year courses are microbiology and immunology, biochemistry, behavioral science, primary care preceptorship, genetics, gross anatomy, histology, embryology, neurobiology, ethical and social issues in medicine, physiology, and clinical skills I. Second-year courses are introduction to medicine, primary care preceptorship, psychopathology and human sexuality, introduction to child development, pathogenic microbiology, pathology, pharmacology, ethical social issues in medicine, clinical skills II, and clinical aspects of lifestyle abuse (addresses behavioral aspects of health maintenance for both patients and physicians). The Academic Support and Counseling Center assists students by providing them with enrichment sessions and tutorials. Most classes take place in the Brody Medical Sciences Building, a modern facility that has classrooms with computer and video technology, large laboratories, auditoriums, and a clinical outpatient center. The presence of a clinical facility in this classroom structure suggests the importance of integrating basic and clinical sciences at East Carolina. Another building used frequently by first- and second-year students is the W. E. Laupus Health Sciences Library, which has 52,900 volumes and 1,550 subscriptions in addition to computer and audiovisual learning aids.

CLINICAL TRAINING

Required clerkships are family medicine (eight weeks), internal medicine (eight weeks), obstetrics/gynecology (eight weeks), pediatrics (eight weeks), psychiatry (eight weeks), and surgery (eight weeks). Students spend at least ten of these forty-eight weeks in an ambulatory setting. Fourth-year students make selections from specified categories that include primary care experiences (two months), surgical selectives (one month), medicine selectives (one month), transition to residency (one month), and electives (four months). Clinical training takes place at sites throughout Eastern North Carolina, with the cooperation of the school's extended faculty members, some of whom practice in remote, rural areas. Training also takes place at the Developmental Evaluation Clinic, Eastern Carolina Family Practice Center, Pitt County Memorial Hospital (731 beds), specialized research institutes, and at rural affiliated hospitals throughout the state.

Students

Virtually all students are North Carolina residents, many of whom attended college outside of the state. More than 20 percent of students are underrepresented minorities, mostly African Americans. Almost half of entering students have taken some time off after completing their undergraduate degrees and before attending medical school. In a recent entering class, the mean age at matriculation was twenty-six. Class size is seventy-two.

STUDENT LIFE

The university has an active student union and facilities such as student lounges, theaters, concert halls, museums, and an athletic center. Medical students are integrated into the greater campus community and also have enjoy a cohesive social life among themselves. Medical student groups are organized around volunteer efforts, professional interests, support groups, and religious affiliations. Examples are the Generalist Physicians in Training Interest Group, the Medical Student Council, peer counseling, the Christian Medical/Dental Fellowship, and the Greenville Community Shelter Clinic. Greenville is known for its gentle climate and low cost of living, which are both assets to medical students. There are plenty of housing options both on and off campus for married or single students.

GRADUATES

The goal of the Generalist Physician Initiative is to have at least half of medical school graduates enter primary care fields. There are at least twelve residency programs and several fellowship programs offered at Pitt County Memorial Hospital, with the majority of positions in internal medicine, family medicine, and emergency medicine.

Admissions

REQUIREMENTS

One year each of physics, biology, general chemistry, organic chemistry, and English are all required. Laboratories are required with all science courses. The MCAT is required and must be no more than three years old. The most recent set of scores is generally considered for students who have retaken the exam. State residency or close affiliation with the state is a requirement for admission.

SUGGESTIONS

Beyond required courses, students are advised to take humanities and social science courses and an additional year of English. Taking classes that are part of the medical school curriculum is not recommended. Extracurricular activities that involve exposure to the medical practice are important. The Admissions Committee looks for applicants who are likely to contribute to meeting the health care needs of North Carolina.

PROCESS

All AMCAS applicants who are state residents (or who demonstrate strong ties to the state) are sent secondary applications, of which about 60 percent are interviewed between August and April. The interview consists of two thirty- to sixty-minute sessions with faculty or student members of the committee. On interview day, applicants have an opportunity to meet with students and to tour the campus. About 15 percent of interviewed candidates are accepted; the remaining candidates are rejected or wait-listed. Candidates awaiting a decision may send additional information to enhance their files.

Admissions Requirements (Required)

MCAT scores, science GPA, non-science GPA, letters of recommendation, interview, state residency, essays/personal statement, extracurricular activities, exposure to medical profession.

COSTS AND AID

In-state tuition	$2,951
Out-of-state tuition	$22,206
Cost of books	$1,750
Fees	$1,113

Financial Aid

Average grant	$8,259
Average loan	$12,720
Average debt	$43,714

EAST TENNESSEE STATE UNIVERSITY

JAMES H. QUILLEN COLLEGE OF MEDICINE

BOX 70580, JAMES H. QUILLEN COLLEGE OF MEDICINE, JOHNSON CITY, TN 37614-1708 • ADMISSION: 423-439-2033 • FAX: 423-439-2110 • E-MAIL: SACOM@ETSU.EDU • WEBSITE: HTTP://COM.ETSU.EDU

STUDENT BODY

Type	Public
Enrollment	236
% male/female	52/48
% underrepresented minorities	12
# applied (total/out)	1,144/679
# accepted (total/out)	60/5
# enrolled (total/out)	60/5
Average age	25

FACULTY

# student/faculty ratio	1:1

ADMISSIONS

Average GPA and MCAT Scores

Overall GPA	3.5
MCAT Bio	9.6
MCAT Phys	9
MCAT Verbal	9.7
MCAT Essay	0

Application Information

Regular application	12/1
Regular notification	7/1
Early application	6/1-8/1
Early notification	10/1
Are transfers accepted?	Yes
Admissions may be deferred?	Yes
Interview required?	Yes
Application fee	$50

Academics

Joint MS/PhD programs are offered through the School of Graduate Studies in anatomy, biochemistry, cell biology, microbiology, pharmacology, and physiology. Most students earn an MD in four years through either the traditional track or the RPCT.

BASIC SCIENCES: With the exception of clinical work, basic science courses are taught primarily in a lecture/lab format. Students are in scheduled sessions for about twenty-four hours per week. First-year courses for all students are anatomy, biochemistry, biostatistics and epidemiology, communication skills for health professionals, cell and tissue biology, physiology, geriatrics, behavorial science and lifespan development, and human development biology and genetics. Traditional students also take case oriented learning, while RPCT students take introduction to rural health, rural and community health, and health assessment/examination. Patient contact begins in case oriented learning for traditional track students and begins as part of weekly visits to rural health providers for RPCT students. The second-year curriculum for all students is geriatrics, neuroscience, microbiology, practicing medicine, immunology, pathology, psychiatry, and pharmacology. Traditional track students take clinical skills and clinical preceptorship while RPCT students take rural health needs, health assessment, and patient/client assessment. Instructional facilities are located in a newly constructed, multimillion dollar basic sciences building on the grounds of the Mountain Home Veterans' Affairs facility. The medical library has almost 100,000 volumes, several online medical databases, educational software programs, computerized access to the university library system, computers for student use, and rooms for audiovisual study, reading, and conferences. Grades of A through F are used to evaluate the students. Students must pass Step 1 of the USMLE for promotion to year three.

CLINICAL TRAINING

Third-year required rotations for traditional track students are family medicine (eight weeks), obstetrics/gynecology (eight weeks), pediatrics (eight weeks), psychiatry (eight weeks), internal medicine (eight weeks), and surgery (eight weeks). RPCT students participate in shorter rotations in the same specialties and are required to complete a sixteen-week primary care clerkship in a rural area. During the fourth year, all students complete a minimum of sixteen weeks of electives. RPCT students have additional rural primary care requirements, and traditional tract students must take internal medicine and senior surgery. Clinical training takes place in three cities (Bristol, Kingsport, and Johnson City) and in neighboring rural towns. Affiliated hospitals are The Johnson City Medical Center, VA Medical Center, Woodridge Psychiatric Hospital, Johnson City Specialty Hospital, Northside Hospital, The Holston Valley Hospital, Indian Path Medical Center, Bristol Regional Medical Center, and Hawkins County Hospital. In total, these hospitals provide 3,000 patient beds. Grades of A through F are used to evaluate the students, and the USMLE Step 2 is required for graduation.

Students

Almost all students are from Tennessee or the immediately surrounding areas. Most students went to college in Tennessee, although undergraduate institutions from around the country are represented in the medical student body. About 15 percent of students are underrepresented minorities, most of them African American. Class size is sixty.

STUDENT LIFE

Medical students take advantage of the extracurricular opportunities at ETSU, such as its theater, films, intramural sports, and athletic and recreational facilities. Campus housing is encouraged as a way of promoting friendship and a sense of community among students. Options include residence halls, efficiency apartments, and larger units suitable for couples or parents. As an urban area, Johnson City offers many services and attractions.

GRADUATES

Of the fifty-eight students who graduated and entered residency programs in 2002, 83 percent chose a residency in primary care family. Other residencies that students choose include anesthesiology, emergency medicine, medicine psychiatry, opthamology, orthopedic surgery, and surgery. A few seniors each year enter the accelerated residency training program (ARTP), which combines the final year of medical school with the first year of residency in family medicine.

Admissions

REQUIREMENTS

Applicants must complete chemistry (eight semester hours), organic chemistry (eight hours), physics (eight hours), biology (eight hours), and communication skills (nine hours). An additional forty-nine hours of course work is required. The MCAT is required and should be no more than two years old. The April MCAT is advised as the August exam will delay application processing.

SUGGESTIONS

Other recommended courses are comparative vertebrate anatomy, histology, mammalian anatomy, advanced mathematics, statistics, biochemistry, microbiology, public speaking, history, economics, philosophy, psychology, social science, and foreign languages. Recent course work is helpful for candidates who have been out of school for a significant period of time. The Admissions Committee looks for traits and experiences that are consistent with primary care practice. Admissions is particularly competitive for out-of-state residents, and with the exception of applicants from the contiguous Appalachian region who are interested in primary care, out-of-state applicants must have extremely strong qualifications to be considered.

PROCESS

About one-third of AMCAS applicants are sent secondary applications, of which the majority are Tennessee residents and about 10 percent are out-of-state residents who are invited to interview between September and March. Applicants receive two one-hour interviews with faculty, medical students, administrators, or community members. About 40 percent of Tennessee residents and 15 percent of out-of-state residents who interview are accepted on a rolling basis. The remaining candidates are either rejected or wait-listed. Generally, only a few students from the wait list are accepted.

Admissions Requirements (Required)

MCAT scores, science GPA, non-science GPA, letters of recommendation, interview, state residency, essays/personal statement, extracurricular activities, exposure to medical profession.

COSTS AND AID

In-state tuition	$14,390
Out-of-state tuition	$29,332
Cost of books	$1,360
Fees	$553

Financial Aid

% students receiving aid	91
Average grant	$8,000
Average loan	$28,000
Average debt	$94,000

Eastern Virginia Medical School

Eastern Virginia Medical School

Office of Admissions, 721 Fairfax Avenue, Norfolk, VA 23507-2000 • Admission: 757-446-5812 • Fax: 757-446-5896 • E-mail: nanezkf@evms.edu • Website: www.evms.edu

STUDENT BODY

Type	Private
Enrollment	432
% male/female	47/53
% underrepresented minorities	12
# applied (total/out)	2,565/1,846
# accepted (total/out)	335/197
# enrolled (total/out)	110/50

ADMISSIONS

Average GPA and MCAT Scores

Overall GPA	3.5
MCAT Bio	10
MCAT Phys	9.8
MCAT Verbal	9.5

Application Information

Regular application	11/15
Early application	6/1-8/1
Early notification	10/1
Are transfers accepted?	Yes
Admissions may be deferred?	Yes
Interview required?	Yes
Application fee	$90

Academics

The curriculum is designed to help students master both the science of medicine and the art of clinical problem solving. A combined MS/PhD program is available for qualified students and leads to the doctoral degree in one of the biomedical science fields. Summer research projects are available for medical students who are interested in medical research. Grades of honors, high pass, pass, and fail are used to evaluate medical students.

BASIC SCIENCES: The first two years are devoted to basic sciences that are fundamental to the practice of medicine. Students also learn the clinical skills of physical diagnosis and interviewing. During the first two years, students are in class or other scheduled sessions for about twenty-five hours per week. Lectures, labs, and small group discussions are the instructional modalities used. First-year courses include biochemistry, gross anatomy, histology, human development, introduction to the patient/longitudinal generalist mentorship, medical ethics, medical molecular and cellular biology, neuroscience, physiology, and the doctor/the patient. Second-year courses include biostatistics, epidemiology, introduction to the patient/longitudinal mentorship, medical ethics, microbiology/immunology, pathology, pathophysiology, pharmacology, and psychopathology.

CLINICAL TRAINING

Required third-year clerkships are family medicine (six weeks), internal medicine (twelve weeks), obstetrics/gynecology (eight weeks), pediatrics (eight weeks), psychiatry (six weeks), and surgery (eight weeks). Fourth-year required clerkships include four weeks of surgical specialties, two weeks of geriatrics, one week of substance abuse, and twenty-five weeks of electives, which may be selected from basic science and clinical offerings. For clinical training, students have access to a wide variety of facilities including the East Coast's largest naval hospital, full-service community hospitals, interdisciplinary primary care centers, one of the largest Level I shock trauma centers in the state, private hospitals, a prestigious children's hospital, and clinics built for the medically underserved.

Students

At least 70 percent of students are Virginia residents. The student body has a number of older or nontraditional students, and the average age of incoming students is often around twenty-six. Underrepresented minorities account for approximately 7 percent of the student body. Class size is 105.

STUDENT LIFE

EVMS supports students' nonacademic lives and puts significant resources into the well-being of its students. Each fall, students and faculty members convene at a nearby resort for the orientation retreat sponsored by the school's Human Values in Medicine program. The retreat provides a relaxed and informal atmosphere and allows incoming students the chance to interact with each other before classes begin. Throughout the year, students are involved in a number of organizations and events, including ongoing community service projects and a monthly Friday night social hour. In general, the school's location in the Hampton Roads area is ideal because it offers urban conveniences, the friendliness of a small town, and the attractions of a beach community. Most medical students live in the section of Norfolk known as Ghent, a beautiful neighborhood of tree-lined streets and Victorian houses, near the medical school. EVMS also owns and operates an apartment complex near the school that offers housing for both married and single students. Washington, DC, has many attractions and recreational opportunities and is only a four-hour drive away.

GRADUATES

Twenty percent to 25 percent of all graduates are accepted into one of the many residency programs sponsored by the Eastern Virginia Graduate School. Other graduating students are successful in securing residency positions at institutions throughout the state and at locations around the country.

Admissions

REQUIREMENTS

Required courses are one year each of biology, chemistry, organic chemistry, and physics all with associated labs. Applicants are expected to earn a B or better in these courses. The MCAT is required, and scores should be from no more than two years prior to the date of application. The best set of scores is weighed most heavily for applicants who have retaken the exam; therefore, there is no advantage in withholding scores.

SUGGESTIONS

In addition to academic transcripts, an applicant's experiences and background are examined. Personal characteristics are evaluated during the interviews, and honesty and spontaneity are considered essential qualities. Interviewers are interested in an applicant's concept of a physician's role, motivation, sensitivity to the needs of others, and communication skills.

PROCESS

After an initial screening of academic credentials, state residency, and other factors, about 50 percent of AMCAS applicants are sent secondary applications. A slightly larger percentage of state resident applicants are asked to submit secondaries. About one-third of returning secondaries are interviewed between September and March. Interviews consist of one session with a small panel of faculty members and medical students. On interview day, candidates also have the opportunity to meet with current students, tour the campus, and attend group information presentations. About one-third of interviewed candidates are accepted on a rolling basis. Alternate paths to admission are possible for students at schools that have special arrangements with EVMS. These schools are Old Dominion University, The College of William and Mary, Norfolk State University, Hampton University, and Hampden-Sydney College.

Admissions Requirements (Required)

MCAT scores, science GPA, non-science GPA, letters of recommendation, interview, extracurricular activities, exposure to medical profession.

Admissions Requirements (Optional)

state residency, essays/personal statement.

COSTS AND AID

Tuition	$18,975
Cost of books	$1,000
Fees	$2,966

Financial Aid

% students receiving aid	90

Emory University

Emory University School of Medicine

1440 Clifton Road NE, Suite 115, Atlanta, GA 30322-4510 • Admission: 404-727-5660 • Fax: 404-727-5456 • E-mail: medadmiss@emory.edu • Website: www.med.emory.edu

STUDENT BODY

Type	Private
Enrollment	454
% male/female	50/50
% underrepresented minorities	26
# applied (total/out)	3,393/3,041
# accepted (total/out)	319/255
# enrolled (total/out)	113/77
Average age	22

FACULTY

Total faculty (number)	1,716
% female	34
% minority	11
% part-time	7
# student/faculty ratio	4:1

ADMISSIONS

Average GPA and MCAT Scores

Overall GPA	3.8
MCAT Bio	11.1
MCAT Phys	11
MCAT Verbal	10.6
MCAT Essay	P

Application Information

Regular application	10/15
Regular notification	rolling
Are transfers accepted?	Yes
Admissions may be deferred?	Yes
Interview required?	Yes
Application fee	$80

Academics

The four-year medical curriculum begins with basic science courses combined with medical problem based learning, medical decision making, preclinical experiences, and patient doctor course work that provides outstanding preparation for the clinical experiences that make up their third and fourth years. Emory offers joint degree programs that allow qualified students to explore interdisciplinary aspects of medicine. Students may enter a combined MD/MPH program organized with the School of Public Health. In conjunction with the Graduate School of Arts and Sciences, medical students may earn the PhD degree concurrently with the MD.

BASIC SCIENCES: The basic science portion of the curriculum is comprehensive and engaging, with an instructional methodology that relies on lectures, small group problem based learning sessions, and labs. Introductory clinical experiences, discussions about the doctor/patient relationship, medical decision making, and the behavioral aspects of medicine are integrated with basic science concepts during the first and second years. First-year (ten months) courses are anatomy, embryology, biochemistry, neuroscience, physiology, cell biology, and histology and genetics. There is also an opportunity for students to take a clinical preceptorship or to engage in summer research projects within the ten-week block between their first and second years. The second year (ten months) includes courses in microbiology/immunology, pathology, human behavior/psychopathology, clincal methods, human values and ethics, pharmacology, pathophysiology, and medical problem solving.

CLINICAL TRAINING

The third and fourth years consist of twenty-one months of required clerkships; however, only nineteen months of actual course work are required for graduation because students can taje vacations or go on residency interviews for two of those months. Required clerkships include clinical gynecology/obstetrics (six weeks), clinical medicine (twelve weeks during junior year taught with radiology and four weeks senior year taught with advanced clinical medicine), clinical pediatrics (six weeks), clinical psychiatry (six weeks), clinical radiology (two weeks), clinical surgery (eight weeks with a clinical anesthesiology component), clinical family medicine (four weeks), clinical neurology (four weeks), clinical medical ethics and professionalism stressed throughout the currriculum, emergency medicine (four weeks), surgery selectives, and elective courses offered in a wide variety of areas. These clerkships take place within the wide scope of Emory-owned hospitals, facilities, and affiliated institutions such as Emory University Hospital, Emory Crawford Long Hospital, Grady Memorial Hospital, Children's Health Care of Atlanta at Egleston, Atlanta Veterans' Administration Medical Center, the Georgia Cancer Center, the Rollins School of Public Health, the Centers for Disease Control (CDC), and the Emory Clinic and offer a diverse patient community and clinical diagnosis.

Students

Students at Emory are encouraged to find time to pursue outside interests while balancing their school schedules.

STUDENT LIFE

Students have access to the organizations, events, and facilities of both the medical and undergraduate schools. As a release from studying, students use the modern and comprehensive athletic center. Students also participate in intramural sports. Medical students organize community service projects and participate in local and national medical student organizations, which serve to integrate students into the greater community and often provide them with additional clinical exposure. Atlanta is an excellent city for students as it is affordable and offers many cultural, recreational, and entertainment opportunities. While many students choose to live off campus because apartments and houses are plentiful and affordable, many students also choose to live in the new Clairmont Campus residential community. Located within walking distance to the main campus, the residential community includes modern luxury apartments, recreational areas, a student center, dining facilities, and much more. In addition, Georgia's climate is conducive to many outdoor recreational amenities since it offers both urban and rural opportunities year-round.

GRADUATES

Graduates and undergraduates intermingle at the dining facilities, athletic center, and campus wide activities.

Admissions

REQUIREMENTS

In addition to the traditional requirements of one year each of biology, chemistry, physics, and organic chemistry, Emory also requires six semester hours of English and eighteen semester hours of humanities and behavioral/social science course work. The MCAT is required. The best set of scores is typically weighed most heavily for applicants who have retaken the exam. Emory operates a rolling admissions process, making it beneficial to submit MCAT scores and application material early in the summer.

SUGGESTIONS

In addition to required courses, genetics and biochemistry are both strongly recommended. It is also important that students have patient contact in a clinical setting and show interests outside of medicine. Research experiences, volunteerism, and evidence of professionalism are also highly valued.

PROCESS

All AMCAS applicants are sent a supplemental application, of which approximately 750 candidates are invited to interview between October and February. Emory conducts group interviews that involve three applicants and two faculty members and a current medical student. An additional one-on-one interview is conducted with a faculty member. On interview day, candidates meet the dean of admissions, tour the campus and affiliated clinical locations, and meet Emory medical students and faculty. Following the interview, accepted students are notified on a monthly basis. Students placed on the alternate list are encouraged to submit new information to update their files.

Admissions Requirements (Required)

MCAT scores, science GPA, non-science GPA, letters of recommendation, interview, essays/personal statement, extracurricular activities, exposure to medical profession, Emory supplemental application.

Admissions Requirements (Optional)

state residency.

Overlap Schools

Duke University, Johns Hopkins University, Medical College of Georgia, University of Pennsylvania, Vanderbilt University, Washington University, Yale University.

COSTS AND AID

Tuition	$32,576
Cost of books	$492
Fees	$492

Financial Aid

% students receiving aid	86
Average grant	$20,281
Average loan	$29,617
Average debt	$102,977

Finch University of Health Sciences

Chicago Medical School

Office of Admissions, 3333 Green Bay Road, North Chicago, IL 60064 • Admission: 847-578-3204 • Fax: 847-578-3284 • E-mail: admissions@finchcms.edu • Website: www.finchcms.edu

STUDENT BODY

Type	Private
Enrollment	738
% male/female	64/36
% underrepresented minorities	8
# applied (total/out)	7,687/6,735
# accepted (total/out)	505/409
# enrolled (total/out)	193/157
Average age	24

FACULTY

Total faculty (number)	674
% female	27
% part-time	44
# student/faculty ratio	1:1

ADMISSIONS

Average GPA and MCAT Scores

Overall GPA	3.4
MCAT Bio	10.36
MCAT Phys	10.13
MCAT Verbal	9.08
MCAT Essay	P

Application Information

Regular application	11/15
Regular notification	10/15
Early application	6/1-8/1
Early notification	10/1
Are transfers accepted?	Yes
Admissions may be deferred?	Yes
Interview required?	Yes
Application fee	$90

Academics

Although most students earn an MD in four years, they can make arrangements to extend the first two years into three. A few students each year enter joint MD/MS or MS/PhD programs in the following fields: anatomy, biochemistry, cell biology, immunology, microbiology, molecular and cell sciences, neuroscience, pathology, physiology, and pharmacology. A joint degree program leading to an MS in the fields of clinical immunology or pathology is also offered. Grades of A through F are used to evaluate medical students, with the exception of some electives for which grades of pass and fail are used.

BASIC SCIENCES: First-year required courses are genetics, biostatistics/epidemiology, molecular cell biology, medical ethics, anatomy, embryology, histology, physiology, biochemistry, neuroscience, and introduction to clinical medicine. Courses are taught using primarily a lecture/lab format, and students are in class for about twenty-three hours per week. Second-year courses are clinical neuroscience, pathology, introduction to clinical medicine, microbiology, pharmacology, electives, and preventive medicine. Tutoring is available to students on an as-needed basis. Classes are held in a modern building reserved for basic science instruction, research, and administration. Students also spend time in the learning resource center, which houses acadenic resources that include the Boxer University Library. The library contains 92,966 volumes, 1,100 current subscriptions, a complete audiovisual center, and three computer labs with Internet access, databases, academic software programs, and computer-based exams. Students must pass the USMLE Step 1 to progress to year three.

CLINICAL TRAINING

Required third-year clerkships include medicine core (two weeks), medicine (eight weeks), surgery (eight weeks), pediatrics (six weeks), obstetrics/gynecology (six weeks), psychiatry (six weeks), ambulatory care (three weeks), family medicine (four weeks), emergency medicine (four weeks), and neurology (three weeks). The fourth year is reserved for electives (eighteen weeks), internal selectives (fourteen weeks), and a subinternship in medicine (four weeks). There is a great deal of flexibility in terms of fulfilling elective requirements. However, no more than half of elective credits may be earned in a single field. Clinical training takes place at Cook County Hospital, Hines Veterans' Affairs Medical Center, Illinois Masonic Medical Center, Lutheran General Hospital, Mount Sinai Hospital (469 beds), North Chicago Veterans' Affairs Medical Center, Norwalk Hospital (in Norwalk, Connecticut), Swedish Covenant Hospital (340 beds), Christ Hospital, and Elgin Mental Health Center.

Students

Underrepresented minorities—mostly African American students—account for about 8 percent of the student body. Of the class entering in 2001, 19 percent were in-state residents. The average age was twenty-four, with a range of nineteen to thirty-six. The entering class size in 2001 was 193.

STUDENT LIFE

Most first- and second-year students live in the vicinity of campus and drive to school. Often, third- and fourth-year students choose to live in Chicago because the city is relatively close to clinical training sites via public transportation. Finch does not offer university-owned housing. Chicago is one of the largest and most culturally rich cities in the country; students can find a wide variety of entertainment, museums, theaters, restaurants, nightlife, indoor and outdoor athletic activities, and spectator sporting events. Students have a voice in school administrative affairs through the University Student Council and through participation on various boards and committees. The Chicago Medical School has chapters of most national medical student associations and has special interest clubs and organizations based on recreational activities, professional interests, and ethnic and social backgrounds.

GRADUATES

Of the 2001 graduating class, the most popular specialty choices were internal medicine (25 percent), family practice (11 percent), surgery (7 percent), transitional (12 percent), emergency medicine (8 percent), obstetrics/gynecology (6 percent), and pediatrics (9 percent).

Admissions

REQUIREMENTS

One year of biology, chemistry, organic chemistry, and physics (all with labs) are required. The MCAT is required and must be no more than three years old at time of matriculation. The most recent set of scores are used for people who have retaken the exam.

SUGGESTIONS

In addition to requirements, courses in math, social sciences, English, and the arts are recommended. A solid preparation in science, accompanied by a broad background in the liberal arts, is recommended. The Admissions Committee also places strong emphasis on other nonacademic factors such as an applicant's motivation, character, personality, experience, and achievements.

PROCESS

All AMCAS applicants receive secondary applications. Typically, about 5 percent of applicants are interviewed. Interviews take place from October through May and consist of two sessions with faculty, administrators, and/or medical students. Notification of acceptance begins in November and is an ongoing process until the class is filled. Candidates awaiting a decision may submit supplemental information about course work, activities, or new MCAT scores.

Admissions Requirements (Required)

MCAT scores, science GPA, non-science GPA, letters of recommendation, interview, exposure to medical profession, 1 year with lab (biology, physics, chemistry, organic chemistry).

Admissions Requirements (Optional)

state residency, essays/personal statement, extracurricular activities.

Overlap Schools

Loyola University Chicago, Rush Medical College of Rush University, University of Chicago.

COSTS AND AID

Tuition	$35,673
Cost of books	$2,073
Fees	$120

Financial Aid

Average debt	$195,000

Florida State University

College of Medicine

College of Medicine, Florida State University, Tallahassee, FL 32306-4300• Admission: 850-644-7904 • Fax: 850-644-9399 • E-mail: MedAdmissions@med.fsu.edu • Website: http://med.fsu.edu/

STUDENT BODY

Type	Public
Enrollment	115
% male/female	61/39
% underrepresented minorities	38
# applied (total/out)	272/5
# accepted (total/out)	57/1
# enrolled (total)	46
Average age	23

FACULTY

Total faculty (number)	194
% female	26
% minority	13
% part-time	64
# student/faculty ratio	1:1

ADMISSIONS

Average GPA and MCAT Scores

Overall GPA	3.6
MCAT Bio	9.4
MCAT Phys	8.9
MCAT Verbal	8.3
MCAT Essay	0

Application Information

Regular application	12/8
Regular notification	4/15
Early application	8/1
Early notification	9/3
Are transfers accepted?	No
Admissions may be deferred?	Yes
Interview required?	Yes

Academics

The FSU College of Medicine is truly a twenty-first century medical school. Created in June of 2000 by the Florida legislature, it is the first new medical school the country has seen in a generation. As such, it is charting a new course for medical education.

BASIC SCIENCES: The basic science component of the training program takes place on the FSU campus and is integrated into the culture and value system of the liberal arts university. The curriculum is based on a bio-psychosocial foundation that balances biomedicine, medical humanities, and social sciences. The emphasis will be on ambulatory care settings such as physician clinics, HMOs, and chronic care facilities in rural, urban, and suburban areas. Because the FSU medical school will partner with existing medical facilities and practitioners throughout the state rather than operate as a teaching hospital, students will have the opportunity to learn on the front lines of our health care system. Community campuses are being developed in Tallahassee, Pensacola, and Orlando and are planned for Jacksonville, Sarasota, and Ft. Myers in partnership with local hospitals and practices. Nonprofit community corporations in each location will provide community representation and input into the medical education program. A campus dean chairs each community corporation, which is also responsible for community education, fund-raising, and advocacy on issues related to medical education.

Students

The Florida State University College of Medicine carefully selects students who are academically outstanding and are committed to the college's mission of service to Florida's medically underserved populations. FSU medical students come from all over Florida and are culturally diverse. Many come from small towns and rural areas, but the state's major metropolitan areas are also well represented. A number of students are older than average for medical school and bring a broad range of professional and life experiences, while others come straight out of undergraduate programs. Most are active in student organizations, community service projects and medical outreach programs.

STUDENT LIFE

In partnership with Florida communities, the FSU College of Medicine is creating a new model of medical education and research that uses interdisciplinary teams and emerging technologies. Building upon the FSU program in medical sciences—a first-year medical school program begun in 1971—the college's educational program is designed to produce compassionate physicians who will practice patient-centered medicine and who are prepared to practice in a rapidly changing health care environment. FSU trains the physicians of tomorrow in such a way that they will become lifelong learners equipped to teach themselves what they need to know in an era of tremendous innovation in knowledge management and information technology.

Admissions

REQUIREMENTS

The College of Medicine is searching for students who have demonstrated through their lifestyle a commitment of service to others. The college encourages applications from traditional students, nontraditional students, and students from rural, inner city, or other medically underserved areas of the State of Florida. FSU College of Medicine is an Early Start Program. Classes begin June 1. Students apply through the AMCAS. Some are invited to submit a secondary application. The school accepts approximately fifty students each year. An applicant should be a legal resident of Florida. An applicant should have completed the required prerequisite courses: English, biology, chemistry, organic chemistry, physics, biochemistry. An applicant should meet academic standards predictive of success in medical school—academic grade point average and MCAT score. An applicant's MCAT score should be dated no more than three years prior to the beginning of the year of the application cycle. A bachelor's degree is required by the time of matriculation to medical school. If an applicant is currently enrolled in a degree program, the program must be completed and final transcripts provided to the College of Medicine Admissions Office prior to the beginning of classes in May. Non-U.S. citizens must possess a permanent resident visa. Undergraduate degree credit that has been granted to the student on the basis of the College-Level Examination Program (CLEP), an International Baccalaureate program (IB), an Advanced Placement program (AP), or participation in dual enrollment will be accepted provided the credit appears on the official transcript.

PROCESS

All applicants must apply online at the AAMC's website at www.aamc.org/students/start.htm. Applicants may begin to certify and submit their AMCAS application beginning June 1. The deadline for submitting applications to AMCAS is December 1. The regular admission process begins in September and continues until late March. Interviews are scheduled between September and March and applicants are discussed and voted upon by the Admissions Committee. Typically about 150 applicants are interviewed each admission cycle. Those candidates who are accepted outright are sent acceptance letters. All others are held until the final meeting at the end of March, when all candidates for whom a decision has not been made are reviewed again and high alternate, alternate, and hold lists are compiled. Letters are sent informing applicants of their status. The Admissions Committee is especially interested in students who have demonstrated through their lifestyle consistent motivation for service to others. Students from under represented minority groups, students from rural and inner city backgrounds, women, and non-traditional students are of particular interest to the Committee. Consideration for students participating in early admission occurs in August before the beginning of the regular admission cycle which begins in September. Students from Florida State University, University of West Florida, and Florida A&M University who have GPA's above a 3.5 and MCAT scores above 25 are eligible to apply for Early Admission. Students selected for interview are interviewed by two members of the Admissions Committee. Candidates who are selected through early admission are admitted to the College of Medicine. Students who are not chosen for early decision interviews or who are not selected in early decision are notified (and AMCAS informed) that their files have been placed in the general application pool and will be reconsidered during the regular admission cycle.

Admissions Requirements (Required)

MCAT scores, science GPA, non-science GPA, letters of recommendation, interview, state residency, essays/personal statement, extracurricular activities, exposure to medical profession.

Overlap Schools

University of Florida, University of Miami, University of South Florida.

COSTS AND AID

In-state tuition	$13,349
Room and board	$6,274
Cost of books	$7,601
Fees	$1,400

Financial Aid

% students receiving aid	90
Average grant	$1,200
Average loan	$22,962

The George Washington University
School of Medicine and Health Sciences

Office of Admissions, 2300 I Street, NW, Ross Hall, 716 Washington, DC 20037 • Admission: 202-994-3506 • Fax: 202-994-1753 • E-mail: medadmit@gwu.edu • Website: www.gwumc.edu/edu/admis

STUDENT BODY

Type	Private
Enrollment	675
% male/female	55/45
% underrepresented minorities	12
# applied (total/out)	7,418/7,378
# accepted (total/out)	402/397
# enrolled (total/out)	167/166
Average age	24

FACULTY

Total faculty (number)	2,354
% part-time	75
# student/faculty ratio	1:1

ADMISSIONS

Average GPA and MCAT Scores

Overall GPA	3.5
MCAT Bio	9.81
MCAT Phys	9.34
MCAT Verbal	9.27
MCAT Essay	P

Application Information

Regular application	12/1
Regular notification	Rolling
Early application	6/1-8/1
Early notification	10/1
Are transfers accepted?	Yes
Admissions may be deferred?	Yes
Interview required?	Yes
Application fee	$90

Academics

The George Washington University School of Medicine and Health Sciences is located in the heart of Washington, DC. Part of the vision of The George Washington University Medical Center is to be a preeminent academic health institution dedicated to improving the health and well-being of our local community, our country, and beyond. The Medical Center works to achieve this goal through its commitment to excellence and its innovative education and research approach.

BASIC SCIENCES: The George Washington University MD curriculum prepares well trained physicians to complete residencies in primary care or specialized areas of concentration. Our medical school also stresses education through cooperation and collaboration rather than competition and encourages students to work with colleagues and coworkers. Courses in anatomy, biochemistry, immunology, microbiology, neurobiology, and physiology constitute the first year classroom study of the cell and organ systems. The second-year curriculum focuses on abnormal human biology through courses in pathology, pharmacology, and an interdisciplinary, organ system introduction to clinical medicine course.

CLINICAL TRAINING

The School of Medicine curriculum contains a unique practice of medicine (POM) course. This revolutionary course spans all four years and allows students to begin clinical training during their first years while they learn the traditional basic sciences. During POM, students learn about the doctor-patient relationship, essential communication skills, basic clinical assessment skills of interviewing and physical examination, professionalism, ethics, and many issues of the medicine-society interface. The GW Clinical Learning and Simulation Skills (CLASS) Center is housed on the sixth floor of the GW Hospital. Dedicated to education and research, the center features cutting edge technology in one of the most innovative settings in the nation. It is in this setting that students gain the comprehensive clinical exposure, feedback, and evaluation that they need to become technically adept doctors and humane caregivers. This hands-on experience proves invaluable in preparation for the USMLE Step II.

Students

The fall 2003 entering class hailed from thirty-six different states and ninety-two different undergraduate institutions. Forty percent of incoming students were nonscience majors and 14 percent held various graduate degrees. Last year's entering class ranged from twenty to forty-three years old.

STUDENT LIFE

The campus is nestled in the Foggy Bottom area of Washington, DC, and is within walking distance of the White House, The World Bank, the Department of State, the National Academy of Sciences, The John F. Kennedy Center for the Performing Arts, and many other governmental, historical, and cultural landmarks. The campus is also accessible by subway; the Foggy Bottom/GWU metro stop sits immediately outside Ross Hall—the hub for the medical school. Students who are interested in athletics can participate in activities such as intramural sports and aerobics classes. The brand new, state-of-the-art Health and Wellness Center, also two blocks from Ross Hall, is an 188,000 square foot facility that hosts a wide variety of fitness and instructional classes; walk-in recreation; and sport club, intramural, and wellness programs and services.

GRADUATES

The GW SMHS maintains a national reputation for placing qualified graduates into quality residency programs. Many students choose to continue their post-graduate work at GW so they can be a part of our new state-of-the-art hospital. In fact, twenty members of the graduating class of 2003 remained at GW to complete their residencies. Some of the other institutions at which members of the class of 2003 were placed include Brown University, Yale University, Mt. Sinai Hospital, UCLA Medical Center, and the Mayo Clinic. The following list indicates some of the specialties and/or programs that were most highly matched by GW graduates: medicine, surgery, pediatrics, emergency medicine, anesthesia, radiology, orthopedics, family practice, obstetrics/gynecology, and psychiatry.

Admissions

REQUIREMENTS

Applicants must have completed ninety semester hours at an accredited U.S. or Canadian college or university prior to matriculation. Applicants must be U.S. or Canadian citizens or U.S. permanent residents. Applicants must have completed six credits of English as well as six credits of lecture and two credits of lab in each of the following sciences at an accredited U.S. or Canadian college or university prior to matriculation: biology (botany or biochemistry courses do not fulfill this requirement), general chemistry, organic chemistry, and physics. Last year's entering class averaged an overall GPA of 3.53 and a science GPA of 3.44. The MCAT is required and should be no more than three years old from the year of medical school matriculation.

SUGGESTIONS

Because interviews and acceptances are offered as applications and because letters of recommendation are received and processed, we strongly urge you to complete your file as early as possible.

PROCESS

Once the Admissions Office receives an AMCAS application, the secondary application is sent to the applicant. GW requires three letters of recommendation (two from science faculty and one from someone who is familiar with your personal traits), a pre-medical adviser letter, or committee advisory letter. It will take four to five weeks to process your application and letters of recommendation after we have received them. The application process is very competitive since there are over 9,000 candidates applying for approximately 160 seats. Interviews and acceptances are offered on a rolling admissions basis (as applications and letters of recommendation are received and processed). The AMCAS application is due December 1, the GW Secondary Application is due January 1 (postmarked), and letters of recommendation are due January 1 (postmarked). Each year the Admissions Office offers interviews via written notification to approximately 1,000 selected applicants. These interviews are blind (the interviewers do not read the applicant's file prior to the interview). Although we offer interviews only from September to March, we may offer acceptances into classes anytime after the initial interview up until the day before classes start in August. We will mail all final decisions to applicants.

Admissions Requirements (Required)

MCAT scores, science GPA, non-science GPA, letters of recommendation, interview, essays/personal statement, extracurricular activities, exposure to medical profession.

Admissions Requirements (Optional)

state residency.

COSTS AND AID

Tuition	$39,005
Cost of books	$8,310
Fees	$280

Financial Aid

% students receiving aid	80
Average grant	$8,300
Average loan	$35,050
Average debt	$127,400

Georgetown University
School of Medicine

Office of Admissions, 3900 Reservoir Road, NW, Washington, DC 20007 • Admission: 202-687-1154 •
E-mail: medicaladmissions@georgetown.edu • Website: www.dml.georgetown.edu/schmed

STUDENT BODY

Type	Private
Enrollment	699
% male/female	47/53
% underrepresented minorities	26
# applied (total)	7,547
# accepted (total)	1,146

ADMISSIONS

Average GPA and MCAT Scores

Overall GPA	3.6

Application Information

Regular application	11/1
Regular notification	10/15
Are transfers accepted?	Yes
Interview required?	Yes
Application fee	$90

Academics

While most students earn the MD through a four-year program, some extend their studies over five years to take part in yearlong research projects between their second and third years. Others participate in combined degree programs that lead to the MD and the PhD in cell biology, biochemistry, molecular biology, microbiology and immunology, pathology, pharmacology, physiology, biophysics, neuroscience, tumor biology, bioethics, or other disciplines. The proximity of the National Institute of Health facilitates student involvement in important research projects either during summers or yearlong periods. Grades of honors, high pass, pass, and fail are used to evaluate medical students in all their classes except their elective courses; grades of satisfactory or unsatisfactory are used to evaluate those. Passing Step 1 of the USMLE is a requirement for promotion to year three, and passing Step 2 is a graduation requirement.

BASIC SCIENCES: The first two years focus on basic science instruction, but also incorporate interdisciplinary courses; principles of patient care; problem-based learning modules; and ethical, social, economic, and religious aspects of health care. Lectures, labs, and small group discussions are the teaching methods used, with students in scheduled sessions for about twenty-two hours per week. A student-run note-taking service assists with the volume of material presented during the first two years. First-year courses are medical data and reasoning, gross anatomy, microscopic anatomy, biochemistry, biostatistics and epidemiology, embryology, endocrinology, ambulatory care, neurobiology, physiology, introduction to health care, and introduction to the patient. Second-year courses are pharmacology, pathology, microbiology and immunology; clinical problem solving, physical diagnosis, psychiatry, and ambulatory care. Also during the second year, two hours each week are reserved for elective courses, some of which may be taken at Georgetown's main campus. Basic science instruction takes place in several science/research buildings that are part of the medical center complex. The Dahlgren Memorial Library houses over 177,000 volumes and subscribes to over 1,800 journals. Within the library is the Biomedical Academic Computer Center (BACC) with a variety of audiovisual, computer, and educational services. Students have access to the Internet, email, medical software, and databases.

CLINICAL TRAINING

Third-year required rotations are medicine (twelve weeks), surgery (twelve weeks), pediatrics (six weeks), obstetrics/gynecology (six weeks), neurology (four weeks), psychiatry (four weeks), and family medicine (four weeks). Fourth-year requirements are medicine (six weeks), surgery (six weeks), emergency medicine (four weeks), selectives (twenty weeks), and electives (twenty weeks). Medical students train at the Georgetown University Hospital (407 beds) and at nine other affiliated federal and community hospitals in the Washington, DC, metropolitan area. Electives may be taken abroad through Georgetown's international programs or through individually arranged clerkships. Examples of possible training sites are the Bahamas, Colombia, and the Dominican Republic.

Students

Virtually all states are represented in the student body. Among students in the 1997 entering class, 49 percent majored in biological sciences, 24 percent in physical sciences, 18 percent in social sciences, and 9 percent in various humanities or other disciplines. Approximately 11 percent of students are underrepresented minorities. Class size is 165.

STUDENT LIFE

Although Georgetown is a Jesuit institution, the school encourages students of all denominations to express their spirituality. In addition to religious organizations, student groups focused on professional interests and community service are active. Outside of the classroom, students socialize at organized events and in common areas such as the new Student Lounge in the Preclinical Science Building. Medical students take advantage of the Yates Memorial Field House, which is conveniently located behind the library. It has a pool, track, squash and tennis courts, a fitness center, and other athletic facilities. At the Leavey Center, students enjoy performing arts, shops, services, and restaurants. Washington, DC, has vast cultural and recreational opportunities. Admission to the Smithsonian museums is free to Georgetown medical students. Other perks include the wide variety of restaurants, the running and biking trails at Rock Creek Park, and the accessibility of other city attractions via the metro system. A free shuttle between the Medical Center and nearby metro stations is provided. Baltimore, Philadelphia, and New York are easily reached by train, and the Appalachian Mountains and the Atlantic coast are within a few hours drive. All students live off campus, within walking or biking distance of campus.

GRADUATES

Graduates are successful in securing residency positions at institutions throughout the country.

Admissions

REQUIREMENTS

Prerequisites are one year each of chemistry, organic chemistry, biology, physics, english, and math. One semester of biochemistry may be substituted for one semester of organic chemistry. Science courses should include associated labs. The MCAT is required, and scores should be from within the past three years. All sets of scores are considered.

SUGGESTIONS

Recommended courses include biochemistry, computer science, cellular physiology, genetics, embryology, biostatistics, quantitative analysis, and physical chemistry. Applications are not processed until MCAT scores are received. Thus, the April MCAT is preferable to the August exam. The Committee on Admissions considers character, maturity, and motivation along with academic achievement.

PROCESS

All AMCAS applicants are sent secondary applications. About 15 percent of returning secondaries are interviewed between September and May. Interviews consist of one session with a faculty member or senior medical student. Also on interview day, candidates have lunch with medical students, tour the campus, and attend informational meetings. About 20 percent of interviewees are accepted. Notification begins after October 15 and continues on a rolling basis. A few highly qualified Georgetown undergraduates may be accepted to the School of Medicine during their sophomore year without MCAT scores.

Admissions Requirements (Required)

MCAT scores, science GPA, non-science GPA, letters of recommendation, interview, state residency, extracurricular activities, exposure to medical profession.

Admissions Requirements (Optional)

essays/personal statement.

COSTS AND AID

Tuition	$33,670
Room and board	$10,560
Cost of books	$1,759
Fees	$1,330

Financial Aid

% students receiving aid	75

HARVARD UNIVERSITY
HARVARD MEDICAL SCHOOL

OFFICE OF ADMISSIONS, 210 GORDON HALL, 25 SHATTUCK STREET, BOSTON, MA 02115 • ADMISSION: 617-432-1550 • FAX: 617-432-3307 • E-MAIL: ADMISSIONS_OFFICE@HMS.HARVARD.EDU • WEBSITE: WWW.HMS.HARVARD.EDU

STUDENT BODY

Type	Private
Enrollment	735
% male/female	51/49
% underrepresented minorities	20
# applied (total)	5,396
# accepted (total)	250
# enrolled (total)	165
Average age	23

FACULTY

Total faculty (number)	9,352

ADMISSIONS

Average GPA and MCAT Scores

Overall GPA	3.8
MCAT Bio	11.6
MCAT Phys	11.8
MCAT Verbal	10.6
MCAT Essay	Q

Application Information

Regular application	10/15
Regular notification	7/3
Are transfers accepted?	No
Admissions may be deferred?	Yes
Interview required?	Yes
Application fee	$75

Academics

Two distinct programs are available at Harvard—the New Pathway and the Health Science and Technology (HST) Program. All entering students are assigned to one of five societies, organizational units used both to structure academic activities and to facilitate interaction among students and between faculty and students. Joint degree opportunities include the MSTP; other MS/PhD programs designed in collaboration with science and nonscience graduate departments; the combined MD/MPH; and an MD/MPP with the Kennedy School of Government. More than half of all students take at least five years to complete their education to take full advantage of scholastic and research opportunities, some of which are off campus and even overseas.

BASIC SCIENCES: Students in the first year of the New Pathway concentrate on biomedical and social sciences. The year is divided into the following six sections: the human body, chemistry and biology of the cell, physiology, pharmacology, genetics, and immunology. Students are also introduced to clinical medicine in their first year. Year two has the following four segments: human nervous system, pathology, human systems I, and human systems II. Concepts of behavioral and community health are integrated into the basic science studies. During the first two years, lectures are scheduled for only one hour out of each day. Lectures are enhanced with tutorials and labs, but most learning takes place outside of the classroom environment. Students are responsible for addressing specific clinical challenges through independent and small group research and analysis. During the fall semester of year one, HST students take the following: functional human anatomy, human pathology, cellular and molecular immunology, molecular biology, and genetics. During spring semester students take endocrinology; cardiovascular, renal, and respiratory pathophysiology; and research. Students take electives in social and clinical medicine throughout the year. Students take neuroscience, microbial pathogenesis, research, reproductive biology, and gastroenterology during the first semester of the second year and pharmacology, clinical medicine, hematology, and psychopathology during the second semester of the second year. HST students complete a thesis as part of their requirements. Computers that are loaded with curriculum-related software and linked with online data sources are considered an important information management tool and are accessible in the Educational Center, the library, and the residence hall. The Countway Library of Medicine has one of the largest biomedical collections in the country. Grades of satisfactory and unsatisfactory are used to evaluate medical students for all courses. Passing Step 1 of the USMLE is required prior to graduation.

CLINICAL TRAINING

Patient contact begins in year one, when students learn to take histories and become familiar with basic elements of the physical exam. Formal clinical instruction begins in year three, when HST and New Pathway students join for required clerkships. These are medicine (four months), neurology (one month), women's and children's health (three months), psychiatry (one month), radiology (one month), and surgery (three months). Throughout years three and four, students take part in ongoing, part-time primary care training. Year four is made up of mostly electives, which can be clinical and/or research oriented. Elective credit may be earned from several departments at Harvard University or from MIT. Clinical training takes place at Harvard-affiliated hospitals, which include Beth Israel Medical Center, Brigham and Women's Hospital, Cambridge Hospital, The Center for Blood Research, The Children's Hospital, The Dana-Farber Cancer Institute,

DVA Medical Center, Harvard Pilgrim Health Care, Joslin Diabetes Center, Judge Baker Children's Center, Massachusetts Eye and Ear, Massachusetts General, Massachusetts Mental Health Center, McLean Hospital, Mount Auburn Hospital, Schepens Eye Research, and Spaulding Rehab Hospital. Evaluation of student performance in clinical settings uses a high honors, honors, satisfactory, and unsatisfactory scale. Narrative comments accompany these marks. In addition to formal rotations, students can gain experience in clinical environments through volunteer activities such as the Urban Health Project, which provides preventive and curative care to community health centers and underserved populations. Students must pass the USMLE Step 2 to graduate.

Students

About 75 percent of students were science majors in college. About 20 percent of the members of a typical class are underrepresented minorities, and about 30 percent took significant time off between college and medical school. Students are from all around the country. Class size is 165, of which thirty are HST participants and 135 are New Pathway participants.

STUDENT LIFE

The compact class schedule allows students to take part in activities of the medical school, the greater university, and the city of Boston. About 50 percent of medical students live in Vanderbilt Hall, a renovated building adjacent to the medical school. Married students live either off campus or in university-owned apartments. Students are active in organizations focused on topics that include support for various minority groups, abortion rights, and soccer.

GRADUATES

Approximately half of each graduating class remains at Harvard for their residencies. The University of California at San Francisco also appears to be a popular choice. Of the 1997 graduating class, the most common specialty choices were internal medicine (34 percent), pediatrics (13 percent), general surgery (9 percent), and orthopedic surgery (7 percent).

Admissions

REQUIREMENTS

Requirements include one year of biology with lab, physics with lab, expository writing, and college-level calculus. Two years of chemistry are required, both of which should involve laboratory experience. For New Pathway applicants, at least sixteen additional credit hours in nonscience courses are required. For HST applicants, calculus through differential equations and calculus-based physics courses are required. The quality of all applicants' undergraduate institutions are assessed when we evaluate their GPAs. The MCAT is required, and all scores are considered.

SUGGESTIONS

Unlike many schools with rolling admissions, decisions at Harvard are made after all interviews are complete. Thus, applicants who submit scores from the August MCAT are not penalized. There is no preference for particular undergraduate majors but demonstration of academic excellence is expected. In addition, most successful applicants have impressive professional, volunteer, community service, or other extracurricular achievements.

PROCESS

In 1998 Harvard began to participate in AMCAS. In the past, about 14 percent of applicants were interviewed. Interviews take place from September through January and consist of two one-hour sessions each with a member of the Admissions Committee. Decisions are made in late February, and all applicants are notified at once. A wait-list is established at that time, but usually only a few candidates are ultimately accepted from that list.

Admissions Requirements (Required)

MCAT scores, science GPA, non-science GPA, letters of recommendation, interview, essays/personal statement, extracurricular activities.

Admissions Requirements (Optional)

state residency, exposure to medical profession.

COSTS AND AID

Tuition	$32,000
Room and board	$10,050
Cost of books	$1,204
Fees	$2,776

Financial Aid

% students receiving aid	70
Average grant	$20,930
Average loan	$22,625
Average debt	$91,000

HOWARD UNIVERSITY
COLLEGE OF MEDICINE

ADMISSIONS OFFICE, 520 WEST STREET, NW, WASHINGTON, DC 20059 • ADMISSION: 202-806-6270 • FAX: 202-806-7934 • E-MAIL: BHLOGAN@ACCESS.HOWARD.EDU • WEBSITE: WWW.MED.HOWARD.EDU

STUDENT BODY

Type	Private
Enrollment	454
% male/female	51/49
% underrepresented minorities	59
# applied (total/out)	5,505/5,460
# accepted (total/out)	9/9
# enrolled (out)	20

ADMISSIONS

Application Information

Regular application	12/15
Regular notification	10/15 until filled
Are transfers accepted?	No
Admissions may be deferred?	Yes
Interview required?	Yes
Application fee	$45

Academics

Although most students earn their MD in four years, some are given permission to complete requirements over a five-year period. The College of Medicine and the Graduate School of Arts and Sciences offer a joint MS/PhD program. The departments that award the PhD are the following: anatomy, biochemistry, biology, chemistry, genetics, microbiology, pharmacology, and physiology.

BASIC SCIENCES: Basic sciences are presented primarily in a lecture/lab format. Students are in scheduled classes from twenty-five to thirty hours per week. First-year courses are anatomy; biochemistry; psychiatry; histology; microbiology; immunology; physiology; neuroscience; introduction to patient care, in which students visit clinics and interact with physicians; and introduction to psychodynamic thinking, which discusses healthy and pathological mental mechanisms. Second-year courses are microbiology, immunology, pathology, genetics, physiology, physical diagnosis, pathophysiology, pharmacology, psychopathology, and epidemiology. Grades of honors, satisfactory, and unsatisfactory are used to evaluate medical students; academic support services such as workshops, tutorials, and summer sessions are available to them. The USMLE Step 1 is required for promotion to year three. Instruction takes place in the Seeley G. Mudd Building, which features auditoriums, laboratories, and audiovisual and computer-assisted study areas. The Health Sciences Library has 260,000 volumes and journals, video equipment, and a computer linkage with the National Library of Medicine.

CLINICAL TRAINING

Patient contact begins in the first year, in introduction to patient care. Throughout medical school, students have the opportunity to gain clinical experience by volunteering and participating in community outreach programs. Others gain research experience through work at NIH or other prominent institutions. Formal clinical training begins in year three (or year four for students in a five-year course of study), with the following required clerkships: medicine (twelve weeks), surgery (eight weeks), obstetrics/gynecology (eight weeks), pediatrics (eight weeks), psychiatry (six weeks), rehabilitation and neurological disease (four weeks), and family practice (four weeks). For two hours per week, during one semester, third-year students attend lectures on ethical and legal issues in health care. Senior year requirements are medicine (four weeks) and surgery (four weeks). In addition, students take from twenty to twenty-four weeks of electives in four-week blocks. Grades of honors, satisfactory, and unsatisfactory are used to evaluate clinical performance, and the USMLE Step 2 is required for graduation. Clinical training takes place largely at Howard University Hospital (300 beds). Other sites used are Howard University Cancer Center, Center for Sickle Cell Disease, Walter Reed Army and National Naval Medical Centers, DC General Hospital, St. Elizabeth's Hospital, VA Medical Center, Providence Hospital, Greater Southeast Community Hospital, Prince George's Hospital Center, Washington Hospital Center, and National Rehabilitation Hospital.

Students

About 60 percent of the students are African American, and about 10 percent are from African or Caribbean countries. An average of thirty states and several foreign countries are usually represented. From 10 percent to 20 percent of the students in each entering class attended Howard for undergraduate, pre-medical studies. About 20 percent of entrants are considered nontraditional, having taken time off between college and medical school and participated in some sort of post-baccalaureate, pre-medical program. Class size is 110.

STUDENT LIFE

Medical students enjoy both an active campus life and involvement in the greater community. They may participate in Howard University activities, such as its radio and television stations, intramural athletic teams and events, conferences, and social or special interest clubs. Washington, DC, is a center for cultural, academic, recreational, and obviously, political activities. In addition to being an international city, DC has a strong local, predominantly African American community that is highly diverse. The College of Medicine is part of Howard's downtown campus, which is metro accessible and conveniently located near lively neighborhoods and interesting parts of the city such as the White House and Smithsonian Museums. Housing for graduate students is available in modern, university-owned apartments. However, most students live off campus and either walk or take public transportation to school.

GRADUATES

About 25 percent of African American physicians practicing in the United States are Howard Alumni. Howard graduates secure post-graduate positions at institutions all over the country. Significant numbers enter one of the sixteen residency programs at Howard University Hospital or at DC General Hospital, where they are also supervised by Howard faculty.

Admissions

REQUIREMENTS

Requirements are biology (eight hours), chemistry (eight hours), organic chemistry (eight hours), physics (eight hours), college math (six hours), and English (six hours). The MCAT is required and must have been taken within the past three years

SUGGESTIONS

Beyond required courses, cell biology, biochemistry, and developmental biology or embryology are recommended. Students who have taken time off after college should show evidence of recent course work because it's helpful to their applications. The Admissions Committee values activities that demonstrate an interest in working with underserved communities.

PROCESS

All AMCAS applicants receive secondary applications, of which about 10 percent are interviewed by faculty or administrators. The remaining applicants are rejected, advised to retake the MCAT, or put in a hold category and considered for interview later in the year. Of those interviewed, 70 percent are accepted on a rolling basis, and the rest are either rejected or wait-listed. Wait-listed candidates may submit supplementary information and grades. A limited number of high school seniors are accepted into a combined BS/MD program organized with Howard's College of Arts and Sciences that allows students to earn both degrees in a six-year period. Through an Early Entrance Program, a few students nationwide may be admitted to the College of Medicine after their college junior year.

Admissions Requirements (Required)

MCAT scores, science GPA, non-science GPA, letters of recommendation, interview, state residency, extracurricular activities, exposure to medical profession.

Admissions Requirements (Optional)

essays/personal statement.

COSTS AND AID

Tuition	$15,980
Fees	$903

Financial Aid

% students receiving aid	85
Average debt	$63,000

INDIANA UNIVERSITY
SCHOOL OF MEDICINE

FESLER HALL 213, 1120 SOUTH DRIVE, INDIANAPOLIS, IN 46202 • ADMISSION: 317-274-3772 • FAX: 317-278-0211 • E-MAIL: INMEDADM@IUPUI.EDU • WEBSITE: WWW.MEDICINE.IU.EDU/

STUDENT BODY

Type	Public
Enrollment	1,128
% male/female	53/47
% underrepresented minorities	7
# applied (total/out)	2,029/1,424
# accepted (total/out)	378/70
# enrolled (total/out)	280/13

FACULTY

Total faculty (number)	1,116
% female	48
% minority	6

ADMISSIONS

Average GPA and MCAT Scores

Overall GPA	3.7
MCAT Bio	10.2
MCAT Phys	9.9
MCAT Verbal	10
MCAT Essay	P

Application Information

Regular application	12/15
Regular notification	10/15
Early application	6/1-8/1
Early notification	10/1
Are transfers accepted?	Yes
Admissions may be deferred?	Yes
Interview required?	Yes
Application fee	$45

Admissions Requirements

Academics

The School of Medicine in Indianapolis is part of the Indiana University (IU) Medical Center, which includes schools of Nursing, Dentistry, and Allied Health Sciences. The medical center complex occupies eighty-five acres and is situated one mile from downtown Indianapolis. In conjunction with the University Graduate School, The School of Medicine offers selected students an opportunity to pursue the MS or PhD degrees along with an MD. Through this program, degrees may be earned in anatomy, biochemistry, biophysics, genetics, neurobiology, microbiology, pathology, pharmacology, physiology, toxicology, and in humanities and social studies disciplines.

BASIC SCIENCES: First-year students select one of the following nine locations for their preclinical studies: IU Bloomington, IU Indianapolis, Lafayette Center at Purdue, University of Notre Dame, Ball State University, Indiana State University, University of Evansville, Indiana University Northwest, and Fort Wayne Center for Medical Education at Purdue. While the curriculum is essentially the same at each campus, the methods of instruction may differ, with some programs relying more or less on case-based learning. At all schools, the core basic science courses are complemented by early clinical correlations. Throughout the first two years, scheduled classes account for twenty-six to twenty-eight hours per week. At the Indianapolis campus, 80 percent of class time is devoted to lectures and labs, and 20 percent is used for small group discussions. First-year courses are anatomy, histology, biochemistry, physiology, microbiology, evidence-based medicine, immunology, patient/doctor relationship, and concepts of health and disease (teaches students how to apply basic science concepts to clinical problems). Second-year courses are biostatistics, pharmacology, pathology, clinical medicine, medical genetics, and neurobiology. With the exception of clinical medicine, during which students join medical teams in hospitals, second-year courses use lectures and labs as instructional techniques. The medical center offers all modern learning tools, including computers and audiovisual equipment. The Ruth Lilly Medical Library (200,000 volumes) is located in the Medical Research Building in Indianapolis and serves the Schools of Medicine and Nursing. All campuses have affiliated library systems, and all libraries are electronically linked. The libraries have access to 400 databases and online informational resources. Grades of honors, high pass, pass, and fail are used to evaluate medical students. Passing the USMLE Step 1 is a requirement for promotion to year three.

CLINICAL TRAINING

All students spend their third year at the Medical Center in Indianapolis, rotating through eleven hospitals in the Indianapolis area. The patient population is drawn from both urban and rural areas. Year three is largely composed of required rotations that include the following: medicine (twelve weeks), surgery (eight weeks), pediatrics (eight weeks), obstetrics/gynecology (six weeks), psychiatry (six weeks), and family medicine (four weeks). Required fourth-year clerkships are surgical subspecialties (eight weeks), neurology (four weeks), and radiology (four weeks). Year four is mostly dedicated to elective study, which may be pursued off campus, around the country, or overseas. Grades of honors, high pass, pass, and fail are used to evaluate clinical performance; this is complemented by narratives. Honors students generally take part in departmental research activities. Passing the USMLE Step 2 is a requirement for graduation.

Students

Typically, 95 percent of an entering class are Indiana residents. About 6 percent are underrepresented minorities, most of whom are African Americans. Approximately 5 percent of students are over thirty at the time of matriculation.

STUDENT LIFE

Students are given a voice in school administration and curriculum development through an elected student government. Although student life differs from one campus to the next, medical students generally benefit from the social and cultural offerings of a large university system. Some students live on campus in residence halls or apartments, other students live off campus. Medical students have access to all campus recreational facilities and events.

GRADUATES

Slightly less than half of the 2000 graduating class entered residency programs in Indiana. Other popular locations for post-graduate training were Michigan, Ohio, and Illinois. The most common specialty choices were family medicine (16 percent of the class), internal medicine (11 percent), pediatrics (11 percent), surgery (10 percent), radiology (9 percent), obstetrics/gynecology (8 percent), and emergency medicine (7 percent), and anesthesia (7 percent). About 60 percent of graduates entered fields considered to be primary care.

Admissions

REQUIREMENTS

Required undergraduate courses are one year each of the following: chemistry, organic chemistry, biology, and physics. All courses must include labs. Beyond GPA, the quality of an applicant's undergraduate course load is considered rather than the quantity of extra course hours. The MCAT is required and must be no more than four years old. If an applicant has retaken the MCAT, the most recent scores are considered.

SUGGESTIONS

Undergraduate course work in social sciences and humanities is important. It is beneficial for applicants who have taken significant time off after college to show evidence of recent course work. The April, rather than August MCAT, is strongly recommended. Out-of-state applicants with strong qualifications and some sort of ties to the state are likely to be admitted. The school aims to admit candidates who are likely to choose careers in primary care.

PROCESS

Almost all Indiana residents receive a secondary application, and about 93 percent of those returning secondaries are interviewed. Among out-of-state applicants, only highly qualified candidates are sent secondary applications, and about 10 percent are invited to interview. Interviews take place on Wednesdays, from September through February, and are scheduled in the order in which completed applications are received. Interviews consist of a one-hour session with a team of faculty members. Notification occurs on a monthly basis, beginning in October. Applicants are either accepted, rejected, or deferred and reevaluated later in the year. In the spring, a wait-list is established. Wait-listed candidates may submit supplementary material if it adds new information to their files.

(Required)

MCAT scores, science GPA, non-science GPA, letters of recommendation, interview, state residency, essays/personal statement, extracurricular activities, exposure to medical profession.

Overlap Schools

Michigan State University, University of Illinois at Chicago, Washington University.

COSTS AND AID

Financial Aid

% students receiving aid	84
Average grant	$45,000
Average loan	$22,000
Average debt	$85,000

Jefferson Medical College of Thomas Jefferson University
Jefferson Medical College

Associate Dean for Admissions, 1015 Walnut Street, Philadelphia, PA 19107 • Admission: 215-955-6983 • Fax: 215-955-5151 • E-mail: JMC.admissions@jefferson.edu • Website: www.tju.edu

STUDENT BODY

Type	Private
Enrollment	901
% male/female	55/45
% underrepresented minorities	6
# applied (total/out)	7,500/6,310
# accepted (total/out)	228/252
# enrolled (total/out)	223/117
Average age	25

FACULTY

Total faculty (number)	2,982
% female	18
% minority	3
% part-time	1

ADMISSIONS

Average GPA and MCAT Scores

Overall GPA	3.5

Application Information

Regular application	11/15
Regular notification	rolling
Early application	6/1-8/1
Early notification	10/1
Are transfers accepted?	Yes
Admissions may be deferred?	Yes
Interview required?	Yes
Application fee	$75

Academics

Along with basic science and clinical training, Jefferson's curriculum emphasizes the social and public health issues related to medicine. The academic year is organized around blocks, with the January block devoted to these nontraditional topics. Students with solid science backgrounds may pursue an MD and a PhD in one of the departments of the College of Graduate Studies. These include biochemistry, developmental biology, genetics, immunology, microbiology, molecular pharmacology, pathology, cell biology, and physiology. A joint MD/MBA degree is offered in conjunction with Widener University in Chester, Pennsylvania, as is a combined MD/MA in hospital administration. Pennsylvania State University and Jefferson Medical College allow students to pursue a combined BS/MD program, which grants both degrees in a six-year period. Jefferson has special arrangements with the University of Pennsylvania's, Bryn Mawr's, and Columbia University's post-baccalaureate programs through which highly qualified students may be admitted to Jefferson prior to completion of their pre-medical requirements. Upon arrival at Jefferson, all students are assigned a faculty adviser.

BASIC SCIENCES: Innovations in instructional techniques have reduced the time spent in lecture. To supplement lectures and labs, students participate in small group discussions. In the first year, block one begins in September and continues through December. Courses include biochemistry and molecular biology, anatomy, and the doctor in health and illness, a course that asks students to apply their developing scientific knowledge to patient problems and to learn fundamental skills in patient interaction, history-taking, examination, and diagnosis. During block two, which occurs entirely in January, first-year students focus on health policy, ethics, biostatistics, and genetics. Block three lasts from February through May and includes physiology, histology, and the doctor in health and illness. Block five lasts from May to June and is reserved for neuroscience. Block one of year two occurs in August and September and consists of pathology, microbiology, pharmacology and elective study. Block two of year two occurs in November and December and includes physical diagnosis and introduction to clinical medicine. The January block curriculum is nutrition, health of the public, law and medicine, physical diagnosis and elective study. The final block lasts from February through May and includes pathology, electives, clinical medicine and physical diagnosis. Grades are on a percentile scale, and the passing score is determined for each course. Preclinical studies take place in the central medical college building complex, which includes administrative offices, labs, lecture halls, common areas, and recreational facilities. The Samuel Parsons Scott Library includes 160,000 volumes, a Learning Resources Center and computer labs in addition to videos, slides, and supplemental learning materials. MEDLINE and other electronic data systems are available. The USMLE is required after completion of year two.

CLINICAL TRAINING

Patient contact officially begins in year one, with doctors in health and illness. There are also ongoing opportunities for medical students interested in volunteer clinical experience or clinical research through summer programs and part-time jobs. Formally, the clinical portion of the curriculum begins in year three with required rotations. These are family medicine (six weeks), general surgery (six weeks), internal medicine (twelve weeks), pediatrics (six weeks), psychiatry and human behavior (six weeks), and obstetrics/gynecology (six weeks). Phase II of clinical rotations are selectives in which students choose specialties within broadly defined categories. Twelve weeks are also designated as purely elective. Training sites include Albert Einstein Medical Center, Bryn Mawr Hospital (383 beds), Bryn Mawr Rehabilitation Hospital, Christiana Care Medical Center, DuPont Hospital for Children, Geisinger Medical Center (in Danville, Pennsylvania, providing rural exposure), Lankenau Hospital (475 beds), Latrobe Hospital (280 beds, family medicine), Magee Rehabilitation Hospital, Mercy Hospital/Pittsburgh, Wills Eye Hospital, and West Jersey Health System. The patients come from several states and represent extremely diverse populations. The USMLE Step 2 is required for graduation.

Students

About thirty states are represented by the students within a class, mostly those of the eastern part of the country. About 40 percent of the students are Pennsylvania state residents. Underrepresented minorities make up about 6 percent of each class, the majority of whom are African American. Class size is 228. Approximately 20 percent of each class is over twenty-five years of age upon matriculation. In recent years, about 10 percent of matriculates have held advanced degrees.

STUDENT LIFE

Student organizations range from the Jefferson Karate Club to the Asian Professional Society. Medical fraternities are relatively popular and sponsor activities such as intramural sports. Beyond campus, the city of Philadelphia provides ample recreational and cultural possibilities and New York is just over an hour away. On-campus housing options include residence halls and apartments of all sizes; housing is guaranteed to first-year students. Having a car is unnecessary because of Jefferson's central and urban location.

GRADUATES

More than half of Jefferson graduates enter residency programs at university-affiliated hospitals around the nation. Jefferson graduates do very well in the residency-matching program, both in primary care and in more specialized fields.

Admissions

REQUIREMENTS

Required course work is one year of biology with lab, chemistry with lab, organic chemistry with lab, and physics with lab. The MCAT is required and applicants' most recent scores are used, along with grades, to determine if they will be interviewed.

SUGGESTIONS

Applicants should demonstrate problem solving capability, success in a range of subjects, and some in-depth knowledge of one or a few subjects. Strong writing skills are also valued. Experience in a medical or research environment is important. State residents are given slight preference, as are children of alumni and applicants from programs that have special arrangements with Jefferson. Because the admissions process is rolling, applicants are advised to take the April MCAT and to submit all materials in a timely fashion.

PROCESS

All AMCAS applicants receive a secondary application. Interviews are conducted from September through March, and about 20 percent of the applicant pool is eventually interviewed. Interviews are approximately thirty to forty-five minutes long and are conducted by a member of the faculty or administration. About 50 percent of candidates who interview are accepted. Others are either rejected or wait-listed. When places become available later in the spring, wait-listed applicants will be notified and offered positions. Indicating interest in Jefferson may help the prospects of wait-listed candidates.

Admissions Requirements (Required)

MCAT scores, science GPA, letters of recommendation, interview, essays/personal statement, extracurricular activities, exposure to medical profession.

Admissions Requirements (Optional)

nonscience GPA, state residency.

COSTS AND AID

Tuition	$34,565
Room and board	$12,520
Cost of books	$4,207

JOHNS HOPKINS UNIVERSITY
SCHOOL OF MEDICINE

733 N. BROADWAY, SUITE G-49, BALTIMORE, MD 21205 • ADMISSION: 410-955-3182 •
WEBSITE: WWW.HOPKINSMEDICINE.ORG

STUDENT BODY

Type	Private
Enrollment	475
% male/female	55/45
% underrepresented minorities	13
# applied (total/out)	6,118/5,720
# accepted (total)	234
# enrolled (total/out)	119/101
Average age	22

ADMISSIONS

Average GPA and MCAT Scores

Overall GPA	3.8
MCAT Bio	11
MCAT Phys	12
MCAT Verbal	11
MCAT Essay	Q

Application Information

Regular application	10/15
Regular notification	10/31
Early application	7/1-8/15
Early notification	10/1
Are transfers accepted?	Yes
Admissions may be deferred?	Yes
Interview required?	Yes
Application fee	$75

Academics

In 1992 Johns Hopkins implemented a revised curriculum that introduced case-based learning, exposure to clinical settings during the first year, and a physicians and society (P & S) course, which integrates social, economic, and ethical perspectives into the four-year basic and clinical science curriculum. Studies leading to both an MD and a PhD or MA/MS in the following fields are possible: biochemistry, cellular and molecular biology, biological chemistry, biomedical engineering, biophysics, biophysics/molecular biophysics, cell biology and anatomy, cellular and molecular medicine, history of medicine, genetics, history of science, medicine and technology, human genetics and molecular biology, immunology, medical and biological illustration, neuroscience, pharmacology, molecular sciences, physiology, and public health. The combined MD/MPH is particularly popular, which is not surprising given the excellent reputation of the School of Public Health.

BASIC SCIENCES: The first year is organized into four blocks, all of which are ten weeks long. They are molecules and cells (block 1), anatomy and developmental biology (block 2), neuroscience and clinical epidemiology (block 3) and organ systems (block 4). The P & S course is a year long. Introduction to clinical medicine is also a year long; students spend two days a month working with a private physician. During the first year, classes end at 1: 00 P.M. four days a week, which gives students ample time to study. Many students take on research projects during the summer between their first and second years. Second-year students study pathology, pathophysiology, and pharmacology, which are offered as yearlong courses. All three courses are integrated and are organized around organ systems. Lectures, discussion , case-study, and labs are all important components of the basic science curriculum. With relatively few hours of scheduled lectures, students generally attend classes and do not rely on student note-taking cooperatives. Grades of honors, high pass, pass, and fail are used to evaluate students. Faculty members who are assigned to incoming students both advise them and monitor their progress. The Welch Medical Library and its three affiliated sites own over 380,000 books and subscribe to about 3,000 journals. It provides resources that support instruction such as extensive database and Internet tools. The USMLE is not used for grading or promotional purposes.

CLINICAL TRAINING

Facilities for clinical training include the Johns Hopkins Hospital complex, which is made up of numerous affiliates, is housed in thirty-seven buildings, and contains over 1,100 beds. In addition to serving the urban population of Baltimore and the surrounding areas, Johns Hopkins hospitals attract patients from around the country and the world. Students are exposed to patient care at renowned institutions such as the Wilmer Eye Institute, Adolf Meyer Center for Psychiatry, Brady Urological Institute, Clayton Heart Center, Meyerhoff Center for Digestive Diseases, the Children's Center, Oncology Center, Halsted Surgical Service, and Osler Medical Service. Students are also encouraged to pursue clinical experiences away from Hopkins, and a significant number do so overseas. With faculty input, students determine the order of their required clerkships and electives. Requirements are the following: medicine (nine weeks), surgery (nine weeks), pediatrics (nine weeks), opthalmology (one week), psychiatry (four weeks), neurology (four weeks), obstetrics/gynecology (six weeks), emergency medicine (four weeks), and ambulatory internal medicine (three weeks). Clinical instruction is generally carried out in small groups, and individual initiative is encouraged. Grades of honors, high pass, pass, and fail are used to evaluate medical students for both required and elective courses. Through its subsidiaries, The Johns Hopkins Health Systems provide statewide health care services to individuals and health plan participants. This integration into managed care operations, coupled with large federal research grants, suggests that the institution is financially stable.

Students

The diversity of the student body reflects the school's national reputation. A typical class has students from thirty-five different states and from seventy or more colleges. As is the case with most top schools, half of the entrants are women. Efforts are made to recruit ethnic minorities, and about 10 percent of the student body is African American. Class size is limited to 120.

STUDENT LIFE

Social life revolves around school for some students who tend to spend a great deal of time there. Other students, particularly those who are from the area or who have families, don't spend additional time at the medical school. Housing is available for single and married students in Reed Hall dorms adjacent to campus. However, most students choose to live in apartments off campus. The housing situation in Baltimore is good for students who are accustomed to New York or Washington, DC. The Housing Office assists students in their apartment searches. Recreational facilities, including a full-size gym, are free to medical students and are located next to Reed Hall. Several medical societies exist, including a Women's Medical Alumni Association, which provides support for female students and physicians. There is also a Student National Medical Association, which is active in both campus and community minority affairs.

GRADUATES

Graduates of Hopkins have their pick of residency programs, even students who graduate with GPAs that are at the lower end of their class. About 50 percent of graduates enter primary care specialties; 20 percent ultimately enter academic medicine or work in research.

Admissions

REQUIREMENTS

The following are required in addition to the typical requirements of one year each: biology, chemistry, organic chemistry, physics, one semester of calculus (high school is acceptable), and 24-semester-hours combined of humanities and social sciences. Johns Hopkins participates in AMCAS. Once the AMCAS application is received, the applicants are sent a password to access the online Hopkins supplement.

SUGGESTIONS

Hopkins is concerned with both the academic and personal records of applicants and notes that intellectual progress through college is important. Extracurricular activities need not be medically related, but should demonstrate humanistic values and perseverance.

PROCESS

About 14 percent of applicants are invited for interviews, which occur between September and March; about 25 percent of candidates who are interviewed are accepted on a rolling basis. Applicants are interviewed by Admissions Committee Members, and regional interviews may be arranged for applicants who live a distance away from Baltimore. At Admissions Committee meetings, decisions are made to admit, reject, or wait-list applicants. In April, wait-listed candidates are notified of their position on the list.

Admissions Requirements (Required)

MCAT scores, science GPA, non-science GPA, letters of recommendation, interview, essays/personal statement.

Admissions Requirements (Optional)

state residency, extracurricular activities, exposure to medical profession.

Overlap Schools

Columbia University, Cornell University, Duke University, Harvard University, Stanford University, Yale University.

COSTS AND AID

Tuition	$30,900
Room and board	$8,386
Cost of books	$1,515
Fees	$2,313

Financial Aid

% students receiving aid	80
Average grant	$15,576
Average loan	$20,000
Average debt	$82,896

Loma Linda University
School of Medicine

Loma Linda University School of Medicine, Loma Linda, CA 92350 • Admission: 909-558-1100 • Fax: 909-824-4146 • E-mail: webmaster@ccmail.llu.edu • Website: www.llu.edu/sm1.html

STUDENT BODY

Type	Private
Enrollment	661
% male/female	59/41
% underrepresented minorities	6
# applied (total/out)	3,990/2,083
# accepted (total/out)	10/9
# enrolled (out)	35

ADMISSIONS

Application Information

Regular application	11/1
Regular notification	12/15
Early application	6/1-8/1
Early notification	10/1
Are transfers accepted?	No
Admissions may be deferred?	Yes
Interview required?	No
Application fee	$55

Academics

Joint degree programs are offered to qualified students. Along with the MD, students may earn the MS or PhD degree in fields such as anatomy, biochemistry, genetics, immunology, microbiology, neuroscience, molecular biology, pharmacology, and physiology. Examinations and other methods of evaluation are given percentile scores, but the courses are graded pass or fail. Passing the USMLE Step 1 is a requirement for promotion to year three.

BASIC SCIENCES: Although Loma Linda's curriculum covers the basic science topics typical of most medical schools, its religious affiliation adds another dimension to it. In addition to learning about human biology, the nature of disease, and the appropriate treatment for disease, first- and second-year students participate in a course called whole person formation, which emphasizes biblical, ethical, and relational aspects of the practice of medicine. Patient contact occurs during the first year, in physical diagnosis and interviewing. Other first-year courses are biochemistry/molecular biology, cell structure and function, gross anatomy and embryology, human behavior, information sciences and population-based medicine, medical applications of the basic sciences, and neuroscience. Second-year courses are human behavior, microbiology, pathology, physiology, pathophysiology and applied physical diagnosis, and pharmacology. First- and second-year instruction takes place in facilities located on the Loma Linda campus and close to the medical center, giving students access to university resources and clinical activities. Computers are available in a comprehensive computer lab and are used for instruction and research.

CLINICAL TRAINING

Third-year required rotations are orientation to clinical medicine/preventive medicine (four weeks), family medicine (four weeks), obstetrics/gynecology (six weeks), internal medicine (twelve weeks), pediatrics (eight weeks), psychiatry (six weeks), and surgery (twelve weeks). Half of the fourth year is reserved entirely for basic science and clinical electives, and half of the year is split between required clerkships and selectives. Required clerkships are subinternship selectives (eight weeks, selected from family medicine, internal medicine, obstetrics/gynecology, pediatrics, and surgery), intensive care unit (four weeks), neurology (four weeks), ambulatory care (four weeks), and electives (sixteen to twenty-two weeks). Training takes place primarily at Loma Linda University Medical Center (500 beds), the Jerry L. Pettis Memorial Veterans' Hospital, Riverside General Hospital, and the White Memorial Medical Center in Los Angeles. Other affiliated sites are San Bernardino County General Hospital, Kaiser Foundation Hospital, and Glendale Adventist Medical Center.

Students

Most students are members of the Seventh-day Adventist Church. About 6 percent of all students are underrepresented minorities, most of whom are African American. Generally, there is a wide age range among incoming students and the average age is twenty-four. Class size is 189.

STUDENT LIFE

For the most part, student life revolves around the medical school and the immediate community. When in need of a change of scenery, Los Angeles and beautiful Southern California beaches are a short drive. Perhaps as a result of a shared religious background, students are cohesive. Alcohol is not a part of the social life, as it is prohibited in the Seventh-day Adventist Church. Beyond extracurricular activities sponsored by the medical school, students are welcome to participate in university-wide events and organizations. Medical students have access to the university's athletic facilities, and are active in intramural sports. Students live both on and off campus, and nearly all them own cars.

GRADUATES

Graduates are successful in securing residencies in all specialty fields. Loma Linda Medical Center is a popular destination for post-graduate training, offering about twenty-five residency programs.

Admissions

REQUIREMENTS

Prerequisite course work is eight semester hours each of biology, general chemistry, organic chemistry, and physics. Applicants should have met the English and religion requirements of their respective undergraduate institutions. The MCAT is required, and scores should be no more than three years old. For applicants who have retaken the exam, all sets of scores are considered.

SUGGESTIONS

Courses in the humanities and social sciences are recommended, and applicants are urged to take the April rather than August MCAT. Applicants who have taken time off after college should show evidence of recent course work because the school considers it important. Some involvement in health care delivery is valued by the Admissions Committee. Preference is given to qualified applicants who are members of the Seventh-day Adventist Church. However, others who demonstrate a commitment to Christian principles are also favorably considered.

PROCESS

All AMCAS applicants are sent secondary applications of which about 10 percent are invited to interview between November and March. Interviews consist of one- or two-hour-long sessions with faculty, students, and/or administrators. Lunch, a campus tour, and the opportunity to meet with current students are all provided on interview day. About 40 percent of interviewed candidates are accepted on a rolling basis; the remaining candidates are rejected or wait-listed. Wait-listed candidates may send updated transcripts.

Admissions Requirements (Required)

MCAT scores, science GPA, non-science GPA, letters of recommendation, state residency, extracurricular activities, exposure to medical profession.

Admissions Requirements (Optional)

interview, essays/personal statement.

COSTS AND AID

Tuition	$24,949

Louisiana State University
School of Medicine in New Orleans

Office of Admissions, 1901 Perdido Street, Box P3-4, New Orleans, LA 70112 • Admission: 504-568-6262 • Fax: 504-568-7701 • E-mail: ms-admissions@lsuhsc.edu • Website: www.medschool.lsuhsc.edu/admissions

STUDENT BODY

Type	Public
Enrollment	712
% male/female	59/41
% underrepresented minorities	15
# applied (total)	1,179
# accepted (total)	231
# enrolled (total)	170

ADMISSIONS

Average GPA and MCAT Scores

Overall GPA	3.5
MCAT Bio	9.5
MCAT Phys	9
MCAT Verbal	9
MCAT Essay	P

Application Information

Regular application	11/15
Regular notification	rolling
Early application	9/1
Early notification	10/1
Are transfers accepted?	Yes
Admissions may be deferred?	Yes
Interview required?	Yes

Academics

The course of instruction that leads to the MD extends over a four-year period. A revised first- and second-year curriculum was introduced in 1995, and changes in the third- and fourth-year clinical curriculum were implemented in 1996. An honors program that involves independent research challenges exceptional students and is thus open to students who excel during their first semester of medical school. A combined MS/PhD program is available for highly qualified students who are interested in research careers. Grades of honors, high pass, pass, and fail are used to evaluate medical students. All students are required to pass Step 1 of the USMLE following completion of year two; fourth-year students must pass Step 2 of the exam.

BASIC SCIENCES: Although most instruction uses a lecture format, small group discussions and tutorials are also part of the curriculum. First-year courses are anatomy, human prenatal development, cell biology and micro-anatomy, biochemistry, physiology, clinical correlation, neuroscience, medicine, medical ethics, introduction to clinical medicine, psychiatry, and social issues in medicine. Electives are offered in geriatrics, problem based learning, community service, and health promotion and wellness. Second-year courses are microbiology, immunology and parasitology, pathology, clinical pathology, pharmacology, and introduction to clinical medicine. Basic sciences are taught in a modern building that is part of the medical center complex. Important educational resources are maintained by the LSU Division of Learning Resources, which provides audiovisual and classroom services to the downtown campus of the LSU Health Sciences Center. The medical library in New Orleans has a total of about 188,000 volumes, nearly 4,000 audiovisual titles, and approximately 2,000 periodicals. The library is fully computerized and houses individual computers that are equipped with educational software programs.

CLINICAL TRAINING

The third and fourth years are primarily devoted to clinical rotations. Lectures, conferences, and small group discussions supplement the hands-on clinical training. Year three consists of eight-and-a-half days of ophthalmology course work in addition to rotations in medicine (twelve weeks), general surgery (eight weeks), otolaryngology (two weeks), urology (two weeks), pediatrics (eight weeks), family medicine (four weeks), obstetrics/gynecology (six weeks), and psychiatry (six weeks). The final year consists of thirty-six weeks divided into nine four-week blocks, which are ambulatory care, general medicine, neural sciences, special topics, and an acting internship. The special topics block includes nutrition, human sexuality, geriatrics, drug and alcohol abuse, office management, and financial planning. The remainder of the year may include electives either in basic or clinical sciences with four weeks of vacation time. Most training takes place at LSU-affiliated hospitals including Charity Hospital, which has a total of 2,200 beds. Elective requirements may be fulfilled at any accredited medical school or teaching hospital in the United States or Canada. With approval, electives may also be taken at foreign institutions.

Students

All students are Louisiana residents. Approximately 15 percent of students are underrepresented minorities, most of whom are African American. The average age of entering students is about twenty-three, and there are usually a number of students in their late twenties and thirties. Class size is 165.

STUDENT LIFE

Some medical students are active in the student government, which works closely with the faculty and the administration on a range of important issues. Others are involved in the student publication or in any number of professional clubs, honor societies, recreational groups, and community service projects. Extracurricular opportunities in New Orleans abound. The restaurants, music scene, historic and cultural sights, and annual festivals and events are world-renowned. Some students opt to live in the school's residence hall, which has its own student center. Others live off campus where housing is generally reasonably priced.

GRADUATES

The school assists and advises graduating students in and about obtaining suitable appointments in hospitals. LSU—New Orleans itself offers a comprehensive graduate medical education program in more than twenty specialty fields.

Admissions

REQUIREMENTS

Louisiana residency is a requirement. Prerequisite courses are eight semester hours each of biology, chemistry, organic chemistry, and physics, all with associated labs. Strength in both written and spoken English is required. The MCAT is required, and scores should be from within the past three years. The most recent set of scores is weighed most heavily for applicants who have retaken the exam.

SUGGESTIONS

A well-rounded undergraduate experience with course work in humanities, social sciences, math, and English is advised. Community service or medically related work or volunteer activities are valued.

PROCESS

All AMCAS applicants who are Louisiana residents are sent secondary applications, of which about 50 percent are invited to interview between October and April. The interview consists of two or three one-on-one sessions, each with a faculty member, student, or administrator. On interview day, candidates also have the opportunity to meet with students, tour the campus, and have lunch. About 60 percent of interviewed candidates are accepted on a rolling basis. Wait-listed candidates may send additional information to update their files.

Admissions Requirements (Required)

MCAT scores, science GPA, non-science GPA, letters of recommendation, interview, state residency, extracurricular activities, exposure to medical profession.

Admissions Requirements (Optional)

essays/personal statement.

LOUISIANA STATE UNIVERSITY
SCHOOL OF MEDICINE IN SHREVEPORT

ADMISSIONS OFFICE, 1501 KINGS HIGHWAY, PO BOX 33932, SHREVEPORT, LA 71130-3932 • ADMISSION: 318-675-5190 • FAX: 318-675-5244 • E-MAIL: SHVADM@LSUMC.EDU • WEBSITE: WWW.LSUMC.EDU

STUDENT BODY

Type	Public
Enrollment	391
% male/female	67/33
% underrepresented minorities	5
# applied (total/out)	1,046/272
# accepted (total)	27

ADMISSIONS

Application Information

Regular application	11/15
Regular notification	10/15 until filled
Early application	6/1-8/1
Early notification	10/1
Are transfers accepted?	Yes
Admissions may be deferred?	Yes
Interview required?	No
Application fee	$50

Academics

The first two years are devoted to basic medical sciences with orientation to clinical applications. The second two years are devoted to clinical training and are spent primarily in hospitals and clinics. In addition to the MD degree, advanced studies that lead to the MS/PhD are possible. The doctorate may be earned in anatomy, biochemistry, microbiology, pharmacology, and physiology. All medical students are encouraged to take advantage of the many research opportunities available during the summers and year-round. Special funds are provided for this purpose, and medical students who complete prescribed research activities are awarded diplomas with the special designation "Honors Research Participant." During summer terms, the school offers opportunities for rural, clinical electives. Grades of A through F are used to evaluate medical students in all courses except elective courses, which are evaluated with grades of pass and fail. Passing both steps of the USMLE is a graduation requirement.

BASIC SCIENCES: During the first year, students are in lectures, small group seminars, labs, or other scheduled sessions for about twenty-five hours per week. Courses are CPR, human anatomy, biometry, ethics, medical neuroscience, library science, family medicine and comprehensive care, radiology, introduction to computer-aided learning, medical genetics, histology, physiology and biophysics, psychiatry, biochemistry and molecular biology, and human embryology. The second year is increasingly clinically oriented. Students are in class or other scheduled sessions for about thirty-five hours per week. Courses are pathology, radiology, perspectives in medicine, psychiatry, family medicine and comprehensive care, microbiology, pharmacology, clinical neurology, clinical diagnosis, clinical pathology, and clinical-pathological conference. A note-taking service, organized by and for students, assists with learning and retaining material. Computer-assisted instruction is a critical component of the basic science education, and all entering students are required to own a computer.

CLINICAL TRAINING

An unusual, longitudinal clerkship called comprehensive care spans both the third and fourth years. In it, students work together and serve as the primary caregivers in a functioning clinic. Other third-year required rotations are medicine (eight weeks), surgery (four weeks), surgery subspecialties (three weeks), pediatrics (four weeks), obstetrics/gynecology (eight weeks), psychiatry (four weeks), and family medicine (eight weeks). A minimum of sixteen weeks during the fourth year are reserved for electives. Required clerkships are medicine (six weeks), surgery (three weeks), pediatrics (three weeks), and neuroscience (three weeks). Most training takes place at the LSU Hospital (650 beds), the Shreveport Veterans' Administration Hospital, and the Comprehensive Care Clinic.

Students

All students are Louisiana residents. About 5 percent of all students are underrepresented minorities. There is a wide age range among entering students and includes students in their late twenties and thirties. Class size is 100.

STUDENT LIFE

Outside of class, LSU offers medical students a rich campus life. The university offers more than sixty student organizations in addition to intramural sports, performing arts events, visiting speakers, and social activities. The University Center has dining facilities, a lounge, student activity rooms, and a bookstore, among other student services. Generally, it serves as a meeting place for students. The Health and Physical Education Building houses an indoor swimming pool; handball and racquetball courts; basketball; tennis, volleyball, and badminton courts; a dance studio; and fitness and weight training rooms. Shreveport is a historic southern city with a population of more than 370,000. Museums, art galleries, parks, gardens, restaurants, bars, and shopping areas are some of its many attractions. The cities of Baton Rouge and New Orleans are easily accessible. Houston, Memphis, Little Rock, and Jackson are also within driving distance. Most medical students live off campus.

GRADUATES

An increasing proportion of graduates are entering primary care fields. The majority of graduates return to Louisiana to practice.

Admissions

REQUIREMENTS

Admission to the School of Medicine is limited to Louisiana residents. Requirements are one year each of biology, chemistry, organic chemistry, physics, and English. All science courses must include laboratory work. The MCAT is required, and scores should be from within three years of application. The most recent set of scores is generally weighed most heavily for applicants who have retaken the exam.

SUGGESTIONS

Once prerequisites are fulfilled, perspective applicants are encouraged to pursue their own interests and to develop their own special talents in gaining a broad educational background. In making admissions decisions, the school assesses the motivation, intellectual ability, and preparation of all candidates. Applicants must show the potential to develope into mature, sensitive physicians who will inspire and deserve trust and confidence.

PROCESS

All AMCAS applicants who are Louisiana residents are sent secondary applications, of which about 30 percent are invited to interview between September and March. Interviews are given by members of the Admissions Committee, which is composed of medical school faculty from the basic and clinical sciences as well as physicians from the community at large. The interview is used to assess personal traits and also allows candidates to see the facilities and to meet current students. Approximately 90 percent of all interviewed candidates are accepted on a rolling basis. The remaining candidates are rejected or wait-listed.

Admissions Requirements (Required)

MCAT scores, science GPA, non-science GPA, letters of recommendation, state residency, extracurricular activities, exposure to medical profession.

Admissions Requirements (Optional)

interview, essays/personal statement.

COSTS AND AID

Out-of-state tuition	$7,900
Fees	$6,826

Financial Aid

% students receiving aid	81

LOYOLA UNIVERSITY CHICAGO

STRITCH SCHOOL OF MEDICINE

OFFICE OF ADMISSIONS, 2160 SOUTH FIRST AVENUE, MAYWOOD, IL 60153 • ADMISSION: 708-216-3229 •
E-MAIL: ADMISSIONS@LUMC.EDU • WEBSITE: WWW.MEDDEAN.LUMC.EDU

STUDENT BODY

Type	Private
Enrollment	539
% male/female	52/48
% underrepresented minorities	17
# applied (total/out)	3,547/2,842
# accepted (total/out)	343/225
# enrolled (total/out)	140/81
Average age	23

FACULTY

Total faculty (number)	1,317
% female	29
% minority	24
% part-time	52
# student/faculty ratio	2:1

ADMISSIONS

Average GPA and MCAT Scores

Overall GPA	3.6
MCAT Bio	10
MCAT Phys	9.7
MCAT Verbal	9.6
MCAT Essay	P

Application Information

Regular application	11/15
Regular notification	10/15
Are transfers accepted?	Yes
Admissions may be deferred?	Yes
Interview required?	Yes
Application fee	$60

Academics

Most students follow a four-year curriculum that leads to the MD degree. A dual degree MD/PhD program accepts up to three students each year. In this program, a doctoral degree may be earned in anatomy, biochemistry, cell biology, immunology, microbiology, molecular biology, neuroscience, pathology, pharmacology, or physiology. Evaluation of student performance uses honors, high pass, pass, and fail. Students must pass USMLE Step 1 and USMLE Step 2 to graduate.

BASIC SCIENCES: Stritch's curriculum relies on small group sessions and problem-based learning as much as it does on traditional lectures and labs. Students are in class or other scheduled sessions for approximately twenty-five hours per week discussing behavioral science and humanistic perspectives along with basic science concepts. First-year courses are host defense, molecular cell biology and genetics; structure of the human body; function of the human body; developmental human biology; and introduction to the practice of medicine I, a two-year continuum that begins with the medical interview and later covers the physical diagnosis, health promotion, medical ethics, health care finance, and legal issues in medicine. As part of the course, each student participates in special mentoring programs, participating on hospital rounds with a primary care physician and chaplain. Second-year courses are neuroscience, mechanisms of human disease, pharmacology and therapeutics, developmental human biology, and introduction to the practice of medicine II. During the second, third, and fourth years, medical humanities and ethics grand rounds take place. The Stritch facility includes classrooms of many different sizes to accommodate different instructional modalities, labs, video equipment, computer laboratories, lounges, study areas, and other spaces. The Health Sciences Library houses about 170,000 volumes and periodicals.

CLINICAL TRAINING

Required third-year rotations are family medicine (six weeks), internal medicine (twelve weeks), obstetrics/gynecology (six weeks), pediatrics (six weeks), psychiatry (six weeks), and surgery (twelve weeks). During the fourth year, requirements are neurology (four weeks), medical humanities (one week), subinternships (eight weeks), and twenty-six weeks of electives. Clinical facilities include the Hines Veterans' Affairs Hospital, Loyola University Hospital and Loyola Outpatient Center, Cardinal Bernardin Cancer Center, and a variety of community hospitals. Elective credits can be earned at other academic or clinical institutions.

Students

About half of Stritch's medical students are Illinois residents. Approximately one-quarter of all students took time off between college and medical school. Underrepresented minorities account for about 5 percent of the student body. Class size is 140.

STUDENT LIFE

At Loyola, there is a very strong sense of indentity among students in each class. Class officers, including social chairs, promote numerous group activities, including small study groups, class specific events, and all-school social events. To help promote the interaction among students of different classes, students are assigned to one of three communities. All students have a wardrobe locker and mailbox within the community and share study spaces, lounge areas, and kitchenettes. Students also get to know one another through the numerous registered student organizations, which include professional, academic, social, and religious based groups. Each organization has a faculty adviser, who in turn helps the student leaders and student members to direct their own organization. During the first two years, most preclinical courses end early enough to allow time students to focus on the introduction to the practice of medicine curiculum, self directed learning, and extracurricular pursuits. Many students use this time to volunteer for public clinics, homeless shelters, senior centers, hospital based pediatrics, school and reading programs, and to present educational health related topics at various local schools. On- and off-campus events and programs are also sponsored by the University Ministry. To help round out the physical well-being of the students, there is a 622,000-square-foot Health and Fitness Center adjacent to the medical school. The center features various cardiovascular equipment, a state-of-the-art aerobic/exercise studio, free weights and variable resistance equipment, basketball and volleyball courts, an aquatics area, an elevated running track, racquetball courts, and spa and massage services. Off-campus activities are plentiful, as Chicago is easily accessible from the medical center. All students live off-campus and most students live within the western suburbs of Chicago.

GRADUATES

Graduates are successful in securing residency positions nationwide in primary care and specialized fields. About 65 percent of graduates remain in the Midwest, 25 percent go to the Western United States, 5 percent to the East, and 5 percent to the South.

Admissions

REQUIREMENTS

Applicants must be U.S. citizens or hold a permanent resident visa. Prerequisites are one year each of biology, chemistry, organic chemistry, and physics, all with associated labs. One semester of biochemistry may be substituted for a semester of organic chemistry. The MCAT is required, and scores should be from within four years of anticipated entrance to medical school. The most recent set of scores is weighed most heavily for applicants who have retaken the exam.

SUGGESTIONS

Although state residents are given some preference, there are no positions reserved for them. Some recent course work is important for nontraditional applicants who have been out of school for a period of time. All students are advised to take the April MCAT so that the exam may be repeated in August if scores are not at the national average. Qualities that the school seeks in applicants are maturity, integrity, the ability to work with diverse populations, dedication to community service, and an awareness of the environment surrounding health care provision.

PROCESS

All applicants who meet minimum qualifications receive secondary applications, of which about 15 percent are interviewed between September and April. Interviews consist of two one-hour sessions each with a faculty member, administrator, or Student Committee on Admissions member. On interview day, candidates also have lunch with current medical students and tour the campus. About 55 percent of interviewed candidates are accepted on a rolling basis; the school begins to notify them in October. Candidates who are wait-listed or in a hold category may send additional information to update their files and indicate their interest in Loyola.

Admissions Requirements (Required)

MCAT scores, science GPA, non-science GPA, letters of recommendation, interview, essays/personal statement, extracurricular activities, exposure to medical profession, baccalaureate degree.

Admissions Requirements (Optional)

state residency.

COSTS AND AID

Tuition	$32,800
Cost of books	$4,148
Fees	$490

Financial Aid

% students receiving aid	92
Average grant	$13,694
Average loan	$37,674
Average debt	$143,582

Marshall University

Marshall University Joan C. Edwards School of Medicine

Office of Admissions, 1600 Medical Center Drive, Huntington, WV 25701 • Admission: 800-544-8514 •
Fax: 304-691-1744 • E-mail: warren@marshall.edu • Website: www.musom.marshall.edu

STUDENT BODY

Type	Public
Enrollment	199
% male/female	56/44
% underrepresented minorities	11
# applied (total/out)	709/502
# accepted (total/out)	96/11
# enrolled (total/out)	53/6
Average age	24

FACULTY

Total faculty (number)	216
% female	30
% minority	14
% part-time	15
# student/faculty ratio	1:1

ADMISSIONS

Average GPA and MCAT Scores

Overall GPA	3.5
MCAT Bio	8.9
MCAT Phys	8.7
MCAT Verbal	8.9
MCAT Essay	0

Application Information

Regular application	12/1
Regular notification	10/15
Are transfers accepted?	Yes
Admissions may be deferred?	Yes
Interview required?	Yes
Application fee	$50

Academics

The academic curriculum is influenced by the needs of rural providers and the priorities of the community and the state; it is geared toward achieving greater retention of West Virginia trained physicians in underserved communities. Although most students complete a four-year course of study that leads to the MD degree, qualified students who are interested in research may concurrently pursue an MS or PhD in biomedical sciences. Grades of A through F are used to evaluate student performance. Passing Step 1 of the USMLE is required for promotion to year three, and passing Step 2 is a requirement for graduation.

BASIC SCIENCES: Basic science is taught primarily by using a lecture/lab format, although some time is spent in small group discussions and clinical settings. Students are in scheduled sessions for about thirty hours per week. First-year courses are gross anatomy and embryology, microanatomy and ultrastructure, neuroscience, biochemistry, physiology, behavioral medicine, human sexuality, medical cell and molecular biology, medical ethics, and introduction to patient care. Second-year courses are pharmacology, microbiology, pathology, physical diagnosis, introduction to clinical medicine, introduction to patient care, community medicine, psychopathology, genetics, medical ethics, and immunology. The medical education building where basic sciences are taught is self-contained; it has a library and other educational resources.

CLINICAL TRAINING

Third-year students participate in the following required third-year clerkships: medicine (eight weeks), obstetrics/gynecology (eight weeks), psychiatry (eight weeks), surgery (eight weeks), pediatrics (eight weeks), family practice (eight weeks), and clinical orientation (one week). During the fourth year, required rotations are medicine (four weeks), surgery (four weeks), and senior symposium (one week). A full twenty-seven weeks are reserved for elective study; during the third and fourth years, a total of three months must be taken in rural areas. Affiliated clinical teaching sites are numerous and include Cabell Huntington Hospital (363 beds), St. Mary's Hospital (440 beds), and the Veterans' Affairs Medical Center (90 beds).

Students

Among entering students in a recent class, 23 percent graduated from Marshall's undergraduate college. A total of twenty-six other undergraduate institutions were represented in the class. Seventy-one percent majored in biology, 10 percent in chemistry, and the remainder in other disciplines. The average age of incoming students is about twenty-six, with an age range of twenty to fifty. About 11 percent of all medical students are minorities, most of whom are Asian. Class size is fifty.

STUDENT LIFE

The small class size at Marshall contributes to a supportive and friendly environment. Students are active in chapters of national organizations and in groups such as the Christian Medical and Dental Society, American Medical Women's Association, and the American Medical Student Association. Huntington is a small city that offers to students the amenities and resources they need and yet provides them with easy access to rural areas. For more recreational and cultural opportunities, the larger cities of Pittsburgh and Cincinnati are each about a four-hour drive away. Medical students have access to the athletic and recreational facilities of the main university, and take part in university-wide events. University-administered housing options include university dormitories and units suitable for families. Off-campus housing is also affordable and readily available.

GRADUATES

Two-thirds of graduates enter primary care fields, which include internal medicine, family medicine, pediatrics, and obstetrics/gynecology. Graduates are successful in securing residencies inside and outside of West Virginia.

Admissions

REQUIREMENTS

Prerequisites are eight semester hours each of biology, chemistry, organic chemistry, and physics. Six semester hours each of social or behavioral science and English are also required. Applicants' GPAs are evaluated with consideration given to their academic institutions and the rigor of courses they took. The MCAT is required, and scores must be from within three years of matriculation. The latest set of scores is weighed most heavily for applicants who have retaken the exam.

SUGGESTIONS

As a state school, Marshall gives preference to West Virginia residents. A maximum of six positions in each year's class are reserved for residents of states that border West Virginia and for candidates with strong ties to the state. The April MCAT is recommended over the August MCAT. In addition to academic records, Marshall considers important personal qualities such as judgment, responsibility, altruism, integrity, and sensitivity. Strong communication skills are also valued.

PROCESS

All West Virginia and bordering state AMCAS applicants receive secondary applications. Almost all West Virginia residents are interviewed, while only about 7 percent of out-of-state applicants are interviewed. Interviews take place between September and February and consist of two thirty-minute sessions with members of the Admissions Committee. Acceptances are issued on a rolling basis. Wait-listed candidates may send information to update their files as the year progresses.

Admissions Requirements (Required)

MCAT scores, science GPA, non-science GPA, letters of recommendation, interview, extracurricular activities.

Admissions Requirements (Optional)

state residency, essays/personal statement, exposure to medical profession.

Overlap Schools

West Virginia University.

COSTS AND AID

In-state tuition	$12,190
Out-of-state tuition	$32,020
Cost of books	$2,000
Fees	$514

Financial Aid

% students receiving aid	94
Average grant	$6,370
Average loan	$31,109
Average debt	$108,464

Mayo Medical School

Mayo Medical School, 200 First Street, SW, Rochester, MN 55905 • Admission: 507-284-3671 • Fax: 507-284-2634 • E-mail: medschooladmissions@mayo.edu • Website: www.mayo.edu/mms

STUDENT BODY

Type	Private
Enrollment	170
% male/female	50/50
% underrepresented minorities	15
# applied (total/out)	2,417/2,134
# accepted (total/out)	77/43
# enrolled (total/out)	44/26
Average age	23

FACULTY

Total faculty (number)	475
# student/faculty ratio	1:1

ADMISSIONS

Average GPA and MCAT Scores

Overall GPA	3.8
MCAT Bio	11.12
MCAT Phys	10.4
MCAT Verbal	9.86
MCAT Essay	Q

Application Information

Regular application	11/1
Regular notification	Rolling
Early application	8/1
Early notification	10/1
Are transfers accepted?	Yes
Admissions may be deferred?	Yes
Interview required?	Yes
Application fee	$75

Academics

Each year, thirty-four students begin a four-year curriculum that leads to the MD degree, and six students pursue a joint MS/PhD program in connection with the Mayo Graduate School. Through this program, a PhD may be obtained in biochemistry, biomedical engineering, immunology, cell biology and genetics, molecular neuroscience, molecular pharmacology and experimental therapeutics, tumor biology, and virology and gene therapy. Two students with DDS degrees are admitted each year for training toward careers in oral and maxillofacial surgery. Courses are grouped into units, which are the organ, the patient, physician and society, the scientific foundation of medical practice, the clinical experience, and the research quarter. All students are required to write a research paper while at Mayo, and 80 percent of these works are published. Grades of honors, high pass, pass, marginal pass, and fail are used to evaluate student performance. Taking the USMLE Steps 1 and 2 are requirements for graduation. Three weeks (prior to the third year) are devoted to preparation for the clinical clerkships in the third and fourth years. Radiology course, ECG course, survival skills workshop, and a breaking bad news lecture.

BASIC SCIENCES: During the first five months of school, students take molecular biology and genetics, pathology and cell biology, immunology, and anatomy. The remainder of year one is organized around the following organ and physiological systems: cutaneous system, respiratory system, hematopoietic system, neuroscience, growth and development, renal system, cardiovascular system, digestive system, endocrine system, allergy, and musculoskeletal system. Patient contact begins in year one, in introduction to the patient and continuity of care. Small groups and problem-based learning enhance the lecture/lab format and account for about one-third of the twenty-eight hours per week of scheduled class time. The second year is split between clinical and basic science education. The first block of year two includes microbiology and infectious disease, psychopathology, and ENT, SAR/sexual medicine, and bioethics. In the next block, second-year students attend lectures and seminars and rotate through several clinical departments evaluating patients under the guidance of a preceptor. Clinical rotations are dermatology (three weeks), family medicine (two weeks), musculoskeletal medicine and rehabilitation (three weeks), medicine (nine weeks), surgery (three weeks), pediatrics (six weeks), and clinical skills aquisition (three weeks). Tutoring and a wide variety of advising services are available to students, and a formal system is in place to identify and assist students who may be experiencing academic difficulties. Scheduled classes and labs take place on the Mayo campus, while independent and computer-aided instruction is offered in the Learning Resource Center located in the Mitchell Student Center. The Mayo Medical Library houses 353,000 volumes and subscribes to 4,300 journals.

CLINICAL TRAINING

The third year is divided into four quarters. The research quarter is a thirteen-week experience in which students participate in a biomedical research project and produce a related scientific paper. Three quarters are spent in clinical rotations: family medicine (two weeks), internal medicine (six weeks), neurology (three weeks), surgery (six weeks), pediatrics (six weeks), obstetrics/gynecology (six weeks), and psychiatry (four weeks), and a three-week elective at Mayo. Training takes place at the Mayo Clinic, Rochester Methodist, and Saint Mary's Hospitals, which together have 2,000 beds.

Students

The student body consists of about 170 students from more than forty states. About 15 percent of a typical class are underrepresented minorities. Class size is forty-two.

STUDENT LIFE

The small class size facilitates cohesion among students. Mitchell Student Center, in addition to housing the Learning Resource Center, provides an area for relaxation and communal study. Students are involved in medically related organizations and societies, community service projects, and groups organized around athletic and cultural interests. Students also play an important role in the school's administration by participating in governing committees. Rochester's population is 80,000; students can enjoy concerts, theaters, museums, golf courses, parks, and other recreational opportunities. All students live off campus.

GRADUATES

In a class of recent graduates, 36 percent of them entered residencies in primary care. Specialties selected by more than one student were as follows: family medicine (5 percent), internal medicine (8 percent), obstetrics/gynecology (5 percent), pediatrics (18 percent), anesthesiology (8 percent), dermatology (5 percent), diagnostic radiology (13 percent), and radiation oncology (5 percent).

Admissions

REQUIREMENTS

Prerequisites are biology with lab (one year), chemistry with lab (one year), organic chemistry with lab (one year), physics with lab (one year), and biochemistry (one course). The MCAT is required and must be no more than three years old.

SUGGESTIONS

Mayo is interested in undergraduate course work that demonstrates both aptitude in science and breadth of knowledge in social science and humanities. Substantial experience in community service and leadership are also very important considerations.

PROCESS

No supplementary application is required. About 15 percent of AMCAS applicants are asked to submit letters of recommendation and participate in a telephone interview. About 65 percent of those screened applicants are invited to an on-campus interview. The interviews are scheduled between September and March. Applicants have two thirty to forty-five minute interviews with faculty, students, community members, or administrators. About 30 percent of interviewed applicants are accepted on a rolling basis. Other applicants are rejected or wait-listed. Additional material from wait-listed candidates is not encouraged.

Admissions Requirements (Required)

MCAT scores, science GPA, non-science GPA, letters of recommendation, interview, essays/personal statement, extracurricular activities, exposure to medical profession.

Admissions Requirements (Optional)

state residency.

COSTS AND AID

Tuition	$22,500
Cost of books	$1,792

Financial Aid

% students receiving aid	100
Average grant	$16,987
Average loan	$18,865
Average debt	$60,823

McGill University
McGill University, Faculty of Medicine

3655 Promenade Sir William Osler #633, Montreal, QC H3G 1Y6 • Admission: 514-398-3517 • Fax: 514-398-4631 • E-mail: admissions.med@mcgill.ca • Website: www.medicine.mcgill.ca/admissions/

STUDENT BODY

Type	Public
# applied (total/out)	980/400
# accepted (total/out)	223/32
# enrolled (total/out)	160/32

ADMISSIONS

Average GPA and MCAT Scores

Overall GPA	3.7

Application Information

Regular application	11/15
Regular notification	3/31
Early notification	1/15
Are transfers accepted?	No
Admissions may be deferred?	Yes
Interview required?	Yes
Application fee	$60

Academics

The curriculum recognizes the importance of a solid database and a multidisciplinary approach to medical education with integration of clinical and basic science experience. It is designed to permit a variety of teaching and evaluation methods that recognize the importance of small group teaching and clinical relevance of material. Flexibility in the program permits opportunities for research and for a range of ongoing clinical inpatient and ambulatory care experience. The curriculum is made up of four components entitled basis of medicine, introduction to clinical medicine, practice of medicine, and back to basics. Although most students complete a four-year program that lead to the MD degree, joint degree programs are also offered. An MS/PhD program is open to qualified students who are interested in a research career in academic medicine. For students interested in both medicine and health management, the faculties of medicine and management offer a five year program that leads to an MD/MBA degree.

BASIC SCIENCES: The first academic period begins in September and continues through December of the second year. The theme of the first academic period is basis of medicine, and courses are organized into blocks. These are: molecules, cells, and tissues (four weeks); gas, fluids, and electrolytes (nine weeks); life cycle (three weeks); endocrinology, metabolism, and nutrition (seven weeks); musculoskeletal and blood (four weeks); nervous system and special senses (eight weeks); host defense and host parasite (eight weeks); and pathobiology, treatment and prevention of disease.

CLINICAL TRAINING

The second academic period, introduction to clinical medicine (ICM), begins in January of the second year and goes through September of the third year. ICM takes place in hospitals and outpatient clinical settings. Topics covered are introduction to clinical sciences, medical ethics, health law, medicine, family medicine, geriatric medicine, neurology, surgery, emergency medicine, anesthesia, radiology, introduction to hospital practice, pediatrics, psychiatry, obstetrics/gynecology, and an elective. During the third academic period—practice of medicine—students rotate through required clerkships. These are medicine (eight weeks), surgery (eight weeks), psychiatry (eight weeks), psychiatry (eight weeks), obstetrics/gynecology (eight weeks), pediatrics (eight weeks), family medicine (four weeks), and electives/selectives (sixteen weeks). The final academic period is back to basics. During this sixteen-week session, students take medicine and society, topics in medical science, and ambulatory care. Teaching hospitals include Montreal General Hospital, Montreal Children's Hospital, Montreal Neurological Hospital, Sir Mortimer B. Davis—Jewish General Hospital, Douglas Hospital, and Royal Victoria Hospital. Training also takes place at a number of affiliated hospitals and other clinical care centers.

Students

Each entering class has about 110 students. Typically, 25 percent of students are non-Canadians, most of whom are from the United States. About 50 percent of students are women.

STUDENT LIFE

McGill is a large and active campus that offers social and recreational activities to a diverse student body. In addition, the city of Montreal itself is an interesting and exciting place for students to live. McGill has four coeducational residences and one women's residence located on the main campus, which are open to medical students. Information concerning apartments or flats located in the vicinity of the campus can be obtained from the Off-Campus Housing Office.

Admissions Requirements (Required)

MCAT scores, science GPA, non-science GPA, letters of recommendation, interview, essays/personal statement, extracurricular activities, exposure to medical profession.

Admissions Requirements (Optional)

state residency.

Admissions

REQUIREMENTS

The Faculty of Medicine offers a four-year undergraduate medical curriculum. Students are ordinarily admitted into the first year of this program, but admission is also available by means of a Med-P program directly after CEGEP. The faculty does not accept students for part-time medical studies. An MD/PhD program is offered for students who are interested in a research career in academic medicine. For students who interested in both medicine and management, the faculties of medicine and management offer a five-year program leading to an MD/MBA degree. The language of instruction is English. Applicants must have received an undergraduate degree or be in the final year of a course of study at a recognized college or university that leads to an undergraduate degree with at least 120 academic credits. Prerequisites include one year with laboratory work in each of general biology, general chemistry, organic chemistry, and physics. The MCAT is required and applicants must have taken the exam no later than August 1999.

SUGGESTIONS

In addition to prerequisite science courses, some course work in biochemistry or molecular biology is strongly recommended. Applicants to the four-year program should have undergraduate GPAs of 3.5 or better and a total of 30 or more in the MCAT scores. In a recent entering class, the average GPA was a 3.7, and the average overall MCAT score was 31.10.

PROCESS

The deadline for receipt of applications to the regular MD program is January 15 for Quebec residents and November 15 for all others. Applicants with strong academic qualifications submit an application that includes an autobiographical letter used to assess personal qualities and achievements. Selection for interview is based on grades, MCAT scores, letters of reference, and autobiographical letter. Once interviews have been completed, all the components of the application are considered in the admissions decisions. Residents of Quebec will be notified after May 1. Nonresidents will be notified as soon as possible after March 31.

McMaster University

McMaster University Undergraduate Medical Programme

1200 Main Street W. Room 1M7, Hamilton, ON L8N 3Z5 • Admission: 905-525-9140 • Fax: 905-546-0349 • E-mail: mdadmit@mcmaster.ca • Website: www.fhs.mcmaster.ca/mdprog

STUDENT BODY

Type	Public
# applied (total)	3,732
# accepted (total)	193
# enrolled (total)	138
Average age	26

ADMISSIONS

Average GPA and MCAT Scores

Overall GPA	3.8

Application Information

Regular application	10/1
Regular notification	5/31
Are transfers accepted?	No
Admissions may be deferred?	Yes
Interview required?	Yes

Academics

The three-year program in Medicine uses a problem-based approach to learning that emphasizes skills, knowledge, critical thinking, independent study, professional behavior, and lifelong learning. The components have been organized in sequential units with early exposure to patients and case management. Flexibility is ensured to allow for the variety of student backgrounds and career goals. In addition to required units, electives form an integral part of the curriculum. Full-time elective blocks, ongoing horizontal electives, and special enrichment electives are all important components of the medical education. The three-year program (130 weeks of instruction) uses an approach to learning that will remain valid throughout a physician's career. Flexibility is ensured to allow for the variety of student backgrounds and career goals. The graduates of McMaster's Undergraduate Medical Programme will have developed the knowledge, ability, and attitudes necessary to qualify for further education in any medical career. The general goals for students in the program include the following: the development of competency in problem-based learning and in problem solving; the development of the personal characteristics and attitudes compatible with effective health care; the development of clinical and communication skills; and the development of the skills to be a lifelong, self directed learner. To achieve the objectives of the Undergraduate Medical Programme, students are presented with a series of health care problems and questions requiring the understanding of principles and data collection. Much of the learning occurs within the setting of the small group tutorial. Faculty members serve as tutors/facilitators or as sources of expert knowledge. The Undergraduate Medical Programme is arranged as a four-unit pre-clerkship sequence followed by a clerkship; there are additional elective opportunities, both in block periods (totaling twenty-seven weeks) and horizontal electives taken concurrently with ongoing units. Unit one is a twelve-week introduction to concepts and information from three knowledge perspectives: population, behavior, and biology. In addition, a major theme of the entire curriculum, the life cycle, is developed as a perspective and anchors the three subunits of unit one: early development, maturation, and aging. Units two and three are fourteen weeks. Unit four is thirteen-weeks and is organized on the basis of organ systems; biomedical and health care problems are analyzed in depth. The clerkship emphasizes the clinical application of concepts learned in the earlier units and consists of experience in inpatient and ambulatory settings. These concepts include internal medicine, family medicine, surgery, psychiatry, obstetrics-gynecology, and pediatrics. Unit six follows the clerkship and is an interactive unit in which students tackle issues derived from societal expectations of a practicing physician.

Students

Each entering class has 138 students. In a recent entering class, 130 were from Ontario, and eight were from the rest of Canada. About one-third of the class is over twenty-five, with an age range of nineteen to forty-nine. In this class, the male/female ratio was 32:106. As of fall 2000, McMaster has admited up to ten students from a new international applicant pool.

STUDENT LIFE

The teaching methodology and general approach at McMaster fosters student interaction, which carries over outside of the classroom. Medical students take part in extracurricular activities including clubs, athletics, and community service. Off-campus housing is available.

GRADUATES

Post-graduate programs are offered at McMaster in anesthesia, community medicine, critical care, emergency medicine, family medicine, internal medicine, laboratory medicine, obstetrics/gynecology, pediatrics, psychiatry, radiology, and surgery.

Admissions

REQUIREMENTS

At the time of entrance, students must have completed a minimum of three years (thirty full credits) of undergraduate work. Additionally, two years (twenty full credits) must be above the year one level courses. Only degree credit courses taken at an accredited university are considered. Applicants must have achieved an overall simple average of at least a 3.0 in their academic work at the time of application. There are no specific prerequisite courses and the MCAT is not required. Students who are granted admission must be proficient in spoken and written English. All students are required to have obtained a current certificate in basic cardiac life support prior to registration in the medical program.

SUGGESTIONS

Priority is given to residents of Ontario and then to applicants from the rest of Canada. International students may choose to apply through this applicant pool.

PROCESS

The application and transcript deadline for submission to OMSAS is October 15. Approximately 400 applicants are invited for interviews at McMaster in March or April. All applicants are notified in writing on the last day of May as to the results of their application.

Admissions Requirements (Required)

science GPA, nonscience GPA, letters of recommendation, interview, extracurricular activities.

Admissions Requirements (Optional)

MCAT scores, state residency, essays/personal statement, exposure to medical profession.

Overlap Schools

University of Ottawa.

Medical College of Georgia

School of Medicine

Office of Admissions, AA-2040 Augusta, GA 30912 • Admission: 706-721-3186 • Fax: 706-721-0959 •
E-mail: sclmed.stdadmin@mail.mcg.edu • Website: www.mcg.edu

STUDENT BODY

Type	Public
Enrollment	720
% male/female	58/42
% underrepresented minorities	11
# applied (total/out)	1,448/623
# enrolled (total/out)	180/3

FACULTY

Total faculty (number)	502
% female	23
% minority	19

ADMISSIONS

Average GPA and MCAT Scores

Overall GPA	3.6
MCAT Bio	10
MCAT Phys	9.4
MCAT Verbal	9.5

Application Information

Regular application	11/1
Regular notification	5/1
Early application	6/1-8/1
Early notification	10/1
Are transfers accepted?	Yes
Admissions may be deferred?	Yes
Interview required?	Yes

Academics

The school emphasizes early patient contact, uses problem-based learning, and strives to educate physicians who will help meet the health care needs of Georgians. Students and applicants who are interested in earning both an MD and a PhD may apply to combined degree programs arranged with the School of Graduate Studies or with departments of the University of Georgia, Georgia Institute of Technology, or Georgia State University. Areas of doctorate study include, but are not limited to, biochemistry, anatomy, biomedical engineering, biophysics, cell biology, genetics, immunology, microbiology, molecular biology, neuroscience, pharmacology, and physiology.

BASIC SCIENCES: During the two preclinical years, students acquire the building blocks of basic science that underlie medical practice and acquire the skills required for clinical decision-making and patient interaction. The modular content of the curriculum is taught in lectures, labs with integrated clinical conferences, and small group activities. In the first semester of year one, the introductory molecular cell biology module provides a foundation for the basic sciences and is followed by the cellular and systems structures module to introduce students to gross anatomy, histology, and development. In the second semester, biochemistry and physiology are taught in the cellular and systems processes module while the brain and behavior module, gives students an understanding of the interplay between psychiatry and neuroscience. Offered concurrently with the basic science modules, the yearlong essentials of clinical medicine emphasizes familial, cultural, and population aspects of health care; communication skills and information retrieval and analysis; health promotion/disease prevention; ethics; history-taking with children and adults; and a community project. The essentials of clinical medicine is a two-year sequence that emphasizes the skills needed for success in the third year. In year two, essentials of clinical medicine addresses interviewing and physical examination, common medical problems, and interdisciplinary topics such as ethics, nutrition, and the impact of behavior on health while highlighting principles of patient care for each stage of life. Teaching strategies, including interactive small groups, preceptor relationships, and lectures are linked to course objectives. On average, students are in scheduled activities for twenty-six hours per week during the first two years. Classes are held in the modern research and education building and the medical student resource area, which include small group rooms with computers and Internet access. Each student is advised to purchase a computer capable of using relevant educational software. The Greenblatt Library maintains more than 1,800 current journal subscriptions and provides access to many external databases. Audiovisual learning aids are used in class and are available to the library. Grades of A through F (with C constituting a passing grade) are used to evaluate medical students. Passing the USMLE Step 1 is a requirement for promotion to year three.

CLINICAL TRAINING

Patient contact begins during year one in the essentials clinical medicine course, which extends through year two. Year three consists of the following required core clerkships: internal medicine (twelve weeks), pediatrics (six weeks), family medicine (six weeks), obstetrics/gynecology (six weeks), surgery (eight weeks), psychiatry (six weeks), and neurology (four weeks). Core clerkships take place at the Medical College of Georgia Hospitals and Clinics, the Children's Medical Center, and various affiliated hospitals and community-based teaching sites throughout the state. Students may rotate to affiliated community hospitals for part of the core curriculum. During year four, students must complete four-week rotations in emergency medicine, critical care, and an acting internship in medicine, family medicine, pediatrics, surgery, or obstetrics and gynecology. The remainder of the fourth year is for elective study, which can include both clinical and research courses. Grades of A through F are used to evaluate students during the clinical years is based on assessment of knowledge, clinical skills, and professional behavior. Passing the USMLE Step 2 is a requirement for graduation.

Admissions Requirements (Required)

MCAT scores, science GPA, non-science GPA, letters of recommendation, interview, state residency, essays/personal statement, extracurricular activities, exposure to medical profession.

COSTS AND AID

In-state tuition	$9,772
Out-of-state tuition	$29,976
Fees	$783

Financial Aid

% students receiving aid	84
Average debt	$74,685

Students

At least 95 percent of students are Georgia residents. Underrepresented minorities account for about 6 percent of the student body. About one-quarter of each class took time off after college, and there is a wide variety of prior experiences within the student body. Class size is 180.

STUDENT LIFE

The campus is close to downtown Augusta, the second-largest metropolitan area in Georgia. Augusta offers a wide variety of activities including museums, theaters, restaurants, music, shopping, water skiing, sailing, tennis, and golf. Many on-campus housing options are available, including residency halls, one- or two-bedroom apartments, and family housing.

GRADUATES

In the past, the majority of graduates have selected specialized fields. As part of their generalist initiative, the medical college encourages students to explore primary care. The goal of the initiative is for at least half of the graduates to enter residencies in family practice, internal medicine, or pediatrics. Students may remain at the Medical College of Georgia for their post-graduate study while other students enter programs elsewhere in the state and the nation.

Admissions

REQUIREMENTS

Undergraduate preparation must include: biology with lab (one year), inorganic chemistry with lab (one year), organic chemistry with lab (one semester), additional upper-level chemistry (one semester), physics with lab (one year), and English (one year). Transcripts should have grades; pass/fail courses are not advised. The MCAT is required and must be no more than three years old.

SUGGESTIONS

The April MCAT is strongly preferred over the August one. Students who have taken time off after college should show evidence of recent course work, as it is recommended. Experiences that involve patient contact is valuable. In addition to academic strength and general personal qualities, the Admissions Committee looks for an individual's potential for meeting the health care needs of Georgia.

PROCESS

All Georgia residents who submit AMCAS application are sent secondary applications, while only selected out-of-state residents receive secondaries. About half of in-state residents and less than 5 percent of out of state residents are interviewed. Interviews consist of two thirty-minute sessions with faculty, administrators, or students. One interview is conducted by a member of the Admissions Committee, and the other interview is conducted by a faculty member who is not a member of the Admissions Commitee. Interviews take place from October through March. Notification is rolling for regular admissions. After enough offers have been made to fill the class, an alternate list is established from which about forty-fifty candidates are usually admitted.

Medical College of Ohio

Medical College of Ohio, Toledo, OH 43699 • Admission: 419-381-4229 • Fax: 419-381-4005 •
Website: www.mco.edu

STUDENT BODY

Type	Public
Enrollment	565
% male/female	70/30
% underrepresented minorities	10
# applied (total/out)	3,698/2,472
# accepted (total/out)	37/6
# enrolled (out)	9

FACULTY

Total faculty (number)	335
% female	23
% minority	15
% part-time	10
# student/faculty ratio	2:1

ADMISSIONS

Application Information

Regular application	11/1
Regular notification	10/15 until filled
Early application	6/1-8/1
Early notification	10/1
Are transfers accepted?	Yes
Admissions may be deferred?	Yes
Interview required?	No
Application fee	$30

Academics

Although most students follow a four-year program, some educationally disadvantaged students enter the flexible curriculum program, which permits extension of the MD curriculum over a five-year period. Joint-degree programs offered in conjunction with affiliated schools are available, including the MD/MS and MS/PhD through which a doctoral degree may be earned in the following areas: anatomy, biochemistry, microbiology, neuroscience, pathology, pharmacology, physiology, and numerous other fields. Grades of honors, high pass, pass, and fail are used to evaluate medical students. Passing Step 1 of the USMLE is a requirement for promotion to year three. To graduate, a score on Step 2 must be recorded.

BASIC SCIENCES: The first two years are devoted to an integrated approach to the basic sciences, behavioral sciences, primary care preceptorships, introductory clinical experiences, and problem-based learning (PBL) for all students. First-year courses are the following: cellular and molecular biology; human structure and development; neuroscience and behavioral science; integrated pathophysiology I (PBL); and physician, patient, and society I. During the first year, students are in classes for about thirty hours per week, most of which are either lecture or lab periods. Second-year courses are introduction to primary care; immunity and infection; organ systems; integrated pathophysiology II (PBL); and physician, patient, and society II. Physician, patient, and society includes introduction to primary care, introduction to clinical medicine, and a series of courses that address topics in medical ethics, managed care, medical decision-making, nutrition, geriatrics, and substance abuse disorders. The ICM course covers practical skills such as taking patient histories and conducting physical examinations. It also serves as a forum for correlating basic science principles with clinical case studies and for discussing ethical issues related to practicing medicine. Second-year students are in class for about twenty hours per week. Basic science instruction takes place in the Health Sciences Teaching and Laboratory Building and the Health Education Building. The Mulford Library holds 125,000 volumes and 1,800 journals; along with the Computer Learning Resource Center, it provides educational and informational resources to students.

CLINICAL TRAINING

Third-year required clerkships are the following: medicine (twelve weeks), surgery (twelve weeks), pediatrics (six weeks), psychiatry (six weeks), family medicine (six weeks), and obstetrics/gynecology (six weeks). During the fourth year, one basic science selective (four weeks) and one neurology clerkship (four weeks) are required. The remaining twenty-eight weeks are reserved for elective study. Three teaching hospitals operate on campus, the Medical College of Ohio Hospital (258 beds), Coghlin Rehabilitation Hospital (thirty-six beds), and Lenore W. and Marvin S. Kobacker Center (a children's psychiatric hospital with twenty-five beds). Other associated hospitals include St. Vincent Mercy Medical Center, The Toledo Hospital/Children's Medical Center of Northwest Ohio, Flower Hospital, and Northwestern Psychiatric Hospital. Through the Area Health Education Center clerkships, MCO students also have the opportunity to train in rural and inner-city communities.

Students

At least 80 percent of students are Ohio residents although many attended undergraduate institutions outside of the state. Underrepresented minorities, mostly African Americans, account for approximately 10 percent of the student body. Among entrants, there are significant numbers of older individuals, some of whom are in their late thirties and early forties. Typically, about 80 percent of medical students were science majors in college.

STUDENT LIFE

In addition to providing academic resources, the Office of Student Affairs supports students in and outside of the classroom, organizing events such as an annual orientation for incoming students. There are countless student associations, ranging from one that administers a community care clinic, to a student-to-student support group, to organizations focused on personal, recreational, religious, cultural, and professional interests. MCO is situated on 475 acres of land, with ponds, streams, trees, and open areas. The campus offers extensive athletic and recreational facilities. Major attractions in Toledo are easily reached on public transportation and include riverside restaurants and bars, museums, parks with golf courses and other facilities, a zoo, theaters, and shopping areas. Further distraction is found in Detroit, Cincinnati, Pittsburgh, Cleveland, and Chicago—all of which are in driving distance of MCO. Students live off campus, usually in the surrounding residential neighborhood.

GRADUATES

About 40 percent of graduates go on to practice in Ohio. In recent years, about 60 percent of graduates have entered primary care fields.

Admissions

REQUIREMENTS

Prerequisites are one year each of biology, general chemistry, organic chemistry, physics, math, and English. All science courses must include labs. The MCAT is required. For applicants who have retaken the exam, the best set of scores is weighted most heavily. Thus, withholding scores is not advantageous.

SUGGESTIONS

As a state-supported institution, MCO gives preference to Ohio residents. Additional preparation in biology is recommended as are courses in the humanities and social sciences. Students who have been out of school for a significant period of time should show evidence of recent course work. Community service and medically related experience involving patient contact are both considered valuable.

PROCESS

About 75 percent of AMCAS applicants are sent secondary applications, of which about 25 percent of Ohio residents and 10 percent of nonresidents are invited to interview between October and April. Interviews consist of two hour-long sessions each with a faculty member, medical student, or school administrator. Also on interview day, candidates tour the campus, hear group informational sessions, and have the opportunity to informally meet with current students. About one-third of interviewees are accepted and are notified throughout the year. Wait-listed candidates may send additional information such as transcripts and test scores to update their files.

Admissions Requirements (Required)

MCAT scores, science GPA, non-science GPA, state residency, extracurricular activities, exposure to medical profession.

Admissions Requirements (Optional)

letters of recommendation, interview, essays/personal statement.

COSTS AND AID

In-state tuition	$10,512
Out-of-state tuition	$22,966
Cost of books	$2,054
Fees	$741

Financial Aid

% students receiving aid	90
Average grant	$6,000
Average loan	$18,500

MEDICAL COLLEGE OF WISCONSIN

OFFICE OF ADMISSIONS, 8701 WATERTOWN PLANK ROAD, MILWAUKEE, WI 53226 • ADMISSION: 414-456-8246 • FAX: 414-456-6505 • E-MAIL: WWW.MEDSCHOOL@MCW.EDU • WEBSITE: WWW.MCW.EDU/MEDSCHOOL/

STUDENT BODY

Type	Private
Enrollment	805
% male/female	65/35
% underrepresented minorities	10
# applied (total/out)	3,929/3,459
# accepted (total/out)	471/298
# enrolled (total/out)	204/101
Average age	23

FACULTY

Total faculty (number)	1,039

ADMISSIONS

Average GPA and MCAT Scores

Overall GPA	3.7
MCAT Bio	10
MCAT Phys	10
MCAT Verbal	9.7
MCAT Essay	P

Application Information

Regular application	11/1
Regular notification	10/15
Early application	6/1-8/1
Early notification	10/1
Are transfers accepted?	No
Admissions may be deferred?	Yes
Interview required?	Yes
Application fee	$60

Academics

Although most students earn the MD degree in four years, an extended curriculum allows students to complete first-year course work over a two-year period and to graduate in five years. This enables students to pursue research or employment opportunities or personal activities. Medical students who are interested in research are also encouraged to take part in research projects during summers and as part of electives. Other degrees offered by MCW are the PhD, MS, MA, and MPH. Qualified students may enter a combined MS/PhD degree program, and four students each year do so through the MSTP. The Graduate School of Biomedical Sciences offers programs in bioethics, biostatistics, biochemistry, biophysics, cellular biology, medical informatics, microbiology, pathology, pharmacology and toxicology, and physiology. Medical students are evaluated by use of a five interval grading system. Passing Step 1 of the USMLE and sitting for Step 2 are requirements for graduation.

BASIC SCIENCES: Basic sciences are taught through a combination of lectures, labs, tutorials, and small group discussions along with computer aided instructing (CAI), problem-based learning (PBL), and independent study options. On average, students are in class or other scheduled sessions for twenty-three hours per week. First-year courses are clinical human anatomy, medical microanatomy, integrated medical neuroscience, human development, biochemistry, physiology, and clinical continuum I. Second-year courses are pathology, pharmacology, microbiology, foundations of clinical psychiatry, and clinical continuum II. In the clinical continuum sequence, a local physician is assigned as a personal mentor who guides the students through clinical studies in one of the primary care specialties. In addition to learning physical examination and evaluation skills, topics of discussion include the doctor-patient relationship, medical ethics, and health care systems. As part of the course, students follow individual patients for the two-year period and observe their treatment and progress. Support services for medical students include individual and group advising, tutorials, preparation for USMLE exams, and career counseling. Educational facilities include the new Health Research Center completed in spring 1999. The HRC features an auditorium with modern electronic capabilities, rooms designated for small group instruction, and an expanded library. In total, MCW libraries house more than 240,000 volumes and 1,800 journal titles.

CLINICAL TRAINING

Third-year required rotations are introductory clinical skills (one week), ambulatory medicine (one month), medicine (two months), surgery (two months), pediatrics (two months), obstetrics/gynecology (two months), psychiatry (six weeks), and anesthesiology (two weeks). The fourth year consists of a medicine or pediatric subinternship (one month), a medicine selective rotation (one month), a surgery selective (one month), and six months of electives. MCW is one of six components of the Milwaukee Regional Medical Center (MRMC), a campus that includes Froedtert Hospital, Children's Hospital of Wisconsin, Curative Rehabilitation Center, Milwaukee County Mental Health Complex, and the Blood Center of Southeastern Wisconsin Research Institute and Eye Institute. MCW is affiliated with over fifteen additional hospitals and clinics in and around Milwaukee, and with rural care centers in other parts of the state. Up to four months of electives may be taken at other academic medical centers and in foreign countries.

Students

MCW is the seventh largest medical school in the country. Of the 204 first year students, approximately 40 percent are Wisconsin residents. Underrepresented minorities account for about 10 percent of the student body. About one-quarter of students took significant time off between college and medical school.

STUDENT LIFE

Student organizations focus on professional and leadership development, community service, support for minority students, and recreational pursuits. The Medical College is involved with over thirty community service activities, including a student-run clinic for uninsured patients, an AIDS intervention research center, and a health education program in high schools. Medical students take part in organized social events such as parties and dinners and ongoing activities such as intramural sports. Located in the medical education building are an expanded fitness center and a lounge. These facilities allow students to relax and socialize or exercise between scheduled classes. The MCW campus is park-like, covering 248 acres. However, it is an easy drive to downtown Milwaukee, a city with a population of over one million. Milwaukee has a wide variety of cuisine, performing arts and musical groups, several professional sports teams, and outdoor sites like Lake Michigan. Most students live off campus.

GRADUATES

In June, 1996, MCW was one of only six medical schools nationwide in which 100 percent of second-year students passed the USMLE. This type of performance, coupled with the school's reputation for excellent clinical training, results in excellent placement records for graduates.

Admissions

REQUIREMENTS

Candidates must have completed ninety or more undergraduate graded credits at an accredited college/university in the United States or Canada. Prerequisites, which must be taken for graded credit, are eight semester hours including lab each of biology, general chemistry, organic chemistry, and physics. In addition, six semester hours of English and one high school or college course in algebra are required. AP credit is only accepted for three graded credits of English. The MCAT is required and must be taken no more than three years prior to matriculation. For applicants who have retaken the exam, the best score in each section from the last two testings are considered.

SUGGESTIONS

Beyond required courses, applicants are encouraged to study public speaking, literature, history, music, philosophy, and social sciences. In addition to academic credentials, qualities such as a mature sense of values, sound motivation, and the willingness to assume responsibility are important.

PROCESS

MCW uses a secondary application. Interviews consist of two thirty-minute sessions, each with a faculty member or medical student. On interview day, applicants hear group presentations, receive a campus tour, and have the opportunity to talk with current students. Applications are reviewed, interviews conducted and offers made on a rolling, first come/first serve basis until the class is filled.

Admissions Requirements (Required)

MCAT scores, science GPA, non-science GPA, letters of recommendation, interview, essays/personal statement, extracurricular activities, exposure to medical profession.

Admissions Requirements (Optional)

state residency.

COSTS AND AID

Tuition	$31,150
Cost of books	$820
Fees	$45

Financial Aid

% students receiving aid	97
Average grant	$9,562
Average loan	$34,637
Average debt	$116,700

Medical University of South Carolina

College of Medicine

96 Jonathan Lucas Street, Suite 601, PO Box 250617, Charleston, SC 29425 • Admission: 843-792-2055 • Fax: 843-792-4262 • E-mail: taylorwl@musc.edu • Website: www2.musc.edu/COM/COM1.html

STUDENT BODY

Type	Public
Enrollment	584
% male/female	55/45
% underrepresented minorities	14
# applied (total/out)	1,746/1,324
# accepted (total/out)	179/5
# enrolled (total/out)	135/2
Average age	26

FACULTY

Total faculty (number)	612
% female	32
% minority	13
# student/faculty ratio	2:1

ADMISSIONS

Average GPA and MCAT Scores

Overall GPA	3.6
MCAT Bio	9.4
MCAT Phys	9.8
MCAT Verbal	9.8
MCAT Essay	Q

Application Information

Regular application	12/1
Regular notification	rolling
Early application	6/1-8/1
Early notification	10/1
Are transfers accepted?	Yes
Admissions may be deferred?	Yes
Interview required?	Yes
Application fee	$55

Academics

The goal of the College of Medicine is to produce caring and competent physicians who are capable of succeeding in their post-graduate career. The four-year program, which leads to an MD degree, is divided into two years of preclinical instruction that consists of education in the basic sciences and an introduction into clinical medicine, followed by years of clinical science education. The curriculum during the first two years addresses four major objectives: provision of basic science concepts, acquisition of problem solving strategies, development of skills that permit the performance of an adequate history and physical examination, and an introduction to the role of the physician in society. Throughout, emphasis is placed on small group instruction. The curriculum was changed in fall 1999 to expand and improve opportunities for independent, self directed learning. As a result, students are being exposed earlier to clinical skills.

CLINICAL TRAINING

The junior year consists of eight clinical core clerkships. The clinical core consists of eight weeks each of internal medicine, obstetrics/gynecology, pediatrics, and surgery, as well as four weeks each of family medicine, psychiatry, dean's rural primary care, and neurology. During the clerkships, emphasis is placed on the development of clinical, interpersonal, and professional competence. In addition, students participate in the foundations in clinical medicine course. This course is designed to integrate basic and clinical sciences utilizing small group discussions and patient case scenarios. During the senior year, students take a minimum of eight four-week rotations. The student is required to take a clinical externship and one month each of surgery, psychiatry, and internal medicine. The remaining four blocks are electives and, depending upon previous academic performance, can be taken at approved sites throughout the state or country. A complete listing of elective courses may be found in the catalog of electives at www.musc.edu/comelectives/index.html. In addition, students are required to complete and satisfactorily pass the Clinical Practice Exam (CPX).

Students

Over 95 percent of students are South Carolina residents. About 15 percent are underrepresented minorities, most of whom are African American. The average age of incoming students is typically around twenty-five, and at least 10 percent of students in entering classes are usually over thirty years old. Class size is 135.

STUDENT LIFE

During orientation, incoming students are assigned to groups made up of first- and second-year students and a faculty member. The groups serve as informational resources for both academic and nonacademic matters. Also during the first week of school, the Activities Fair is held and introduces various student activities, groups, and events. Organizations that are popular with medical students include chapters of national medical fraternities, professionally oriented interest groups, and groups focused on health care related community service. Intramural sports are also popular. The Harper Student Center (HSC) houses student service offices, a student lounge, and a comprehensive fitness center with indoor and outdoor tracks, rooftop tennis courts, and a swimming pool, among other features. HSC is also a gathering site for students, offering happy hours and other social events. Beyond the campus, Charleston is a city known for its beauty and charm. Students enjoy the nearby beaches and other outdoor attractions. All students live off campus.

GRADUATES

Graduates are successful in securing residencies in all medical fields, with a significant number entering family medicine. MUSC itself offers over twenty post-graduate training programs. More than 95 percent pass USMLE Step 2.

Admissions

REQUIREMENTS

No prerequisites are specified. An applicant's GPA is evaluated with consideration given to the undergraduate institution attended and the difficulty of the course load. The MCAT is required, and scores must be from within the past five years. For applicants who have retaken the exam, the best set of scores is used.

SUGGESTIONS

South Carolina residents are given strong preference. The MCAT requirement suggests that applicants should have a basic science background. However, the school also values the breadth of course work, including courses in the humanities and social sciences. Since the best set of MCAT scores is used, there is no advantage to withholding scores. Extracurricular activities, specifically activities that are medically, community-service, or research related are important. During the interview, noncognitive traits such as emotional stability, integrity, honesty, and enthusiasm are evaluated.

PROCESS

All applicants are asked to submit secondary applications, of which about 65 percent of state residents and 3 percent of out-of-state residents are interviewed if they are academically qualified. Interviews are conducted from September through March and consist of three sessions each with a faculty member or MUSC alumni. About one-third of interviewees are accepted on a rolling basis. The remaining candidates are rejected or wait-listed.

Admissions Requirements (Required)

MCAT scores, science GPA, non-science GPA, letters of recommendation, interview, essays/personal statement, extracurricular activities, exposure to medical profession, Preference is given to SC residents.

Admissions Requirements (Optional)

state residency.

Overlap Schools

Duke University, Emory University, University of South Carolina.

COSTS AND AID

In-state tuition	$13,302
Out-of-state tuition	$37,622
Cost of books	$3,890
Financial Aid	
% students receiving aid	81
Average grant	$2,000
Average loan	$25,865
Average debt	$92,883

MEHARRY MEDICAL COLLEGE

SCHOOL OF MEDICINE

1005 DR. D. B. TODD JR. BOULEVARD, NASHVILLE, TN 37208-3599 • ADMISSION: 615-327-6223 • FAX: 615-327-6228 • E-MAIL: ADMISSIONS@MMC.EDU • WEBSITE: WWW.MMC.EDU

STUDENT BODY

Type	Private
Enrollment	343
% male/female	48/52
% underrepresented minorities	48
# applied (total/out)	3,542/3,323
# accepted (total/out)	145/120
# enrolled (total/out)	80/60
Average age	26

FACULTY

Total faculty (number)	184
# student/faculty ratio	2:1

ADMISSIONS

Application Information

Regular application	12/15
Regular notification	10/15
Early application	6/1-8/1
Early notification	10/1
Are transfers accepted?	No
Admissions may be deferred?	No
Interview required?	Yes
Application fee	$60

Academics

Meharry benefits from its proximity to Fisk University and Tennessee State University. The three schools share certain facilities and together provide an active academic community. Most medical students at Meharry complete their studies in four years, although some extend their first year over a longer period of time and complete medical training in five years. A combined MS/PhD program is offered in biochemistry, biomedical science, microbiology, pharmacology, and physiology. Grades of A, B, C, and F are used to evaluate medical students. All medical students must pass Step 1 of the USMLE to be promoted to year three and must pass Step 2 of the USMLE to graduate.

BASIC SCIENCES: First-year courses are anatomy, biochemistry, physiology, and introduction to clinical medicine I. Students are in class or other scheduled sessions for twenty to twenty-five hours per week. Most instruction uses a lecture format, supplemented by labs and small group discussions. second-year courses are microbiology, general and clinical pathology, behavioral sciences, genetics, pharmacology, and introduction to clinical medicine II. During the second year, students are in class for about thirty hours per week, a significant proportion of which is devoted to small group discussions. The Teaching and Learning Resource Center is located in the Student Center; it serves as a comprehensive academic support unit where students can go for tutoring and board review. The library holds over 50,000 volumes and 1,000 journals and is located in the same complex.

CLINICAL TRAINING

Third-year required rotations are medicine (twelve weeks), surgery (twelve weeks), pediatrics (eight weeks), obstetrics/gynecology (eight weeks), family and preventive medicine (eight weeks), and psychiatry (four weeks). Fourth-year subinternships are medicine (four weeks), surgery (four weeks), family and preventive medicine (four weeks), radiology (four weeks), and psychiatry (four weeks). Twelve weeks are reserved for electives. Major teaching hospitals are Metropolitan Nashville General Hospital, Alvin C. York Veterans' Administration Medical Center, and Blanchefield Army Community Hospital. Other affiliated health care institutions are Centennial Medical Center, Vanderbilt Medical Center, Middle Tennessee Mental Health Hospital, and numerous clinics and health centers throughout the state. All students complete an ambulatory rotation in an underserved area.

Students

About 70 percent of students are African American. Students come from around the country, with about 20 percent of students from Tennessee. Class size is eighty.

STUDENT LIFE

Students are supportive and cooperative, usually opting to study together in groups. There are a large number of student organizations, including honor societies, medical fraternities, support groups such as the Meharry Wives Club, groups focused on professional interests, such as the Family Practice Club, and societies focused on a common religion or ethnicity. The Daniel T. Rolfe Student Center accommodates student activities and organizations and provides a focal point for extracurricular life. Many students are involved in community activities such as serving as mentors for high school students. Medical students interact with other Meharry students and also with peers at nearby universities. Nashville offers restaurants, nightlife, outdoor activities, and a generally student-friendly atmosphere. On-campus housing options are residence halls and apartment complexes with both one- and two-bedroom units.

GRADUATES

The College of Medicine has graduated more than 5,000 African American physicians, almost half of the total number of African American physicians who studied and who practice in the United States. About three-quarters of graduates go on to work in medically underserved rural and inner-city areas. Some graduates enter residency programs at Meharry, which has a total of thirty post-graduate positions in family practice, internal medicine, occupational medicine, preventive medicine, and psychiatry.

Admissions

REQUIREMENTS

Required course work is eight semesters hours each of biology, general chemistry, organic chemistry, and physics, all with associated labs. Six semester hours of English are also required. The MCAT is required, and scores should be from within the past three years. The April MCAT is strongly preferred over the August MCAT. For applicants who have taken the exam on multiple occasions, all sets of scores are considered.

SUGGESTIONS

Special consideration is given to underrepresented minority students and students from disadvantaged backgrounds. Meharry is interested in applicants who are dedicated to improving health care for the underserved. In addition to academic credentials, medically related or community service activities are important.

PROCESS

All qualified AMCAS applicants are sent secondary applications. Of those returning secondaries, about 10 percent are interviewed between September and May. Interviews consist of two sessions, each with a faculty member, administrator, or current medical student. On interview day, applicants also have the opportunity to informally meet with students. About one-third of interviewed candidates are accepted on a rolling basis. Others are rejected or placed on a wait-list. Wait-listed candidates may send additional information if it serves to update their files.

Admissions Requirements (Required)

MCAT scores, science GPA, non-science GPA, letters of recommendation, interview, extracurricular activities, exposure to medical profession.

Admissions Requirements (Optional)

state residency, essays/personal statement.

COSTS AND AID

Tuition	$23,208
Cost of books	$1,528
Fees	$3,916

Financial Aid

% students receiving aid	79
Average grant	$1,000
Average loan	$28,893
Average debt	$125,339

Memorial University Newfoundland

Faculty of Medicine, Memorial University

Room 1751, Health Sciences Center, St. John's, NF A1B 3V6 • Admission: 709-777-6615 • Fax: 709-777-8422 • E-mail: munmed@mun.ca • Website: www.med.mun.ca/admissions/

STUDENT BODY

Type	Public
Enrollment	244
% male/female	48/52
# applied (total)	648
# accepted (total)	77
# enrolled (total)	60

FACULTY

Total faculty (number)	186
% female	31
% part-time	60

ADMISSIONS

Average GPA and MCAT Scores

Overall GPA	3.7
MCAT Bio	9
MCAT Phys	9
MCAT Verbal	9
MCAT Essay	0

Application Information

Regular application	11/15
Regular notification	3/1
Are transfers accepted?	No
Admissions may be deferred?	Yes
Interview required?	Yes
Application fee	$75

Academics

Each of the first two years is organized into three terms. Although the emphasis of the course work is on basic science, clinical medicine is also introduced. During the second two years, students perform clerkships in affiliated hospitals that provide both undergraduate and graduate medical education. In addition to the four-year MD degree, MSc and PhD degree programs are also open to qualified students. Areas of academic strength include endocrinology and metabolism; gastroenterology, human genetics; immunology; molecular biology; neurosciences, and cardiovascular sciences, including epidemiology; and community medicine.

BASIC SCIENCES: An important component of the first year is basic science of medicine. This course introduces students to the biology of the normal human and integrates biochemistry, physiology, immunology, cell biology, genetics, microbiology, nutrition, pharmacology, pathology, and anatomy. Teaching methods include lectures, small group sessions, laboratories, seminars, and open discussions. Students have the opportunity to initiate basic science research, which can be pursued throughout medical school. First-year students also take integrated study of disease, which teaches pathology and pharmacology through the study of diseases of the major organ systems. In clinical skills, students are first introduced to the medical interview and techniques of counseling. The physical exam and important ethical issues are also part of the course. Community medicine is a unique course, which focuses on the contextual aspects of disease and introduces preventive medicine, biostatistics, epidemiology, social and organizational factors in health, environmental and occupational health, community nutrition, and behavioral sciences. The course includes visits to community-based hospitals and clinics. All courses continue in the second year, building on principles learned during the first year. On average, preclinical students are in class or other scheduled sessions for twenty-three hours per week.

CLINICAL TRAINING

Year three is of twelve months duration beginning in September and continuing to the following fall. It is made up of the core clerkships and some electives. Core clerkships, typically eight weeks in length, are internal medicine, surgery, psychiatry, pediatrics, and obstetrics/gynecology. A four-week rural family medicine rotation is also required. The fourth year consists of electives and selectives, some of which may be completed at institutions other than those affiliated with the university. Teaching hospitals include General Hospital (531 beds), Grace General Hospital, Dr. Charles A Janeway Child Health Centre, St. Clare's Mercy Hospital, Waterford Hospital, and a number of institutions that are not under the Health Care Corporation of St. John's.

Students

The school's class size is relatively small at sixty students. The male/female ratio within the student body is about 50:50.

STUDENT LIFE

On-campus housing is available for both single and married students. In addition, the university provides assistance in locating off-campus housing. Medical students benefit from an active counseling center, child care services, learning enhancement programs, a career planning office, and a student health service. The Student's Union promotes artistic, educational, charitable, and social activities, and the graduate student union provides common areas for social and other activities. Medical students have access to the services and resources of the greater university.

GRADUATES

A significant proportion of graduates enter residencies at affiliated hospitals in areas such as anesthesia, internal medicine, neurology, obstetrics/gynecology, orthopedics, anatomic pathology, general pathology, pediatrics, psychiatry, radiology, and surgery. Most graduates enter clinical medicine, often in primary care fields.

Admissions

REQUIREMENTS

To be eligible for admission, a bachelor's degree is required in almost all circumstances. Requirements include two courses in English. The MCAT is also required, and must be taken prior to the application deadline, which is normally November 15. Transcripts and letters of reference must be submitted by November 29. Interviews are required of some candidates. The majority of places in each class are reserved for applicants who are residents of Newfoundland and Labrador. There are a limited number of places available for applicants from New Brunswick and other Canadian provinces and for non-Canadians (who pay higher fees).

SUGGESTIONS

There are approximately 650 applications received for sixty places each year. Therefore, competition is high. Material submitted after the stated deadlines will not be considered. Academic achievement, MCAT scores, work or other experiences, and personal traits are all reviewed in admissions decisions. Although age itself is not used as a basis for selection, time away from academic studies may be taken into consideration.

PROCESS

Requests for applications should be directed to the address above. Applications are accepted until November 15 in the year preceding anticipated matriculation. Decisions are made in the spring. Notification of the committee's decision will be made to candidates by letter from the Admissions Committee. Applicants have fourteen days in which to confirm that they accept the place offered to them.

Admissions Requirements (Required)

MCAT scores, letters of recommendation, interview, essays/personal statement, extracurricular activities.

Admissions Requirements (Optional)

science GPA, nonscience GPA, state residency, exposure to medical profession.

COSTS AND AID

In-state tuition	$6,250
Out-of-state tuition	$30,000
Cost of books	$1,593
In-state Fees	$457
Out-of-state Fees	$645

Financial Aid

% students receiving aid	90
Average grant	$800
Average debt	$150,000

MERCER UNIVERSITY
MERCER UNIVERSITY SCHOOL OF MEDICINE

1550 COLLEGE STREET, MACON, GA 31207 • ADMISSION: 478-301-2542 • FAX: 478-301-2547 •
E-MAIL: FAUST_EK@MERCER.EDU • WEBSITE: WWW.MERCER.EDU

STUDENT BODY

Type	Private
Enrollment	221
% male/female	54/46
% underrepresented minorities	4
# applied (total/out)	738/180
# accepted (total)	60
# enrolled (total)	60
Average age	25

ADMISSIONS

Average GPA and MCAT Scores

Overall GPA	3.4
MCAT Bio	8.65
MCAT Phys	7.8
MCAT Verbal	8.88
MCAT Essay	N

Application Information

Regular application	11/1
Regular notification	Rolling
Early application	6/1-8/1
Early notification	10/1
Are transfers accepted?	Yes
Admissions may be deferred?	Yes
Interview required?	Yes
Application fee	$50

Academics

All entering students are assigned to a faculty adviser who assists them with the transition to medical school, with strategies for preclinical studies, and later with decisions involved in electives and specialty selections. Almost all students complete the MD curriculum in four years. Grades of satisfactory and unsatisfactory are used to evaluated first- and second-year medical students, and grades of honors, satisfactory, and unsatisfactory are used to evaluate third- and fourth-year students. Self and peer evaluations are also used in some situations. Passing both steps of the USMLE are requirements for graduation.

BASIC SCIENCES: Basic sciences are presented during the first two years as part of the biomedical problems program, which uses case-based instructional techniques and computer-assisted, self directed study. The curriculum is organized around physiological systems or phases, which are cells and metabolism, genetics and development, host defense, hematology, neurology, brain and behavior, musculoskeletal, cardiology, pulmonology, gastrointestinal, renal endocrinology, biology of reproduction, and infectious disease. Issues related to medical ethics are also discussed in the context of case studies. Community Science is another important part of the first two years. Courses included in this category are community epidemiology, rural preceptorship, managed care and physician workforce, clinical biostatistics, and research design and the medical literature. Clinical training begins during the first year, when students learn interviewing and examination skills by working with simulated patients. Actual patient contact occurs through the community office practice program (COPP) in which students work directly with community physicians. Most basic science instruction takes place in the medical education building, which, in addition to classrooms, houses the medical library, Mercer Health Systems (which provides clinical services), the Health Education Center, and the school's administrative offices. This physical arrangement, with basic science and clinical facilities in the same building, guarantees to first- and second-year students an integrated educational experience. The library has over 90,000 volumes, 2,500 audiovisuals, and 850 current subscriptions. The Learning Resource Center offers computers and labs.

CLINICAL TRAINING

Third-year required rotations are internal medicine (twelve weeks), surgery (eight weeks), pediatrics (eight weeks), obstetrics/gynecology (six weeks), family medicine (eight weeks), and psychiatry (six weeks). During the fourth year, students choose among fields within surgical subspecialities (four weeks) and also complete clerkships in community science (four weeks), substance abuse (two weeks), and critical care (two weeks). The remainder of the year is reserved for elective study. The primary teaching hospitals are the Medical Center of Central Georgia in Macon (518 beds) and the Memorial Health University Medical Center in Savannah (530 beds). Other major affiliates are Floyd Medical Center in Rome, Phoebe Putney Memorial Hospital in Albany, and the Medical Center in Columbus. Training also takes place outside of major hospitals, at sites such as community hospitals, clinics, and physicians' offices throughout the state.

Students

All students are Georgia residents. About 4 percent are underrepresented minorities. The average age of incoming students is around twenty-four, and at least 20 percent of a typical entering class took significant time off between college and medical school.

STUDENT LIFE

Medical students have access to the facilities of the greater university. These include cafeterias, athletic facilities, and recreational centers. Medical students also have their own student center, which has a snack bar and functions as a meeting place. Students may join chapters of national medical student organizations, including organizations that focus on the needs of women and minority medical students. Mercer offers conveniently located, campus-owned apartments to medical students on a limited basis. Affordable accommodations are also available in and around Macon. The Office of Admissions and Student Affairs helps students find suitable housing.

GRADUATES

Most graduates enter residency programs in Georgia and go on to practice in primary care fields within the state.

Admissions

REQUIREMENTS

Generally, only residents of Georgia are accepted. Required course work is one year each of biology, physics, chemistry, and organic chemistry. The MCAT is required and scores must be no more than two years old.

SUGGESTIONS

In addition to required preparatory courses, biochemistry is recommended. The April MCAT is strongly advised as files are not reviewed until MCAT scores are available. The Admissions Committee is interested in students who are strongly motivated to work with underserved populations and in rural areas. Students who have taken time off after college are advised to demonstrate recent course work.

PROCESS

Secondary applications are sent to AMCAS applicants who meet minimum requirements. Typically, about 70 percent of Georgia residents who apply receive secondary applications, of which about 20 percent are invited to interview between October and March. Interviews consist of two sessions with faculty members. About one-third of interviewees are accepted. All decisions are made before March 15, at which point a wait-list is created.

Admissions Requirements (Required)

MCAT scores, science GPA, non-science GPA, letters of recommendation, interview, state residency, essays/personal statement, extracurricular activities, exposure to medical profession, practice vision statement.

COSTS AND AID

Tuition	$26,372
Cost of books	$1,700

Financial Aid

% students receiving aid	95
Average grant	$5,452
Average loan	$27,149
Average debt	$135,438

Michigan State University

College of Human Medicine

Admissions Office, A-239 Life Sciences East, Lansing, MI 48824 • Admission: 517-353-9620 • Fax: 517-432-0021 • E-mail: MDAdmissions@msu.edu • Website: www.chm.msu.edu

Student Body

Type	Public
Enrollment	438
% male/female	42/58
% underrepresented minorities	36
# applied (total/out)	2,850/1,825
# accepted (total/out)	222/63
# enrolled (total/out)	106/21
Average age	25

Faculty

Total faculty (number)	326
% part-time	28

Admissions

Average GPA and MCAT Scores

Overall GPA	3.5
MCAT Bio	10
MCAT Phys	9.2
MCAT Verbal	9.4
MCAT Essay	P

Application Information

Regular application	11/15
Regular notification	Rolling
Early application	8/1
Early notification	10/1
Are transfers accepted?	Yes
Admissions may be deferred?	Yes
Interview required?	Yes
Application fee	$60

Academics

The four-year curriculum is modern and highly innovative. While the first two years are spend at MSU's main campus in East Lansing, during the third and fourth years, students are assigned to one of six community-based programs for clinical training. These communities are Kalamazoo, Upper Peninsula, Grand Rapids, Flint, Lansing, and Saginaw. Along with its focus on primary care, the College of Human Medicine is dedicated to research programs leading to a master's or PhD. Fields in which graduate degrees may be earned are biochemistry/molecular biology, bioethics/humanities/society, epidemiology, health communication, microbiology/molecular genetics, pharmacology/toxiocology, and physiology. Medical students are evaluated with a modified pass or fail system.

BASIC SCIENCES: In addition to mastering basic science concepts, first-year students address the doctor/patient relationship in clinical skills. A unique mentor program assigns small groups of students to a preceptor, allowing the groups to explore patient care and the complex roles of the physician. Students accompany their mentor for hospital rounds and patient visits. The course integrative clinical correlations, taught by basic science faculty members and clinicians, develops problem solving skills and allows students to apply basic science concepts to clinical case studies. Other first-year courses are gross anatomy, biochemistry, genetics, microbiology, neuroscience, pathology, biostatistics and epidemiology, clinical skills, pharmacology, physiology, histology, human behavior and development, and radiology. The second year is organized around body systems and general disease categories. These are infectious diseases, disorders of development and behavior, hematopoietic/neoplasia, cardiovascular, urinary tract, pulmonary, metabolic endocrine reproductive, digestive, neurological/musculoskeletal, and major mental disorders.In the social context of clinical decisions, students take part in a series of small group seminars dealing with the concepts of medical ethics; epidemiology; biostatistics; critical reasoning; humanities; and social, economic, and organizational issues in medicine. The primary mode of instruction during the second year is small group discussions/tutorials. Students are in scheduled sessions for less than twenty hours per week, allowing ample time for individual and group study. Academic facilities include the Echt Computer Lab, which offers computer-based instructional programs and audio/visual aids; a twenty-four-hour exclusive and comprehensive student learning center; and MSU's main library.

CLINICAL TRAINING

Most clerkship requirements are fulfilled during the third year and the early part of year four. Students move to one of six communities during the summer of their third year. They then rotate through eight weeks of each of the following: family practice, internal medicine, pediatrics, surgery, obstetrics/gynecology, and psychiatry. Four weeks of advanced medicine and advanced surgery are also required. Throughout the period in which students complete required clerkships, students also participate in a core competency seminar, which requires two hours per week and provides a forum for discussion of interdisciplinary topics important to the care and health management of patients. A total of twenty weeks are reserved for elective experiences. Students may rotate to other communities in the state, to hospitals and academic centers in other states, and to clinical sites overseas.

Students

At least 80 percent of students are Michigan residents. Class size is 106. In a recent class, the average age of incoming students was twenty-five.

STUDENT LIFE

First- and second-year students enjoy the activities, facilities, resources, and social life of a big ten university. Medical students are also involved in the greater community, volunteering at clinics and as health educators in schools. Professionally focused and special-interest organizations are numerous, as are athletic opportunities such as intramural sports. A variety of campus-owned housing options are available. Some single students live in a graduate/professional student residence hall. Apartments of all sizes are also available, accommodating single and married students, and students with larger families. Where students spend their third and fourth years is largely determined by a lottery, with consideration given to special circumstances and preferences.

GRADUATES

Students typically score above the national average on the USMLE, contributing to their success in securing top-choice residency positions. A recent three year average of residency choices resolved: family practice (27 percent), internal medicine (15 percent), obstetrics/gynecology (10 percent), surgery (13 percent), pediatrics (15 percent), psychiatry (3 percent), other programs (17 percent). About 50 percent of graduates remained in Michigan for residency programs.

Admissions

REQUIREMENTS

Prerequisites are eight semester credits of biology, chemistry, organic chemistry, and physics, all with associated labs. Eight semester credits in English and social science, one upper level biology course, and college algebra or statistics and probability are also required. The MCAT is required, and scores must be no more than three years old. For applicants who have retaken the exam, the most recent set of scores is used. Thus, there is no advantage in withholding scores.

SUGGESTIONS

Although Michigan residents are given preference, about 20 percent of the positions in an entering class are available to highly qualified nonresident applicants. MSU is focused on training generalist physicians and seeks applicants with an interest in primary care and community-based medicine. Applicants should have medical/clinical experience. Important personal traits are competence, honesty, social responsibility, and compassion.

PROCESS

About one-quarter of AMCAS applicants are sent secondary applications, of which about one-third are interviewed. Interviews are conducted on Thursdays between September and March. Interviews consist of two sessions: one with a faculty member and the other with a current medical student. On interview day, candidates attend informational sessions, have lunch with medical students, and tour the campus. About one-third of interviewees are accepted on a rolling basis.

Admissions Requirements (Required)

MCAT scores, science GPA, non-science GPA, letters of recommendation, interview, essays/personal statement, extracurricular activities, exposure to medical profession, U.S. resident, U.S. permanent resident, visa, or Canadian.

Admissions Requirements (Optional)

state residency.

Overlap Schools

University of Michigan, Wayne State University.

COSTS AND AID

In-state tuition	$19,726
Out-of-state tuition	$43,526
Room and board	$11,184
Cost of books	$2,605
Fees	$1,225

Financial Aid

% students receiving aid	94
Average grant	$3,500
Average loan	$23,310
Average debt	$130,100

MOREHOUSE
SCHOOL OF MEDICINE

ADMISSIONS AND STUDENT AFFAIRS, 720 WESTVIEW DRIVE, SW, ATLANTA, GA 30310 • ADMISSION: 404-752-1650 • FAX: 404-752-1512 • WEBSITE: WWW.MSM.EDU

STUDENT BODY

Type	Private
Enrollment	182
% male/female	37/63
% underrepresented minorities	87
# applied (total/out)	2,047/1,736
# accepted (total/out)	116/43
# enrolled (total/out)	52/25
Average age	23

FACULTY

Total faculty (number)	260
% female	43
% minority	85
% part-time	14
# student/faculty ratio	1:1

ADMISSIONS

Application Information

Regular application	12/1
Regular notification	11/1
Early application	6/1-8/1
Early notification	10/1
Are transfers accepted?	Yes
Admissions may be deferred?	Yes
Interview required?	Yes
Application fee	$50

Academics

Most students follow a four-year curriculum leading to the MD, although some students pursue joint degree programs of MD/MPH or MS/PhD. To be considered for these programs, applications must be submitted to the appropriate graduate department at the time of application to medical school. Grades of A through F are used to evaluate medical students. Passing the USMLE Step 1 is a requirement for promotion to year three and passing Step 2 is a requirement for graduation.

BASIC SCIENCES: Instruction uses a lecture/lab format, and students are in class or laboratories for about thirty hours per week. First-year courses are human morphology, medical biochemistry, neurobiology, medical physiology, biostatistics and epidemiology, human behavior, human values in medicine, community health, and a weekly preceptorship with a community physician. Community health promotion is an examination of preventive medicine, while human values in medicine addresses the behavioral, socioeconomic, and ethical aspects of medicine. Second-year courses are introduction to primary care, pathophysiology, human values in medicine, psychopathology, microbiology and immunology, pathology, pharmacology, and nutrition. During the second year, students learn patient interview and examination techniques. Instruction takes place in the Basic Medical Sciences Building, which contains classrooms, laboratories, and administrative offices, and in the adjacent Medical Education Building. In 1996, a new Multidisciplinary Research Center opened.

CLINICAL TRAINING

Third- and fourth-year required clerkships are internal medicine (two months), pediatrics (two months), obstetrics/gynecology (two months), psychiatry (seven weeks), radiology (one week), surgery (two months), family medicine (one month), ambulatory medicine (one month), maternal child health (one month), and rural primary care (one month). Five months are reserved for electives. Third-year rotations take place primarily at Grady Memorial Hospital (1,000 beds), a full-service facility for indigent patients that, for training purposes, is shared with Emory University. Other clinical sites include the Tuskegee Veterans Hospital (900 beds), Georgia Regional Hospital—Ridgeview Institute, West Fulton Community Mental Health Center, Brawner Psychiatric Institute and HCA West Paces Ferry Hospital, and Southwest Hospital and Medical Center. A portion of elective credit may be earned at accredited medical schools other than Morehouse, and at a wide variety of clinical institutions.

Students

Approximately 95 percent of students are African American. About 70 percent of students are from Georgia, and the remaining students come from a wide geographic area. Class size is thirty-five.

STUDENT LIFE

Community service is an important part of student life, and virtually all students are involved in some sort of volunteer activity while in medical school. Students are cohesive both in and out of the classroom. The large percentage of students who are in study groups demonstrates the cooperation that exists between students. Students participate in local chapters of national medical school organizations and in student groups focused on professional interests. Atlanta is the cultural, financial, and industrial hub of the Southeastern United States, and offers a wide variety of activities and attractions including arts, sports, recreation, dining, and entertainment. The city is accessible by public transportation. Although there is no school-owned housing, students are able to locate affordable housing off campus.

GRADUATES

Graduates are successful in securing residencies in prestigious programs nationwide. Approximately 75 percent of graduates enter primary care fields, one of the highest percentages among medical schools. Most go on to work with underserved populations, either in inner cities or in rural areas.

Admissions

REQUIREMENTS

Required courses are biology (one year), general chemistry (one year), organic chemistry (one year), physics (one year), college-level math (one year), and English (one year). All science courses must include associated labs. Grades are assessed with consideration of academic improvement, balance and depth of academic program, difficulty of courses taken, and overall achievement. The MCAT is required, and scores must be from within the past two years. Applicants who have retaken the exam are not penalized, but the most recent set of scores is weighed most heavily.

SUGGESTIONS

Of the forty spots in a class, at least twenty are reserved for Georgia residents. Thus, competition for out-of-state residents can be intense. The April MCAT is preferred over the August. Beyond academic achievement, the committee is interested in extracurricular activities, research projects and experiences, and interests and talents. Compassion, honesty, motivation, and perseverance are qualities that are considered important to the practice of medicine.

PROCESS

About 80 percent of AMCAS applicants are sent secondary applications, of which about 8 percent are invited to interview between October and March. About 25 percent of Georgia residents are invited to interview. Interviews generally consist of one thirty-minute session with a faculty member. On interview day, candidates receive a campus tour, group orientation sessions, lunch, and the opportunity to meet with current medical students. About 10 to 20 percent of interviewees are accepted and are notified beginning in December. Wait-listed candidates may send supplementary material to update or strengthen their files.

Admissions Requirements (Required)

MCAT scores, science GPA, non-science GPA, letters of recommendation, interview, essays/personal statement, extracurricular activities, exposure to medical profession.

Admissions Requirements (Optional)

state residency.

COSTS AND AID

Tuition	$20,966
Room and board	$10,970
Cost of books	$8,779
Fees	$4,405

Financial Aid

% students receiving aid	96
Average grant	$18,477
Average loan	$30,384
Average debt	$118,091

NEW YORK MEDICAL COLLEGE

NEW YORK MEDICAL COLLEGE

OFFICE OF ADMISSIONS, ADMINISTRATION BUILDING, VALHALLA, NY 10595 • ADMISSION: 914-594-4507 • FAX: 914-594-4976 • E-MAIL: MDADMIT@NYMC.EDU • WEBSITE: WWW.NYMC.EDU

STUDENT BODY

Type	Private
Enrollment	767
% male/female	49/51
% underrepresented minorities	8
# applied (total/out)	6,495/5,134
# accepted (total/out)	785/550
# enrolled (total/out)	189/124
Average age	26

FACULTY

Total faculty (number)	2,805
% female	28
% minority	31
% part-time	4

ADMISSIONS

Average GPA and MCAT Scores

Overall GPA	3.5
MCAT Bio	10.4
MCAT Phys	10.3
MCAT Verbal	9.2
MCAT Essay	Q

Application Information

Regular application	12/15
Regular notification	Rolling
Early application	8/1
Early notification	10/1
Are transfers accepted?	Yes
Admissions may be deferred?	Yes
Interview required?	Yes
Application fee	$100

Academics

Students have an opportunity to earn joint degrees, combining the MD with an MPH, which is of great value considering the increased awareness of public health issues, or a PhD in the basic medical sciences. Grades of honors, high pass, pass, and fail are used to evaluate medical students. Passing Steps 1 and 2 of the USMLE are graduation requirements. In recent years, the pass rate has been at or near 100 percent.

BASIC SCIENCES: The curriculum of the first two years, although focused on the basic sciences, maintains a consistent clinical orientation. The program has been revised to bring clinical relevance and small group teaching into all courses. During the first two years, students focus on developing a thorough understanding of the sciences basic to clinical medicine. The core of the first-year curriculum—anatomy, histology, biochemistry, physiology, neural science, and behavioral science—is supplemented by clinical case correlations and courses in epidemiology and biostatistics. The second-year curriculum, with its strong focus on pathology/pathophysiology, emphasizes small group discussion, problem-based learning, and self-study; students spend only 25 percent of their class time in large lectures. Clinical skills training, pharmacology, and medical microbiology prepare students for the clerkship experience of the next two years.

CLINICAL TRAINING

While immersed in the basic science curriculum, all first-year students work in primary care physician offices and thus have ongoing direct patient contact. This one-on-one placement gives to students the necessary clinical exposure and allows them to develop personal mentor relationships. This preceptorship experience can be continued throughout the second year to fulfill the clinical skills requirement. Third-year clinical clerkships are the following: medicine (twelve weeks), surgery (eight weeks), pediatrics (eight weeks), obstetrics/gynecology (six weeks), psychiatry (six weeks), neurology (four weeks), family medicine clerkship (four weeks), and community and preventive medicine (one week). The school's location in the suburban New York area and large hospital network afford clinical-training opportunities in demographically and clinically diverse settings. About half of the third-year class moves into New York City during their clinical years; many live in college-owned housing in Manhattan. Fourth-year requirements are the following: medicine or pediatrics subinternship (four weeks), ambulatory surgical subspecialties (four weeks), geriatrics or chronic care pediatrics (four weeks), and anesthesiology/rehabilitation medicine (two weeks). The eighteen weeks of electives can be taken anywhere. About fifteen to twenty students take international electives each year.

Students

The school's student body is generally representative of the demographic diversity of the country. The first-year class size is 190 students; in recent years it has been fairly equally divided by gender, with the proportion of females increasing incrementally. About half of all students come from public colleges and universities.

STUDENT LIFE

Most first- and second-year students live on campus in attractive, unfurnished garden apartments or furnished suite-style apartment shares in suburban settings that encourage a sense of community. Students gather for pick-up football, soccer, and basketball games outdoors when weather permits. Many third- and fourth-year students live in safe, comfortable, and affordable college-owned apartments in New York City. Students can participate in more than forty clubs and organizations groups that focus on professional, cultural, social, educational, and athletic interests. These include The Arrhythmias, an a cappella singing group; a chamber music club; and other cultural groups. Project Sunshine works to better the lives of children in hospitals, and AMSA, AMA, AMWA, and SMNA—student chapters of major professional organizations—let students represent the school at regional and national student conferences.

GRADUATES

The School of Medicine encourages students to aim high when they apply for residency matches. While a large number of students are choosing to match in primary care disciplines, there are equally impressive matches in highly competitive specialty programs. Matches for the current year can be viewed on the school's website. Some 10,000 alumni are supported by alumni association chapters in major cities. Alumni can track university announcements of upcoming events on the website; a special alumni section allows them to post news and read about other alumni. Alumni can also keep current on their classmates' activities via the university magazine, Chironian, which is mailed to all alumni and is also available for viewing on the Web.

Admissions

REQUIREMENTS

All applicants must have taken the MCAT within the last three years and must have completed or have in progress the following prerequisites: two semesters of biology, chemistry, organic chemistry, and physics, all with their required labs. Two semesters of English are also required. The most recent MCAT scores are given greatest weight. While most students have majored in the sciences, the school encourages those with strong humanities backgrounds and the necessary science requirements to apply.

SUGGESTIONS

We look for students who not only meet the academic requirements but also show clear evidence through their activities of strong motivation toward medicine and a sense of dedication to the service of others. Personal qualities of character and personality are evaluated from letters of recommendation, from the personal statement, and from the interview. New York Medical College does not deny admission to any applicant on the basis of race, gender, religion, national origin, age, or handicap.

PROCESS

All AMCAS applicants are requested to complete an online secondary application. After the completed secondary application and all letters of recommendation have been processed, the applicant's file is reviewed for consideration. Interviews are by invitation and are conducted on campus. We generally interview from October through April, and decisions are made on a rolling basis.

Admissions Requirements (Required)

MCAT scores, science GPA, non-science GPA, letters of recommendation, interview, essays/personal statement, extracurricular activities, exposure to medical profession.

Admissions Requirements (Optional)

state residency

COSTS AND AID

Tuition	$34,040
Room and board	$10,512
Cost of books	$1,602
Fees	$2,880

Financial Aid

% students receiving aid	90
Average grant	$18,000
Average loan	$42,000
Average debt	$142,000

New York University
Mount Sinai School of Medicine

Annenberg 5-04A, Box 1002, One Gustave L. Levy Place, New York, NY 10029-6574 • Admission: 212-241-6696 • Fax: 212-828-4135 • E-mail: admissions@mssm.edu • Website: www.mssm.edu

STUDENT BODY

Type	Private
Enrollment	712
% male/female	51/49
% underrepresented minorities	10
# applied (total)	3,178
# accepted (total)	416
# enrolled (total/out)	160/73
Average age	21

FACULTY

Total faculty (number)	1,332
% female	32
% minority	15
% part-time	27

ADMISSIONS

Average GPA and MCAT Scores

Overall GPA	3.6
MCAT Bio	11
MCAT Phys	11
MCAT Verbal	10
MCAT Essay	0

Application Information

Regular application	11/1
Regular notification	12/1
Are transfers accepted?	No
Admissions may be deferred?	Yes
Interview required?	Yes
Application fee	$85

Academics

Mount Sinai's approach to medical education emphasizes cooperative rather than competitive learning to prepare students for the lifelong learning that is essential to the modern medical career. Group study, small classes and, for the past thirty years, a pass/fail grading system for the first- and second-year students help to emphasize the cooperative environment. The majority of the students spend some of their first two (preclinical) years focused on the core biomedical knowledge and the basic skills of the doctor-patient relationship. Through direct patient contact during the third and fourth (clinical) years in inpatient and ambulatory settings, students develop the skills necessary for the practice of medicine. Joint degree programs, such as the MS/MD, are possible. Eight students each year pursue an MSTP-sponsored PhD degree along with the MD in conjunction with the Mount Sinai Graduate School of Biological Sciences. The PhD may be earned in biochemistry, biomathematical sciences, cell biology and anatomy, genetics, immunobiology, microbiology, molecular biology, neuroscience, pharmacology, or physiology/biophysics. Grades of pass and fail are used to evaluate medical students in preclinical courses, and grades of honors, high pass, pass, and fail are used to evaluate medical students in clinical training. Students must pass Step 1 of the USMLE for promotion to year three and Step 2 to graduate.

BASIC SCIENCES: Basic sciences are taught through a combination of lectures, small group discussions, labs, and clinical correlates. Lecture time is kept to two hours per day and students typically have three mornings or afternoons per week of study time. Beginning on day one, the art and science of medicine, taught in both the first and second years, introduces students to the skills they need to care for patients. Throughout both years the emphasis is on case-based learning. Integrated with every course are numerous means for providing clinical relevance for the basic science being studied. Topics such as ethics, radiology, and palliative care that overlap many areas are incorporated into the curriculum of all four years through courses without walls. First-year courses are genetics, first aid, embryology, molecules and cells, histology and physiology, and pathogenesis and host defense mechanisms. The year ends with an integrative core that focuses on translational topics and therefore allows students to work with faculty from the bench to the bedside on a selected and structured topic. Extensive study of mechanisms of disease and therapy is the major focus of the second year. This sequence of courses addresses each of the major pathophysiology topics essential to the practice of medicine. Organs and systems covered include respiratory, cardiovascular, renal/genitourinary, breast, skin, gynecologic, hematologic, endocrine, and musculoskelatal. A section on brain and behavior encompasses both psychopathology and neurology; at the end of the year, the focus shifts to epidemiology and biostatistics.

CLINICAL TRAINING

The curriculum in the third year is composed of four twelve-week modules of clinical clerkships. The modules are pediatrics, obstetrics, nursery, and gynecology; medicine and geriatrics; surgery and psychiatry; and neurology, anesthesia, and family practice. Four weeks of electives are also offered in the third year. As in the first two years, an integrated case-based curriculum enriches the learning opportunities throughout the year. The fourth year begins with a four-week preparation period for Step 2 of the USMLE, followed by an emergency rotation and a subinternship in medicine. A clinical translational fellowship combines the clinical practice of medicine with the relevant basic science. A four-week required post-match integrated selective addresses issues essential for students to explore before they going on to their residencies. A significant portion of clinical training takes place at The Mount Sinai Hospital, which includes the 625-bed Guggenheim Pavilion and a primary care building with an expansive ambulatory care program. Affiliated teaching facilities include, but are not limited to, Bronx Veterans' Affairs Medical Center (561 beds), Elmhurst Hospital Center (Queens, 526 beds), Englewood Hospital and Medical Center (New Jersey, 520 beds), North General Hospital (Central and East Harlem), and Maimonedes Medical Center.

Students

The 2002 entering class represented fifty-six different undergraduate institutions and pursued thirty-nine different undergraduate majors. Underrepresented minorities accounted for 17 percent of the students. The average age of incoming students was twenty-three.

STUDENT LIFE

Mount Sinai provides a healthy environment and encourages the development of lifelong healthy habits. Cultural diversity is respected and supported both in and out of the classroom. Students are active in a wide variety of school-related organizations, particularly organizations that focus on community service activities. Furthermore, New York City is a rich source of extracurricular life. The Recreation Office provides discounted tickets to theater, movies, sporting events, and concerts. The Aron Residence Hall offers over 600 furnished suites for single students. It is conveniently located and features a fitness center, among other amenities. School-owned housing for couples is also available.

GRADUATES

Among graduates of the 2001 class, 28 percent entered internal medicine, 16 percent entered pediatrics, 17 percent entered surgical specialties, and 7 percent entered obstetrics/gynecology. The remainder entered a broad range of other post-graduate programs.

Admissions

REQUIREMENTS

Prerequisites are one year each of general chemistry, organic chemistry, biology, college-level math, English, and physics. The MCAT is required, and scores from 2000 onward are acceptable.

SUGGESTIONS

Students who have taken significant time off after college should have some recent course work. No particular extracurricular activities are specified, although successful applicants usually have participated in community service, research, or medically-related activities.

PROCESS

All AMCAS applicants receive secondary applications, of which about 17 percent are interviewed. Interviews are conducted from September through April and consist of two thirty-minute sessions, either with two faculty members or a faculty member and a medical student. Some candidates are notified of the committee's decision shortly after the interview, while others may not hear until later in the year. About 30 percent of interviewees are ultimately accepted. Wait-listed candidates may send supplementary material to update their files. An early assurance program admits a limited number of sophomores with admission contingent upon completing undergraduate requirements.

Admissions Requirements (Required)

MCAT scores, science GPA, non-science GPA, letters of recommendation, interview, essays/personal statement, extracurricular activities.

Admissions Requirements (Optional)

state residency, exposure to medical profession.

Overlap Schools

Columbia University, Cornell University, Harvard University, Johns Hopkins University, New York University, UMDNJ, University of Pennsylvania.

COSTS AND AID

Tuition	$26,750
Room and board	$9,900
Cost of books	$1,000
Fees	$3,750

Financial Aid

% students receiving aid	80
Average grant	$3,000
Average loan	$22,000
Average debt	$92,000

NEW YORK UNIVERSITY

NEW YORK UNIVERSITY SCHOOL OF MEDICINE

PO BOX 1924, NEW YORK, NY 10016 • ADMISSION: 212-263-5290 • FAX: 212-263-0720 •
E-MAIL: ADMISSIONS@MED.NYU.EDU • WEBSITE: WWW.MED.NYU.EDU/HOMEPAGE.HTML

STUDENT BODY

Type	Private
Enrollment	450
% male/female	49/51
% underrepresented minorities	40
# applied (total/out)	4,308/3,225
# accepted (total/out)	310/191
# enrolled (total/out)	120/70
Average age	23

FACULTY

Total faculty (number)	1,922
% female	36
% minority	25
% part-time	13

ADMISSIONS

Average GPA and MCAT Scores

Overall GPA	3.6
MCAT Bio	10.9
MCAT Phys	11
MCAT Verbal	10
MCAT Essay	Q

Application Information

Regular application	11/1
Regular notification	Rolling
Early application	8/1
Early notification	10/1
Are transfers accepted?	Yes
Admissions may be deferred?	Yes
Interview required?	Yes
Application fee	$100

Academics

The goal of the curriculum is to train physician-scholars who will approach the profession of medicine with intellectual rigor and who also understand the humanistic and ethical aspects of the field. Selected students may pursue a curriculum that leads to both the MD and PhD degrees in a minimum of six years. The PhD may be earned in a basic medical science field or in a social science discipline. An honors program permits students who are following the standard four-year MD curriculum to supplement formal classwork with summer research or ongoing projects for which they receive credit. Grades of pass and fail are used to evaluate medical students in their preclinical years. Letter grades are used to evaluate medical students during their clinical clerkships.

BASIC SCIENCES: In the fall of 1997, the School of Medicine implemented a new basic science curriculum organized into interdisciplinary modules. Year one has three modules. The first module consists of molecular biology/ genetics and biochemistry, anatomy, and embryology. The second module includes cellular biology, physiology, histology, and immunology. The third module is organ physiology, histology of tissues/organs, microbiology, immunology, and parasitology. Throughout the first year, students take behavioral science/introduction to clinical medicine, which addresses the interrelationship among patients, their families, their environments, their particular illness, and their care. The first year also includes a new course, the skills and science of doctoring. This includes a preceptorship in the office of a practicing physician and serves to integrate basic science concepts with clinical applications. First-semester, second-year courses are neuroscience, general pathology, and psychopathology. In the second semester, pathophysiology, systemic pathology, pharmacology and biostatistics/epidemiology are integrated in a human organ system module. During the first two years, class time is divided between lectures and small group discussions. Laboratory work and computer-assisted instruction enhance learning. In total, first- and second-year students are in class or other scheduled sessions for about twenty hours per week. There is a newly established division of academic computing, which has resulted in increased integration of bioinformatics into the curriculum. Each of the courses has a Web page where students can access all course materials, including lecture slides. Instruction takes place in the medical science building and adjacent facilities, which provide laboratory space, lecture halls, rooms for small group discussions, and conference rooms. The Frederick L. Ehrman Medical Library occupies three stories in the medical science building and has areas that are open to students twenty-four hours a day. Its collection includes over 160,000 volumes and 2,000 current serial titles.

CLINICAL TRAINING

Required clerkships must be completed during year three and the first part of year four. Clerkships are as follows: medicine (ten weeks), pediatrics (eight weeks), surgery (ten weeks), obstetrics/gynecology (six weeks), psychiatry (six weeks), neurology (four weeks), and ambulatory care medicine (four weeks). During the fourth year, all students take six weeks of advanced medicine. The remainder of the year is reserved for elective study, which typically involves a research project. Clinical training takes place at Bellevue Hospital Center and New York University Medical Center Complex and at affiliated institutions. In total, the complex has a capacity of 5,400 beds. A portion of electives may be taken at other hospitals in the United States or abroad.

Students

Approximately 50 percent of students are New York residents. Other students come from all regions of the country. About 7 percent of students are underrepresented minorities, most of whom are African American. Though the majority of students are in their early twenties, each class has several nontraditional students who have pursued careers or other activities between college and medical school. Class size is 160.

STUDENT LIFE

Because most students live in university-owned housing, they interact outside of class and are able to enjoy a real student community. The neighborhood around NYU is filled with restaurants, cafés, bars, shops, galleries, and other attractions. New York is a cultural, artistic, commercial, and entertainment center with virtually unlimited recreational opportunities. The entire city is accessible by public transportation. The School of Medicine operates housing facilities for students, thereby assuring that all NYU medical students can afford convenient and comfortable housing. Both residence halls and apartments are available.

GRADUATES

Of 1999 graduates, the most prevalent fields for post-graduate training were the following: categorical internal medicine (37 percent), general surgery (10 percent), obstetrics/gynecology (9 percent), pediatrics or medicine/pediatrics (8 percent), psychiatry (8 percent), radiology (8 percent), and dermatology (4 percent). Many graduates enter residency programs at top institutions nationwide.

Admissions

REQUIREMENTS

Prerequisites are six semester hours each of general chemistry, organic chemistry, physics, biology, and English; all science courses must include laboratory work. The MCAT is required, and scores should be from the post-1997 version of the test. For applicants who have retaken the exam, the best set of scores is considered.

SUGGESTIONS

Biochemistry is strongly recommended. Other recommended courses are calculus, quantitative and physical chemistry, genetics, embryology, and Spanish, particularly if the applicant intends on practicing in the New York area. Experience in a health care setting is considered valuable.

PROCESS

NYU Medical School participates in the AMCAS program. About 20 percent of applicants are invited to interview between November and February. Interviews consist of one session with a faculty member or administrator. On interview day, applicants also tour the campus and have lunch with medical students. About 25 percent of interviewed candidates are accepted, and they are notification about one month after the interview. Remaining candidates are rejected or put on hold and either accepted or wait-listed later in the year. Wait-listed candidates may send information to update their files.

Admissions Requirements (Required)

MCAT scores, science GPA, non-science GPA, letters of recommendation, interview, essays/personal statement, extracurricular activities, exposure to medical profession.

Admissions Requirements (Optional)

state residency.

COSTS AND AID

Tuition	$31,250
Room and board	$10,500
Cost of books	$1,220
Fees	$2,650

Financial Aid

% students receiving aid	85
Average gr ant	$18,968
Average loan	$26,446
Average debt	$85,042

Northeastern Ohio Universities College of Medicine

PO Box 95, Rootstown, OH 44272-0095 • Admission: 330-325-6270 • Fax: 330-325-8372 •
E-mail: admission@neoucom.edu • Website: www.neoucom.edu

STUDENT BODY

Type	Public
Enrollment	430
% male/female	46/54
% underrepresented minorities	6
# applied (total/out)	794/286
# accepted (total/out)	61/6
# enrolled (total)	23
Average age	22

FACULTY

Total faculty (number)	1,905
% female	19
% minority	15
% part-time	86

ADMISSIONS

Average GPA and MCAT Scores

Overall GPA	3.6
MCAT Bio	8.8
MCAT Phys	8.8
MCAT Verbal	9
MCAT Essay	P

Application Information

Regular application	12/1
Regular notification	3/21
Early application	6/1-8/1
Early notification	10/1
Are transfers accepted?	Yes
Admissions may be deferred?	No
Interview required?	Yes
Application fee	$30

Academics

While most students participate in the six- or seven-year BS/MD program, about fifteen to twenty-five students each year enter the four-year MD program. A combined MS/PhD program is offered in collaboration with either Kent State or the University of Akron, which leads to the doctoral degree in biomedical engineering or a number of medically related science fields. A summer fellowship program provides a stipend to selected medical students who undertake research or clinical education projects related to community health. Medical students are evaluated with grades of honors, satisfactory, conditional-unsatisfactory, or unsatisfactory for most courses. Passing the USMLE Step 1 is a requirement for promotion to year three, and passing Step 2 is a requirement for graduation.

BASIC SCIENCES: Basic sciences are taught primarily in a lecture/lab format, although some courses also utilize small group discussions and tutorials. On average, students are in class or other scheduled sessions for thirty-two hours per week. First-year courses are human anatomy/embryology, microscopic anatomy, medical neuroscience, biochemistry and molecular pathology, physiology, behavioral science, infectious diseases, developmental medicine, immunobiology, introduction to physical exam and ambulatory care experience, and problem-based learning. Second-year courses are introduction to clinical medicine (ICM), systemic pathology, pharmacology, principles of medical sciences, infectious disease-2, M2 ambulatory care experience, and radiology. The ICM course focuses on clinical problems, fundamental doctor-patient communication skills, the physical examination, and clinical evaluation. NEOUCOM's approach to instruction in this transitional year allows for extensive clinical exposure and patient contact. As part of ICM, students spend time each week in family practice centers. Students benefit from academic support and counseling services offered by the Office of Academic Affairs. The Oliver Ocasek Regional Medical Information Center on the Rootstown campus houses more than 91,000 books and journals, in addition to computerized information systems. The center is electronically linked to libraries in the teaching hospitals and consortium universities.

CLINICAL TRAINING

Third-year required rotations are internal medicine (ten weeks), surgery (ten weeks), general pediatrics (eight weeks), obstetrics/gynecology (eight weeks), psychiatry (six weeks), and family medicine (six weeks). During the fourth year, additional requirements are primary care preceptorship (four weeks), medical humanities (four weeks), community medicine clerkship (four weeks), and twenty weeks of electives. Training takes place at affiliated hospitals, which include Lodi Community Hospital, Wadsworth-Rittman Hospital, Akron General Medical Center, Barberton Citizens Hospital, Children's Hospital Medical Center, Edwin Shaw Hospital, Summa Health System, Robinson Memorial Hospital, Hillside Rehabilitation Hospital, Trumbull Memorial Hospital, St. Elizabeth Health Center, Western Reserve Care System, Salem Community Hospital, Aultman Hospital, Massillon Psychiatric Center, and Columbia Mercy Medical Center. In addition, students train at community-based centers that are part of the Area Health Education Center Program.

Students

Approximately 95 percent of students are Ohio residents. About 105 students in each class are admitted through the BS/MD program, and up to twenty-five of them are admitted through the traditional route. Although most entering students are in their early twenties, there are a few older or nontraditional students in each class. Underrepresented minorities account for about 4 percent of the student body.

STUDENT LIFE

Rootstown is a small town located about fifteen miles east of Akron. The medical school campus has recreation and exercise centers, student lounges, a picnic area, and tennis, basketball, and volleyball courts. Student groups include chapters of national medical student organizations, groups focused on professional interests, student-to-student support groups, and a recreation club. On-campus housing such as residence halls and apartments is available on all three campuses.

GRADUATES

NEOUCOM graduates usually score well above the national average on the USMLE. Of the 1,350 graduates currently in residency or practice, 55 percent of them have remained in Ohio. About half of all graduates enter primary care fields.

Admissions

REQUIREMENTS

Prerequisites are one year each of organic chemistry and physics, although success on the MCAT probably requires preparation in biology and general chemistry as well. The MCAT is required, and scores must be no more than two years old. For applicants who have retaken the exam, the most recent set of scores is considered. Therefore, there is no advantage to withholding scores.

SUGGESTIONS

Ohio residents are given strong preference in the admissions process, and slight preference is given to graduates of consortium schools. Highly qualified applicants are encouraged to apply to the early decision program. Beyond requirements, recommended course work includes biochemistry, calculus, community health, embryology, general biology, general chemistry, humanities, microbiology, molecular biology, physiology, psychology, sociology, and statistics. Applicants who have taken time off after college should show evidence of some recent course work.

PROCESS

High school students interested in the combined BS/ MD program apply in the fall of the senior year to NEUOCOM, and complete a condensed undergraduate experience at Kent State, University of Akron, or Youngstown State before arriving at the Rootstown campus. As a result of attrition from this program, a limited number of seats are available for college graduates who are interested in the four-year MD program. These applicants must apply through AMCAS. About 30 percent of AMCAS applicants are sent secondary applications, of which about 40 percent are interviewed between November and March. On interview day, candidates receive one interview with a panel of members of the Admissions Committee, a tour of the campus, lunch with current students, and a group informational session. Of interviewed candidates, about 10 percent are accepted on a rolling basis. Wait-listed candidates may update their files with transcripts.

Admissions Requirements (Required)

MCAT scores, science GPA, non-science GPA, letters of recommendation, interview, essays/personal statement.

Admissions Requirements (Optional)

state residency, extracurricular activities, exposure to medical profession.

COSTS AND AID

In-state tuition	$18,225
Out-of-state tuition	$33,993
Cost of books	$1,250
Fees	$1,004

Financial Aid

% students receiving aid	95
Average grant	$2,350
Average loan	$15,000
Average debt	$80,916

Northwestern University
Feinberg School of Medicine

Admissions, Room 606, 303 East Chicago Ave., Chicago, IL 60611-3008 • Admission: 312-503-8206 • Fax: 312-503-0550 • E-mail: med-admissions@northwestern.edu • Website: http://med-admissions.northwestern.edu

STUDENT BODY

Type	Private
Enrollment	696
% male/female	55/45
% underrepresented minorities	9
# applied (total)	6,054
# accepted (total/out)	322/255
# enrolled (total/out)	170/135
Average age	23

FACULTY

Total faculty (number)	3,265
% female	33
% minority	4
% part-time	51
# student/faculty ratio	4:1

ADMISSIONS

Average GPA and MCAT Scores

Overall GPA	3
MCAT Bio	11.3
MCAT Phys	11.6
MCAT Verbal	10.2
MCAT Essay	Q

Application Information

Regular application	10/15
Regular notification	12/15
Are transfers accepted?	Yes
Admissions may be deferred?	Yes
Interview required?	Yes
Application fee	$70

Academics

The medical curriculum retains the best aspects of traditional medical education and incorporates innovative, interactive methods designed for the independent adult learner. Students benefit from clinical exposure that begins on day one. Although most students complete studies in four years, some enter joint degree programs such as the MD/MPH and MD/MBA offered in conjunction with other graduate and professional schools at Northwestern. Qualified students who are interested in careers in medical research can pursue a PhD along with the MD in the medical scientist training program. A medical student research program facilitates the arrangement of post-first-year summer research experiences. Students are also encouraged to seek extended, yearlong research opportunities.

BASIC SCIENCES: The first- and second-year curriculum consists of four major courses, each presented in a series of discreet, topically focused units. Each course and nearly every unit is interdisciplinary and draws faculty from a number of departments. Two courses are in the basic medical sciences. Each involves approximately ten hours of lecture per week for the entire academic year, complemented by problem-based learning sessions, laboratories, and small group discussions and tutorials. Structure-function, the first-year course, begins with a review of cell and molecular biology, genetics, and signal transduction, then addresses gross and microscopic anatomy, biochemistry, and physiology in a consecutive sequence of organ systems. The scientific basis of medicine in the second year begins with an overview of immunology, microbiology, and infectious diseases and then details the pathology, pathophysiology, and pharmacology specific to each organ system. The medical decision-making course occupies three short blocks of time: the initial week of the first year, one week later in the first year, and the final portion of the second year. This innovative course allows students to develop the knowledge and skills in information management, epidemiology and biostatistics, and clinical problem solving essential to the contemporary practice of medicine. The patient, physician, and society course is devoted to the development of clinical skills and professional perspectives, and provides each student the opportunity to develop mentoring relationships with a variety of faculty preceptors. The class is divided into four colleges, each of which is led by an experienced clinician.

CLINICAL TRAINING

The third year consists of forty-nine weeks of required clerkships. Students gain experience in medicine (twelve weeks), surgery (twelve weeks), pediatrics (six weeks), obstetrics/gynecology (six weeks), psychiatry (four weeks), neurology (four weeks), and primary care (four weeks). A one-week introduction to clinical clerkships provides students with orientation to the clerkship teaching format. During the fourth year, students complete a six-week acting internship in medicine, pediatrics, or surgery and a two-week clerkship in physical medicine and rehabilitation. The remainder of the fourth year is elective. The majority of clinical rotations are taught at Northwestern Memorial Hospital, one of the major tertiary care facilities in Chicago. Other affiliated health care centers include the Rehabilitation Institute of Chicago, VA Chicago Health Care System, Evanston Northwestern Health Care, and Children's Memorial Hospital.

Students

The 170 students in Feinberg's entering class are usually approximately half women and half men. Ages have ranged from twenty to forty-five years old. For the last few years about one-fourth of each class has been made up of students who took off at least one year between undergraduate school and medical school matriculation. The student body usually represents students form nearly sixty undergraduate instituitions, over thirty states, and several foreign countries. The myriad of races and ethnicities are seen in the classes.

STUDENT LIFE

Northwestern students spend less time in class than students at many other schools and more time in outside preparation and group and independent learning. Students are also encouraged to pursue supplemental academic interests, community service endeavors, and other activities. The school's location, in one of the most vibrant cities in the country, is an important asset. A good public transportation system makes Chicago's museums, shopping areas, parks, restaurants, clubs, theaters, and other attractions easily accessible.

GRADUATES

Northwestern graduates are accepted to competitive residencies throughout the nation. Today, there are more than 12,000 medical school alumni living in the United States and around the world. Northwestern alumni are particularly well represented in academic medicine.

Admissions

REQUIREMENTS

At minimum, one full year of biology, organic chemistry, and physics (all with required labs) and one year of English are recommended. However, students accepted to Feinberg have traditionally gone beyond the recommended course work and taken additional science courses in preparation for the rigors of the medical school curriculum. The MCAT with scores not more than three years old and exposure to clinical medicine and/or community service are required.

SUGGESTIONS

Feinberg looks for students who have strong academic performance, a demonstrated motivation for a career in medicine, and a well-rounded and distinguished background. Applicants who have involved themselves in research, majored in nonscience areas, and have had varied life experiences are appreciated.

PROCESS

Approximately 70 percent of AMCAS applicants who apply to Feinberg are sent a supplemental application, of which about 10 percent are interviewed between October and March. The medical school uses a combined interview approach, both individual and panel interview. The individual interview is conducted by a member of the dean's administration or admissions committee, and the panel is conducted by three members of the interview committee (usually two faculty and one medical student). Three to four candidates are interviewed in a panel. The interview day further includes a campus tour, lunch, and a financial aid session. Notification of final decisions occurs two to three times during the interview season. Applicants are accepted, declined, or placed on an alternate waiting list.

Admissions Requirements (Required)

MCAT scores, science GPA, non-science GPA, letters of recommendation, interview, essays/personal statement, extracurricular activities, exposure to medical profession.

Admissions Requirements (Optional)

state residency.

Overlap Schools

Case Western Reserve University, Columbia University, Rush Medical College of Rush University, University of Chicago, University of Illinois at Chicago, University of Michigan, Washington University.

COSTS AND AID

Tuition	$34,998
Room and board	$11,862
Cost of books	$2,529
Fees	$2,020

Financial Aid

% students receiving aid	67
Average grant	$16,705
Average loan	$38,653
Average debt	$86,174

Ohio State University

College of Medicine and Public Health

209 Meiling Hall, 370 West 9th Avenue, Columbus, OH 43210 • Admission: 614-292-7137 • Fax: 614-247-7959 • E-mail: medicine@osu.edu • Website: http://medicine.osu.edu

STUDENT BODY

Type	Public
Enrollment	839
% male/female	57/43
% underrepresented minorities	26
# applied (total/out)	3,276/2,275
# accepted (total/out)	369/167
# enrolled (total/out)	210/80
Average age	22

FACULTY

Total faculty (number)	2,511
% female	28
% minority	19
% part-time	42
# student/faculty ratio	1:1

ADMISSIONS

Average GPA and MCAT Scores

Overall GPA	3.6
MCAT Bio	10.8
MCAT Phys	10.6
MCAT Verbal	9.9
MCAT Essay	P

Application Information

Regular application	11/1
Regular notification	10/15
Early application	8/1
Early notification	10/1
Are transfers accepted?	Yes
Admissions may be deferred?	Yes
Interview required?	Yes
Application fee	$60

Academics

As part of one of the most comprehensive health science campuses in the nation, Ohio State offers medical students great opportunities and flexibility. Students train alongside research faculty who are unlocking the promise of the human genome to attack diseases such as cancer and Parkinson's disease. They don't just read about tomorrow's technologies; they employ them every day in their training. Ohio State students see the spectrum of pathology—the common and the rare—in rural family practice clinics and robotic surgical suites. They expand their education to the global classroom by immersing themselves in international health programs.

BASIC SCIENCES: In the first year at Ohio State, students study gross anatomy and embryology as part of a six-member student team during the first twelve weeks of medical school. After anatomy, students choose one of two curricular pathways to learn about the body systems: integrated pathway or the independent study pathway. The integrated pathway features body systems oriented content that fuses the basic and clinical sciences. It combined the proven educational methods of student centered active learning, small group case-based discussion, and lectures. The independent study pathway allows students to utilize highly structured objectives, resource guides, and Web- and computer-based materials to learn on their own. Patient centered medicine and physician development are courses that are also taken regardless of the pathway selected. These courses combine small group roleplaying settings, lectures, and experiences with senior citizens and physicians in the community.

CLINICAL TRAINING

Ohio State has a strong reputation for rigorous clinical training programs and breadth of educational settings. In the first year, students might choose to do their community project at a retirement community, free clinic, or homeless shelter; they may also choose to do their project with the Alzheimer's Association, the OSU High Risk Perinatal Teen Program, or the Columbus Health Department. Physician development and patient centered medicine spans both the Med 1 and Med 2 years. These courses provide students with the opportunity to gain clinical experiences early in their education and master skills prior to the clinical years. During the third year of medical school, students spend twelve months in a range of experiences, including ambulatory primary care medicine, obstetrics and gynecology, surgery, internal medicine, psychiatry, neurology, and pediatrics. The fourth year of medical school features four differentiation of care selectives (DOCS) covering the undifferentiated patient, chronic care, subinternship in internal medicine, and a subinternship in surgical care. Students have great flexibility in the fourth year, with four months of elective rotations and three months of vacation.

Students

Columbus is Ohio's largest city and one of the fastest growing metropolitan areas in the United States. As Ohio's capital, Columbus offers great diversity in the arts, cultural events, festivals, restaurants, sports, and nightlife, all of which are within close proximity to the medical center. Arts and leisure activities range from the avant garde Short North Gallery Hops to nationally acclaimed performances by the Columbus Symphony Orchestra, Ballet Met, and Opera Columbus. Columbus offers a fresh blend of clubs, concerts, comedy, Broadway productions, and movies.

STUDENT LIFE

Receiving a medical education at Ohio State connects students to one of the United State's great institutions of higher learning. Founded in 1870, The Ohio State University has one of the nation's largest single college campus enrollments and, more importantly, the vast resources that go with it. In the College of Medicine, there are student chapters of all of the national medical groups, plus an assortment of others, including COMA (Comedy to Overcome Medical Anxiety); Medical Scientist Student Organization; mEDnOTES, a student-directed a cappella vocal group; and Student Council. Students have over forty choices of extracurricular activities just within the medical rubric.

GRADUATES

College of Medicine students receive not only excellent training in the basic sciences but also have a large amount of patient responsibility during their third and fourth years of medical school. The rigorous training program and breadth of educational settings prepare Ohio State students for selection to competitive residency programs across the country. Nearly 90 percent of residency program directors surveyed nationally rate Ohio State College of Medicine graduate better prepared for residency than graduates of other medical schools. Graduates match is a wide variety of disciplines, including family medicine, general internal medicine, pediatrics, obstetrics and gynecology, surgery, orthopedic surgery, and ophthalmology.

Admissions

REQUIREMENTS

Applicants are expected to embody high ethical standards, especially honesty and concern for others, and must be free of substance abuse, addictions, and violent behaviors. Applicants must also possess the skills required to practice direct patient care. No specific undergraduate curriculum or college major is required, but the following science courses are required: general chemistry with qualitative analysis, organic chemistry with laboratory, physics with laboratory, and biology (each should be a full academic year or equivalent sequence).

SUGGESTIONS

In addition to the required courses, course work in biochemistry or cellular and molecular biology is strongly recommended. We encourage applicants to include such subjects as philosophy, literature, writing, history, arts, and languages in their traditional premedical curriculum.

PROCESS

Application is initiated through the American Medical College Application Service (AMCAS), available online at www.aamc.org/students/applying/. Students designating The Ohio State University on the AMCAS application will receive information directing them to the Web-based secondary application. AMCAS applications are accepted from June 1 to November 1 of the year prior to anticipated matriculation.

Admissions Requirements (Required)

MCAT scores, science GPA, non-science GPA, letters of recommendation, interview, essays/personal statement, extracurricular activities, exposure to medical profession.

Admissions Requirements (Optional)

state residency.

COSTS AND AID

In-state tuition	$19,323
Out-of-state tuition	$25,462
Room and board	$6,850
Cost of books	$4,326

Financial Aid

% students receiving aid	98
Average grant	$4,465
Average loan	$33,935
Average debt	$79,527

OREGON HEALTH & SCIENCE UNIVERSITY

SCHOOL OF MEDICINE

OFFICE OF EDUCATION AND STUDENT AFFAIRS, 3181 SW SAM JACKSON PARK ROAD, L102, PORTLAND, OR 97239 • ADMISSION: 503-494-2998 • FAX: 503-494-3400 • E-MAIL: MDADMISS@OHSU.EDU • WEBSITE: WWW.OHSU.EDU/SOM/

STUDENT BODY

Type	Public
Enrollment	396
% male/female	52/48
% underrepresented minorities	14
# applied (total/out)	2,693/2,406
# accepted (total/out)	184/110
# enrolled (total/out)	104/47
Average age	25

FACULTY

Total faculty (number)	1,066
% female	40
% minority	3
% part-time	4
# student/faculty ratio	4:1

ADMISSIONS

Average GPA and MCAT Scores

Overall GPA	3.6
MCAT Bio	10.16
MCAT Phys	10.2
MCAT Verbal	10.15
MCAT Essay	P

Application Information

Regular application	10/15
Regular notification	Rolling
Are transfers accepted?	Yes
Admissions may be deferred?	No
Interview required?	Yes
Application fee	$75

Academics

Although most students complete a four-year MD curriculum, others follow alternative courses of study, including joint degree programs. The five-year MD/MPH degree program is offered by the School of Medicine's Department of Public Health and Preventive Medicine in conjunction with appropriate departments at Oregon State University and Portland State University. Generally, students indicate their interest in this program when they apply to the School of Medicine. First-year medical students may pursue an epidemiological and biostatistical track, which also serves as preparation for careers in public health. The joint degree program is the MS/PhD in the following fields: biochemistry and molecular biology, cell biology and anatomy, molecular and medical genetics, medical psychology, molecular microbiology and immunology, pharmacology and physiology, and neuroscience. Grades of honors, near honors, satisfactory, marginal, and fail are used to evaluate medical students. Taking both steps of the USMLE are a requirement for graduation.

BASIC SCIENCES: Students spend two hours per day in lecture. An additional two hours each day are used for small group sessions and/or laboratory activities. One afternoon each week is devoted to principles of clinical medicine in which students work one-on-one with physicians and spend an additional afternoon studying issues related to public health, behavioral sciences, history-taking, and learning physical diagnosis skills. First-year courses are anatomy, embryology, and imaging; cell structure and function; systems process and homeostasis; biological basis of disease; and principles of clinical medicine, which continues into the second year. The second year is organized around organ systems and physiological concepts, which include blood, circulation, neuroscience and behavior, metabolism, and human development and life cycle. The first two years are spent largely in the basic sciences and education buildings, which have facilities for lectures, discussions, computer learning, and laboratories. The library contains over 150,000 volumes and 2,500 periodicals.

CLINICAL TRAINING

Required third-year rotations are transition to clerkship (one week), medicine (twelve weeks), primary care (six weeks), obstetrics/gynecology (six weeks), child health (six weeks), psychiatry (six weeks), family medicine (six weeks), and surgery (six weeks). During the fourth year, students fulfill advanced clerkship requirements in medicine, surgery, child health, and neurology (four weeks each) in addition to selectives and electives. The fourth year culminates in transition to physician, a weeklong experience. Clinical training takes place at the University Hospital and Clinics and at affiliated institutions, which include Doernbecher Children's Hospital and Portland's Veterans' Affairs Medical Center. The School of Medicine's research touches all realms of modern medical sciences. Some students investigate the causes and treatments of learning disorders, addiction, heart disease, stroke, cancer, infertility, movement disorders, and emotional disorders. Other students work at the molecular and cellular levels to unravel the most basic aspects of human health.

Students

About 6 percent of students at OHSU are from underrepresented minority backgrounds. The average age of incoming students is around twenty-five. Class size is ninety-six.

STUDENT LIFE

Portland is an ideal location for students because it offers the comforts of a midsize city that is located near spectacular outdoor destinations. Close to campus are parks and other places where students can run, walk, or ride bikes. A bit further are mountains for hiking and skiing. For an urban area, Portland is relatively affordable and safe. On-campus activities are also popular with medical students. The newly renovated Fitness and Sports Center includes a full weight room, racquetball and squash courts, aerobics classes, swimming pools, and a spa. The Office of Multicultural Affairs supports students of ethnic and international backgrounds with supplemental counseling services, recreational activities, workshops, and classes. Numerous clubs and organizations bring students together around professional or extracurricular interests. Although student housing is available on a limited basis in the residence halls, most students opt to live off campus.

GRADUATES

Graduates are successful in securing residency positions at prestigious institutions all over the United States. However, most of them enter programs in the Western United States. Over half of them enter primary care residencies.

Admissions

REQUIREMENTS

Required courses are chemistry/organic chemistry (two years), biology (one year), physics (one year), college-level math (one semester), English (one year), humanities (one year), and social science (one year). GPAs from all four year undergraduate institutions are evaluated equally, although factors such as the breadth of education, rigor of major, GPA trends, course load, and extracurricular activities are considered. The MCAT is required, and scores must be from within three years of the year of matriculation.

SUGGESTIONS

Preference is given to residents of Oregon and certified WICHE states. Applicants with exceptional qualifications, applicants from underrepresented ethnic/racial groups, and applicants to the MS/PhD and MD/MPH programs are considered even if they are not residents of preferred states. For students who apply to the MS/PhD program, advanced course work in chemistry and biology and courses in psychology and statistics are recommended, in addition to requirements for MD/MPH. It is important for all applicants to show some medically related experience.

PROCESS

About half of all AMCAS applicants receive secondaries, and about 40 percent of candidates in this group are interviewed. Interviews consist of two thirty-minute sessions with members of the faculty or Admissions Committee. Interviewees are invited to lunch with medical students and are given a tour of the campus. Approximately 20 percent of interviewees are accepted on a rolling basis. Wait-listed candidates are ranked and have a fairly good chance of being accepted later in the spring.

Admissions Requirements (Required)

MCAT scores, science GPA, non-science GPA, letters of recommendation, interview, essays/personal statement, extracurricular activities, exposure to medical profession.

Admissions Requirements (Optional)

state residency, Preference is given to Oregon residents.

Overlap Schools

University of Washington.

COSTS AND AID

In-state tuition	$21,000
Out-of-state tuition	$31,500
Cost of books	$2,800
Fees	$3,517

Financial Aid

% students receiving aid	90
Average grant	$2,000
Average loan	$30,000
Average debt	$112,000

PENNSYLVANIA STATE UNIVERSITY
COLLEGE OF MEDICINE

OFFICE OF STUDENT AFFAIRS, PO BOX 850, HERSHEY, PA 17033 • ADMISSION: 717-531-8755 • FAX: 717-531-6225 • E-MAIL: HMCSAFF@PSU.EDU • WEBSITE: WWW.HMC.PSU.EDU/

STUDENT BODY

Type	Private
Enrollment	423
% male/female	56/44
% underrepresented minorities	28
# applied (total/out)	6,615/5,509
# accepted (total/out)	8/6
# enrolled (out)	15
Average age	23

FACULTY

Total faculty (number)	155
% female	18
% minority	23

ADMISSIONS

Application Information

Regular application	11/15
Regular notification	10/1 until filled
Early application	6/1-8/1
Early notification	10/1
Are transfers accepted?	Yes
Admissions may be deferred?	Yes
Interview required?	No
Application fee	$40

Academics

Penn State was one of the first medical schools in the country to institute departments of humanities and behavioral science and to incorporate these perspectives into the basic science and clinical education programs. The College of Medicine was also among the first to develop a separate family and community medicine department. The college offers a combined MS/PhD program that allows students to earn the doctoral degree in biochemistry, biomedical engineering, cell biology, genetics, immunology, microbiology, molecular biology, pharmacology, and physiology. There are also numerous opportunities for students to pursue discreet research projects as electives or during summers. Grades of honors, high pass, pass, and fail are used to evaluate medical students. Students must pass USMLE Step 1 after the preclinical years and Step 2 to graduate.

BASIC SCIENCES: During the first and second years, students are in class or other scheduled sessions for approximately twenty-three hours per week. This schedule gives students the opportunity for independent and collaborative study. Clinical problems are used as a means of applying and correlating the basic science information that is presented in lectures or discussions. Labs and computer-assisted learning are also important parts of the curriculum. First-year courses are structural basis of medical practice; cellular and molecular basis of medical practice; biological basis of disease; and physicians, patients and society, which touches on the psychological, social, ethical, legal, and humanistic aspects of medicine. Second-year courses are pharmacology, microbiology, immunology, psychiatry, pathology, introduction to medicine III and IV, physical diagnosis, and issues in medical practice. Instruction takes place in the medical sciences building, which houses classrooms and laboratories. The Harrell Library is open twenty-four hours a day, and holds approximately 125,000 volumes and 2,000 periodicals, in addition to modern computer and audiovisual resources.

CLINICAL TRAINING

Third-year required clerkships are internal medicine (eight weeks), surgery (eight weeks), pediatrics (six weeks), obstetrics/gynecology (six weeks), psychiatry (four weeks), family and community medicine (four weeks), selectives (eight weeks), and primary care (four weeks). The fourth year is devoted to electives and selectives, which are chosen from clinical or research departments. An overseas elective program allows a number of fourth-year students to fulfill elective requirements at clinical sites in Asia, Africa, and Latin America. Generally, clinical training takes place at the University Hospital (463 beds), Children's Hospital, the Rehabilitation Center, and at other hospitals and clinics affiliated through an organized health network called Alliance Health. Additional facilities on campus are a sports medicine center, the general clinical research center, an animal research center, and a trauma center.

Students

About 40 percent of students are Pennsylvania residents. Over 25 percent of students are underrepresented minorities, a tribute to the school's commitment to recruiting a diverse student body. The average age of incoming students is twenty-three, with a wide age range. Class size is 110.

STUDENT LIFE

Educational facilities, clinical teaching sites, campus housing, and recreational centers are within walking distance of one another. The College of Medicine is an attractive campus, occupying 550 acres. Hershey provides a comfortable, student friendly community that is relatively safe. As a tourist destination, Hershey offers a variety of dining and entertainment possibilities. Medical students are involved in organizations such as honor societies, professional interest groups, local chapters of national organizations, and groups focused on community service or recreational pursuits. When in need of urban distractions, the state capital, Harrisburg, is twelve miles away, and both Philadelphia and Pittsburgh are easily accessible. On-campus housing options include one-, two-, and three-bedroom apartments.

GRADUATES

Graduates are successful at securing residencies nationwide. Penn State emphasizes primary care and encourages students to consider post-graduate training programs in primary care fields.

Admissions

REQUIREMENTS

Prerequisites are one year each of biology, physics, chemistry, organic chemistry, and college-level math. All science courses should have associated labs. One semester each of social sciences and humanities is also required. The MCAT is required, and scores must be no more than two years old. For applicants who have retaken the exam, all sets of scores are considered.

SUGGESTIONS

Beyond requirements, course work in calculus, psychology, statistics, sociology, genetics, and anthropology are recommended. The college advises candidates to submit the April MCAT scores over the August one. Health care related experience is valued, as are interpersonal and communication skills. State residency is not a consideration in the application process.

PROCESS

All AMCAS applicants are sent secondary applications, of which about 10 percent are interviewed between September and March. Interviews consist of two or three sessions each with a faculty member. On interview day, candidates also tour the campus and have lunch with current medical students. About one-third of interviewees are accepted on a rolling basis. Another group is wait-listed. Wait-listed candidates are not encouraged to send supplementary material.

Admissions Requirements (Required)

MCAT scores, essays/personal statement, extracurricular activities, exposure to medical profession.

Admissions Requirements (Optional)

science GPA, nonscience GPA, letters of recommendation, interview, state residency.

COSTS AND AID

Room and board	$6,144
Cost of books	$1,205

Financial Aid

% students receiving aid	91
Average grant	$10,248
Average loan	$23,500
Average debt	$98,061

Ponce School of Medicine

School of Medicine

PO Box 7004, Ponce, PR 00732 • Admission: 787-840-2575

STUDENT BODY

Type	Private
# applied (total/out)	729/408
# accepted (total/out)	144/36

ADMISSIONS

Average GPA and MCAT Scores

Overall GPA	3.4
MCAT Bio	6.7
MCAT Phys	6.7
MCAT Verbal	7.2
MCAT Essay	K

Application Information

Regular application	12/1
Regular notification	rolling
Are transfers accepted?	No
Admissions may be deferred?	No
Interview required?	Yes
Application fee	$50

Academics

The primary goal of the School of Medicine is to provide quality medical education to bilingual students, with an emphasis on primary care and family medicine. The curriculum includes a strong emphasis on basic sciences, which enables students to get the most out of their clinical training. Longitudinal programs in preventive medicine and medical ethics are integrated into the four-year curriculum.

BASIC SCIENCES: Basic sciences are taught during the first two years. Year one courses include gross anatomy imaging and embryology, cellular biology and histology, neuroscience, biochemistry, microbiology and immunology, behavioral science, physiology, general pathology, bioethics, human genetics, and a yearlong session devoted to clinical correlation. Second year courses are pathophysiology, pathology, pharmacology, psychiatry, introduction to clinical medicine, infectious diseases, family and community medicine, and bioethics. Instructional methods include computer-assisted learning, lectures, labs, and problem-based learning. Standardized patients are used for teaching and evaluation of basic clinical skills. During the first two years, students are in class or other scheduled sessions for about thirty hours per week. Students must pass Step I of the USMLE for promotion to year three.

CLINICAL TRAINING

The third year begins in July with two weeks of a course called introduction to hospital life. After this orientation, students begin the following required clerkships: internal medicine (ten weeks), surgery (ten weeks), pediatrics (ten weeks), obstetrics/gynecology (five weeks), psychiatry (five weeks), and family medicine (five weeks). The third year also includes a Dean's Hour, which emphasizes medical humanities, health economics, law, bioethics, and literature. In the fourth year, students participate in a required clerkship in medicine (four weeks), a sub-internship (medicine, obstetrics/gynecology, pediatrics, or family medicine), a clerkship in emergency medicine (four weeks), and a primary care selective (four weeks). Students are also required to complete sixteen weeks of elective rotations, of which five weeks may be completed at sites other than Ponce. USMLE Step II must be passed prior to graduation.

STUDENT LIFE

The relatively small class size of sixty students encourages communication between students and faculty. The school's location is an asset because it offers a pleasant environment for living and studying.

REQUIREMENTS

Required undergraduate course work includes eight semester credits in biology, general chemistry, organized chemistry, and physics in addition to six credits in advanced math and Spanish. Twelve credits in both behavioral sciences and English are also required. Behavioral science includes psychology, sociology, anthropology, political sciences, economics, and anthropology. Applicants must have a minimum overall grade point average of 2.7 and an average of 2.5 in science courses. The MCAT is required, and scores should be from within one year of application. Applicants should have at least the mean score on all sections of the MCAT.

SUGGESTIONS

In evaluating applicants, the Admissions Committee considers academic achievements, MCAT scores, interview reports, letters of recommendation, and other supplementary information. Preference is given to residents of Puerto Rico.

PROCESS

Ponce takes part in the AMCAS application process. The deadline for submission to AMCAS is December 15. Secondary applications are sent to all qualified applicants, and interviews are conducted throughout the spring.

Admissions Requirements (Required)

interview.

Admissions Requirements (Optional)

MCAT scores, science GPA, non-science GPA, letters of recommendation, state residency, essays/personal statement, extracurricular activities, exposure to medical profession.

COSTS AND AID

Tuition	$25,304
Fees	$1,761

Financial Aid

Average grant	$8,000
Average loan	$35,954
Average debt	$96,931

QUEEN'S UNIVERSITY
SCHOOL OF MEDICINE

68 BARRIE STREET, KINGSTON, ON K7L 3N6 • ADMISSION: 613-533-2542 • FAX: 613-533-6190 •
E-MAIL: JEB8@POST.QUEENSU.CA • WEBSITE: HTTP://MEDS.QUEENSU.CA

STUDENT BODY

Type	Public
Enrollment	100
% male/female	52/48
% underrepresented minorities	2
# applied (total)	1,388
# accepted (total)	175
# enrolled (total)	100

ADMISSIONS

Average GPA and MCAT Scores

Overall GPA	3.6
MCAT Bio	11
MCAT Phys	11.11
MCAT Verbal	10.84
MCAT Essay	P

Application Information

Regular application	10/1
Regular notification	5/31
Are transfers accepted?	No
Admissions may be deferred?	Yes
Interview required?	Yes
Application fee	$250

Academics

Most students follow a four-year curriculum leading to an MD degree. Master's and doctoral degree programs are also offered in biochemistry, biostatistics, environmental and occupational health, epidemiology, general community health, health care systems, pathology, and preventive medicine. Although there are no formally structured combined programs, superior students may be permitted the flexibility to work toward an MSc or a PhD concurrently with the MD. Grades of honors, pass, and fail are used to evaluate medical students.

BASIC SCIENCES: Most basic science instruction takes place during the first three years. First-year course starts with phase I, introduction to the sciences relevant to medicine, an introduction to the fundamental language and concepts of medical science, and communication/clinical skills. Phase IIA includes dermatology/musculoskeletal systems, hematology and oncology, microbiology and infectious diseases, allergy and immunology, and clinical skills. Second-year courses are psychiatry/neuroscience/ophthalmology/ent, genitourinary/cardiovascular/respirology, and clinical skills. In addition, eight weeks are left open for an elective. Third-year courses are endocrine/metabolism/reproduction, gastrointestinal, and clinical skills. In addition to problem-based learning, teaching methods include lectures, seminars, small group discussions, laboratory experience, and computer-based instruction. Basic science instruction takes place primarily at Botterell Hall, which also houses administrative offices and Bracken Library. The Clinical Learning Center is an important educational facility within the Faculty of Health Sciences specifically designed for the teaching, learning, and evaluation of important clinical skills, and is used during both preclinical and clinical years. The Health Sciences Library subscribes to approximately 844 serials and its total collection consists of 156,000 volumes. In the library is the Multimedia Learning Center, which offers both video- and computer-assisted instruction.

CLINICAL TRAINING

Clerkships begin in January of the third year. They are medicine (twelve weeks), surgery (eight weeks), psychiatry (six weeks), obstetrics/gynecology (six weeks), pediatrics (six weeks), family medicine (four weeks), geriatrics (two weeks), and emergency medicine (two weeks). Four weeks of selectives and twelve weeks of electives are also required. Clerkships takes place at a number of affiliated hospitals including Kingston General Hospital, Hotel Dieu Hospital, St. Mary's of the Lake Hospital, Kingston Psychiatric Hospital, and Ongwanada Hospital. The provision of health care services in Kingston is presently being restructured and will change over the next few years.

Students

Each class has ninety students, about fifty of whom are typically from the province of Ontario. The student body is approximately 50 percent women.

STUDENT LIFE

Medical students enjoy the recreational, cultural, and social activities of the greater university and the city of Kingston. On-campus attractions include museums, concert halls, cinema, and an observatory. Student services include a child care resource center, a foundation supporting women, comprehensive health services, an international center, a physical education center and a student center. The university provides accommodations in single and double occupancy rooms for approximately 300 graduate students. In addition, the Apartment and Housing office manages university-owned rentals in the area.

Admissions

REQUIREMENTS

To apply, students must have completed three years of full-time study at a university. In addition, one year each of Biological sciences, physical sciences, and humanities/social sciences are required. The MCAT is required. To be eligible for admission, applicants must be Canadian citizens, Canadian permanent residents, or children of Queen's University alumni.

SUGGESTIONS

The Admissions Committee looks for both academic abilities such as commitment, achievement, critical thinking, and self directed learning, and personal characteristics such as communication skills, creativity, and sensitivity. No preference is given to a particular undergraduate program of studies, and college students who seek admission are encouraged to pursue studies in their area of interest.

PROCESS

Applicants who seek further information about admission should contact the School of Medicine. Applications are made through Ontario Medical School's Application Service, 70 Research Lane, Guelph, Ontario N1G 5E2. The deadline is October 15. The first admissions cutoff is based on the cumulative converted grade point average, and the second is made on the basis of MCAT scores. Applicants who qualify are interviewed. Applicants are then ranked according to evaluation of letters of reference, autobiographic sketch, and interview results.

Admissions Requirements (Required)

MCAT scores, science GPA, non-science GPA, letters of recommendation, interview, essays/personal statement, extracurricular activities.

Overlap Schools

McMaster University, University of Ottawa, University of Toronto, University of Western Ontario.

COSTS AND AID

Tuition	$13,500

Ross University
School of Medicine

499 Thornall Street, 10th Floor, Edison, NJ 08837 • Admission: 732-978-5300 • Fax: 732-978-5304 •
E-mail: admission@rossmed.edu • Website: www.rossmed.edu

STUDENT BODY

Type	Private
Enrollment	2,012
% male/female	60/40
% underrepresented minorities	30
# applied (total)	1,054
# accepted (total)	491
# enrolled (total)	301
Average age	26

FACULTY

# student/faculty ratio	17:1

ADMISSIONS

Average GPA and MCAT Scores

Overall GPA	3.2
MCAT Bio	7
MCAT Phys	6.8
MCAT Verbal	6.4
MCAT Essay	N

Application Information

Regular application	rolling
Regular notification	rolling
Are transfers accepted?	Yes
Admissions may be deferred?	Yes
Interview required?	Yes
Application fee	$75

Academics

Ross University challenges and empowers students to achieve their full professional and personal potential as physicians. In accordance with this philosophy, the School of Medicine was established to teach qualified students who are pursuing a medical curriculum patterned on the type offered in the United States.

The Ross University School of Medicine's (RUSM) objective is to provide an educational program that incorporates the best features of Western medical education. Courses are taught in English by experienced faculty members recruited primarily from medical schools in the United States and the United Kingdom.

BASIC SCIENCES: The basic science segment offers an in-depth, comprehensive program of basic medical sciences that have traditionally been deemed appropriate for future medical practitioners and is completed by passing the NBME Basic Sciences Comprehensive Examination. It provides clinical correlations and examples of clinical relevance throughout the instructional program in sciences and presents a physical diagnosis course that provides the practical experience needed by students to adequately prepare for their clerkships.

CLINICAL TRAINING

Ross University has over forty affiliated teaching hospitals throughout the United States for core rotations and many more for electives. As a result, RUSM has the largest United States clinical presence of any foreign medical school. The majority of third and fourth year students complete their entire clinical program in United States teaching hospitals. RUSM also maintains a clinical program in Dominica at Princess Margaret Hospital.

Ross University maintains clinical affiliations with hospitals in the states of California, Connecticut, Florida, Illinois, Massachusetts, Maryland, Missouri, New Jersey, New York, Ohio, and Washington, DC.

Students

The university's basic science campus is located in the country of Dominica, West Indies—not the Dominican Republic. Dominica is a beautiful, English-speaking island in the Caribbean. Ross University's administrative headquarters is located in New York City. Ross University also maintains regional offices in Florida, California, and Michigan. The university does not have a dormitory. Housing in Dominica is plentiful and is available close to campus. Housing ranges from apartment-style units to dorm-like facilities. We always recommend that our students visit the housing website at www.rossmed.edu.dm so they can view current samples of available housing; they can also contact Joy Adrian, the housing director, at 767-445-5355.

STUDENT LIFE

Dominica is known for some of the best snorkeling and scuba diving in the world. Simple hiking may be the most chosen activity of those who truly appreciate the beauty of the island. If you would just like to relax, the Student Government Association recently opened a new lounge with cable television, foosball, air hockey, ping-pong, pool, and two Sony Playstations. Students participate in weight lifting, aerobics, volleyball, tennis, football, basketball, Frisbee, and baseball.

GRADUATES

To be eligible for residency programs, which usually begin on July 1 of every year, students must graduate by June and have their Educational Commission for Foreign Medical Graduates (ECFMG) certification in hand by June 30 of that year. Most residency programs accept applications from August to December for entry the following July. Non-U.S. citizens who are not permanent residents must obtain the appropriate visa to be eligible for U.S. residencies. A major avenue to securing a residency position is participation in the National Resident Matching Program (NRMP). Students and graduates of RUSM who are seeking post-graduate residency positions in the United States are eligible to enroll with the NRMP, provided that they have submitted proof of having passed the examinations required to obtain certification from the ECFMG by February of the relevant year. ECFMG certification must be obtained before residency training can begin. The NRMP matches applicants with appropriate institutions offering residency positions. Approximately one year prior to graduation from Ross University, students need to begin planning for the residency process. The Department of Graduate Affairs is dedicated to helping students through this process.

Admissions

REQUIREMENTS

Applicants who have completed their undergraduate studies in countries that have an educational system different from that of the United States will be evaluated on their merits but will be expected to have completed a pre-medical curriculum comparable to that described above. All required documents, if originally in a foreign language, must be accompanied by a notarized English translation. All transcripts documenting post-secondary course work completed in institutions outside the United States must also be evaluated by an approved international credential evaluation service. Contact the Admissions Office for more information on these matters. Applicants who present less than sixty upper-division credits from an English language college or university must provide the official record of the scores for the Test of English as a Foreign Language (TOEFL). The minimum acceptable score is 550 on the paper-based test or 213 on the computer-based test. The Ross University TOEFL Institutional code number is #9614. Ross University requires that MCAT scores be submitted by the applicant prior to enrollment. Applicants who have retaken the test must submit all the results prior to enrollment. The Ross University code number is #906. MCAT scores are not an admissions requirement, but accepted applicants must submit MCAT scores before they are allowed to register for classes. Inquiries concerning application, test dates, and locations for the MCAT should be directed to the following:

Medical College Admission Test Registration
The American College Testing Program
PO Box 4056
Iowa City, IA 52243
319-337-1357

Admissions Requirements (Required)

MCAT scores, science GPA, non-science GPA, letters of recommendation, interview, essays/personal statement.

Admissions Requirements (Optional)

state residency, extracurricular activities, exposure to medical profession.

Overlap Schools

Boston University, SUNY at Stony Brook, University of Florida, University of Illinois at Chicago, University of Miami.

COSTS AND AID

Tuition	$20,280
Cost of books	$1,700

Financial Aid

% students receiving aid	85

Rush Medical College of Rush University

Rush Medical College

Office of Admissions, 524 AAC, 600 South Paulina Street, Suite 440, Chicago, IL 60612 • Admission: 312-942-6913 • Fax: 312-942-2333 • E-mail: RMC_Admissions@rush.edu • Website: www.rushu.rush.edu

STUDENT BODY

Type	Private
# applied (total)	2,023
# accepted (total)	290
# enrolled (total/out)	120/25
Average age	23

ADMISSIONS

Average GPA and MCAT Scores

Overall GPA	3.5
MCAT Bio	10
MCAT Phys	10
MCAT Verbal	9.5
MCAT Essay	P

Application Information

Regular application	11/15
Regular notification	Rolling
Early application	6/1-8/1
Early notification	10/1
Are transfers accepted?	No
Admissions may be deferred?	Yes
Interview required?	Yes
Application fee	$65

Academics

Students follow a four-year curriculum, except those who are pursuing a PhD along with the MD degree. Joint MS/PhD programs are offered in many disciplines, including anatomy, biochemistry, immunology, microbiology, neuroscience, pharmacology, and physiology. Medical students are evaluated with honors, pass, and fail. Passing the USMLE Step 1 is a requirement for promotion to year three. Entering students are assigned a faculty member as an academic adviser to assist with education and career development.

BASIC SCIENCES: Students learn basic sciences through the traditional curriculum, which relies on lectures and labs for instruction, or the alternate curriculum, which is entirely case-based and emphasizes self directed learning and problem solving skills. About twenty-four students enter the alternate curriculum each year. All students participate in the generalist curriculum, which involves one-on-one mentorships with physician preceptors. Topics covered in the first year are anatomy, behavioral science, biochemistry, ethics and law in medicine, histology, neurobiology, physiology, general pathology, health and the public, primary care preceptorship, physical diagnosis, and interviewing and communication. Second-year subjects are psychopathlogy, clinical pathophysiology, pathology, pharmacology, preventive medicine, immunology, microbiology, primary care preceptorship, physical diagnosis, and interviewing and communication. To enhance classroom instruction, the McCormick Learning Resource Center offers audiovisual and computer-based learning aids. Academic Computer Resources operates a personal computer laboratory and a computer-assisted instruction laboratory that is available twenty-four hours a day. The tutoring program provides additional instruction and study tips from faculty, classmates, or upper-class students.

CLINICAL TRAINING

All students fulfill the same clerkship requirements during the third and fourth years. Third-year rotations are internal medicine (twelve weeks), surgery (twelve weeks), obstetrics/gynecology (eight weeks), pediatrics (eight weeks), psychiatry (six weeks), family practice (six weeks), and neurology (four weeks). Fourth-year students participate in an advanced, primary care subinternship and choose from family medicine, internal medicine, or pediatrics (four weeks). At least eighteen weeks are reserved for electives. Most clinical training takes place at Rush-Presbyterian-St. Luke's Hospital (903 beds), a nonprofit hospital with over thirty specialty areas. Other affiliated institutions in urban, suburban, and rural locations are Illinois Masonic Medical Center, Rush North Shore Medical Center, Rush-Prudential Health Plans, Cook County Hospital, Hinsdale Hospital, LaGrange Memorial Hospital, MacNeal Memorial Hospital, and Westlake Hospital.

Students

Approximately 85 percent of students are Illinois residents. About 10 percent of students are underrepresented minorities, and about 30 percent are older or nontraditional, since they have taken time off between college and medical school. Class size is 120.

STUDENT LIFE

Student life, both on and off campus, is varied and exciting. Campus facilities are designed to encourage student interaction. For example, student lounges provide space for socializing, relaxing between classes, or special events. The Academic Facility is open to Rush students twenty-four hours a day and is a good spot for group or individual study. Student organizations are numerous and range from the Rush Golf Club to the Multicultural Affairs Coalition to chapters of national medically oriented organizations. The Rush community service initiative program (RCSIP) is a student-run umbrella organization for many projects and activities, all of which allow students to contribute to the community. RCSIP activities include free clinics, health education programs, and big sibling relationships with children who have HIV. Students have access to athletic and recreational facilities at Rush and at the University of Illinois, including indoor tennis courts, swimming pools, a bowling alley, and pool tables. Chicago is an ideal city for students, as it is relatively affordable and can be accessed with public transportation. Convenient and comfortable housing options are available both on and off campus.

GRADUATES

Rush has met its stated goal that at least 50 percent of graduates will enter primary care fields. Graduates are successful in securing residencies all over the country. Rush graduates practice in fifty states and in a number of foreign countries.

Admissions

REQUIREMENTS

Prerequisites are eight semester hours each of biology, general chemistry, organic chemistry, and physics. The MCAT is required, and scores must be from within the past four years. For applicants who have retaken the exam, recent scores are most heavily weighed.

SUGGESTIONS

Preference is given to residents of Illinois, although up to twenty to thirty out-of-state applicants are accepted each year. Beyond requirements, Rush suggests undergraduate courses in math, social sciences, and English. The committee looks for social and intellectual maturity, personal integrity, motivation, and concern in applicants. Applicants are encouraged to take the MCAT in April of the year of application.

PROCESS

All AMCAS applicants receive secondary applications. About 500 applicants, or 10 percent of the applicant pool, are interviewed between September and March. Interviews consist of two sessions with faculty members, in addition to a tour of the campus and the opportunity to meet with current students. Of interviewed candidates, about half are accepted on a rolling basis. Wait-listed candidates may submit supplementary material to update their files.

Admissions Requirements (Required)

MCAT scores, science GPA, non-science GPA, letters of recommendation, interview, state residency, essays/personal statement, extracurricular activities, exposure to medical profession.

COSTS AND AID

Tuition	$32,268
Cost of books	$1,050
Fees	$1,530

Financial Aid

% students receiving aid	80

ST. GEORGE'S UNIVERSITY
SCHOOL OF MEDICINE

ONE EAST MAIN STREET, BAY SHORE, NY 11706-8399 • ADMISSION: 800-899-6337 • FAX: 631-665-5590 •
E-MAIL: SGUINFO@SGU.EDU • WEBSITE: WWW.SGU.EDU

STUDENT BODY

Type	Private
Average age	25

ADMISSIONS

Average GPA and MCAT Scores

Overall GPA	3.3
MCAT Bio	9
MCAT Phys	9
MCAT Verbal	8
MCAT Essay	0

Application Information

Regular application	rolling
Regular notification	rolling
Are transfers accepted?	No
Admissions may be deferred?	No
Interview required?	Yes
Application fee	$75

Academics

Founded as an independent school of medicine in Grenada over twenty-five years ago, St. George's University has evolved into a top international center of education, offering medical, pre-medical, veterinary, and pre-veterinary programs. The School of Medicine also offers advanced research degrees in the biomedical sciences, a master of public health, and a variety of combined degree programs. Almost 5,000 physicians have graduated from the School of Medicine and are practicing medicine in over thirty-five countries and every state in the United States. They practice in virtually every specialty and subspecialty and in positions in academic medicine, as well as public health and institutional practice. Their scores on standardized tests over the years attest to the academic excellence of our curriculum. St. George's University has a five-year average pass rate of 90 percent for first time takers of the USMLE Step I, far exceeding the 62 percent average pass rate of all non-U.S. schools during the same period. State Education Departments across the United States and various government councils around the world have conducted site visits and extensive evaluations of our medical program, and St. George's University has received a favorable review each time, meeting or exceeding all standards.

BASIC SCIENCES: The first two years of study concentrate on the traditional basic science disciplines, and the curriculum incorporates small group discussions designed for problem-based learning, lectures, and laboratory experiences. Clinical skills are introduced into the first term and enhanced by hospital visits to the Kato Memorial Hospital in St. Vincent during terms five and six, emphasizing integration of basic science into the clinical experience.

CLINICAL TRAINING

St. George offers a highly integrated system of affiliated hospitals and clinical centers in the United States, all of whose core rotations have ACGME-approved residency training programs running concurrently. Our program in the United Kingdom is similar to that in the United States, providing students with clinical opportunities at over fifty affiliated hospitals in the United States and United Kingdom. Although clinical training may be completed in one country, students may combine clinical experiences in the United States and the United Kingdom for a more international experience.

Students

Over the last ten years, over forty-two new buildings have been beautifully blended into the Caribbean environment on the True Blue campus in Grenada. The brand new administrative, residential, academic, and scientific buildings include a 45,000 square-foot, fully electronic library; gross anatomy laboratory with ample supply of cadavers; microbiology, pathology, and histology laboratories with extensive microscopic and gross preparations collections; and an up-to-date array of audiovisual and computerized materials in all subjects. The student center is home to two restaurants, a fully equipped weight room, and exercise facilities. After classes and on weekends, students can also be found on the new sports fields and basketball courts, participating in many sporting activities and team sports. To accommodate our growing population we have expanded our on-campus housing to include a wide variety of comfortable, attractive, and convenient living arrangements. In addition, there are numerous choices for living off-campus that can be accessed by the university bus system.

STUDENT LIFE

Students attend their basic science years on our campuses in Grenada and the neighboring island of St. Vincent. The inhabitants of both islands are English-speaking, and all course work is delivered in English. Students have options of taking clinical rotations in the U.S. and/or in the U.K. The community at St. George's University gathers there from all four corners of the world—it is extremely diverse. Over ninety nations are represented in the student population and over twenty-five student organizations are organized around various interests—cultural, religious, avocational, and community service—fostering a sense of belonging as well as collegiality. Students participate in many types of sporting activities and team sports.

Admissions

REQUIREMENTS

Applicants are advised that the Board of Admissions requires an academic indicator within the three years prior to making application. MCAT scores must be from within the three years prior to application and may be used as a recent academic indicator. Applicants from the North American model of education need a bachelor's degree from an accredited university. In rare instances, an unusually well qualified applicant is considered for admission with only three years of post-secondary education completed toward a bachelor's degree. All North American applicants must submit MCAT scores. Our MCAT code is 904. Applicants from the British system of education need a bachelor's degree with a strong science background. If English is not the applicant's main language, he or she must submit an official record of a score of at least 600 from the Test of English as a Foreign Language (TOEFL). Our TOEFL code is 2864. Applicants from other systems of education must have achieved the successful completion of secondary school (twelve years post-kindergarten, make up four years post-primary/elementary, that, in itself, is at least eight years long), preferably in a science curriculum or track.

PROCESS

The curriculum is a series of integrated educational experiences that facilitate growth and aim to develop the student's capacity for self directed and self-motivated learning. The School of Medicine begins first-term classes in mid-August and again in mid-January of each year. The Board of Admissions utilizes a rolling admissions policy in the School of Medicine; therefore, applications are accepted on an ongoing basis. The board reserves the right to defer an application to the following semester if there are no available seats. The Office of Admissions will acknowledge receipt of a candidate's application within two weeks of its arrival. A candidate will be informed of any required supporting documents missing at that time. Within one month after receipt of all application materials, a candidate will receive notice that the application is complete and is being reviewed to determine whether an interview will be granted. Candidates are advised that being granted an interview is no guarantee of acceptance; the interview itself plays a significant part in the decision by the Board of Admissions. For information or to speak to an admissions counselor, interested students may call 1-800-899-6337 or visit our website at www.sgue.edu

Admissions Requirements (Required)

MCAT scores, science GPA, non-science GPA, letters of recommendation, interview, essays/personal statement.

Admissions Requirements (Optional)

state residency, extracurricular activities, exposure to medical profession.

COSTS AND AID

Tuition	$29,837

Saint Louis University
School of Medicine

Committee on Admissions, 1402 S. Grand Boulevard, Room 226, St. Louis, MO 63104 • Admission: 314-977-9870 • Fax: 314-977-9825 • E-mail: slumd@slu.edu • Website: http://medschool.slu.edu/admissions

STUDENT BODY

Type	Private
Enrollment	616
% male/female	53/47
% underrepresented minorities	12
# applied (total/out)	3,120/2,859
# accepted (total/out)	483/410
# enrolled (total/out)	158/112

FACULTY

Total faculty (number)	1,739
% female	24
% minority	1
% part-time	66

ADMISSIONS

Average GPA and MCAT Scores

Overall GPA	3.6
MCAT Bio	10.27
MCAT Phys	9.9
MCAT Verbal	9.82
MCAT Essay	P

Application Information

Regular application	12/15
Regular notification	10/15
Early application	6/1-8/1
Early notification	10/1
Are transfers accepted?	Yes
Admissions may be deferred?	Yes
Interview required?	Yes
Application fee	$100

Academics

The medical curriculum is continually evolving to respond to the rapid changes in the health care field and to reflect national trends in medical education. Current students enjoy a program of study that uses problem-based learning and emphasizes small group and independent study. SLU offers several options for students who are interested in research. Qualified students may enter an MS/PhD program, which allows them to complete both degrees within six to seven years. The doctorate is offered in anatomy, biochemistry, cell biology, genetics, immunology, microbiology, molecular biology, neuroscience, pathology, pharmacology, and physiology. Students who are interested in summer or elective research experiences may graduate in four years, earning an MD with distinction in research. Medical students are evaluated with honors, pass, or fail throughout all four years. Passing the USMLE Step 1 is a requirement for promotion to year three and passing Step 2 is a requirement for graduation.

BASIC SCIENCES: The first and second years each consist of thirty-six weeks of instruction, which includes laboratories, demonstrations, discussion groups, didactic lecture sessions, and preceptorships at clinical sites. Students are in class or other scheduled sessions for about twenty hours per week, which provides them with ample time for self directed learning. First-year courses are introduction to human anatomy; cell biology; metabolism; microbes and host responses; molecular biology and genetics; principles of pharmacology; health information resources; and patient, physician, and society, which covers topics such as bioethics, community medicine, medical communication, and the physical diagnosis. Second-year courses are introduction to clinical psychiatry; introduction to medicine; microbiology; neuroscience; pathology; pharmacology; preventive and social medicine; and patient, physician, and society, which includes both clinical and sociological/psychological topics. An important resource for students is the Learning Resources Center, which houses both the Health Sciences Center Library and the Clinical Skills Center, where both diagnostic and treatment skills are taught.

CLINICAL TRAINING

The third year consists of core clerkships in most basic medical fields. These are internal medicine (twelve weeks), surgery (eight weeks), obstetrics/gynecology (six weeks), pediatrics (eight weeks), family medicine (four weeks), psychiatry (six weeks), and neurology (four weeks). The fourth year is flexible and allows students to pursue elective opportunities in both clinical and research areas. A minimum of thirty-six weeks of instruction must be completed. Required rotations are in intramural floor service (four weeks) and surgery subspecialty selective (four weeks). Most training is conducted at the St. Louis University Hospital, a 365-bed tertiary care facility. It is also a level I trauma center. Other affiliated institutions include the Cardinal Glennon Children's Hospital, the Anheuser-Busch Eye Institute, and the St. Louis Veterans' Affairs Medical Center. A portion of electives may be taken at other academic and clinical institutions.

Students

Although students come from all regions of the United States, a large number are from the Saint Louis area. About 10 percent of students are underrepresented minorities and about 10 percent are nontraditional students who have pursued other careers or interests between college and medical school.

STUDENT LIFE

SLU students can pursue their health related interests by taking part in research forums or by participating in the school's many organizations. The campus ministry is particularly strong. Those who need a break from academic and career pursuits can take advantage of the resources of the main campus, including the award-winning Simon Recreational Center or the well subscribed intramural sports program. St. Louis also offers a wide variety of extracurricular activities. Tower Grove Park and the Missouri Botanical Gardens are a few blocks from the medical school. Nearby Forest Park, one of the nation's largest metropolitan parks, is the home of the St. Louis Zoo, the Art Museum, and the Science Center. St. Louis also has its own opera, theater, and ballet, in addition to professional baseball and hockey teams. Although the school has some housing facilities, most medical students choose to live off campus, where housing is affordable and comfortable.

GRADUATES

The majority of graduates enter primary care residencies. Students are competitive applicants for specialty fields as well.

Admissions

REQUIREMENTS

Requirements are one year each of chemistry, biology, organic chemistry, and physics. In addition, six semester hours of English and twelve hours of humanities or behavioral science are expected. The MCAT is required, and scores must be from the new version of the test. For applicants who have retaken the exam, the best set of scores is considered. Thus, there is no advantage to withholding scores.

SUGGESTIONS

Students should apply early in the application cycle as interviews and acceptances are given on a rolling basis. Both hospital and research experience is highly valuable. Activities that demonstrate a commitment to serving others are also useful.

PROCESS

All AMCAS applicants receive secondary applications. Of the approximately 4,200 students who return secondaries, about 21 percent are interviewed on a rolling basis. Interviews are one hour long and are conducted by a faculty member. The remainder of the interview day includes a tour of the campus, group informational sessions, and lunch with current students. Applicants are notified of committee decisions within a few weeks of the interview and are either accepted, rejected, or put into a hold category. Approximately 35 percent of the interviewed group is accepted. For wait-listed applicants, additional grades or new MCAT scores are useful supplementary information

Admissions Requirements (Required)

MCAT scores, science GPA, non-science GPA, letters of recommendation, interview, essays/personal statement.

Admissions Requirements (Optional)

state residency, extracurricular activities, exposure to medical profession, exposure to research, volunteer experience.

COSTS AND AID

Tuition	$36,190
Cost of books	$707
Fees	$1,820

Financial Aid

% students receiving aid	87
Average grant	$8,000
Average loan	$32,000
Average debt	$128,482

SOUTHERN ILLINOIS UNIVERSITY
SCHOOL OF MEDICINE

PO BOX 19624, SPRINGFIELD, IL 62794-9624 • ADMISSION: 217-545-6013 • FAX: 217-545-5538 •
E-MAIL: ADMISSIONS@SIUMED.EDU • WEBSITE: WWW.SIUMED.EDU

STUDENT BODY

Type	Public
Enrollment	292
% male/female	48/52
% underrepresented minorities	8
# applied (total/out)	1,139/312
# accepted (total/out)	148/2
# enrolled (total)	72
Average age	23

FACULTY

Total faculty (number)	329
% female	21
% minority	16
% part-time	8
# student/faculty ratio	1:1

ADMISSIONS

Average GPA and MCAT Scores

Overall GPA	3.6
MCAT Bio	9.31
MCAT Phys	8.79
MCAT Verbal	9.11
MCAT Essay	0

Application Information

Regular application	11/15
Regular notification	10/15
Are transfers accepted?	Yes
Admissions may be deferred?	Yes
Interview required?	Yes
Application fee	$50

Academics

SIU offers a case-based, small group-oriented curriculum with an abundance of patient contact and early clinical exposure. In cooperation with the SIU School of Law, a joint MD/JD degree program is also offered. Medical students are evaluated with grades of pass, fail, and honors. The USMLE Step 1 must be passed as a graduation requirement.

BASIC SCIENCES: The instructional format emphasizes small group instruction, self directed study, and a case-based approach, but also incorporates lectures and an organ system organizational scheme. Topics covered in the first year are cardiovascular, respiratory, renal, endocrine, reproductive, gastrointestinal, and sensorimotor systems and behavior. In Carbondale, basic science instruction takes place in Lindegren Hall. Early clinical experiences are offered at Memorial Hospital in Carbondale (151 beds), the Carbondale Clinic, offices of local physicians, and at the VA Hospital (171 beds). In Springfield, the Medical Instructional Facility contains lecture halls, classrooms, labs, and a teaching museum. A four-year doctoring curriculum (physician conduct and attitude, clinical skills development, and medical humanities issues) begins immediately. Both simulated and real patients are used. Topics covered in the second year include circulation, infection, and host diseases, neoplasia, population health and preventitive medicine, neuromuscular, and medicine and behavior. Computer assisted instruction is used as a learning aid, and computers are available in the student computer lab and at other sites. The Morris Library at Carbondale houses more than 100,000 volumes, while the Medical Instruction Facility in Springfield contains 113,000 volumes.

CLINICAL TRAINING

Third-year required multidisciplinary rotations are internal medicine, surgery, family and community medicine, psychiatry, neurology, obstetrics, gynecology, and pediatrics. The doctoring curriculum continues during this year. At the conclusion of the third year, students must pass an examination that evaluates their skills in assessing and managing patient problems. During the fourth year, students complete two additional required clerkships anesthesiology (two weeks) and neurology (two weeks). Thirty-one weeks are reserved for elective studies. Clinical training sites include Memorial Medical Center (580 beds), St. John's Hospital and Pavilion (715 beds), and the clinics and offices of faculty and community physicians. Electives may be taken off compus, and SIU has an institutional agreement with overseas universities—including locations in Germany and the Netherlands—that facilitate training overseas.

Students

At least 95 percent of students are Illinois residents. The average age of incoming students is twenty-three. Underrepresented minorities account for about 8 percent of the student body. Class size is seventy-two.

STUDENT LIFE

On-campus recreational facilities at Carbondale include a complete fitness room, swimming pools, racquetball courts, and a student center. Taking part in intramural sports and attending intercollegiate sporting events are popular extracurricular activities for medical students. St. Louis, with the amenities of a large city, is a two-hour drive. The surrounding area features a state park and the Shawnee National Forest, where the students can hike, bike, camp, canoe, or enjoy the beach. In Springfield, medical students enjoy discounts to health clubs such as the YMCA. Lake Springfield offers fishing, swimming, boating, and sailing. Parks, golf courses, and cultural and historical sites are other local attractions. All students live off campus in both Carbondale and Springfield.

GRADUATES

Among the 2001 graduating class, the most prevalent fields for post-graduate training were internal medicine (26 percent), family medicine (40 percent), and general surgery (10 percent). Students generally score around the national mean on the USMLE Part 1, and above the mean on Part 2, making them well-positioned for securing residency positions.

Admissions

REQUIREMENTS

To do well on the MCAT, students should have taken at least one year each of biology, chemistry, organic chemistry, physics, English, and math, the last of which should have included some statistics. The MCAT is required and scores must be no more than two years old. For applicants who have taken the exam on multiple occasions, the most recent set of scores is considered.

SUGGESTIONS

As a state school, preference is given to applicants from Central and Southern Illinois who are interested in practicing in the region. Applicants are expected to have a good foundation in the natural sciences, social sciences, and humanities in addition to sound English skills. The Admissions Committee looks beyond scholastic achievement for evidence of responsibility, integrity, compassion, motivation, interest in medicine, community service, and sound interpersonal skills. The medical education preparatory program (MEDPREP) is a nondegree post-baccalaureate program that assists disadvantaged students with meeting the requirements for the SIU School of Medicine.

PROCESS

About one-fifth of AMCAS applicants are interviewed, the vast majority of them Illinois state residents. Interviews are conducted between August and April, and consist of two sessions with individual faculty and/or administrators. About 33 percent of interviewed candidates are accepted on a batch basis. The other candidates are rejected or wait-listed. Wait-listed candidates may send supplemental material to update their files.

Admissions Requirements (Required)

MCAT scores, science GPA, non-science GPA, letters of recommendation, interview, state residency, essays/personal statement, extracurricular activities, volunteer/employment experience.

Admissions Requirements (Optional)

exposure to medical profession.

Overlap Schools

Loyola University Chicago, Rush Medical College of Rush University, University of Illinois at Chicago.

COSTS AND AID

In-state tuition	$16,148
Out-of-state tuition	$48,444
Cost of books	$1,554
Fees	$2,008

Financial Aid

% students receiving aid	89
Average grant	$13,809
Average loan	$25,386
Average debt	$97,008

SPARTAN HEALTH SCIENCES

SCHOOL OF MEDICINE

PO BOX 324 VIEUX FORT, ST. LUCIA, WI • ADMISSION: 758-454-6128 • FAX: 758-454-6811 • E-MAIL: SPARTAN-MED@AOL.COM • WEBSITE: HTTP://SPARTANMED.ORG

STUDENT BODY

Type	Private
Enrollment	300
% male/female	70/30
% underrepresented minorities	80
# applied (total)	100
# accepted (total)	50
# enrolled (total)	50
Average age	28

FACULTY

Total faculty (number)	17
% female	18
% minority	100
% part-time	20
# student/faculty ratio	7:1

ADMISSIONS

Average GPA and MCAT Scores

Overall GPA	3.0

Application Information

Regular application	7/15
Are transfers accepted?	Yes
Admissions may be deferred?	Yes
Interview required?	Yes
Application fee	$60

Academics

Spartan Health Sciences University, School of Medicine, offers a four academic years (thirty-six calendar month) program leading to the doctor of medicine degree (MD), and is taught on a trimester (four months) schedule. The curriculum of the university's doctor of medicine degree program encompasses a comprehensive course of basic sciences (BS), preclinical and clinical sciences (CS) that lasts for four academic years. The trimester periods start in January, May, and September of each year. A student may elect to enter in any one of the three trimesters. To provide the best possible medical education to the students, the curriculum is under continuous review by the deans of basic and clinical sciences in conjunction with the faculty. All students are required to demonstrate competency in the basic medical sciences before being permitted to begin clinical rotations. Competency is assessed from the university administered and required Comprehensive Exit Examination at the end of basic sciences program. No student will be eligible for graduation until all academic requirements and financial obligations to the university have been fulfilled.

BASIC SCIENCES: The initial four trimesters of the program represent an integrated course presentation of the basic sciences (BS) which include anatomy, physiology, pharmacology biochemistry, immunology, pathology, microbiology, behavioral sciences, neuroanatomy, general introduction to medicine, including physical diagnosis. Didactic lectures in internal medicine, pediatrics, psychiatry, obstetrics/gynecology, and surgery are offered. Clinical correlated conferences are conducted for related basic sciences to clinical medicine.

CLINICAL TRAINING

The final five trimesters are committed to broad clinical exposure in the major clinical disciplines of internal medicine (twelve weeks), surgery and its subspecialties (twenty weeks), pediatrics (six weeks), obstetrics and gynecology (eight weeks), psychiatry (six weeks), family medicine (six weeks), radiology (four weeks), pathology (four weeks), and clinical electives (fourteen weeks).

Students

The university's student body is made up of multiracial backgrounds. Some of the students were professionals in their fields before they were admitted; some were pharmacists, biochemists, and researchers with post-graduate degrees. The university is a microcosm of the United Nations in the pursuit of eradication of diseases that plague the human race. Students come from different continents around the world (eighty-seven countries).

STUDENT LIFE

Spartan Health Sciences University, School of Medicine, is located in the former British Colony of Saint Lucia. The people of Saint Lucia are English speaking, friendly, and very accommodating. The population of St. Lucia at the end of 2000 was 163,819. The local language is Creole (or Patois, an adulterated French) emerged as a result of British and French influences with English as the official language. Outside of the classroom, students involve in various community health care events. Medical students take advantage of the fitness center, tennis courts, on school premises, and cricket and soccer fields behind the school. All students live off campus, within walking or biking distance of campus.

Admissions

REQUIREMENTS

The minimum requirement for admission is ninety semester credit hours of college-level work. Prerequisites are one year each of general chemistry, organic chemistry, biology, physics, English, and mathematics. The MCAT is not required. Applicants from the United Kingdom, British Commonwealth of Nations, and other countries with similar educational standards must possess a baccalaureate degree and have completed courses in biology, chemistry, mathematics, and physics. However, applicants with high grades in the general certificate of education (GCE) advanced level with courses in the sciences may be considered. Prospective students from other countries with educational systems different from the British or U.S. will be evaluated on their merits.

SUGGESTIONS

The Mission of Spartan Health Sciences University, School of Medicine, is to train doctors of all races, nations for the world rather than indulgence in parochialism of medical education. The primary objective of the university is to provide qualified students an opportunity to fulfill their lifelong ambition of serving humanity with medical education, prolongation of human life through medical care and research. The university strives hard to attain a high standard of education with affordable tuition fees ever since its inception. This does not in any way compromise the standard of medical education offered by this institution. The university is dedicated to train its graduates with an excellent medical knowledge and competent skills to assure the society and the medical profession to meet the health care demands of the societies to which they belong.

PROCESS

In evaluating individual applicant's credentials, Admissions Committee looks for the applicant's capacity to do academic work for absorption of the material needed for sound foundation in the basic medical sciences. Evaluation is also carried out on GPA from individual colleges and universities and letters of recommendation. However, academic background is not the main criterion for selection; character and motivation to become a physician are essential determinants for admission.

Admissions Requirements (Required)

science GPA, nonscience GPA, letters of recommendation, interview, essays/personal statement.

Admissions Requirements (Optional)

MCAT scores, state residency, extracurricular activities, exposure to medical profession.

COSTS AND AID

Tuition	$7,100
Cost of books	$500

Financial Aid

% students receiving aid	60
Average loan	$20,000

Stanford University

Stanford University School of Medicine

Office of MD Admissions, 251 Campus Drive, MSOB XC301, Stanford, CA 94305-5404 • Admission: 650-723-6861 • Fax: 650-725-7855 • E-mail: admissions@med.stanford.edu • Website: www.med.stanford.edu

STUDENT BODY

Type	Private
Enrollment	462
% male/female	49/51
% underrepresented minorities	23
# applied (total/out)	5,445/3,421
# accepted (total/out)	186/115
# enrolled (total/out)	87/53
Average age	23

FACULTY

Total faculty (number)	710
% female	33
% minority	5

ADMISSIONS

Average GPA and MCAT Scores

Overall GPA	3.8
MCAT Bio	11.83
MCAT Phys	11.56
MCAT Verbal	10.18
MCAT Essay	R

Application Information

Regular application	10/15
Regular notification	Rolling
Early application	6/1-8/1
Early notification	10/15
Are transfers accepted?	Yes
Admissions may be deferred?	Yes
Interview required?	Yes
Application fee	$75

Academics

Generally, about 60 percent of Stanford students receive their MD in five rather than four years, which allows for individual research and elective study. In addition to the MD, departmental joint degrees include an MS/PhD in biochemistry, developmental biology, genetics, microbiology and immunology, molecular and cellular physiology, molecular pharmacology, and structural biology. Interdepartmental joint degrees are also possible, and include an MS in biomechanical engineering and health services research, an MS and PhD in epidemiology and medical information sciences, and a PhD in biophysics, cancer biology, immunology, and neuroscience. There are about six to eight MSTP slots available. In addition to formal degree programs, students may take electives in nonmedical departments. Through the medical student scholars program and other programs, students enjoy a range of research opportunities, most of which are remunerated.

BASIC SCIENCES: Stanford operates on a quarter system, and preclinical studies are organized into six quarters. During this period of rigorous science course work, students are gradually introduced to clinical care and have clinical training opportunities throughout. Classes demand twenty to thirty-five hours per week, with considerable variation from quarter to quarter. During the fall (first) quarter of the first year, students typically take human anatomy and development, which includes an introduction to the physical examination, structure of cells and tissues, and introduction to psychiatry, which involves patient interviews. Winter (second) quarter offers biochemistry, biostatistics and epidemiology, neurobiology, health systems/policy, clinical psychiatry, and physicians and patients, a course exploring interdisciplinary topics and continuing medical interviews. During the spring (third) quarter, students take molecular biology, genetics, cardiovascular physiology, pathology, and host parasites and defense are taken. The second-year fall (fourth) quarter introduces students to infectious basis of disease, physiology, pharmacology, and more pathology. In addition, preparation for clinical medicine begins. In the fifth quarter, students take endocrine physiology, pathophysiology, and more pharmacology and pathology. Students make the transition into their clinical studies during this quarter and the second year (sixth quarter) with clinical problem solving, presented in a case-based, small group format and a preceptor program, including general and psychiatric patient care. The Lane Medical Library, which is soon to benefit from substantial remodeling and enlargment, currently houses 3,000 journal titles, 350,000 volumes, and online data management services. Computer, audiovisual, and other learning aids are accessible to students at the Fleischmann Learning and Resource Center. Videotapes of most preclinical courses are available and appear to substitute for student-organized note services. Grading is strictly pass/fail, and mid-quarter exams are optional. A weeklong reading period prior to final exams allows students uninterrupted study time. Step 1 of the USMLE must be passed no later than one year prior to graduation and Step 2 must be passed to graduate.

CLINICAL TRAINING

Patient contact begins in the fall quarter of the first year, and there are opportunities for clinical experiences during the first two years. Third- and fourth-year clerkships take place at the major affiliated teaching hospitals, which include Stanford Hospital (479 beds), the Lucile Salter Packard Children's Hospital (162 beds), Santa Clara Valley Medical Center (644 beds), three VA Hospitals, Kaiser Permanente (336 beds), and

Columbia San Jose Medical Center (529 beds). These facilities serve both rural and urban populations with diverse needs. Students complete fifteen months of clinical clerkships, including nine months of required core clerkships in medicine, surgery, pediatrics, obstetrics/gynecology, psychiatry, and family medicine. Three months are spent training in areas related to required clerkships through selectives, in which students choose from basics in clinical care, ambulatory care, and subinternship. The final three months are designated as elective clerkships.

Students

Stanford students are often characterized as being less cut throat than those attending other top-ranked schools, perhaps because the flexible curriculum encourages students to focus beyond the classroom. Special effort is made to recruit students from underrepresented minority backgrounds, and student organizations support these and other student groups. With eighty-six students per class, Stanford is relatively small.

STUDENT LIFE

The campus and the surrounding areas offer excellent sports and other outdoor activities. San Francisco is an hour away and is accessible by train. Numerous on-campus housing options exist, including family housing, apartments, dormitories, and co-ops. However, high rent in the vicinity of Stanford makes student housing competitive.

GRADUATES

Stanford itself offers excellent residency programs, and many graduates opt for postgraduate training at Stanford. Perhaps as a result of the teaching and research experience students gain while in school, many go on into academic medicine. Increasingly, graduates are entering primary care fields.

Admissions

REQUIREMENTS

Biology with lab (one year), chemistry/organic chemistry with labs (two years), and physics with lab (one year). The MCAT must be no more than three years old. The most recent set of scores is used.

SUGGESTIONS

Biochemistry, calculus, and behavioral sciences are recommended, as is knowledge of a second language. No preference is given to California residents or to Stanford undergraduates. Successful applicants generally have significant medical, health related, research, or community service experience.

PROCESS

Secondary applications are sent out on a rolling basis, with information due in two weeks. Interviews involve two semistructured, one-hour sessions, one with a faculty member and one with a medical student. Of interviewed candidates, about one-third are accepted, one-third are rejected, and one-third are wait-listed; candidates receive responses within four to six weeks of the interview. During the past few years, up to fifteen applicants were eventually accepted off of the wait-list.

Admissions Requirements (Required)

MCAT scores, science GPA, non-science GPA, letters of recommendation, interview, essays/personal statement, extracurricular activities, exposure to medical profession.

Admissions Requirements (Optional)

state residency.

Overlap Schools

Harvard University, University of California at Hastings.

COSTS AND AID

Tuition	$34,716
Room and board	$14,500
Cost of books	$1,500

Financial Aid

% students receiving aid	66
Average grant	$28,705
Average loan	$14,849
Average debt	$63,695

SUNY at Buffalo
School of Medicine and Biomedical Sciences

131 BEB, Buffalo, NY 14214-3013 • Admission: 716-829-3466 • Fax: 716-829-3849 •
E-mail: jjrosso@acsu.buffalo.edu • Website: www.smbs.buffalo.edu/ome

STUDENT BODY

Type	Public
Enrollment	757
% male/female	56/44
% underrepresented minorities	15
# applied (total/out)	3,505/1,159
# accepted (total/out)	7/1
# enrolled (out)	1
Average age	23

ADMISSIONS

Application Information

Regular application	12/15
Regular notification	10/15 until filled
Early application	6/1-8/1
Early notification	10/1
Are transfers accepted?	No
Admissions may be deferred?	Yes
Interview required?	No
Application fee	$65

Academics

In addition to the MD, the School of Medicine and Biomedical Sciences awards the PhD, MA, MS, and the combined MS/PhD. There are four MSTP-sponsored MS/PhD positions available each year. Departments awarding graduate degrees include anatomy, biochemistry, biophysics, cell biology, genetics, immunology, microbiology, molecular biology, neuroscience, pathology, pharmacology, and physiology. A new joint degree program that leads to the MD/MBA began in 1997. Grades of honors, pass, and fail are used to evaluate medical students. Passing the USMLE Step 1 is required before matriculants can enter third year.

BASIC SCIENCES: Basic sciences are taught through a combination of lectures, labs, small group sessions, problem-based learning, and clinical experiences. On average, students are in class or scheduled sessions for about twenty hours per week. First-year courses are gross anatomy; biochemistry; human behavior; histology; embryology; physiology; neuroscience, medical genetics; scientific basis of medicine; social and preventive medicine; and clinical practice of medicine, which provides early patient-contact experiences. Second-year courses are hematology, pathology, microbiology, pharmacology, scientific basis of medicine, social and preventive medicine, genetics, human behavior, and the continuation of clinical practice of medicine. Summer externships, which allow up to sixty first- and second-year medical students to shadow primary care physicians, are available with stipends. Stipends are also available on a limited basis for summer research projects. The Health Sciences Library features a Media Resources Center with approximately 2,000 multimedia items, a History of Medicine Collection with 12,000 volumes, and a comprehensive general medicine/scientific book and journal collection.

CLINICAL TRAINING

Third-year required rotations are internal medicine (eight weeks), surgery (eight weeks), obstetrics/gynecology (seven weeks), pediatrics (seven weeks), psychiatry (seven weeks), and family medicine (seven weeks). The family medicine clerkship includes six sessions in a community-based family physician's office, two sessions in a problem-based learning format, one session focusing on a community project, and one session devoted to independent learning. During the third year, students also choose a weeklong seminar from diverse selective offerings. Fourth-year requirements are four weeks each of neurology, medicine, and surgery, and four weeks of an ambulatory experience. Four-year electives are also available. Training takes place at The Buffalo General Hospital, Children's Hospital of Buffalo, Erie County Medical Center, Mercy Hospital, Millard Fillmore Health System, Sisters of Charity Hospital, Roswell Park Cancer Institute, and the Buffalo VA Medical Center. The community academic practice program identifies community-based sites for clinical training. With faculty approval, up to sixteen weeks of electives may be taken at other academic institutions.

Students

All but five or six students in each class are New York residents. About 20 percent of entering students are over twenty-five years old. Approximately 5 percent of students are underrepresented minorities. Class size is 135.

STUDENT LIFE

The first year begins with a relaxed orientation week that allows students to get acquainted with each other and their new surroundings. Several student centers serve as focal points for student life on campus. The Student Union houses more than seventy-five clubs and organizations in addition to recreational facilities, dining areas, and a theater. The Oasis Recreation Center features pool tables, music, and a TV room. The Harriman Student Activities Center is an alternate student union, and the Creative Craft Center provides ongoing craft programs and courses. The Living Well Center (LWC) is dedicated to improving students' overall health and wellness. It offers a range of services to students, including counseling, health education, fitness assessments, seminars on personal health issues, relaxation services such as massage, and special events with outside speakers. For medical students, the LWC also provides opportunities for volunteer work in areas related to preventive medicine. Buffalo is an affordable and student-friendly community. Residence halls and graduate student apartments close to campus are available.

GRADUATES

Among graduates in a recent class, the most prevalent specialty fields were internal medicine (28 percent), pediatrics (25 percent), family practice (15 percent), obstetrics/gynecology (10 percent), surgery (11 percent), and emergency medicine (5 percent). Approximately half of graduates entered residency programs in New York State.

Admissions

REQUIREMENTS

Prerequisites are biology (two semesters), chemistry (four semesters, including two of organic chemistry), physics (two semesters), and English (two semesters). The MCAT is required and must be from after 1998. For applicants who have retaken the exam, the best set of scores is generally considered. Thus, there is no advantage in withholding scores.

SUGGESTIONS

In addition to science requirements, two years of course work in social sciences and one year in the humanities are advised. Students who have taken time off after college are advised to demonstrate recent course work. Medically related experience is important.

PROCESS

All applicants are sent secondary applications. Between 400 and 500 applicants are interviewed from September through February. These candidates are selected from a pool of about 2,000, meaning that about 20 percent of applicants make it to the interview stage. Interviews consist of two sessions each with a faculty member or medical student. On interview day, there are also group informational sessions, a campus tour, and the opportunity to have lunch with current medical students. The first acceptance letters are mailed in October, with subsequent batches of letters sent at four- to six-week intervals throughout the year. Approximately 30 percent of interviewees are accepted initially. Others are rejected or placed on a wait-list. Supplementary material from wait-listed candidates is not encouraged. Usually 60 to 70 percent of interviewees are eventually offered an acceptance before orientation begins.

Admissions Requirements (Required)

MCAT scores, science GPA, non-science GPA, letters of recommendation, state residency, extracurricular activities, exposure to medical profession.

Admissions Requirements (Optional)

interview, essays/personal statement.

COSTS AND AID

In-state tuition	$10,840
Out-of-state tuition	$21,940
Fees	$220

Financial Aid

Average debt	$59,906

SUNY Downstate Medical Center

Office of Admissions, 450 Clarkson Avenue, Box 60M, Brooklyn, NY 11203 • Admission: 718-270-2446 • Fax: 718-270-7592 • Website: www.hscbklyn.edu

STUDENT BODY

Type	Public
*Enrollment	757
*% male/female	56/44
*% underrepresented minorities	15
# applied (total/out)	3,505/1,159
Average age	23

ADMISSIONS

Application Information

Regular application	12/15
Regular notification	10/15 until filled
Early application	6/1–8/1
Early notification	10/1
Are transfers accepted?	No
Admissions may be deferred?	Yes
Interview required?	No
Application fee	$65

Academics

The curriculum emphasizes the development of clinical reasoning and problem solving skills, integrates basic and clinical sciences, and exposes students from the first year to patient care. Each student spends one afternoon biweekly in a physician's private office or clinic; the practicing physician serves as the student's clinical mentor for the entire year. Students are also encouraged to participate in research. Opportunities are available throughout the four years of medical school. Those who make a significant research contribution are eligible to graduate with distinction in research. A MS/PhD program is open in one of two modern biomedical science areas, neuroscience, or molecular and cell biology. Medical students are evaluated with grades of honors, high pass, pass, and fail. Students must pass Step 1 of the USMLE to be promoted to year three. Students are encouraged to take Step 2 prior to graduation, but it is not a requirement.

BASIC SCIENCES: Basic science courses have been integrated into topics or blocks. Each block is taught using a combination of traditional lectures, case-based, small group sessions, laboratories, conferences, and a weekly clinical experience. First year topics are genes to cells, skin and connective tissue, musculoskeletal system, blood/hematopoiesis/lymphoid, cardiovascular system, respiratory system, gastrointestinal system/ intermediary metabolism, renal/urinary system, endocrine and reproduction systems, head and neck, and neuroscience. The current second-year curriculum includes courses in pathology, pathophysiology, pharmacology, microbiology and immunology, preventive medicine, preparation for clinical medicine, psychopathology, and nutrition. With the exception of the last two, each course runs throughout the full academic year; each discipline presents material related to specific organ systems. The Office of Academic Development promotes students' academic success through seminars, workshops, and individual tutoring. The Health Science Education Building holds two floors of study carrels, which serve as home base to students during the first two years. In the same building are the Medical Research Library (one of the largest medical school libraries in the country) and a 500-seat auditorium. A Learning Resource Center has ninety computer work stations loaded with an array of medical applications.

CLINICAL TRAINING

The current clerkships are medicine (ten weeks), surgery (eight weeks, anesthesia (two weeks), pediatrics (six weeks), obstetrics/gynecology (six weeks), psychiatry (six weeks), neurology (four weeks), primary care, a subinternship (four weeks), and at least twenty weeks of electives. Training takes place at a number of major affiliates, University Hospital, and Kings County Hospital. Electives can be completed at those institutions or at extramural hospitals or medical centers.

Students

The 2004 first-year class has 185 students from more than sixty individual colleges. About 93 percent are New York State residents. Approximately 13 percent of students are underrepresented minorities. The age range of the 2001 entering class was twenty to thirty-five, with a median of twenty-two.

STUDENT LIFE

All entering students are assigned a clinical faculty mentor who provides guidance and support throughout the first year. The focal point for recreational, social, and cultural activities on campus is the Student Center, which has lounges, a piano room, an athletic center, a swimming pool, squash courts, and a spa. Student organizations focus on professional, ethnic, service related, social, and recreational interests, and also provide support for groups of students. For example, the Daniel Hale Williams Society, named for a prominent Black physician, is a voice for minority students on campus and also brings students together to participate in educational, social, and service related goals. Brooklyn is a culturally rich, active community that provides an exciting extracurricular life for medical students. Manhattan is easily accessible by subway. On-campus housing options are single or shared studios or dormitory rooms. Students who live off campus often reside in the nearby neighborhood of Park Slope.

GRADUATES

Graduates perform above the national average in terms of securing residency positions at top institutions nationwide. Alumni hold faculty positions at universities such as Harvard, Case Western, Stanford, Yale, Hopkins, Columbia, Cornell, and the University of Pennsylvania, among other prestigious institutions. Forty percent of 2002 graduating students entered residency programs in primary care. More than 69 percent of graduates chose to stay within New York State.

Admissions

REQUIREMENTS

Fifteen positions in each class are reserved for students in a BA/MD program organized with Brooklyn College. Five positions are reserved for early assurance applicants from Queens College and the College of Staten Island. New York residents are given strong preference for the remaining spots. Prerequisites are eight semester credits each of biology, chemistry, organic chemistry, and physics, all with associated labs. Six semester hours of English are also required. The MCAT is required and scores must be from within three years of the date of anticipated enrollment. Component scores for each MCAT series are looked at individually.

SUGGESTIONS

In addition to required courses, one year each of college-level math, biochemistry, and another advanced science are recommended. Medically related experience and demonstrated commitment to social service and community outreach activities are important factors in admission.

PROCESS

All AMCAS applicants are sent secondary applications, of which about 20 percent are interviewed between September and April. Interviews consist of a one-hour session with a faculty member. On interview day, candidates also have a group orientation session, lunch with current students, and a campus tour. Of interviewed candidates, about 40 percent are accepted on a rolling basis. Wait-listed candidates are not encouraged to send supplementary information.

COSTS AND AID

Tuition & Fees

Tuition (in/out)	$10,840/$21,940
Fees	$220

Financial Aid

Average debt	$59,906

SUNY at Stony Brook

Stony Brook University, School of Medicine

Committee on Admissions, Level 4, Room 147, Health Sciences, Stony Brook, NY 11794 • Admission: 631-444-2113 • Fax: 631-444-6032 • E-mail: somadmissions@stonybrook.edu • www.hsc.sunysb.edu/som/

STUDENT BODY

Type	Public
Enrollment	428
% male/female	47/53
% underrepresented minorities	14
# applied (total/out)	2,523/643
# accepted (total/out)	266/8
# enrolled (total/out)	101/2
Average age	23

FACULTY

Total faculty (number)	465
% female	30
% part-time	13

ADMISSIONS

Average GPA and MCAT Scores

Overall GPA	3.6
MCAT Bio	11
MCAT Phys	10
MCAT Verbal	10
MCAT Essay	P

Application Information

Regular application	11/15
Regular notification	10/15
Early application	6/1-8/1
Early notification	10/1
Are transfers accepted?	Yes
Admissions may be deferred?	Yes
Interview required?	Yes
Application fee	$75

Academics

Most students earn their MDs in four years. Students who engage in relevant projects or course work may be eligible for the MD with recognition in research, the MD with recognition in primary care, or the MD with recognition in humanities. A combined MS/PhD program is offered as part of the MSTP. The doctoral degree may be earned in anatomy, biochemistry, biomedical engineering, cell biology, genetics, immunology, microbiology, molecular biology, neuroscience, pathology, pharmacology, and physiology. Medical students are evaluated with grades of honors, pass, and fail and must take both steps of the USMLE to graduate.

BASIC SCIENCES: Taken throughout all four years, the medicine in contemporary society course addresses a range of social issues as they relate to medical training. Other first-year courses are preventive medicine; the body; cell, genes and molecules; organ systems; neuroscience; introduction to human behavior; pathology; nutrition; and introduction to clinical medicine, which teaches fundamental clinical skills and provides early patient contact. Second-year courses are microbiology/infectious diseases; pharmacology; introduction to clinical medicine II; and a systems approach to medicine, which is organized around body systems. Students are in class or scheduled sessions for twenty to twenty-five hours per week. Class time is divided between lectures, labs, small group discussions, and clinical experiences, which serve to enrich learning and to motivate students. The Health Sciences Center Library houses approximately 273,000 volumes and 2,750 health science related periodicals, in addition to networked and online computer resources.

CLINICAL TRAINING

Third-year required clerkships are medicine (twelve weeks), surgery (eight weeks), pediatrics (eight weeks), obstetrics/gynecology (six weeks), psychiatry (four weeks), family medicine (six weeks), radiology (two weeks), and emergency medicine (two weeks). During the fourth year, a one month subinternship, a one month rotation in neurology, one month of a didactic course, one month of surgical specialties, and two weeks of psychiatry in medicine are required. The remainder of the year is reserved for electives. Most training takes place at the University Hospital (504 beds), the Northport Veterans' Affairs Medical Center (698 beds), Nassau University Medical Center (615 beds), and Winthrop-University Hospital (501 beds). As a way of learning about and relating to the community, all health sciences students must spend some time working with a Long Island health and welfare agency. Generally, students enjoy considerable flexibility in how and where they earn clinical elective credits.

Students

Typically, close to 100 percent of students are New York residents. About 13 percent are underrepresented minorities. There is a wide age range among students, and at least five to ten students in each class are in their thirties. Class size is 100.

STUDENT LIFE

Stony Brook is located on the North Shore of Long Island, just over an hour's train ride from Manhattan. Students enjoy both the comfort of their school's suburban location and its proximity to the city. The campus offers a vast sports complex, and the immediate area offers bike trails, beaches, and parks. The Stony Brook Union is the campus center for hundreds of activities, including eating, socializing, watching TV, taking art and other noncredit classes, playing billiards and table tennis, and shopping. It is also the home of student organizations, student government, and informational services. On-campus child care is available to students. university-owned housing includes residence halls and several apartment complexes with units of all sizes. Most students own cars, which are particularly important during the clinical years.

GRADUATES

Among 2002 graduates, the most prevalent fields for residencies were medicine (35 percent), surgery (5 percent), pediatrics (13 percent), family medicine (6 percent), obstetrics/gynecology (7 percent), and emergency medicine (7 percent). About 27 percent entered programs at university-affiliated hospitals.

Admissions

REQUIREMENTS

With the exception of MSTP applicants, New York residency is virtually a requirement. Academic prerequisites are one year each of biology, physics, chemistry, organic chemistry, and English. Science courses must include associated labs. The MCAT is required, and scores must be no more than five years old. For applicants who have retaken the exam, the best scores are considered. Thus, there is no advantage in withholding scores.

SUGGESTIONS

Applicants who have taken significant time off after college should have some recent course work. For all applicants, some medically related experience is important, and patient contact is particularly valued.

PROCESS

All AMCAS applicants receive secondary applications, of which about 25 percent are interviewed between September and March. Interviews consist of one session with a member of the Admissions Committee in addition to a group orientation session, tour, and the opportunity to meet with current medical students. About 40 percent of interviewed candidates are accepted, with notification occurring on a rolling basis. An alternate admissions path is through the BA/MD scholars for medicine program, which admits a limited number of high school students via the honors college into an eight year combined program. In addition, seven post-baccalaureate programs, including Bryn Mawr, Goucher, Stony Brook, NYU, Queens, Hunter, and Columbia have admission arrangements with Stony Brook through a linkage program.

Admissions Requirements (Required)

MCAT scores, science GPA, non-science GPA, letters of recommendation, interview, essays/personal statement, extracurricular activities, exposure to medical profession.

Admissions Requirements (Optional)

state residency.

Overlap Schools

Brown University, Columbia University, Cornell University, New York University, State University of New York, SUNY Upstate Medical University, Yale University.

COSTS AND AID

In-state tuition	$16,800
Out-of-state tuition	$29,800
Cost of books	$1,500
Fees	$670

Financial Aid

% students receiving aid	85
Average grant	$2,200
Average loan	$33,000
Average debt	$88,000

SUNY Upstate Medical University

College of Medicine

Office of Student Admissions, 766 Irving Avenue, Syracuse, NY 13210 • Admission: 315-464-4570 • Fax: 315-464-8867 • E-mail: studadmis@upstate.edu • Website: www.upstate.edu

STUDENT BODY

Type	Public
Enrollment	631
% male/female	55/45
% underrepresented minorities	31
# applied (total/out)	2,441/754
# accepted (total/out)	366/59
# enrolled (total/out)	152/21
Average age	23

FACULTY

Total faculty (number)	2,666

ADMISSIONS

Average GPA and MCAT Scores

Overall GPA	3.6
MCAT Bio	10.03
MCAT Phys	9.88
MCAT Verbal	9.35
MCAT Essay	P

Application Information

Regular application	11/1
Regular notification	10/15
Early application	8/1
Early notification	10/1
Are transfers accepted?	Yes
Admissions may be deferred?	Yes
Interview required?	Yes
Application fee	$100

Academics

An alternative track that involves clinical training in Binghamton is geared toward students who are interested in primary care and ambulatory medicine. About one-third of entering students participate in this track and diverge from the rest of the group for their third and fourth years. Opportunities for research include the academic research track, electives that are research-based, summer research projects, and the combined MS/PhD program. The PhD is offered in anatomy, biochemistry, cell biology, immunology, microbiology, molecular biology, neuroscience, pharmacology, and physiology. Each year, two MSTP positions are available in addition to other funding options. A joint MD/MBA program is also possible. Medical students are evaluated with grades of honors, high pass, pass, and fail, and they must pass both steps of the USMLE to graduate.

BASIC SCIENCES: First-year courses are embryology, human anatomy, microscopic anatomy, physiology, biochemistry, cell and molecular biology, neuroscience, genetics, and medicine and society I. During the first year, students are in class or other scheduled sessions for thirty-five hours per week. The majority of class time is devoted to lectures and labs, supplemented with small group discussions. Second-year courses are medicine and society II, microbiology and immunology, nutrition, pathology, pharmacology, epidemiology, introduction to clinical medicine, family practice, and behavioral sciences. During the second year, students are in class for about thirty hours per week, with less emphasis on laboratory work and more time spent in small group sessions. Basic science instruction takes place in Weiskotten Hall, which is adjacent to the school's main clinical affiliates. The library houses over 171,000 volumes and features online reference services. Microcomputers and audiovisual equipment are available as learning resources.

CLINICAL TRAINING

The third and fourth years are considered as a continuum. For students at the Syracuse campus, required clerkships are medicine (twelve weeks), general surgery (six weeks), pediatrics (six weeks), obstetrics/gynecology (six weeks), neurology/neurosurgery/ophthalmology (six weeks), psychiatry (six weeks), radiology (three weeks), orthopedic surgery/ent/anesthesia (four weeks), preventive medicine (two weeks), and urology (two weeks). Training takes place at State University Hospital (350 beds), U.S. Veterans' Administration Medical Center (379 beds), Crouse-Irving Memorial Hospital (490 beds), Community-General Hospital (350 beds), Richard H. Hutchings Psychiatric Center, and St. Joseph's Hospital and Health Center (472 beds). Students who are interested in a community-oriented clinical experience may opt to spend their third and fourth years in Binghamton, referred to as the Clinical Campus. Students establish close working relationships with community physicians and have enhanced opportunities for training in ambulatory care settings. Required clerkships are advanced skills (two weeks), ambulatory surgery (four weeks), general surgery (six weeks), internal medicine (twelve weeks), neuroscience (two weeks), psychiatry (six weeks), obstetrics/gynecology (six weeks), pediatrics (six weeks), and radiology (two weeks). Other elements of the curriculum include a longitudinal primary care clerkship (one half day per week) and a course dealing with social aspects of medicine. Typically, two required clerkships, gerontology/geriatric medicine and preventive medicine/community health, are taken during the fourth year. Affiliates in Binghamton are Wilson Memorial Hospital (350 beds), Binghamton General Hospital (250 beds), Our Lady of Lourdes Memorial Hospital (acute care/hospice), and Robert Packer Hospital (366 beds). In both tracks, a minimum of twenty-four weeks of electives are required. A portion of these may be taken in nonuniversity settings in the area, around the country, and overseas.

Students

From 90 to 95 percent of students are New York residents. About 12 percent of students are underrepresented minorities, and about 15 percent took some significant time off between college and medical school. Class size is 156.

STUDENT LIFE

SUNY Upstate recognizes the need for nonacademic opportunities and encourages a range of student activities. The Campus Activities Building is a hub for extracurricular pursuits and student interaction. Its athletic facilities include a comprehensive gym, a swimming pool, squash courts, tennis courts, running tracks, and pool tables. Other attractions are the snack bar, lounge, bookstore, and outdoor patio. Intramural sports, and campus-sponsored events such as movies and happy hours provide further distractions to medical students who need a break from studying. Student organizations include chapters of national associations, in addition to a number of groups based on ethnic or religious background, professional goals, or recreational interests. Syracuse is a midsize city surrounded by countryside. It is a one-hour drive to Lake Ontario's beaches, and four hours to New York City. Binghamton is conveniently situated about three hours from New York City, Philadelphia, and Buffalo. Modern residence halls at the Syracuse campus provide dormitory rooms, studios, and one-bedroom apartments for single and married students. In Binghamton, students live off campus.

GRADUATES

Graduates are successful in securing residencies in all fields.

Admissions

REQUIREMENTS

Prerequisites are chemistry (six to eight semester hours), organic chemistry (six to eight hours), biology (six to eight hours), physics (six to eight hours), and English (six hours).

SUGGESTIONS

Academic work in the humanities and social sciences is considered as important as science course work.

PROCESS

All applicants are sent secondary applications, of which about 20 percent are invited to interview between September and February. Interviews consist of two sessions each with faculty members, administrators, students, or alumni. About 20 percent of interviewed candidates are accepted on a rolling basis, and others are admitted later in the year.

Admissions Requirements (Required)

MCAT scores, science GPA, non-science GPA, letters of recommendation, interview, essays/personal statement, extracurricular activities, exposure to medical profession.

Admissions Requirements (Optional)

state residency.

Overlap Schools

SUNY at Buffalo, SUNY at Stony Brook.

COSTS AND AID

In-state tuition	$16,840
Out-of-state tuition	$28,940
Cost of books	$1,935
Fees	$1,060

Financial Aid

% students receiving aid	90
Average grant	$7,195
Average loan	$21,626

TEMPLE UNIVERSITY
SCHOOL OF MEDICINE

3340 NORTH BROAD STREET, SFC SUITE 305, PHILADELPHIA, PA 19140 • ADMISSION: 215-707-3656 • FAX: 215-707-6932 • E-MAIL: MEDADMISSIONS@TEMPLE.EDU • WEBSITE: WWW.MEDSCHOOL.TEMPLE.EDU

STUDENT BODY

Type	Private
Enrollment	786
% male/female	54/46
% underrepresented minorities	17
# applied (total/out)	7,239/6,326
# accepted (total/out)	493/197
# enrolled (total/out)	177/70
Average age	24

FACULTY

Total faculty (number)	452
% female	27
% minority	5
% part-time	18
# student/faculty ratio	2:1

ADMISSIONS

Average GPA and MCAT Scores

Overall GPA	3.5
MCAT Bio	10
MCAT Phys	10
MCAT Verbal	9
MCAT Essay	Q

Application Information

Regular application	12/15
Regular notification	10/15
Early application	8/1
Early notification	10/1
Are transfers accepted?	Yes
Admissions may be deferred?	Yes
Interview required?	Yes
Application fee	$55

Academics

The academic program has options that appeal to all students, whether they are interested in research, intensive clinical training, or both. Summer research projects in both basic and clinical sciences are encouraged and are often funded. Qualified students may pursue an MPH, MBA or PhD concurrently with an MD. PhD degrees may be obtainted in the following fields: anatomy, biochemistry, immunology, microbiology, molecular biology, pathology, pharmacology, and physiology. Grades of honors, high pass, pass, conditional, and fail are used to evaluate medical students. A grade of pass or higher is required for promotion, and passing both steps of the USMLE is a graduation requirement.

BASIC SCIENCES: During the first two years, students are assigned to basic science faculty advisers who are available to discuss academic matters as well as personal issues. Students are in class for about twenty-five hours per week, with about half of scheduled sessions utilizing a lecture format. Other instructional methods include small group discussions, labs, and interactive clinical training. There is a student-run note service, wherein each student takes responsibility for course notes on specified days and then shares them with the other participants. First-year courses are anatomy, behavioral science, biochemistry, physiology, fundamentals of clinical care I, and a choice of electives. second-year courses are pathology, microbiology, fundamentals of clinical care II & III, pharmacology, pathophysiology, behavioral medicine, genetics, and a wide choice of electives. The current library system includes clinical and research journals and texts, an electronic reference/information center, a microcomputer learning center, and access to online Internet informational services. Plans are in progress for a new academic building.

CLINICAL TRAINING

Students are introduced to clinic experiences in the first year, as an adjunct to basic science studies. In the third year, students are assigned to a clinical faculty adviser who assists with decisions about electives and post-graduate training. Third-year required rotations are anesthesiology (one week), internal medicine (twelve weeks), obstetrics/gynecology (six weeks), pediatrics (six weeks), family medicine (six weeks), psychiatry (six weeks), surgery (eight weeks), and surgical subspecialties (three weeks). During the fourth year, twenty weeks of electives are required, in addition to clerkships in emergency medicine (four weeks) and neuroscience (four weeks), and a subinternship in internal medicine, pediatrics, or surgery (eight weeks). Training takes place at the Temple University Hospital (500 beds), a busy emergency room, and several specialized centers such as a sports medicine center and one of the nation's largest heart transplantation programs. The new Temple University Children's Medical Center opened in January, 1998. Other affiliated hospitals include the Crozer Chester Medical Center, Scranton Mercy Hospital, the Western Pennsylvania Medical Center, the Fox Chase Cancer Center, the Reading Hospital and Medical Center, Abington Memorial Hospital, St. Luke's Hospital, Mercy Hospital, Lehigh Vally Hospital, and Moss Rehabilitation Hospital.

Students

Approximately 60 percent of students are Pennsylvania residents. About 15 percent of students in a typical class are underrepresented minorities. In particular, Temple has a strong contingent of African American and Latino students. Class size is 180.

STUDENT LIFE

Temple students benefit from rich extracurricular offerings both on and off campus. Both Temple Medical School and the main Temple campus have comprehensive athletic and recreational facilities. Medical students are active in school governance and are members of the curriculum, financial affairs, and admissions committees. There are numerous student organizations that range from support groups for minority medical students, to community outreach organizations, to a rugby club. Philadelphia is a historically and culturally rich city. It is also a very student-friendly city, where medical students in particular abound. Most students live off campus.

GRADUATES

About half of Temple's graduates enter residency programs in Pennsylvania. Among students who graduated in 2001, the most prevalent specialty choices were internal medicine (35 percent), surgery (9 percent), transitional (9 percent), pediatrics (8 percent), emergency medicine (6 percent), family medicine (6 percent), orthopedics (4 percent), psychiatry (4 percent) and obstetrics/gynecology (3 percent).

Admissions

REQUIREMENTS

One year each of biology, chemistry, organic chemistry, and physics are required as well as six semester hours of humanities. The MCAT is required, and scores must be no more than three years old.

SUGGESTIONS

As a state-related school, Temple gives some preference to Pennsylvania residents, although significant numbers of out-of-state applicants are admitted. For applicants who have been out of college for a period of time, some recent course work is important. The April MCAT is preferred over the August one. Medically related and community service activities are valued, and the Admissions Committee is serious about selecting students who will make supportive class members and caring physicians.

PROCESS

There is no GPA or MCAT cut off, and all applications are reviewed by a member of the Admissions Committee. All AMCAS applicants receive requests for secondary application materials, and about 15 percent of those are invited to interview. Interviews take place between September and May and consist of a one-hour session with a faculty member or administrator. On interview day, applicants receive a campus tour and have lunch with current medical students. About one-third of interviewees are accepted and are notified on a rolling basis. Admission may also be gained through programs with post-baccalaureate, pre-medical programs at Temple, Goucher, Duquesne, Bryn Mawr, Columbia, Scripps, Brandies, West Chester, Scranton, and the University of Pennsylvania. Early assurance programs exist with pre-medical programs at Duquesne and Washington-Jefferson. Uniquely qualified high school students may apply for BA/BS or MD Programs with Temple, Washington-Jefferson, Duquesne, Scranton, and Widener.

Admissions Requirements (Required)

MCAT scores, science GPA, non-science GPA, letters of recommendation, interview, essays/personal statement, extracurricular activities, exposure to medical profession.

Admissions Requirements (Optional)

state residency.

COSTS AND AID

Tuition	$30,020
Cost of books	$1,598
Fees	$460

Financial Aid

% students receiving aid	89
Average grant	$8,240
Average loan	$37,874
Average debt	$140,652

TEXAS A&M UNIVERSITY SYSTEM HEALTH SCIENCE CENTER
COLLEGE OF MEDICINE

159 JOE H. REYNOLDS MEDICAL BUILDING, COLLEGE STATION, TX 77843-1114 • ADMISSION: 979-845-7743 • FAX: 409-847-8663 • E-MAIL: FGMALDONADO@TAMU.EDU • WEBSITE: HTTP://TAMUSHSC.TAMU.EDU

STUDENT BODY

Type	Public
Enrollment	272
% male/female	48/52
% underrepresented minorities	44
# applied (total/out)	1,779/122
# accepted (total/out)	64/0
# enrolled (total/out)	64/1
Average age	23

FACULTY

Total faculty (number)	831
# student/faculty ratio	1:1

ADMISSIONS

Application Information

Regular application	10/15
Regular notification	1/15
Are transfers accepted?	Yes
Admissions may be deferred?	Yes
Interview required?	Yes
Application fee	$45

Academics

Students may pursue a joint MS/PhD in conjunction with graduate departments of the university in the following fields: anatomy, biochemistry, biomedical engineering biophysics, cell biology, genetics, immunology, microbiology, molecular biology, neuroscience, pathology, pharmacology, and physiology. Clinical instruction is integrated into the basic science curriculum, as are sessions that emphasize the social and ethical aspects of medicine.

BASIC SCIENCES: The first year is organized into semesters. Fall semester of the first year consists of the following: gross anatomy (lecture/lab), biochemistry and genetics (lecture), humanities in medicine (small group), and introduction to patients (small group, which discusses clinical care). In the spring, students take microanatomy (lecture/lab), neuroscience (all methods of instruction), physiology (lecture/small group), and physical diagnosis (small group). Throughout the year, students participate in an innovative leadership in medicine (small group) course that encourages community involvement. Working with patients, which introduces the patient interview, spans part of each semester. During year one, students are in class for about twenty-seven hours per week. The second year is divided into trimesters; students take pathology (lecture/lab), pediatrics (lecture), obstetrics/gynecology (lecture), and the primary care preceptorship (clinical). Humanities (small group) is taken during the first trimester. For the duration of the first two trimesters, microbiology (lecture/lab) and pharmacology (lecture/small group) are studied. Clinical medicine and psychiatry (lecture) are taken during the final trimester. Students are in class for about twenty-nine hours per week during year two. Tutoring is available to all students and is conducted by professors and qualified students. Study facilities include the Learning Resources Unit, which contains instructional videos and computer programs and 1,200 basic science text and reference books; the Medical Sciences Library, which houses over 100,000 books and numerous computer databases; and Evans Library, which has over two million books. Grades of A through F are used to evaluate medical students during the first two years. Passing the USMLE Step 1 is required for promotion to year three. The passing rate for Texas A&M medical Students exceeds the national average.

CLINICAL TRAINING

Patient contact begins in year one, in working with patients and continues through year two, in the preceptorship for primary care program. Early informal patient contact is possible for those who engage in certain community service or volunteer activities. The third year begins with a weeklong orientation, followed by required rotations: obstetrics/gynecology (six weeks), pediatrics (six weeks), family medicine (twelve weeks), and surgery (twelve weeks). The fourth year consists of electives plus four required clerkships: neurology (four weeks), alcohol and drug dependence (two weeks), acting internship in a ten case, ten care specialty (four weeks), and becoming a clinician (three weeks). Training takes place at several sites including Scott & White Hospital (based in Temple with seventeen affiliated rural clinics), Central Texas Medical Centers (a consortium of hospitals totaling 2,271 beds), Teague Veterans' Center (serves veterans in a thirty-five county service area), the Darnall Army Community Hospital (serves the largest armored installation in the United States), and Driscoll Children Hospital (serves the children of Corpus Christi and South Texas). Libraries are available for third- and fourth-year students at the Teague Veterans' Center and the Scott & White Hospital.

During the third year, grades of A through F are used to evaluate students; during three fourth year, grades of pass and fail are used to evaluate most rotations. Passing the USMLE Step 2 is required for graduation.

Students

The vast majority of students are from Texas. About 10 percent of students are underrepresented minorities, most of whom are of Mexican American descent. About 90 percent of the student body were science majors of some type as undergraduates.

STUDENT LIFE

Each medical school class selects and sponsors human service organizations, at which students volunteer. This, along with social activities sponsored by the school and the university, unifies the class and gives students extracurricular activities to pursue with each other. The university's recreational facilities are outstanding and offer every possible athletic activity. Students live off campus, generally in apartments.

GRADUATES

Of those who graduated between 1991 and 1995, the following residencies were the most popular: family practice (21 percent of graduates), internal medicine (13 percent), surgery (12 percent), obstetrics/gynecology (9 percent), pediatrics (9 percent), psychiatry (7 percent), anesthesiology (7 percent), and radiology (6 percent). Half of the graduates enter residency training programs at university-affiliated hospitals or elsewhere in the state.

Admissions

REQUIREMENTS

The College of Medicine considers for enrollment individuals who have completed at least ninety credit hours of undergraduate course work. By state mandate, enrollment of out-of-state residents may not exceed 10 percent. Each year sixty-four entering students enroll. The following courses are required with at least a grade of C: general biology with lab (eight hours), additional biological sciences (three hours), general chemistry with lab (eight hours), organic chemistry with lab (eight hours), general physics with lab (eight hours), english (six hours), and calculus (three hours). The MCAT is required and must have been taken no earlier than five years before the expected date of enrollment. The most recent set of test scores is considered in the evaluation process. Applicants should not withhold previous test scores.

SUGGESTIONS

Although the MCAT is offered twice each year, in April and August, we strongly encourage applicants to take the MCAT in April. Official scores must be released directly to the Texas Medical and Dental Schools Application Service in Austin, Texas. Involvement in community service and health related work that involves patient and physician contact are helpful. For applicants who have been out of school for several years, some recent course work is recommended.

PROCESS

Approximately 30 percent of Texas applicants are interviewed, and 20 percent of those interviewed are offered a place in the class. About 5 percent of out-of-state residents are interviewed, and only a few are accepted each year. Interview sessions typically are scheduled from August to December. Each applicant is given two thirty-minute interviews. Tender of acceptance is made on January 15. The College of Medicine participates in the Texas Medical Schools Matching Program employed by the Texas Medical and Dental Schools Application Service. A ranked wait-list is established in February. The Texas Medical and Dental Schools Application Service (TMDSAS) processes all applications. Application materials may be obtained after May 1 online at http://dpweb1.dp.utexas.edu/mdac/.

Admissions Requirements (Required)

MCAT scores, science GPA, non-science GPA, letters of recommendation, interview, state residency, essays/personal statement.

COSTS AND AID

In-state tuition	$6,550
Out-of-state tuition	$19,650
Cost of books	$1,150
Fees	$860

Financial Aid

% students receiving aid	90
Average grant	$4,000
Average loan	$23,000
Average debt	$28,000

TEXAS TECH UNIVERSITY

TTU HEALTH SCIENCES CENTER SCHOOL OF MEDICINE

3601 4TH STREET, 2B116, LUBBOCK, TX 79430 • ADMISSION: 806-743-2297 • FAX: 806-743-2725 •
E-MAIL: AMANDA.MCSWEEN@TTUHSC.EDU • WEBSITE: WWW.TTUHSC.EDU

STUDENT BODY

Type	Public
Enrollment	490
% male/female	70/30
% underrepresented minorities	22
# applied (total/out)	2,202/166
# accepted (total)	145
# enrolled (total)	145
Average age	24

FACULTY

Total faculty (number)	527
% female	29
% minority	31
% part-time	9
# student/faculty ratio	1:1

ADMISSIONS

Average GPA and MCAT Scores

Overall GPA	3.7
MCAT Bio	9.7
MCAT Phys	9.5
MCAT Verbal	9.5
MCAT Essay	0

Application Information

Regular application	11/1
Regular notification	2/1
Early application	8/1
Early notification	10/1
Are transfers accepted?	Yes
Admissions may be deferred?	Yes
Interview required?	Yes
Application fee	$40

Academics

Most students complete a four-year curriculum designed to prepare physicians with a broad base of medical knowledge and sound analytic and problem solving skills. It is organized in two stages—basic science and clinical training. Some students devote an additional year to research and earn the MD degree in five years. Others are involved in summer research projects. Qualified students interested in biomedical research or academic medicine can earn a PhD along with the MD degree. To address the needs of a rapidly changing health care system, students can participate in an MD/MBA joint degree program in which both degrees are earned in four years. Medical students are graded on a numerical system and must maintain a weighted average of seventy-five for promotion and graduation.

BASIC SCIENCES: First-year courses are gross anatomy, histology, biochemistry, physician in society, neuroscience, physiology, and concepts in community and ambulatory care, which serves as an introduction to clinical medicine and uses physician community mentors. First-year students also have the opportunity to take an elective. Second-year courses are microbiology, pharmacology, pathology, integrated approach to patient care, introduction to medicine, and introduction to psychiatry. During the first and second years, instruction primarily uses a lecture/lab format. However, some concepts are addressed in small group sessions. Students are in classes or other scheduled sessions for about twenty-seven hours per week. All instruction takes place in medical education buildings on the Lubbock campus.

CLINICAL TRAINING

Third-year required rotations are internal medicine (twelve weeks), surgery (twelve weeks), pediatrics (six weeks), family medicine (six weeks), obstetrics/gynecology (six weeks), and psychiatry (six weeks). Fourth-year requirements are neurology (four weeks), selectives (eight weeks), a subinternship (four weeks), and sixteen weeks of electives. After successful completion of years one and two, approximately thirty-five students go on to Amarillo for clinical training, thirty-five students stay in Lubbock, and fifty students go to El Paso. Amarillo, El Paso, and Lubbock all serve both urban and rural populations. Multiple clinical affiliations of each site provide a wealth of training opportunities for students. El Paso serves an urban border population of more than 700,000 and provides a unique multicultural educational opportunity. Training sites include Thomason Hospital and other community and military facilities. In Lubbock, students benefit from recreational and cultural opportunities available on the Texas Tech University campus of the main university. The primary teaching hospital is University Covanant Health—Lakeside. Other affiliated hospitals include Mary of the Plains Hospital, Charter Plains Hospital, and the Veterans' Administration Outpatient Clinics. Amarillo provides exposure to medicine primarily from a private hospital perspective. Teaching hospitals include Northwest Texas Health Care System, Baptist-St. Anthony Health Care System, and Veterans' Administration Hospital. In total, Texas Tech affiliates provide almost 3,000 teaching beds.

Students

The 1998 entering class had the following characteristics: 100 percent Texas residents, 23 percent underrepresented minorities, 75 percent science majors. Typically, about 20 percent of students in an entering class are a bit older and have therefore taken time off after college. Class size is 120.

STUDENT LIFE

During their first two years, students benefit from the resources of the Health Science Center and from being adjacent to Texas Tech University, a major undergraduate institution. Medical students are supportive of one another, as demonstrated by a student-initiated, peer-tutoring program. First- and second-year students are often involved in community service projects, which provide early clinical exposure. Student life during the third and fourth years varies according to location.

GRADUATES

Approximately 21 percent of graduates enter Texas Tech residency programs, which operate on all four campuses. Other graduates are successful in obtaining positions throughout Texas and at institutions in other regions of the country. Eighty-one percent of 1998 graduates matched with one of their top three residency choices.

Admissions

REQUIREMENTS

Requirements are biology (twelve semester hours), biology lab (two semester hours), general chemistry with lab (eight semester hours), organic chemistry with lab (eight semester hours), physics with lab (eight semester hours), english (six semester hours), and calculus (three semester hours). All prerequisite courses require a grade of C or better. The MCAT is required and should be taken within the past five years. For applicants who have retaken the exam, the most recent set of scores is weighed most heavily; however, students must report all scores. Texas residents and residents of neighboring counties in New Mexico and Oklahoma, which make up the service areas of the school, are given preference in admission. Only nonresident applicants with GPAs of 3.60 or higher and MCAT scores of 29 or higher will be considered for admission.

SUGGESTIONS

The April MCAT is preferred over the August one. In addition to high intellectual ability and a record of strong academic achievement, the committee looks for qualities and traits such as compassion, motivation, communication skills, maturity, and personal integrity.

PROCESS

Texas Tech does not participate in AMCAS. Texas Tech participates with five other state-supported medical schools in the Texas Medical and Dental Application Service (TMDAS). A single application is sent to the TMDAS for processing and then is forwarded to any or all of the participating schools as requested by the applicant. A secondary application is also required by Texas Tech. Both applications will be available via the Internet. In addition, application forms may be requested from Texas Medical and Dental Application Service, 702 Colorado Street, Suite 6400, Austin, TX 78701. About 38 percent of applicants are interviewed between September and January. Interviews consist of two sessions, each with an admissions committee/faculty member. On interview day, applicants tour the campus, attend group information sessions, meet current students, and have the opportunity to attend classes. Notification begins on October 15 and continues until the class is filled.

Admissions Requirements (Required)

MCAT scores, science GPA, non-science GPA, letters of recommendation, interview, essays/personal statement, extracurricular activities, exposure to medical profession.

Admissions Requirements (Optional)

state residency.

COSTS AND AID

In-state tuition	$7,654
Out-of-state tuition	$20,754
Cost of books	$1,271
Fees	$1,226

Financial Aid

% students receiving aid	85
Average grant	$1,600
Average loan	$20,084
Average debt	$100,000

TUFTS UNIVERSITY
SCHOOL OF MEDICINE

OFFICE OF ADMISSIONS, 136 HARRISON AVENUE, STEARNS 1, BOSTON, MA 02111 • ADMISSION: 617-636-6571 •
E-MAIL: SGP@COR.CDM.NEMC. • WEBSITE: WWW.TUFTS.EDU/MED

STUDENT BODY

Type	Private
Enrollment	695
% male/female	52/48
% underrepresented minorities	11
# applied (total/out)	8,207/8,336
# accepted (total)	491
# enrolled (total/out)	170/113

ADMISSIONS

Average GPA and MCAT Scores

Overall GPA	3.5
MCAT Bio	10.5
MCAT Phys	10.3
MCAT Verbal	9.9

Application Information

Regular application	11/1
Regular notification	10/15
Early application	8/1
Early notification	10/1
Are transfers accepted?	Yes
Interview required?	Yes
Application fee	$95

Academics

The majority of students follow a four-year curriculum that leads to the MD degree. Students with an interest in public health have the opportunity to earn an MPH along with their MD. This combined MD/MPH program may be completed in four years. Other combined-degree programs include the four year MD/MBA in health management in partnership with Brandeis University and Northeastern University, the MS/PhD in conjunction with the Sackler School of Graduate Biomedical Sciences, and the BS in engineering and combined MS/MD in engineering degree program, a collaborative effort of the Tufts College of Engineering and the Tufts University School of Medicine. The doctorate may be earned in the following fields: anatomy, biochemistry, biophysics, cell biology, genetics, immunology, microbiology, molecular biology, neuroscience, pathology, pharmacology, and physiology. Each year, four funded MS/PhD positions are available. A primary care preceptorship program allows students with a particular interest in primary care to experience early patient contact.

BASIC SCIENCES: In addition to required courses, first and second-year students choose among preclinical selectives. These are graded as pass/fail and allow students to explore their interests early on in the program. A new principles and practice of medicine program (PPM) was developed to enhance the first- and second-year curriculum. PPM integrates basic science topics with interdisciplinary subjects such as information management, computer literacy, negotiation/team building skills, health care economics, and ethics. PPM also introduces important clinical techniques such as the patient interview, examination, and physical diagnosis. First-year courses are the following: gross anatomy, histology, biochemistry, genetics, epidemiology biostatistics, molecular biology, physiology, cell biology, immunology, hematology, problem-based learning, preclinical selectives, and PPM. Second-year courses are the following: pathology, pathophysiology/infectious disease, neuroscience, psychopathology, pharmacology, microbiology, problem-based learning, addiction medicine, preclinical selectives, and PPM (focuses on clinical skills and serves as an important transition to third-year clerkships). During the first and second years, instruction involves lectures, labs, and small group sessions. As an important learning aid, Tufts Health Sciences Library developed the Health Sciences Database. It contains the full text of many syllabi, lecture slides, reserve slide collections, lecture recordings, and other multimedia and resource materials.

CLINICAL TRAINING

Third-year required clerkships are the following: medicine (twelve weeks), surgery (twelve weeks), obstetrics/gynecology (six weeks), pediatrics (six weeks), and psychiatry (six weeks). About four weeks are available for elective study during the third year. Fourth-year requirements are a four-week primary care clerkship and a four-week neurology elective. At least thirty-two weeks of electives are also required, twenty of which must be completed at Tufts facilities. Twelve weeks of electives may be taken at other academic and clinical institutions. Some students fulfill a portion of elective requirements overseas.

Students

In last year's entering class, about 28 percent of students were Massachusetts residents, and about 14 percent of students went to Tufts as undergraduates. Another 28 percent of students were California residents, and 10 percent were New York residents. Approximately 30 percent of students were at least twenty-three years old, and 15 percent of them were twenty-five years old or older. Women accounted for 41 percent of the class, and underrepresented minorities accounted for about 11 percent.

STUDENT LIFE

Medical students at Tufts are generally cohesive and supportive of one another. Some students are involved in clubs or in local chapters of national medical student organizations. Off campus, students enjoy the offerings of Boston, a city filled with students, bookstores, coffee shops, restaurants, parks, and cultural activities. Residence facilities are available on a limited basis in Posner Hall, located close to the medical school campus. Students who live off campus generally share apartments in neighborhoods that are conveniently located by the school.

GRADUATES

Graduates are successful in securing residency positions at institutions in all regions of the country. Tufts prepares graduates for careers in both primary care and specialty areas.

Admissions

REQUIREMENTS

Requirements are eight semester credits of biology, chemistry, organic chemistry, and physics all with associated labs. Applicants must possess the ability to speak and write English correctly. The MCAT is required, and scores should be from within the past three years. For applicants who have retaken the exam, the best scores are used.

SUGGESTIONS

In addition to prerequisite courses, recommended course work includes calculus, statistics, computer science, English, and biochemistry. The selection of candidates for admissions is based not only on performance in the required pre-medical courses but also on the applicant's entire academic record and extracurricular experiences.

PROCESS

All AMCAS applicants are sent secondary applications, of which about 12 percent are invited to interview between November and March. Interviews consist of two sessions, each with a faculty member, school administrator, or senior medical student. On interview day, applicants also attend informational sessions and a reception with current medical students. Approximately half of interviewed candidates are accepted and are notified on a rolling basis with the final notifications occurring in May. Wait-listed candidates are generally not encouraged to send additional information.

Admissions Requirements (Required)

MCAT scores, science GPA, non-science GPA, letters of recommendation, interview, state residency, extracurricular activities, exposure to medical profession.

Admissions Requirements (Optional)

essays/personal statement.

COSTS AND AID

Tuition	$39,579
Room and board	$9,864
Cost of books	$1,500
Fees	$2,679

Financial Aid

% students receiving aid	75
Average grant	$6,867
Average loan	$24,383

TULANE UNIVERSITY
SCHOOL OF MEDICINE

OFFICE OF ADMISSIONS, 1430 TULANE AVENUE, SL67, NEW ORLEANS, LA 70112 • ADMISSION: 504-588-5187 • FAX: 504-599-6735 • E-MAIL: MEDSCH@TMCPOP.TMC.TULANE.EDU • WEBSITE: WWW.MCL.TULANE.EDU

STUDENT BODY

Type	Private
Enrollment	599
% male/female	55/45
% underrepresented minorities	12
# applied (total/out)	8,439/7,916
# accepted (total/out)	22/7
# enrolled (out)	16

ADMISSIONS

Application Information

Regular application	12/15
Regular notification	10/15 until filled
Early application	6/1-8/1
Early notification	10/1
Are transfers accepted?	Yes
Admissions may be deferred?	Yes
Interview required?	No
Application fee	$95

Academics

The School of Medicine is one part of the Tulane University Health Sciences Center. In addition to the School of Medicine, the Health Sciences Center includes the School of Public Health and Tropical Medicine, the Tulane University Hospital and Clinic, the Tulane Hospital for Children, the University Health Service, the Primate Research Center and the U.S.-Japan Biomedical Research Laboratories. The following programs and centers of excellence are located within the Health Sciences Center: Center for Gene Therapy, the Center for Infectious Diseases, General Clinical Research Center, the Hayward genetics Center, Hypertension and Renal Center, Tulane Center for Clinical Effectiveness and Prevention, the Center for Bioenvironmental Research at Tulane and Xavier University, DePaul-Tulane Behavioral Health Center, Tulane Cancer Center, the Tulane Center for Abdominal Transplant, the Tulane Institute of Sports Medicine, the Tulane-Xavier National Women's Center, and Tulane Cardiovascular Center of Excellence.

BASIC SCIENCES: First-year courses include anatomy, histology, embryology, neuroscience, physiology, and biochemistry. Multimedia lectures, problem-based learning sessions, small group discussions, laboratories, and clinical correlations are all employed by these first year courses. An emphasis is placed upon the clinical application of the basic science material. The second year takes a systems-oriented approach that integrates pharmacology, pathology, microbiology, immunology, pathophysiology, and physical diagnosis. During the second semester of the first year and throughout the entire second year, students choose from an extensive offering of both basic and clinical science electives, including many research opportunities. Each year, many students will use some of their elective time to take courses in the School of Public Health and Tropical Medicine; approximately thirty to thirty-five students each year graduate with the MD and the MPH degrees, having earned both degrees over a four year period. Grades of honors, high pass, pass, conditional, and fail are used to evaluate medical students. Students are required to record a grade on USMLE Step 1, but are not required to pass for promotion. The USMLE Step 2 is not required for graduation.

CLINICAL TRAINING

During the first two years, clinical training is integrated with the basic science curriculum, with patient contact beginning immediately in year one through the foundations in medicine program. During these two years, students work with actual patients in hospitals near the school (the Tulane University Hospital, the Medical Center of Louisiana, University Hospital, and the Veterans' Affairs Hospital) and with surrogate, or standardized, patients. Formal clinical training begins with the third year and consists of the following required eight-week rotations: family/community medicine, internal medicine, obstetrics and gynecology, pediatrics, psychiatry and neurology, and surgery. During the fourth year, students do a four-week clerkship that focuses on the undifferentiated patient; this internship allows students to experience ambulatory care medicine in several settings. Also in the fourth year, students do a four-week subinternship in ward management. Fourth year students also have six selectives, which may include locations either domestically or internationally. Established international rotations are available in Africa, South and Central America, and Asia. A formal exchange program exists with organizations in Sweden, Germany, and Japan.

Students

Students of the class of 2005 entering class represented thirty-one states and five countries. Of a class of 155 students, thirty-two came from Louisiana, twenty-seven from California, and seven each from Massachusetts and Utah. The average age range is twenty-one to thirty-four, with an average age of 24. About 14 percent of the class is from an underrepresented minority population.

STUDENT LIFE

Students are very much involved in life both on- and off-campus. Medical school extracurricular groups dedicated to student social life include medart, music & medicine, the tulane chorale, and students against right brain atrophy. Organizations based upon academics, specialty interests, religion, hobbies, ethnicity, and athletics bring medical students together around shared interests. An expansive support program is available for students experiencing problems, whether academic or personal. A housing facility, located adjacent to the Tulane University Health Sciences Center, makes over 250 apartments available to medical students, although most students choose to live off-campus.

GRADUATES

Of the 2002 graduating class, the most popular residencies were internal medicine, surgery, pediatrics, family practice, and psychiatry. Approximately 50 percent of the class entered specialties considered to be primary care. Graduates from the class of 2002 will be pursuing residency training in twenty-nine different states, with thirty-three of them staying in the State of Louisiana. Other popular states for residency training were Texas, California, Washington, Pennsylvania, Massachusetts, and Maryland.

Admissions

REQUIREMENTS

All students must have completed the following prerequisites prior to matriculation: English (six semester hours), general chemistry (six semester hours), organic chemistry (six semester hours), physics (six semester hours), and biology (six semester hours). While an undergraduate degree is not required, it is preferred. All required sciences courses must include labs. The MCAT is required and should be no more than three years old; if the MCAT is taken more than once, the best set of scores is considered.

SUGGESTIONS

It is strongly advised that applicants take the MCAT in April of the year in which they intend to apply to medical school and not wait until the August administration. Activities that demonstrate strong interpersonal skills and/or evidence of self-discipline are valued, as are leadership positions.

PROCESS

Tulane University is an AMCAS school; therefore, the process begins with the student submitting an AMCAS application. All who submit an AMCAS application receive a Tulane secondary application, of which about 20 percent are interviewed from September through February. Interviews consist of three one-on-one interviews; two with faculty and one with a Tulane medical student. After the interview, the applicant's file is submitted to the Committee on Admissions, which is an action committee. Notification of the committee's action occurs on a rolling basis with every effort made to inform the applicant of the committee's decision within two weeks of the interview. Of those interviewed, about 30 percent are offered a place in the class; candidates who are wait-listed are invited to send additional information if they feel it will strengthen their files.

Admissions Requirements (Required)

MCAT scores, science GPA, non-science GPA, letters of recommendation, state residency, extracurricular activities, exposure to medical profession.

Admissions Requirements (Optional)

interview, essays/personal statement.

COSTS AND AID

Cost of books	$1,000

Financial Aid

% students receiving aid	87
Average grant	$10,000
Average loan	$29,704
Average debt	$90,000

UNIFORMED SERVICES UNIVERSITY OF THE HEALTH SCIENCES
F. EDWARD HEBERT SCHOOL OF MEDICINE

4301 JONES BRIDGE ROAD, BETHESDA, MD 20814 • ADMISSION: 301-295-3101 • FAX: 301-295-3545 •
E-MAIL: ADMISSIONS@USUHS.MIL • WEBSITE: WWW.USUHS.MIL

STUDENT BODY

Type	Public
Enrollment	681
% male/female	70/30
% underrepresented minorities	8
# applied (total)	1,686
# accepted (total)	262
# enrolled (total)	167
Average age	24

FACULTY

Total faculty (number)	3,059
% female	20
% minority	6
% part-time	41
# student/faculty ratio	5:1

ADMISSIONS

Average GPA and MCAT Scores

Overall GPA	3.5
MCAT Bio	9.7
MCAT Phys	9.3
MCAT Verbal	9.2
MCAT Essay	0

Application Information

Regular application	11/3
Regular notification	rolling
Are transfers accepted?	No
Admissions may be deferred?	Yes
Interview required?	Yes

Academics

Incoming students without prior uniformed service experience attend a professional orientation course during the summer before entering the School of Medicine. Most classes and rotations are evaluated with grades of A through F. Students must pass both steps of the USMLE to graduate.

BASIC SCIENCES: Lectures and labs are the primary means of instruction during the first two years, and students are in scheduled sessions for about twenty-five hours per week. In addition to a solid grounding in the basic sciences, students receive interdisciplinary instruction that includes sociological, historical, ethical, and legal perspectives on medicine. First-year courses are anatomy and physiology I; biochemistry; diagnostic parasitology and medical zoology; fundamentals of epidemology and biometrics; head, neck, and CNS anatomy; human context in health care; introduction to clinical medicine I; medical psychology; medical history; military medical field studies (summer); organ system microanatomy; and physiology II. During the summer following the first academic year, students take part in a hands-on field experience that serves as an introduction to military operations. Students who have a background in this area use the summer for research or other activities. Second-year courses are clinical concepts; clinical pharmacology; ethical, legal, and social aspects of medical care; human behavior; introduction to clinical medicine II and III; medical microbiology and infectious diseases; military studies II; pathology; pharmacology; preventive medicine; and radiographic interpretation. Instruction takes place on the grounds of the National Naval Medical Center, in Bethesda, Maryland. Educational resources include the multidisciplinary laboratories and the anatomical teaching laboratories, both of which are open twenty-four hours a day. The Learning Resource Center serves as the library and has 120,000 volumes, journals, slides, videotapes, CDs, microcomputer programs, and online informational programs.

CLINICAL TRAINING

Third-year required clerkships are family practice (six weeks), medicine (twelve weeks), obstetrics/gynecology (six weeks), pediatrics (six weeks), psychiatry (six weeks), and surgery (twelve weeks). During the fourth year, twenty weeks are reserved for clinical electives or research. Required fourth-year clerkships are military contingency medicine, military emergency medicine, military preventive medicine, neurology, and a subinternship. The main teaching hospitals are Walter Reed Army Medical Center, National Naval Medical Center, and Malcolm Grow USAF Medical Center, which are all in the Washington, DC, area, and the Wilford Hall USAF Medical Center, in San Antonio, Texas. In total, these hospitals provide over 3,000 beds. Electives may be fulfilled at clinical sites nationwide and overseas.

Students

In a recent class, 60 percent of all students had no prior military experience. Other students had backgrounds in service academies, ROTC activities, and as active and prior duty officers, enlisted service members, and Reservists. Students are from all over the country and represent a large number of undergraduate institutions. The most prevalent undergraduate majors were biology (35 percent), biochemistry (7 percent), and chemistry (13 percent). About 8 percent of students are underrepresented minorities. The average age of entering students is about twenty-four. Class size is 167.

STUDENT LIFE

USUHS student groups include chapters of national organizations, in addition to organizations that are focused on professional or service oriented goals. These organizations are devoted to activities such as journalism, providing support to women medical students or spouses of medical students, and recreational pursuits. The school sponsors intramural athletic programs for men and women, and offers comprehensive athletic facilities. Nearby military posts and bases provide recreational and social activities for students and their families. Washington, DC, with its museums, sites, parks, events, and diverse population, is an important resource and enriches the lives of medical students. All students live off campus, most in the immediate vicinity of the school or in Metro-accessible areas.

GRADUATES

Graduates must select residency programs at military hospitals, and often enter programs at the hospitals where they performed clerkships. Residencies vary in length, depending on the medical specialty. The residency period does not fulfill the seven-year commitment involved in attending USUHS. The military branch in which graduates will serve is determined when they enter the School of Medicine; it reflects each student's preference and the needs of the organization.

Admissions

REQUIREMENTS

Applicants must be citizens of the United States, be at least eighteen years old at the time of matriculation (but no older than thirty as of June 30) in the year of admission, meet military regulations related to physical health, possess a baccalaureate degree by June 15 in the year of admissions, and fulfill academic prerequisites. These are one year each of biology, physics, general chemistry, and organic chemistry with lab. One year of English composition and/or literature and one semester of calculus are required. The MCAT is required, and scores must be from within three years of desired matriculation. For applicants who have retaken the exam, the best set of scores is used.

SUGGESTIONS

A broad undergraduate background, with courses in history, philosophy, literature, economics, political science, foreign languages, sociology, and psychology, are considered valuable. Applicants must be dedicated both to the medical profession and to the idea of serving the country.

PROCESS

About 80 percent of AMCAS applicants are sent secondary applications, of which about 25 percent are invited to interview between September and February. Interviews consist of two thirty-minute sessions with practicing physicians. About one-third of interviewees are accepted and notified on a rolling basis. Wait-listed candidates may send supplementary material to enhance their files.

Admissions Requirements (Required)

MCAT scores, science GPA, non-science GPA, letters of recommendation, interview, essays/personal statement, exposure to medical profession.

Admissions Requirements (Optional)

state residency, extracurricular activities.

COSTS AND AID

Financial Aid

% students receiving aid	100

UNIVERSIDAD AUTÓNOMA DE GUADALAJARA

UNIVERSIDAD AUTÓNOMA DE GUADALAJARA

4715 FREDERICKSBURG ROAD, 3RD FLOOR, SAN ANTONIO, TX 78229-3642 • ADMISSION: 800-531-5494 • FAX: 210-377-2975 • E-MAIL: UAGSAT@UAG.EDU • WEBSITE: WWW.UAG.MX/MEDICINE/DEFAULT.HTML

STUDENT BODY

Type	Private
% male/female	51/49
# applied (total)	16,000

ADMISSIONS

Application Information

Regular application	rolling
Regular notification	rolling
Are transfers accepted?	No
Admissions may be deferred?	No
Interview required?	No
Application fee	$30

Academics

The curriculum is comprehensive and helps the student to develop the skills of problem solving and the discipline of self-education. The curriculum is diversified enough for students to make knowledgeable decisions about what specialty area or areas they to pursue after graduation. Students learn to adapt to the different environments in which they will have to practice medicine. Yet, the curiculum is structured in such a way that students obtain sufficient depth in each basic science and clinical area of study. In the block system of education, student intensively learn one clinical subject for a period of several weeks. This approach is extremely effective in the clinical years where the students can concentrate on one subject at a time. The typical class day of five to six hours consists of lectures, with audiovisual presentations in one of the lecture halls. These are followed by laboratory studies, discussions of specific clinical problems, highly personalized small group seminars, and question-and-answer sessions guided by supervising professors and teaching assistants. Two additional carefully constructed programs have become a tremendous help to student progress within the curriculum. In the medicine in the community program, students begin seeing patients during their first semesters in the various community clinics around Guadalajara. The second program is the integrated course in the basic sciences—a review course for students who have completed two years.

BASIC SCIENCES: The sciences basic to medicine are presented at the Institute of Biological Sciences (ICB) during the first two years of medical education at the UAG. The courses that students will attend during the sixteen weeks of the first semester include introduction to medical practice, biochemistry, gross anatomy, cell biology, embryology, and genetics. The nineteen weeks in the second semester include development of clinical skills, histology, immunology, general pathology, physiology, behavioral sciences, public health and preventive medicine, nutrition and medical ethics. Second year of basic sciences include microbiology and parasitology, pathophysiology, propedeutics, pharmacology and toxicology, neurosciences, systemic pathology, surgical education, and techniques. In all four semesters of the first two years the student also participates in the medicine in the community program (PMC), where they will do rotations in community clinics, Red Cross units and participate in the medical brigades to rural areas. This program provides the opportunity for students to begin development of a physician-patient relationship with Spanish-speaking patients from their first semester. The PMC helps students develop sensitivity to and an understanding of the social and economic problems that prevail in the care of the sick.

CLINICAL TRAINING

The UAG strives to ensure that students in the third and fourth years meet the academic and clinical requirements to be licensed in the United States and other countries. As required by many state boards, the third year is done at the parent university. During the third and fourth years, students complete clerkships in the following clinical subjects: cardiology, dermatology, ENT, ER medicine, endocrinology, forensic medicine, gastroenterology, hematology, infectious diseases, neurology, nutrition, obstetrics/gynecology, ophthalmology, orthopedics, pediatrics, pneumology, psychiatry, pain management, and psychiatry. The fourth year can be done in either Mexico or in the United States either through electives/selectives that students acquire throughout the United States or through our unique co-op program (cooperative medical education program). These rotations must receive prior approval from the assistant dean for clinical sciences.

Students

The UAG is the oldest private university in Mexico. Founded in 1935 the university is multidisciplinary, coeducational, nondenominational, nonprofit, and independent. The UAG School of Medicine offers the course work that leads to a medical degree and to training in medical specialties. To support these medical education programs the UAG has two separate medical campuses, plus numerous supporting clinical facilities in the Guadalajara area and elsewhere. Our university strives to produce bilingual and bicultural physicians who are compassionate as well as capable of treating illnesses. The faculty recognizes that a physician's performance requires not only intellectual skills but also certain personal characteristics and behavior that are sensitive to human needs. The curriculum and instructional methods are designed to develop and enhance these qualities in each student.

STUDENT LIFE

Our classes are made up of students from all fifty states, Puerto Rico, and Canada. There is no on-campus housing, and all students live either in apartments or houses. Many students live minutes away from the basic sciences campus. The UAG has a myriad of extracurricularactivities that include folkloric ballet, theater, symphonic orchestra concerts, professional sports teams in soccer and basketball, and many recreational activities. Students can also visit nearby historical towns or enjoy the beautiful resort town of Puerto Vallarta.

GRADUATES

Since 1935 the UAG international program has graduated 13,000 bilingual and bicultural physicians. They are licensed, board certified, and practicing in all fifty states and other countries. Our residency match rates run from 98 percent to 100 percent each year with some graduates receiving placement before the match. Residency spots include internal medicine, radiology, emergency medicine, trauma, obstetrics/gynecology, pediatrics, and many more. Numerous graduates are also professors in U.S. medical schools such as UCLA, Yale, Harvard, and the University of Texas system.

Admissions

REQUIREMENTS

A minimum of ninety semester credit hours (a baccalaureate is strongly recommended) with at least eight hours of biology, physics, organic and inorganic chemistry. Additionally, for Puerto Rican applicants we require twelve hours in social sciences. The UAG School of Medicine has two entering classes—one in January and one in August. We have a rolling admissions policy that allows us to receive applications year-round. Interviews can be conducted in Guadalajara, Puerto Rico, Albany (New York), or at our main office in San Antonio, Texas.

Admissions Requirements (Optional)

MCAT scores, science GPA, non-science GPA, letters of recommendation, interview, state residency, essays/personal statement, extracurricular activities, exposure to medical profession.

COSTS AND AID

Tuition	$17,580
Fees	$180

UNIVERSIDAD CENTRAL DEL CARIBE

AVENIDA LAUREL, URB. SANTA JUANITA, PO BOX 60327, BAYAMÓN, PR 00960-6032 • ADMISSIONS: 787-798-6732 • WEBSITE: WWW.UCCARIBE.EDU

STUDENT BODY

Type	Private
Enrollment	240
% male/female	49/51
% underrepresented minorities	5
# applied (total)	726
# accepted (total)	123
# enrolled (total)	62
Average age	22

FACULTY

Total faculty (number)	353
% female	36
% minority	12
# student-faculty ratio	1:1

ADMISSIONS

Overall GPA	3.3
MCAT Bio	7.0
MCAT Phys	7.0
MCAT Verbal	7.0
MCAT Essay	L

Application Information

Regular application	12/15
Regular notification	02/15
Are transfers accepted?	Yes
Admissions may be deferred?	No
Interview required?	Yes
Application fee	$50

Academics

The mission of the SOM is to develop competent physicians with an outstanding preparation within a humanistic and holistic framework. A guiding principle of our mission is to ensure that our graduates possess a strong sense of professionalism and commitment to social duties and service to Puerto Rico and Hispanic communities throughout the U.S. mainland. The curriculum emphasizes techniques and values related to the provision of primary medical care. The first two years primarily teach basic medical sciences with a strong introduction to the clinical sciences through a longitudinal primary care preceptorship, human behavior, and clinical skills. The second two years are devoted to clinical rotations and to continuing interdisciplinary instruction.

BASIC SCIENCES: Basic sciences are primarily taught through lectures. Labs and small group sessions are also utilized. First-year courses consist of human gross anatomy, histology, LPCP I, physiology, neurosciences, behavioral sciences, bioethics and humanities in medicine I, problem base learning I, and introduction to clinical skills. Second-year courses are microbiology and immunology, psychopathology, pharmacology, pathology, pathophysiology, clinical skills, LPCP II, bioethics and humanities in medicine II, and problem based learning II. Most instruction during the first two years takes place in the new biomedical sciences building, which also houses laboratories and research facilities.

CLINICAL TRAINING

Clinical clerkships begin in the third year. These consist of radiology (one week), internal medicine (ten weeks), family medicine (six weeks), surgery (six weeks), pediatrics (six weeks), psychiatry (six weeks), and obstetrics/gynecology (six weeks). Major teaching hospitals are the Dr. Ramon Ruiz Arnau University Hospital, San Pablo Hospital, First Hospital Panamericano, San Jorge Children's Hospital, and San Juan Veterans' Administration Hospital.

Students

Around 50 percent of students are women. Virtually all students are from underrepresented minority groups.

STUDENT LIFE

To help students acclimate to medical school, an orientation is given to the entering first-year class. This also serves as an opportunity for students to interact with each other and with faculty members and administrators. Students are encouraged to develop an interest in culture and the arts. With this in mind, the Dean of Student Affairs sponsors an extracurricular activities program for medical students. Counseling services are aimed at helping students take advantage of the extensive educational opportunities at the medical school. A comprehensive health plan is offered to all medical students. Housing facilities are available through individual arrangements in areas adjacent to the medical school and the university hospital.

GRADUATES

The medical school has graduated about 1,750 physicians who serve the Commonwealth of Puerto Rico and Hispanic communities in the United States.

Admissions

REQUIREMENTS

Applicants must demonstrate proficiency in both Spanish and English. This is essential, as lectures are conducted in the language preferred by the respective professor, most often Spanish. In addition, Spanish is necessary for most clinical work. Applicants must complete a minimum of ninety credits at an institution of higher education. A baccalaureate degree is highly recommended. Required premedical course are general biology (eight credit hours), general chemistry (eight hours), organic chemistry (eight hours), physics (eight hours), college-level math (six hours), English (twelve hours), Spanish (six hours), and behavioral sciences and social sciences (twelve hours). The MCAT is required. Officials exam results from within the past two years must be submitted to the School of Medicine.

PROCESS

The Universidad Central del Caribe School of Medicine participates in the American Medical College Application Service (AMCAS). All applicants must file an AMCAS application. In addition, applicants should contact the School of Medicine for additional application materials and a processing fee, photographs, an essay, and a certificate of Good Conduct. After applications, MCAT scores, and transcripts are given an initial review, applicants who are under consideration will be invited for personal interviews with members of the faculty.

Admissions Requirements (Required)

MCAT scores, science GPA, non-science GPA, letters of recommendation, interview, essays/personal statement

Admissions Requirements (Optional)

extracurricular activities,state residency, exposure to medical profession.

COSTS AND AID

Out-of-state tuition	$18,000
Cost of books	$15,000
Fees	$3,500

Financial Aid

Average grant	$37,600
Average loan	$37,600

Université Laval
Faculté de Médecine

Pavillon Vandry U. Laval, Ste Foy, ON G1K 7P4 • Admission: 418-656-4141 • Fax: 418-656-2733 •
E-mail: denis.verret@fmed.ulaval.ca • Website: www.fmed.ulaval.ca

STUDENT BODY

Type	Public
# applied (total/out)	1,525/123

ADMISSIONS

Application Information

Regular application	3/1 in Quebec 2/1 others
Regular notification	5/15
Admissions may be deferred?	No
Interview required?	Yes
Application fee	$65

Academics

Laval offers a four-year curriculum that leads to the MD degree. In addition, academic programs are available in a number of health and medical science fields, including molecular biology, community health, epidemiology, occupational health and safety, and physiology. Research is an important part of the academic experience at Laval, and students are encouraged to pursue research during summers and throughout the academic year.

BASIC SCIENCES: The first two years involve basic science instruction and opportunities for addressing clinical problems. The first year includes courses in biochemistry, physiology, pharmacology, microbiology-immunology, histology-pathology, and introduction to problems. During the second part of the first year, instruction is organized around anatomical systems and medical concepts such as cardiovascular system, respiratory system, uro-nephrology, microbiology/infectious disease, and physiological/sociological. Introduction to problems continues during the second semester. Students also study endocrinology, obstetrics/gynecology, and growth/development during their first year. Year two subjects are nervous system, locomotor system, medical ethics, problem discussion, the art of interviewing, ENT, ophthalmology, hematology, gastroenterology, psychopathology, preventive medicine, and skin. Laval's library system is an important academic resource for students; it holds millions of volumes and periodicals.

CLINICAL TRAINING

Years three and four are devoted to clinical rotations. Required clerkships are introduction to clinical medicine (nine weeks), medicine (eight weeks), surgery (eight weeks), pediatrics (eight weeks), psychiatry (eight weeks), obstetrics/gynecology (eight weeks), preventive medicine (four weeks), geriatrics/rehabilitation medicine (four weeks), family practice (four weeks), and emergency medicine (four weeks). In addition, up to twenty weeks are open for various clinical and basic science electives. Training takes place at a number of affiliated hospitals including Centre Hospitalier de l'Universite Laval, Hopital Laval, Hopital de l'Enfant-Jesus, Hotel-Dieu de Levis, Hotel-Dieu de Quebec, Hopital du Saint-Sacrement and Hopital Saint-Francois d'Assie.

Students

Each entering class at the Faculty of Medicine is made up of about 112 students. Typically, all but a few are from within the province of Quebec. Students from other provinces must be French speakers. Within the student body are a limited number of international, French-speaking students. Women make up about 60 percent of the students.

STUDENT LIFE

Laval supports medical students both inside and outside the classroom. Programs offered include orientation and counseling services, religious organizations, career placement services, social and athletic organizations, child care, and attractive, low cost student housing. The Laval campus is situated in an urban environment.

GRADUATES

Graduates of Laval Faculty of Medicine enter both clinical and academic medicine. The teaching hospitals affiliated with Laval offer many programs for graduate medical training.

Admissions

REQUIREMENTS

Generally, all applicants must have completed at least two years of college to be considered for admission. Required undergraduate courses are biology (eight semester hours), general chemistry (eight semester hours), organic chemistry (eight semester hours), general physics (two hours), and mathematics including calculus (two hours). In addition, some course work in French, humanities, and social sciences is required. Fluency in French is a requirement for admission.

SUGGESTIONS

Priority is given to residents of the province of Quebec. Candidates are evaluated on the basis of academic achievement, interpersonal skills, experience, and personal characteristics. Although two years of college is the minimum requirement, additional schooling serves to strengthen applications.

PROCESS

Applications are coordinated in part by the organization of Quebec Colleges and Universities. For entrance in the fall, the application deadline is March 1. In addition to a written application, interviews are an important part of the selection process. Generally, about ten to fifteen percent of applicants are accepted in a given year.

COSTS AND AID

Tuition & Fees

Tuition (in/out)	$1,964/7,927
Fees	$200

UNIVERSITY OF ALABAMA AT BIRMINGHAM
UNIVERSITY OF ALABAMA SCHOOL OF MEDICINE

MEDICAL STUDENT SERVICES, VH 100, 1530 3RD AVENUE, SOUTH BIRMINGHAM, AL 35294-0019 • ADMISSION: 205-934-2433 • FAX: 205-934-8724 • E-MAIL: MEDSCHOOL@UAB.EDU • WEBSITE: WWW.UAB.EDU/UASOM/

STUDENT BODY

Type	Public
Enrollment	692
% male/female	59/41
% underrepresented minorities	23
# applied (total/out)	1,365/947
# accepted (total/out)	228/56
# enrolled (total/out)	160/16
Average age	23

FACULTY

Total faculty (number)	1,250
% female	28
% minority	21
% part-time	14

ADMISSIONS

Average GPA and MCAT Scores

Overall GPA	3.7
MCAT Bio	9.9
MCAT Phys	9.7
MCAT Verbal	9.8
MCAT Essay	N

Application Information

Regular application	11/1
Regular notification	10/15
Early application	8/1
Early notification	10/1
Are transfers accepted?	Yes
Admissions may be deferred?	Yes
Interview required?	Yes
Application fee	$65

Academics

Basic sciences are taught during the first two years, primarily through lectures and small group case studies. Clinical techniques are introduced early and are often taught in small groups. The curriculum is particularly rich in relevant humanities and social sciences courses such as ethics and behavioral sciences. Joint MS/MD degrees are offered in many fields, notably the master's in public health/MD combination. About eight students a year are accepted into joint MS/PhD programs, usually as MSTP candidates. A combined undergraduate/medical school program is offered at the University of Alabama at Birmingham, which high school seniors who are Alabama residents may apply to.

BASIC SCIENCES: The academic year is organized into quarters. During the fall quarter of the first year, students take the following: biochemistry, gross anatomy, medical ethics, behaviorial sciences, and human sexuality. Winter quarter includes the following: medical cell and tissue biology and physiology. Spring curriculum is pharmacology, neurosciences, and nutrition. Throughout the first year, students participate in a course call introduction to clinical medicine, which covers the patient interview and addresses doctor/patient interaction. During the fall of year two, pharmacology continues and microbiology/immunology is introduced. Pathology is a yearlong course that students take during their second year. Clinical medicine continues in the second year and focuses on physical diagnosis. The Lister Hill Library at the Birmingham campus houses 240,000 volumes and uses computer online search services. Preclinical performance is evaluated with grades of A through F. The USMLE Step 1 is required following completion of the preclinical studies and before promotion to the third year.

CLINICAL TRAINING

Clinical training begins well before the required clerkships of the third year. In addition to the introductory clinical course work of the first two years, some students are involved in community programs that provide patient exposure to public health programs such as the AIDS Care Team and other projects aimed at young or homeless populations. The final two years are essentially combined—required clerkships fill all of the third year and part of the fourth year. Students choose a primary campus for clerkships; a few students will ultimately rotate to all three campuses. Each campus has unique strengths. Required clerkships are medicine, surgery, pediatrics, obstetrics/gynecology, family medicine, rural medicine, neurology, and psychiatry. Each campus is affiliated with several teaching hospitals, and rotations take students to a variety of learning environments ranging from large Veterans' Affairs Hospitals to small, rural clinics. Grades of A through F are used to evaluate required rotations, and grades of pass and fail are used to evaluate electives. The School of Medicine established a medical student enrichment program in 1995, which encourages and facilitates overseas clinical experience. In addition to providing elective opportunities to medical school seniors, medical students may apply to the program or placements during the summer between their first and second years. In 1996, fourteen out of twenty-two applicants were accepted into the program, which took them to Russia, Guatemala, Jamaica, and South and West Africa. The USMLE Step 2 is required for graduation.

Students

One-seventh of the members of a typical class are considered out-of-state residents, but a much greater percentage of the student body went to college out of state. About 75 percent of the matriculates majored in a scientific field during their undergraduate studies.

STUDENT LIFE

Outside of class, students are often involved in recreational and volunteer activities. Some are active in student organizations such as national medical groups. The Student Government Association consists of elected members of each class. The Birmingham campus with its many departments provides a community beyond that of medical students alone. Most students choose to live off campus, where housing is ample and relatively affordable. Most students have cars.

GRADUATES

Family practice and internal medicine are the particularly popular fields among graduates. Although graduates are competitive for residencies nationwide, a significant number enter residency programs in Alabama at university-affiliated hospitals or other locations in the state.

Admissions

REQUIREMENTS

Undergraduate requirements are biology or zoology (eight semester hours), chemistry with lab (eight semester hours), organic chemistry with lab (eight semester hours), physics with lab (eight semester hours), math (six semester hours), and English (six semester hours). Academic work accomplished overseas may be acceptable, depending on the institution and the course. The MCAT is required, and it must not be more than two years old at the time of application. The spring MCAT is strongly recommended. The AMCAS application is required.

SUGGESTIONS

The Admissions Committee values experience with patient care and exposure to health care environments. The University of Alabama School of Medicine welcomes nontraditional applicants and has admitted several students who are older than forty. Due to the state-mandated preference for Alabama residents, out-of-state applicants are required to have an overall GPA of 3.5 or higher and MCAT scores of 30 or higher.

PROCESS

All AMCAS applicants receive a secondary application. Generally, about 70 percent of in-state applicants are interviewed. About 10 to 12 percent of out-of-state applicants are interviewed. In 2000, about 55 percent of the in-state applicants interviewed were accepted, while about 32 percent of the out-of-state applicants interviewed were accepted. Notification begins in October, and the class is generally filled by April. Interviews consist of three thirty-minute sessions with faculty members.

Admissions Requirements (Required)

MCAT scores, science GPA, non-science GPA, letters of recommendation, interview, essays/personal statement, extracurricular activities, exposure to medical profession.

Admissions Requirements (Optional)

state residency.

Overlap Schools

Emory University, University of South Alabama, Vanderbilt University.

COSTS AND AID

In-state tuition	$7,829
Out-of-state tuition	$23,487
Cost of books	$1,200
Fees	$3,852

Financial Aid

% students receiving aid	89
Average grant	$3,500
Average loan	$17,461
Average debt	$84,040

UNIVERSITY OF ALBERTA
FACULTY OF MEDICINE AND DENTISTRY

2-45 MEDICAL SCIENCES BUILDING, EDMONTON, ALBERTA T6G 2H7 • ADMISSION: 780-492-6350 •
WEBSITE: WWW.MED.UALBERTA.CA

STUDENT BODY

Type	Public
# applied (total/out)	1,095

ADMISSIONS

MCAT Bio	10.8
MCAT Phys	11.3
MCAT Verbal	9.7

Application Information

Regular application	1/31
Admissions may be deferred?	Yes
Interview required?	Yes
Application fee	$60

Academics

Alberta's curriculum reflects the school's emphasis on clinical care and research. The preclinical curriculum has been revised and is largely centered on organ systems. It is multidisciplinary, including both biological and social science perspectives. Although basic sciences are the focus of study during the first two years, courses are taught with clinical applications in mind. The second two years integrate classroom and hospital-based instruction. While most medical students earn an MD degree in four years, qualified students may pursue joint degrees such as the MD/PhD or MD/MPH in a longer period of study.

BASIC SCIENCES: Basic sciences are taught in a variety of forums, including lectures, small-group discussions, laboratories, problem-based learning, independent study, and computer-based instruction. The academic period begins in August, covers thirty-five weeks, and includes courses in introduction to medicine; immunity, infection and inflammation; practice of medicine (part I); cardiology, renal, and pulmonary; and endocrine and metabolism. On average, students are in class or other scheduled sessions for about twenty-five hours per week. The second academic period also begins in August and includes gastroenterology, reproduction and urology, musculoskeletal, neurosciences, oncology, and practice of medicine (part II) in addition to a systems-based curriculum. Systems studied are cardiovascular, endocrinology, gastrointestinal, hematology, medical ethics, nephrology, ophthalmology, pediatrics, pulmonary, surgery, and urology. Basic science instruction takes place mainly at the medical sciences building and uses the resources of the John W. Scott Health Sciences Library. Medical students may use all university libraries and computer facilities. All enrolled students have access to free online service.

CLINICAL TRAINING

The third and fourth academic periods primarily teach clinical skills and consist of classroom instruction, required rotations, electives, and selectives. Required clerkships are anesthesia (two weeks), geriatrics (two weeks), medicine (ten weeks), obstetrics/gynecology (eight weeks), pediatrics (eight weeks), psychiatry (eight weeks), radiology (two weeks), rural family medicine (four weeks), and surgery (ten weeks). Selectives include two weeks in internal medicine and two weeks in surgery. Training takes place at University of Alberta hospitals, the Royal Alexandra Hospital, Edmonton General Hospital, Misericordia Hospital, Alberta Hospital, Glenrose Hospital, Cross Cancer Institute, and Grey Nuns Hospital. A certain number of electives may be taken at nonaffiliated institutions.

Students

Among 102 students in the 1998 entering class, 42 percent are female. About 15 percent are from outside of Alberta. A total of eighty-one students completed at least four years of university.

STUDENT LIFE

Campus housing is available, although most students opt to live off campus in the surrounding area. The students' union provides a registry informing students of available housing. Medical students participate in clubs, events, and recreational activities geared toward medical students and the student body in general. Counseling and other support services are available to students, as are groups focused on special interests and minority groups. Edmonton is a midsize city, offering plenty of restaurants, shops, parks, theaters, sporting events, and outdoor activities. Although public transportation is available, most medical students own cars.

GRADUATES

Graduates enter both clinical medicine and research-oriented careers.

Admissions

REQUIREMENTS

Only Canadian applications are accepted. All applicants should have completed at least sixty units of university course work (approximately two years of full-time studies). Requirements are six units each of general chemistry, organic chemistry, biology, physics, and English, along with three units each of statistics and biochemistry. The MCAT is required and scores are valid for three years after the exam is taken. In addition to an application form, an autobiographical essay and two letters of reference are required.

SUGGESTIONS

Residency is an important consideration in admissions decisions. For admissions purposes, a resident of Alberta is defined as a Canadian Citizen or Permanent Resident who has lived in the Province of Alberta or Yukon or Northwest Territories for at least one continuous year immediately prior to the date of intended matriculation. At least 85 percent of available positions in an entering class are reserved for Alberta residents. The remaining 15 percent are available to other Canadians. Typically, successful applicants have completed four years of university with a grade point average of 7.0 on the University of Alberta's nine point grading system. An MCAT score of less than 7 in any category is not accepted.

PROCESS

Requests for applications should be directed to the address above. Applications are accepted between July 1 and November 1 in the year preceding anticipated matriculation. The essay and reference letters must be received by January 15, and transcripts must be submitted by January 31. Interviews are conducted between February and March, and admissions decisions are made between May and July. For the 1998 entering class, 1,011 students applied for 102 positions. Applicants who feel that they may merit special consideration (because of studies in a nontraditional area or unusual pattern) should write to the Admissions Officer outlining their situation and goals. All native (Aboriginal) students who are interested in medical studies are encouraged to contact Coordinator, Native Health Care Careers Program in care of the address above.

COSTS AND AID

In-state tuition	$6,066
Cost of books	$900
Fees	$6,000

University of Arizona
College of Medicine

Admissions Office, Room 2209, PO Box 245075, Tucson, AZ 85724 • Admission: 520-626-6214 • Fax: 520-626-4884 • Website: www.ahsc.arizona.edu/pre-med

STUDENT BODY

Type	Public
Enrollment	406
% male/female	52/48
% underrepresented minorities	15
# applied (total/out)	608/71
# accepted (total/out)	51/1

ADMISSIONS

Application Information

Regular application	11/1
Regular notification	1/30 until filled
Are transfers accepted?	No
Admissions may be deferred?	Yes
Interview required?	Yes

Academics

Students may apply to joint PhD/MD programs in the following: anatomy, biochemistry, cell biology, genetics, immunology, microbiology, molecular biology, neuroscience, pharmacology, and physiology. Combined studies in other fields are possible as well, including a collaborative program of Arizona State University, Northern Arizona University, and the College of Medicine at the University of Arizona. This program focuses on the health needs of underserved communities and leads to a master's in public health along with the MD. Through this and other venues, medical students at the University of Arizona take advantage of the resources of the academic and medical institutions throughout the state.

BASIC SCIENCES: The basic sciences are taught in the basic science building of the Tucson campus. Traditional lectures with labs are the primary mode of instruction and occupy about twenty-four hours per week. Alternative teaching methods, including small group and case-based learning, account for the remaining six hours per week of structured classroom time. First-year courses are anatomy, histology and cell biology, physiology, neuroscience, biochemistry, medical and molecular genetics, preparation for clinical medicine, and social and behavioral science. During year two, students take microbiology, pathology, pharmacology, preparation for clinical medicine, and social and behavioral science. In the course preparation for clinical medicine, students focus on clinical problem solving and learn patient evaluation skills. This course links basic science principles with clinical applications. Computers, located in the Learning Resource Center, supplement lectures and are an important component of the basic science education. The Arizona Health Science Library houses nearly 200,000 volumes, operates extensive online database and informational services, and is electronically connected to the library system of the greater university. To accommodate the study schedules of all students, the library is open twenty-four hours a day. Students are evaluated with grades of honors, pass, and fail. The USMLE Step 1 is required upon completion of basic science course work.

CLINICAL TRAINING

Patient contact begins during year one in preparation for clinical medicine. Throughout the four years, there are opportunities for clinical exposure through volunteer and outreach programs. In addition, clinical research is often community based and gives medical students a chance to help others while they learn. The commitment to underserved people (CUP) is a program through which many medical students volunteer. In CUP, students are involved in health education for—and supervised treatment of—people in underserved communities. The formal clinical curriculum begins in year three, when students rotate through the following clerkships: medicine (twelve weeks), pediatrics (six weeks), family medicine (six weeks), obstetrics/gynecology (six weeks), psychiatry (six weeks), surgery (six weeks), specialty surgery (three weeks), and neurology (three weeks). Year four is made up of electives, many of which can be taken at alternate locations throughout the state. Clinical facilities in Tucson are the University Medical Center, the University Outpatient Clinic, the Children's Research Center, and the Arizona Cancer Center. The hospitals serve managed care participants, and the medical school seeks to respond to the ongoing changes in the economics of health care, as seen in the public health/health policy components of medical school training. Evaluation of clinical performance use grades of honors, pass, and fail. Passing the USMLE Step 2 is a requirement for graduation.

Students

Students are either Arizona residents or are from western states that do not have their own medical schools. Generally, about 15 percent of the student body are underrepresented minorities, most of whom are of Mexican American descent. Older students make up about one-third of each class. A wide variety of undergraduate institutions and majors are represented in a typical class. Class size is 100.

STUDENT LIFE

With access to both the campus community of over 36,000 students and the midsize urban community, students have active social lives. Recreational facilities are extensive at the university. The medical school's emphasis on community involvement promotes extracurricular activities that are medically related. Student clubs also provide mechanisms for support and social interaction. The Chicano/Latino Club is linked to similar organizations at California universities, providing a larger network for those involved. On-campus housing options include apartments and dorms. Most students, however, opt to live off campus.

GRADUATES

At least 60 percent of graduates enter primary care fields, which include family medicine, obstetrics/gynecology, internal medicine, and pediatrics. About 50 percent of all graduates enter residency programs within the state.

Admissions

REQUIREMENTS

Applicants should have completed one year of each of the following subjects: biology, physics, chemistry, organic chemistry, and English. In addition, at least thirty hours of upper-division course work as part of the undergraduate record is required. For older applicants, recent science course work is necessary. The MCAT is required. The best scores are considered; therefore, applicants should not withhold scores. Together, the MCAT and college record are used for initial screening.

SUGGESTIONS

Hands-on clinical experience is important, as are other activities that demonstrate an applicant's commitment to community service. The Admissions Committee is interested in applicants whose undergraduate records include significant course work in the humanities and social sciences. Applicants are advised to take the April rather than August MCAT.

PROCESS

All AMCAS applicants receive secondary applications, and virtually all who meet residency requirements are interviewed. Interviews are conducted from September through March and consist of three short meetings with faculty members and one longer session with a practicing clinician from the area. About one-quarter of those who interview are accepted and are notified on a rolling basis. A ranked wait-list is established, but candidates who find themselves on this list are not encouraged to send additional information.

Admissions Requirements (Required)

MCAT scores, science GPA, non-science GPA, letters of recommendation, interview, state residency, extracurricular activities, exposure to medical profession.

Admissions Requirements (Optional)

essays/personal statement.

COSTS AND AID

In-state tuition	$7,860
Fees	$72

Financial Aid

% students receiving aid	87

UNIVERSITY OF ARKANSAS FOR MEDICAL SCIENCES
COLLEGE OF MEDICINE

4301 WEST MARKHAM STREET, SLOT 551, LITTLE ROCK, AR 72205-7199 • ADMISSION: 501-686-5354 • FAX: 501-686-5873 • E-MAIL: SOUTHTOMG@UAMS.EDU • WEBSITE: WWW.UAMS.EDU

STUDENT BODY

Type	Public
Enrollment	576
% male/female	56/44
% underrepresented minorities	10
# applied (total/out)	675/343
# accepted (total/out)	171/6
# enrolled (total/out)	140/2
Average age	24

ADMISSIONS

Average GPA and MCAT Scores

Overall GPA	3.6
MCAT Bio	9
MCAT Phys	9
MCAT Verbal	9
MCAT Essay	0

Application Information

Regular application	11/1
Regular notification	2/15
Are transfers accepted?	Yes
Admissions may be deferred?	Yes
Interview required?	Yes
Application fee	$100

Academics

The College of Medicine, along with the schools of Nursing, Pharmacy, Public Health, Health Related Professions, and Graduate Studies, make up the University of Arkansas for Medical Sciences, one of six campuses of the University of Arkansas system. Most students complete the MD curriculum in four years, but a few students each year take part in joint MS/PhD or MD/MPH and MD/MBA programs. Joint degrees can be pursued in the following fields: anatomy, biochemistry, immunology, microbiology, neuroscience, pharmacology, and physiology.

BASIC SCIENCES: Throughout year one, students learn skills related to patient care in introduction to clinical medicine. Fall semester courses are cell biology, genetics, gross anatomy, and microscopic anatomy. Spring semester courses are biochemistry, neuroscience, and physiology. In the fall semester of year two, students take behavioral sciences, medical ethics, microbiology, and pathophysiology I. In the spring, classes are introduction to clinical medicine II, pathophysiology II, and pharmacology. Scheduled class time accounts for about twenty hours per week, most of which is devoted to lecture and lab. Alternately, for perhaps two hours per week, small groups are used as the instructional format. Grades of A through F are used to evaluate students. Passing the USMLE Step 1 is a requirement for promotion to year three, and passing the USMLE Step 2 is a requirement for graduation. Basic science teaching facilities, including libraries and labs, are part of the medical complex, which includes the main hospitals and residence halls.

CLINICAL TRAINING

Patient contact begins the first year in Introduction to clinical medicine. The third year consists of required clerkships in the following: internal medicine (twelve weeks), surgery (eight weeks), obstetrics/gynecology (six weeks), psychiatry (six weeks), pediatrics (eight weeks), specialties (four weeks), geriatrics (unspecified), and family medicine (four weeks). During year four, students choose among primary care selectives (eight weeks) and specialties clerkships (four weeks). The remainder of the year is designated as elective study, some of which may be taken off campus, out of state, or overseas. Training takes place primarily at the University Hospital (400 beds), located in the medical center complex. Other training sites are the Arkansas Children's Hospital (the sixth largest children's hospital in the country) and two VA hospitals (500 and 2000 beds). In addition, outreach training sites in small communities around the state provide students with exposure to rural medicine. The primary care clerkships involve rotations to these sites, located in El Dorado, Fayetteville, Fort Smith, Jonesboro, Pine Bluff, and Texarkana. Specialized research institutes in Little Rock include The Child Study Center, The Ambulatory Care Center, The Arkansas Cancer Research Center, and the Jones Eye Institute. Evaluation of clinical progress in required clerkships uses grades of A through F, and evaluation of electives uses grades of pass and fail. Students must pass the USMLE Step 2 as a requirement for graduation.

Students

Virtually all students are Arkansas residents. About 70 percent of students earned undergraduate degrees in Arkansas. Approximately 79 percent of incoming students in a recent class had undergraduate majors in science disciplines. Classes include a significant number of older students, including some who were older than fifty years old at the time of admission. Class size is 150.

STUDENT LIFE

Little Rock is a small but lively city, with indoor and outdoor recreational activities. Students take part in volunteer and community activities. Many single first- and second-year students live on campus in residence halls. Most upper-class students and married students live off campus.

GRADUATES

Many graduates enter post-graduate programs in Arkansas. Programs in about twenty specialty areas are offered at university-affiliated hospitals in Little Rock. In addition, a number of family practice residencies are available at rural locations around the state. At least half of the graduates of the School of Medicine enter primary care fields.

Admissions

REQUIREMENTS

Within each class, 70 percent of students must be equally divided from among the four congressional districts in the state. The College of Medicine is allowed to admit a few out-of-state applicants each year only if they do not displace Arkansas residents with equal qualifications. Out-of-state applicants should be highly qualified and have close ties to Arkansas. Students must have successfully completed the following courses prior to matriculation: biology (one year), chemistry (one year), organic chemistry (one year), physics (one year), English (one year), and math (one year) or through calculus I. The MCAT is required, and scores must be no more than three years old. Scores from all sections of the MCAT, including the writing sample, are considered.

SUGGESTIONS

Other courses deemed helpful are biochemistry, zoology, botany, embryology, genetics, histology, calculus, physical chemistry, statistics, sociology, speech, anthropology, psychology, human ecology, composition, literature, history, and logic. For students who graduated from college several years ago, some recent course work is useful. All medically related extracurricular activities are valued.

PROCESS

All AMCAS applicants are asked to submit secondary applications. All Arkansas residents and highly qualified out-of-state residents are interviewed, with interviews taking place between October and January. Team interviews consist of a one-hour session with faculty. All applicants are notified by February 15. A ranked wait-list is established, and about twenty-five students from the list are usually admitted. Wait-listed candidates who commit to practicing in underserved areas of Arkansas may improve their chances of admission.

Admissions Requirements (Required)

MCAT scores, science GPA, non-science GPA, letters of recommendation, interview, state residency, essays/personal statement, extracurricular activities, exposure to medical profession.

COSTS AND AID

In-state tuition	$11,642
Out-of-state tuition	$23,284
Cost of books	$1,600

Financial Aid

Average grant	$3,000
Average loan	$25,000
Average debt	$88,000

UNIVERSITY OF BRITISH COLUMBIA

FACULTY OF MEDICINE

317-2194 HEALTH SCIENCES MALL, BRITISH COLUMBIA, BC V6T 1Z3 • ADMISSION: 604-822-2421 • FAX: 604-822-6061 • E-MAIL: ADMISSIONS.MD@UBC.CA • WEBSITE: WWW.MED.UBC.CA

STUDENT BODY

Type	Public
*Enrollment	120
# applied (total/out)	621/145
Average age	23

ADMISSIONS

Average GPA and MCAT Scores

Overall GPA	82%
MCAT Bio	10.4
MCAT Phys	10.1
MCAT Verbal	9.5
MCAT Essay	Q

Academics

The four-year curriculum that leads to the MD degree is integrated and comprehensive; it is designed to take advantage of the vast resources of the Faculty of Medicine. A new case-based curriculum that emphashizes problem solving and lifelong learning was introduced during fall 1998. In addition to the MD program, graduate programs that lead to master's, doctoral, and combined degrees are available.

BASIC SCIENCES: Basic sciences are taught along with introductory clinical concepts during the first two years. First-year courses include introductory clinical skills and systems 1; doctor/dentist; patient and society; family practice continuum; principles of human biology; host defenses and infection; cardiovascular systems; pulmonary; and fluids, electrolytes, and renal. Second-year courses include clinical skills and systems II, doctor/dentist, patient and society, family practice continuum, blood and lymphatic, musculoskeletal and locomotor, GI/nutrition, metabolism and endocrine, integument, brain and behavior and reproduction, and growth and development. Basic sciences are taught primarily through small group forums, lectures, computer-based instruction, and labs.

CLINICAL TRAINING

The third academic period begins with courses in health care epidemiology, radiology, and therapeutics. Following these three courses, students enter a sequence of required clerkships that include orientation (four weeks), anesthesia (two weeks), deratology (one week), emergency medicine (four weeks), medicine (ten weeks), obstetrics/gynecology (eight weeks), ophthalmology (one week), orthopedics (two weeks), pediatrics (eight weeks), psychiatry (eight weeks), and surgery (eight weeks). Six weeks are left open for electives during the third academic period. Sixteen weeks are left open for electives during the fourth academic period. A portion of electives may be completed at sites outside of the network of affiliated institutions including the University Hospital, St. Paul's Hospital, British Columbia Children's Hospital, Vancouver General Hospital, British Columbia Women's Hospital and Health Center, British Columbia Cancer Center Agency, G. F. Strong Rehabilitation Center, and the Canadian Arthiritus and Rheumatism Society Center.

Students

Each entering class has about 120 students. Approximately 50 percent of students are women. Typically, all but a handful of students in each class are from British Columbia.

STUDENT LIFE

Beyond a rich academic life, medical students enjoy the resources, facilities, and surroundings of the Health Science Center, the University of British Columbia, and the city of Vancouver. The Faculty of Medicine and greater university offer a wide variety of support services including counseling, special interest clubs and organizations, resources for minorities and international students, and day care. There are ample opportunities for athletic, social, and recreational activities on campus. Students also enjoy the cultural and recreational aspects of Vancouver.

GRADUATES

A significant number of graduates enter residency programs at hospitals affiliated with the University of British Columbia. Although most graduates enter clinical medicine, others successfully pursue research and academic medicine.

Application Information

Regular application	10/1
Regular notification	3/1
Transfers accepted?	Yes
Admissions may be deferred?	Yes
Interview required?	Yes
Application fee (in/out)	$105/$155

COSTS AND AID

Tuition	$4,000
Cost of books	$1,200
Fees	$256

Admissions

REQUIREMENTS

Applicants should have successfully completed a minimum of ninety credits or the equivalent of three years of full-time course work in any degree program at an accredited university. A minimum of 70 percent academic average is required and all undergraduate courses are included in this average. Prerequisites are one year each of university-level biology, biochemistry, chemistry, organic chemistry, and English literature and composition. The MCAT is required. The exam should be taken no later than August of the year of application.

SUGGESTIONS

There is no preferred program of study for preperation for medical school. Often, due to the large number of applicants, the competitive average for successful applicants is much higher than 70 percent. MCAT scores of a recently admitted class averaged about 10. In addition to excellent academic qualifications, the school bases its admissions decision on personal characteristics such as motivation and integrity. Last year, 695 applications were received for 120 positions.

UNIVERSITY OF CALGARY

FACULTY OF MEDICINE

3330 HOSPITAL DRIVE NW, CALGARY, ALBERTA, T2N 4N1 • ADMISSION: 403-220-4262 •
WEBSITE: HTTP://FACULTY.MED.UCALGARY.CA/

STUDENT BODY

Type	Public
Enrollment	234
% male/female	48/52
# applied (total/out)	1,314/784
Average age	25

ADMISSIONS

Average GPA and MCAT Scores

Overall GPA	3.50
MCAT Bio	10.67
MCAT Phys	10.48
MCAT Verbal	9.77
MCAT Essay	Q

Academics

Medical students follow an intensive, eleven-month curriculum for a period of three years. Learning is based in part on clinical case presentations. In addition to the standard MD course of study, programs are offered in conjunction with the Faculty of Graduate Studies in Biomedical and Health Sciences with the objective of training clinician-scientists for academic medical research and training those who will design, manage, and implement health care delivery programs. MS/PhD and MD/MSc programs are available in biochemistry and molecular biology, cardiovascular/respiratory sciences, community health sciences, gastrointestinal sciences, medical science, microbiology and infectious diseases, and neuroscience.

BASIC SCIENCES: First year courses are based on organ systems and are taught primarily through lectures and small group discussions. Subjects are principles of medicine, blood, muscoskeletal and skin, cardivascular, respiratory, renal-electrolyte, endocrine metabolic, medical skills program, and intergrative. The second academic period begins in July. Subjects are neuroscience, the mind, gastrointestinal, reproduction, human development, and medical skills program. Throughout the first and second years, students also take part in independant research projects. Courses are taught in the Calgary Health Sciences Center, which is about one-and-a-half kilometers from the main campus of the University of Calgary. The medical library is fully computerized, receives more than 1,000 serials, and has approximately 130,000 books. It serves medical and nursing students as well as the greater university and the medical community. Other important facilities include the Medical Learning Resource Center that houses instructional tools geared toward learning anatomical systems and the Medical Skills Center for improving clinical skills and techniques.

CLINICAL TRAINING

Required clerkships are anesthesia (two weeks), family medicine (four weeks), internal medicine (twelve weeks), obstetrics/gynecology (six weeks), pediatrics (six weeks), psychiatry (six weeks), and surgery (eight weeks). Ten weeks are available for clinical electives. Training takes place primarily at the facilities of the Foothills Hospital, the Peter Lougheed Center, the Alberta Children's Hospital, and the Rockyview Hospital. In addition, the University of Calgary Medical Clinic allows medical students to learn about outpatient service delivery, preventative programs, and travel medicine.

Students

While medical students are primarily Canadian, the student body at the University of Calgary includes several hundred international students. Women make up about 50 percent of students within the Faculty of Medicine. The majority of medical students are from within the province of Alberta.

STUDENT LIFE

Student life is enhanced by campus activities, the resources of the community and city of Calgary, and the wide variety of available outdoor activities. Nearby national parks, such as Banff and Jasper, offer skiing and hiking. The region also has vibrant wildlife and areas for fishing, swimming, and canoeing. In addition to its academic facilities, the Health Sciences Center includes a medical bookstore, exercise room, student lounge, cafeteria, and mall area. Medical students also have access to the resources of the greater university, including complete athletic and recreational facilities, intramural sports programs, outdoor programs, arts, and theater. The university student union organizes events and activities and operates a bookstore, cafe, bar, and other such services. On-campus housing is available for single and married students. An off-campus registry is managed by the student union.

GRADUATES

Although most graduates enter post-graduate training that leads to careers in clinical medicine, some go on to pursue research and academic medicine. Increasingly, graduates are entering primary care fields.

Application Information

Regular application	11/15
Regular notification	5/14
Transfers accepted?	Yes
Admissions may be deferred?	Yes
Interview required?	Yes
Application fee	$65

COSTS AND AID

Tuition & Fees

Tuition (in/out)	$6,519/$30,000
Cost of books	$1,200
Fees	$333

Admissions

REQUIREMENTS

Students must have completed at least two full years of university education before being considered for admission. The minimum grade requirement for a Canadian citizen or landed immigrant resident of Alberta is an average of 3.0, which translates to a grade of B or at least 78 percent of each year of study. The minimum grade point average required of Canadians from other provinces is 3.5. The MCAT is required, and applicants should have at least an average score of 8. In addition to transcripts and a completed application form, three letters of reference are required.

SUGGESTIONS

Although the faculty has no prescribed prerequisites, one year of each of the following courses is strongly recommended: English, biology, general chemistry, organic chemistry, biochemistry, physics, physiology, calculus, and pyschology/sociology. Presently, spaces for international students are limited to students who come from institutions and/or countries with which the Faculty of Medicine at the University of Calgary has a formal, contractional agreement. All international students must sign an acknowledgment stating that the MD program would not lead to an opportunity for post-graduate training through the Canadian Resident Matching Service.

PROCESS

The application is available at www.med.ucalgary.ca/admissions. It requires information about all university courses taken, MCAT test dates and results, employment history, extracurricular activities, and an essay. The completed application is due November 15. The deadline for receipt of the three letters of reference, all official transcripts, and official MCAT scores is January 4. Applicants will be notified by March 15 whether they will be invited for an interview. In a recent year, there were 1,300 applicants for 100 positions.

University of California—Davis
School of Medicine

One Shields Avenue, Davis, CA 95616-8661 • Admission: 530-752-2717 • Fax: 530-754-6252 •
E-mail: medadmsinfo@ucdavis.edu • Website: www.som.ucdavis.edu

STUDENT BODY

Type	Public
Enrollment	406
% male/female	50/50
% underrepresented minorities	13
# applied (total/out)	3,741/735
# accepted (total/out)	203/2
# enrolled (total/out)	93/1
Average age	26

FACULTY

Total faculty (number)	572
% female	26
% part-time	11
# student/faculty ratio	1:1

ADMISSIONS

Average GPA and MCAT Scores

Overall GPA	3.5
MCAT Bio	11
MCAT Phys	11
MCAT Verbal	10
MCAT Essay	P

Application Information

Regular application	11/1
Regular notification	10/15
Are transfers accepted?	Yes
Admissions may be deferred?	Yes
Interview required?	Yes

Academics

The School of Medicine is well integrated into the UC—Davis campus and benefits from the academic programs of the university. About 20 percent of each class extend their first two years into three, extend their fourth year, or take time off from the standard curriculum at some point. This enrichment option allows students to pursue research or attend to other academic and personal goals. Joint-degree programs organized in conjunction with graduate departments at UC—Davis lead to an MBA, MA, or PhD along with the MD degree. In addition, the MPH degree may be earned at UC—Berkeley School of Public Health or through the School of Medicine's epidemiology and preventive medicine department. Students who are interested in careers as physician-scientists may apply for programs that lead to doctorates in the following fields: biochemistry, biomedical engineering, cell biology, genetics, immunology, molecular biology, neuroscience, pathology, pharmacology, physiology, and in the humanities or social sciences.

BASIC SCIENCES: Davis operates on a quarter system; each quarter is separated into two segments by a midterm week during which students study and take exams. The two-year preclinical program has a heavy clinical emphasis—more than 60 percent of all courses are taught by physicians. The more typical basic science courses are primarily taught in the first year. The fall-quarter courses are anatomy and biochemistry. Winter-quarter courses are histology, biochemistry, and physiology. Spring-quarter courses are immunology, endocrinology, and neurobiology. Throughout the first year, patient communication, physical examination, and history-taking are taught in introduction to patient evaluation and in the first-quarter psychiatry course. The six-week summer quarter is a transition between basic and clinical sciences with a continuation of the pathology program initiated in the spring quarter: human reproduction and dermatology. Clinician-based courses in the second year include hematology/oncology, musculoskeletal system, cardiovascular medicine, pulmonary medicine, neurology, clinical psychiatry, nephrology, gastrointestinal system, nutrition, and clinical endocrinology. Physical diagnosis also continues throughout the entire second year. During the first year, the students are in class approximately thirty hours per week, with an approximately equal distribution between lecture, student-centered discussion, and laboratory. The preclinical courses are taught in Tupper Hall, central to the UC—Davis campus. The Health Science Library is adjacent to the complex, houses 142,000 volumes, and is fully computerized. The resources for the curriculum are provided by the Office of Curricular Support. Academic support for individual students is provided by the Office of Student Learning and Educational Resources (OSLER). Grades of pass and fail are used to evaluate students. Passing the USMLE Step 1 is a requirement for promotion to year three. In the last three years, the passing rate has been 100 percent. In addition to the formal courses, students gain clinical experience from volunteering in clinics such as Asian Clinic, Clinica Tepati, Imani Clinic, and Shifa Clinic.

CLINICAL TRAINING

Third-year required clerkships are surgery (eight weeks), medicine (eight weeks), pediatrics (eight weeks), obstetrics/gynecology (eight weeks), psychiatry (eight weeks), and primary care plus (eight weeks), which includes four weeks in a family-practice setting and introduces primary care components of certain specialties. Required fourth-year clerkships are emergency medicine (four weeks), physical medicine and rehabilitation (two weeks), ophthalmology (two weeks), neurology (two weeks), and otolaryngology (two weeks). A two-week course that discusses the legal, ethical, and economic issues related to medicine is also required. Most of the fourth year is reserved for selectives, which students choose within the directives of an oversight committee, and electives, which are unrestricted. Required clerkships take place at UC—Davis Medical Center in Sacramento (528 beds), Kaiser Permanente Hospital, David Grant Hospital (Travis Air Force Base), Sutter Hospital, Highland General (Oakland), and at community physician sites. Other clinical facilities include a new Shriners Hospital, which opened on the Sacramento campus to provide care to children with orthopedic and other disorders; an expanded hospital; the Ellison Ambulatory Care Center; and the establishment of the Mather VA Hospital. Among these sites, students serve a diverse patient population. Selectives may be taken at any LCME-accredited medical school. Overseas clinical activities may be taken as electives with programs organized by the departments of family practice and epidemiology and preventive medicine and through individual student efforts. Students must take the USMLE Step 2 to graduate.

Students

All but a few students in each class are California residents. There is also significant diversity in the age of incoming students, the average being twenty-five or twenty-six. Class size is ninety-three.

STUDENT LIFE

Although students live both on and off campus, student life is focused around the school. Recreational facilities on campus include the recreation hall; two swimming pools; a craft center; an equestrian center; a bowling alley; and tennis, handball, racquetball, volleyball, and basketball courts. On-campus housing options include a residence hall with a dining room, one- and two-bedroom units, and student family housing for married students. The Housing Listing Service assists students who are searching for off-campus accommodations.

GRADUATES

About 60 percent of graduates enter primary care fields. UC—Davis Medical Center has at least twenty residency programs. Davis graduates are successful at obtaining residency positions in prestigious programs all over the United States.

Admissions

REQUIREMENTS

The following courses must be completed prior to matriculation: English (one year), biology with lab (one year), chemistry with lab (one year), organic chemistry (one year), physics (one year), and math (up to differential calculus). The MCAT is required and should have been taken within the past three years. For those who have retaken the MCAT, the best scores are considered.

SUGGESTIONS

Additional helpful courses are biochemistry, genetics, and embryology. For students who have been out of school for a period of time, some recent course work is recommended. While no activities or qualities are specified, successful applicants demonstrate interpersonal skills, leadership potential, and the ability to work with diverse populations.

PROCESS

About 2,000 applicants, or roughly 50 percent of AMCAS applicants, receive secondaries. Secondary applications must be returned within a month. From 400 to 500 applicants are interviewed from October through April. Interviews consist of two one-hour sessions with faculty members and/or medical students. About one-third of those who are interviewed are accepted on a rolling basis. Other candidates are rejected or put on a wait-list that is split into thirds, depending on the candidate's prospect for admission. Wait-listed candidates are not advised to send supplementary material.

Admissions Requirements (Required)

MCAT scores, science GPA, non-science GPA, letters of recommendation, interview, state residency, essays/personal statement, extracurricular activities, exposure to medical profession.

COSTS AND AID

Cost of books	$2,152
In-state Fees	$12,115
Out-of-state Fees	$23,247

Financial Aid

% students receiving aid	89
Average grant	$4,000
Average loan	$23,000
Average debt	$60,100

University of California—Irvine
College of Medicine

Medical Education Building 802, Room 100, Irvine, CA 92697-4089 • Admission: 949-824-5388 • Fax: 949-824-2485 • E-mail: medadmit@uci.edu • Website: www.ucihs.uci.edu/admissions

STUDENT BODY

Type	Public
Enrollment	372
% male/female	54/46
% underrepresented minorities	8
# applied (total/out)	3,400/369
# accepted (total)	244
# enrolled (total)	92
Average age	23

FACULTY

Total faculty (number)	788
% female	29
% minority	6
% part-time	18
# student/faculty ratio	2:1

ADMISSIONS

Average GPA and MCAT Scores

Overall GPA	3.7
MCAT Bio	11
MCAT Phys	11
MCAT Verbal	10
MCAT Essay	P

Application Information

Regular application	11/1
Regular notification	Rolling
Are transfers accepted?	No
Admissions may be deferred?	Yes
Interview required?	Yes
Application fee	$60

Academics

Each year, six students who meet the school's requirements are accepted into the Medical Scientist Training Program (MSTP) that leads to a combined MS/PhD degree. The PhD can be earned in a number of fields, including all of the biological sciences, engineering sciences, physical sciences, and information and computer sciences. Students who meet the requirements can pursue a joint MBA/MD program in conjunction with UCI's Graduate School of Management. Most students follow a four-year curriculum and take the patient-doctor course, which integrates clinical, social, and basic science concepts.

BASIC SCIENCES: For the duration of two years, the patient-doctor course gives students an opportunity to interact with real patients in a clinical setting and with simulated patients in a closely monitored learning environment. During the first year, students also take anatomy and embryology, medical biochemistry, histology, neurosciences, physiology/pathophysiology, medical genetics, molecular cell biology, and immunology, which are all taught primarily in a lecture/lab format. The patient-doctor course continues throughout year two and places students in clinical service experiences within community physician offices. During the second year, students also take general and systematic pathology, clinical pathology, topics in medicine, medical microbiology, and medical pharmacology. Tutorial programs, academic monitoring, and study skills workshops promote student success in the basic sciences. The Medical Center Library (MCL) is located at the UCI Medical Center and meets the research, education, and patient care needs of the medical center staff and the UCI College of Medicine. The College of Medicine is fully computerized; it has an internal electronic informational network. Students are evaluated with grades of honors, pass, or fail.

CLINICAL TRAINING

Patient contact begins during the first year when students participate in the patient, doctor and society course and the patient-doctor course. Standardized patients and surrogate patients are employed—throughout the four years—to enhance interactive experience. During the fourth year, the patient-doctor course continues and teaches students to apply basic science concepts to clinical situations. Required clerkships begin during year three and include inpatient and ambulatory medicine (twelve weeks), obstetrics/gynecology (eight weeks), pediatrics (four weeks), psychiatry (six weeks), family medicine (four weeks), and surgery (eight weeks). Year four rotations are intensive care unit (four weeks), substance abuse (two weeks), neuroscience (four weeks), emergency medicine (two weeks), radiology (two weeks), and a musculoskeletal elective (two weeks). The primary training sites are UCI Medical Center in the City of Orange, which includes several specialized clinical and research centers, the Veterans' Administration Medical Center in Long Beach, and the College of Medicine's affiliated hospitals and clinics. Affiliates are located in Orange, Los Angeles, and San Bernardino counties and serve both rural and urban communities. During the clinical years, narrative evaluations supplement the honors, pass, and fail grading system. Students must pass the USMLE Step 1 and Step 2 to graduate.

Students

On and off campus, medical students can find a wide variety of recreational and extracurricular activities to help keep overall balance in their lives.

STUDENT LIFE

UCI has many student-interest groups, including groups that provide support to minority students and to students who have children. Other groups are geared toward volunteer and community activities. Medical students have access to a wide variety of resources at UCI, including cultural events, intramural athletics, and all facilities. On-campus, graduate student housing is affordable, comfortable, and allows medical students to interact with students from other departments. Apartments, residence halls, and residential communities that feature living spaces of all sizes are available. The city of Irvine and the surrounding communities such as Newport Beach provide recreational opportunities and attractive housing options.

GRADUATES

A large proportion of graduates enter post-graduate programs at UCI, which has one of the nation's largest residency programs in primary care disciplines and internal medicine. Most graduates enter programs in California, but seniors have been successful in obtaining residencies all over the United States.

Admissions

REQUIREMENTS

The following must be completed prior to matriculation: general chemistry (two semesters), organic chemistry (two semesters), physics (two semesters), biology (three semesters, with a minimum of one upper-division biology class), biochemistry (one semester), and calculus (one semester). The MCAT is required, and scores should be no more than three years old. For those who have retaken the exam, the most recent set of scores is considered.

SUGGESTIONS

No specific major is required. In addition to the requirements for admission the following classes are also recommended: molecular biology, genetics, cell biology, vertebrate embryology, psychology, and Spanish.

PROCESS

The UCI College of Medicine seeks to admit students who are highly qualified to be trained in the practice of medicine and whose backgrounds, talents, and experiences contribute to a diverse student body. The Admissions Committee carefully reviews all applicants whose undergraduate record and scores on the MCAT indicate that they will be able to handle the rigorous curriculum of medical school. Careful consideration is given to applicants from disadvantaged backgrounds (socially, culturally, and/or economically disadvantaged). In addition to scholastic achievement, attributes deemed desirable in prospective students include leadership ability and participation in extracurricular activities such as exposure to clinical medicine and/or medically related research and community service. Preference is given to California residents and applicants who are either U.S. citizens or permanent residents. The College of Medicine does not accept transfer students. Information provided by the AMCAS application is used for the preliminary screening. Based on decisions reached by the Admissions Committee, applicants may be sent a secondary application. A limited number of applicants (approximately 500) are invited to be interviewed. The Admissions Committee reviews the academic records, letters of recommendation, and the results of personal interviews before making its final selections.

Admissions Requirements (Required)

MCAT scores, science GPA, non-science GPA, letters of recommendation, interview, essays/personal statement.

Admissions Requirements (Optional)

state residency, extracurricular activities, exposure to medical profession, research.

COSTS AND AID

Out-of-state tuition	$12,245
Room and board	$10,913
Cost of books	$1,799
Fees	$16,202

Financial Aid

% students receiving aid	92
Average grant	$4,200
Average loan	$27,122
Average debt	$79,186

University of California—Los Angeles

David Geffen School of Medicine at UCLA

Center for Health Sciences Los Angeles, CA 90095-1720 • Admission: 310-825-6081 • Fax: 310-825-6081 •
E-mail: somadmiss@mednet.ucla.edu • Website: www.medstudent.ucla.edu

STUDENT BODY

Type	Public
Enrollment	674
% male/female	58/42
% underrepresented minorities	30
# applied (total/out)	5,244/1,733
# accepted (total/out)	15/8
# enrolled (out)	13

ADMISSIONS

Application Information

Regular application	11/1
Regular notification	1/15
Are transfers accepted?	Yes
Interview required?	Yes
Application fee	$40

Academics

Each year, ten students are admitted to an Extended Curriculum Program, which spreads out the first two years of the standard curriculum over three years, thus creating opportunities for special projects or supplemental instruction. In each class, as many as twenty-four students who are interested in practicing in underserved communities spend their first two years at UCLA School of Medicine and then complete clinical requirements at Drew University facilities. Drew University is a predominantly African American medical institution. Several joint degree programs are offered to medical students, including an MD/MPH with the School of Public Health, an MD/MBA with the School of Management, and an MSTP-sponsored MS/PhD. All entering students are required to purchase a computer because both the basic science and clinical curriculum emphasize its applications.

BASIC SCIENCES: During the first two years, students are in scheduled sessions for about twenty-six hours per week. In addition to required courses, selectives give students an opportunity to explore topics of interest such as health care reform, addiction, and AIDS. First-year courses are micro-anatomy and cell biology, topics in physiology, biological chemistry, anatomy, organ system physiology, basic neurology, biomathematics, doctoring I, and clinical applications of basic sciences (CABS). Doctoring I is the beginning of the doctoring curriculum, which uses a case-based approach and addresses the interdisciplinary issues that pertain to practicing medicine. In this course, the cultural, ethical, legal, economic, and social perspectives on medicine are considered. In CABS, students participate in community-based, health education, or health care projects and learn to apply basic science concepts to real life clinical problems. Second-year courses are microbiology, pathology, pharmacology, pathophysiology, psychopathology, doctoring II, genetics, and clinical fundamentals (covers physical diagnosis and takes place largely at clinical sites). Both university-sponsored and student-initiated study and tutorial groups are available. Most classes are taught in the health sciences building, a large structure on the UCLA campus in Westwood. The Biomedical Library is nearby and serves faculty, students, and the community with a collection of 500,000 volumes and 6,000 current journals. Grades of pass and fail are used to evaluate students; written citations are used to evaluate outstanding achievement. Promotion to year three requires a passing score on the USMLE Step 1.

CLINICAL TRAINING

Outside of traditional clerkships, students gain experience with patients in doctoring and through the extensive volunteer opportunities. Some students identify volunteer opportunities with the assistance of the Community Service Compendium, a list of community outreach sites. Formal clinical training takes place during the third and fourth years, which are treated as a continuum. Fifty-seven weeks of the third and fourth years are reserved for the following required rotations: medicine (twelve weeks), surgery (twelve weeks), pediatrics (six weeks), obstetrics/gynecology (six weeks), psychiatry (six weeks), family medicine (six weeks), radiology (four weeks), neurology (two weeks), and ophthalmology (two weeks). Clerkships take place primarily at the University Hospital (517 beds). Other affiliated sites are Harbor General (800 beds), Cedars-Sinai, Kaiser Sunset, Kaiser West LA, Kern Medical Center (Bakersfield), King/Drew Medical Center, Olive View-UCLA Medical Center (Sylmar), Sepulveda Veterans' Affairs, St. Mary Medical

Center (Long Beach), and West LA Veterans' Affairs Medical Center. Doctoring III is taken throughout the years, occupying students for one full day every other week. This segment of the course takes students to community-based medical sites and uses a small group format to discuss various patient problems. Twenty-seven weeks remain for electives. Some of the elective requirement may be fulfilled around the country or overseas. Grades of pass and fail are used to evaluate medical students and are supplemented with written evaluations. The USMLE Step 2 is required for graduation.

Students

The students reflect the multicultural population of Los Angeles, with underrepresented minorities accounting for one-third of the student body. In entering classes, the average age is twenty-two, and there are usually no more than a few students over twenty-eight years old. Eighty-five percent of the students are California residents. Class size is 145.

STUDENT LIFE

In addition to the beaches and beautiful weather of Southern California and Los Angeles, the UCLA campus itself offers excellent athletic facilities and plenty of entertainment. Student-led groups and activities within the medical school are numerous, ranging from the Iranian/American Medical Organization to the Salvation Army Outreach Clinic. The medical school also sponsors activities that encourage cohesion between faculty and students. Although residence halls and married-student housing are available, most medical students opt to live off campus.

GRADUATES

Graduates are well-prepared for careers in primary care, more specialized clinical fields, and research. About half of the graduates enter primary care fields, which is roughly the current national average. Many enter residencies at UCLA or affiliated hospitals.

Admissions

REQUIREMENTS

Admissions requirements are: English (one year), college math (one year, to include calculus and statistics), physics (one year), chemistry (two years, including inorganic and organic), and biology (one year). Science courses must have associated labs, and AP credits are not counted. The MCAT is required, and scores must be no more than three years old. Generally, if a student has retaken the exam, the best set of scores is used.

SUGGESTIONS

Courses in humanities and social sciences, as well as Spanish and computer skills are highly recommended. Undergraduate courses that overlap with those in the medical school curriculum, such as anatomy, are not recommended. For applicants who graduated college several years ago, recent course work is expected. The April MCAT is preferred over the August one. Extracurricular activities that are medically related or that involve research or patient contact are useful. UCLA is unusual among state-affiliated medical schools in California in that it welcomes applications from well-qualified nonresidents.

PROCESS

Typically, 55 percent of AMCAS applicants are asked to submit supplementary information, of which about 20 percent are invited for interviews. Interviews take place from November through May and consist of one or two sessions with faculty members and/or medical students. Notification begins in January and continues until enough offers have been made to fill the class. About 25 percent of interviewees are accepted, and another group is wait-listed. Wait-listed candidates may send additional information about academic or extracurricular achievements. The UCLA/UC—Riverside Biomedical Sciences Program allows twenty-four admitted students to obtain both the BS and MD degrees in seven years. In this program, students enter UCLA School of Medicine after completing three years of undergraduate preparation at UC—Riverside.

Admissions Requirements (Required)

MCAT scores, science GPA, non-science GPA, letters of recommendation, interview, state residency, extracurricular activities, exposure to medical profession.

Admissions Requirements (Optional)

essays/personal statement.

COSTS AND AID

In-state tuition	$15,173
Out-of-state tuition	$27,418
Room and board	$14,000
Cost of books	$4,360

University of California—San Diego
School of Medicine

9500 Gilman Drive, MC 0621, La Jolla, CA 92093-0621 • Admission: 858-534-3880 • Fax: 858-534-5282 • E-mail: somadmissions@ucsd.edu • Website: http://meded.ucsd.edu/admissions/

STUDENT BODY

Type	Public
Enrollment	493
% male/female	57/43
% underrepresented minorities	13
# applied (total/out)	4,297/1,297
# accepted (total/out)	274/27
# enrolled (total/out)	121/10
Average age	23

ADMISSIONS

Average GPA and MCAT Scores

Overall GPA	3.7
MCAT Bio	11.6
MCAT Phys	11.4
MCAT Verbal	9.9
MCAT Essay	Q

Application Information

Regular application	11/1
Regular notification	10/15
Are transfers accepted?	No
Admissions may be deferred?	Yes
Interview required?	Yes
Application fee	$40

Academics

In addition to fulfilling course requirements, students must complete an independent study project to graduate. These projects allow students to explore and define their own interests and to collaborate with faculty members who share these interests. The medical school benefits from the resources of other parts of UCSD. Joint MS/PhD programs are possible with UCSD Graduate Departments in biochemistry, biomedical engineering, biophysics, cell biology, genetics, immunology, microbiology, molecular biology, neuroscience, pathology, pharmacology, and physiology. Normally, these degrees are MSTP sponsored. Students can earn an MPH in conjunction with nearby San Diego State University Graduate School of Public Health.

BASIC SCIENCES: The first two years are organized into quarters. Electives are an important supplement to basic science requirements and account for about 20 percent of scheduled course time. During the fall quarter of the first year, cell biology and biochemistry is the main endeavor. This lecture course is referred to as a block, which means that the material is covered intensely during one or two quarters. Students also begin a sequence in social and behavioral sciences, taught mostly through small group sessions. Winter-quarter courses are physiology, pharmacology, and introduction to clinical medicine (continues throughout the basic science curriculum and prepares students for third-year rotations). Spring-quarter courses are neurology, pharmacology, reproductive biology, metabolism, and endocrinology, all of which are taught primarily through lectures. The second year begins with anatomy, histology, biostatistics, and a social/behavioral science course on health care systems. Winter quarter consists of human disease, psychopathology, and hematology. The second year, spring-quarter courses are human disease, neurology, and lab medicine. During the basic science years there are, on average, thirty-four scheduled hours per week. Instruction takes place in the modern basic science building, which is adjacent to the Biomedical Library (100,000 volumes). Computers with access to online informational services and curricular programs are available for student use in the library and in the School's Learning Resource Center. Grades of honors, pass, and fail are used to evaluate medical students. The USMLE Step 1 is required for promotion to year three.

CLINICAL TRAINING

Supervised patient contact begins in January of the first year, in introduction to clinical medicine. The physical examination is taught in conjunction with the study of individual organ systems in the first year, and together with the history, refined in the second basic science year. In addition, a simulated-patient program provides students with the opportunity to improve their history-taking and physical examination skills, as well as to obtain feedback from faculty mentors and view videotapes of their patient interaction. Required third-year rotations are medicine (twelve weeks), neurology (4weeks), obstetrics/gynecology (six weeks), pediatrics (eight weeks), psychiatry (six weeks), surgery (twelve weeks), and primary care (one afternoon per week, all year). Students design their fourth-year curricula by selecting courses from within broad subject areas. Twelve weeks are selected from direct patient care clerkships, four weeks must be a primary care experience, four weeks inpatient training, and four weeks outpatient training. An additional twelve weeks of pure elective clinical clerkships are also required. Clinical training takes place at large hospitals and small clinics, including UCSD Medical Centers (577 beds total), VA Hospital (606 beds), Navy Hospital (750 beds), Children's Hospital (154 beds), Kaiser Foundation Hospital (1,285 beds), Sharp Memorial Community Hospital (1,415 beds), Clinica De Salubridad de Campesinos, and the U.S. Public Health Service Outpatient Clinic. Electives may be taken from the various departments of UCSD or may be carried out in conjunction with community organizations. Most students take advantage of additional clinical training opportunities through volunteer work, some of which takes them across the border in Mexico. The USMLE Step 2 is required for graduation. UCSD students do exceptionally well on both parts of the USMLE.

Students

Students are predominantly Californians. There is a wide age range among students, and it is very common for them to have taken a year or two off after college for research or other activities. About 60 percent of incoming students in a recent class were science majors. Class size is 122.

STUDENT LIFE

On-campus housing is convenient, attractive, and popular with students. Modern apartments of all sizes are available for single and married students and for those who have children or pets. Some students rely on bicycles or shuttle buses, while others own cars. UCSD's location affords many recreational possibilities. Year-round outdoor activities include swimming, surfing, biking, sailing, rollerblading, running, and walking. Other activities are the San Diego Symphony, the zoo, and the Padres professional baseball team. Medical student organizations and events also organize extracurricular activities for students.

GRADUATES

Of the graduating class of 1997, the most popular fields for post-graduate training were internal medicine (twenty-two graduates), family medicine (eighteen), pediatrics (seventeen), obstetrics/gynecology (eleven), emergency medicine (eleven), surgery (eight), radiology (four), otolaryngology (three), dermatology (two), and ophthalmology (two). Many entered programs in San Diego, Oakland, San Jose, Los Angeles, and other California locations.

Admissions

REQUIREMENTS

One year of chemistry, organic chemistry, biology, physics, and math are all required. Strong written and spoken English is a requirement, and the ability to communicate in a second language is preferred. The rigor of an applicant's undergraduate institution is considered in assessing GPA. The MCAT is required, and the spring exam is advised.

SUGGESTIONS

Breadth of academic experience is important. Extracurricular activities are also important, particularly activities that involve some sort of medical exposure, community involvement, or leadership.

PROCESS

About 40 percent of applicants receive a secondary application, of which about 500 are interviewed. Interviews take place from October through May and consist of two one-hour sessions with faculty members. Following interviews, candidates are accepted, rejected, or put on hold for later notification. About half of those candidates who are interviewed are eventually accepted. An extensive wait-list is established.

Admissions Requirements (Required)

MCAT scores, science GPA, non-science GPA, letters of recommendation, interview, essays/personal statement.

Admissions Requirements (Optional)

state residency, extracurricular activities, exposure to medical profession.

COSTS AND AID

Out-of-state tuition	$12,245
Room and board	$826
Cost of books	$1,416
In-state Fees	$15,288
Out-of-state Fees	$12,245

Financial Aid

% students receiving aid	90
Average grant	$17,100
Average loan	$18,741
Average debt	$62,806

UNIVERSITY OF CALIFORNIA—SAN FRANCISCO
SCHOOL OF MEDICINE

SCHOOL OF MEDICINE ADMISSIONS, C-200, BOX 0408, SAN FRANCISCO, CA 94143-0408 • ADMISSION: 415-476-4044 • E-MAIL: ADMISSIONS@MEDSCH.UCSF.EDU • WEBSITE: MEDSCHOOL.UCSF.EDU/ADMISSIONS

STUDENT BODY

Type	Public
Enrollment	629
% male/female	44/56
% underrepresented minorities	43
# applied (total/out)	4,045/1,693
# accepted (total/out)	226/66
# enrolled (total/out)	141/26
Average age	24

FACULTY

Total faculty (number)	1,558
% female	35
% minority	19
% part-time	4
# student/faculty ratio	2:1

ADMISSIONS

Average GPA and MCAT Scores

Overall GPA	3.7
MCAT Bio	11.7
MCAT Phys	11.4
MCAT Verbal	10.4
MCAT Essay	Q

Application Information

Regular application	11/1
Regular notification	rolling
Are transfers accepted?	No
Admissions may be deferred?	Yes
Interview required?	Yes
Application fee	$60

Academics

While the majority of students earn an MD in four years, some students devote an additional year to research activities. Twelve students each year enter a five-year program organized in collaboration with the School of Public Health at the University of California—Berkeley. These students earn a master's degree from Berkeley along with an MD from UCSF. Up to twelve students enter the Medical Science Training Program (MSTP) joint PhD/MD program yearly. Participants may earn a PhD from the following UCSF programs: biochemistry, biophysics, cell biology, developmental biology, endocrinology, genetics, immunology, neuroscience, cancer biology, stem cell biology, chemistry, vascular and cardiac biology, virology and medical anthropology.

BASIC SCIENCES: The first two years form the essential core, and they are organized into eight block courses, each about eight weeks long. These courses deal with major themes and draw together a range of interdisciplinary topics. First year courses are prologue; major organ systems; cancer; and brain, mind, and behavior. Second year courses are infection, inflammation, and immunity; metabolism; life cycle; and consolidation cases. Essential core lectures, labs, and small group sessions account for about twenty hours a week, and they integrate subjects from the basic, social, and clinical sciences. All courses include supplementary resources on a Web-based system that forms the e-curriculum. The essential core includes a course called foundations of patient care, which offers students exposure to clinical settings. This course also allows students to explore issues of professional development, ethics, and doctor-patient interaction.

CLINICAL TRAINING

Patient contact begins during the first year in foundations of patient care and in the weeklong immersion in the hospital wards (called the clinical interlude). Clinical elements are wholly integrated into the basic science curriculum, which allows students to smoothly transition into the third year. Likewise, the clinical years include segments of classroom instruction that focus on basic and social science concepts. For example, the third year includes three intersessions, which occur between clerkship rotations, and offers lectures and small group discussions about basic science connections to the clinical experiences, ethics, evidence-based medicine, and health policy. Required third-year core clerkships are anesthesia (two weeks), family and community medicine (six weeks), medicine (eight weeks), neurology and psychiatry (eight weeks), obstetrics/gynecology (six weeks), pediatrics (six weeks), surgery (eight weeks), and surgical subspecialties (two weeks). Teaching sites are primarily in San Francisco, Oakland, and Fresno and include California Pacific Medical Center, Children's Hospital, Kaiser Foundation Hospitals, UCSF Medical Center (including Mount Zion Hospital), San Francisco City Clinics, San Francisco General Hospital, Veterans' Affairs Medical Centers in San Francisco and Fresno, University Medical Center (Fresno), and Langley Porter Neuropsychiatric Institute. The fourth year consists primarily of elective study, which may entail international work or research in addition to traditional advanced clinical rotations. Evaluation of students during the third and fourth years uses grades of honors, pass, and fail and supplements these with narrative comments. Outside of clerkships, students gain clinical experience through volunteer work and community service at any number of UCSF-affiliated projects.

Students

Twenty percent of the students are out-of-state residents. More than half are nonwhite, and approximately 17 percent are underrepresented minorities, mostly African and Hispanic Americans. Virtually all undergraduate majors are represented in the student body. Class size is 141.

STUDENT LIFE

University-owned housing appropriate for both married and single students is available. Many students take part in community programs, which provide not only an opportunity to contribute but also a chance for student-student and student-faculty interaction in an extracurricular setting. Students have access to school athletic facilities and to many local, outdoor activities, including running in Golden Gate Park, surfing at Ocean Beach, mountain biking in Marin County, and skiing around Lake Tahoe.

GRADUATES

Of the graduating class of 2003, the following specialties were selected by the indicated number of students: family practice (eight), internal medicine (twenty-two), internal medicine/primary care (eleven), pediatrics (nine), emergency medicine (thirteen), psychiatry (twelve), obstetrics/gynecology (five), surgery (three), orthopedic surgery (six), neurology (six), ophthalmology (six), dermatology (four), anesthesiology (ten), neurosurgery (two), otolaryngology (five), radiology (ten), oral surgery (two), pathology (four), physical medicine (two), plastic surgery (one), radiation oncology (two), urology (two), and other (six). In total, 33 percent entered residencies in fields classified as primary care. For more information, see medschool.ucsf.edu/medstudents/resources/match/2003_stats.asp for details.

Admissions

REQUIREMENTS

To be considered for admission, applicants must complete the following by June of the year they expect to matriculate: general chemistry with lab (three quarters, equal to one year), organic chemistry (two quarters), physics, and biology (equal to one year). Applications are welcome from candidates who have taken time off after college. The MCAT is required; the spring MCAT is strongly advised. For those who retake the test, the most recent scores are considered. MCAT scores must be no more than three years old. California residents are given preference.

SUGGESTIONS

Beyond requirements, applicants should have taken college-level math, humanities, and English courses. Upper-division biology is also recommended. All extracurricular activities that demonstrate interests and commitment strengthen the application. Some exposure to medical issues or to patient care is also valuable.

PROCESS

GPA, MCATs, residency, and the AMCAS application are used to screen for secondary applications. The secondary application is straightforward and does not require additional essays for the MD program. Applicants have three weeks from the date of receipt of the secondary application to return it and to send their letters of recommendation. Letters of recommendation sent prior to receipt of the secondary application will be destroyed. About 30 percent of all applicants receive a secondary application, of which about one-third are invited to interview. There is also a hold category for applicants who are not in the top group but who have a chance to be interviewed as the year progresses. Interviews take place between September and March and consist of two one-hour blind sessions, each with a faculty member or one faculty member and one student. After offers have been made to fill the class, some remaining candidates are placed on a ranked wait-list and may be offered a spot as late as August, depending on the matriculation rate of accepted students.

Admissions Requirements (Required)

MCAT scores, science GPA, non-science GPA, letters of recommendation, interview, essays/personal statement.

Admissions Requirements (Optional)

state residency, extracurricular activities, exposure to medical profession.

Overlap Schools

Harvard University, Stanford University, University of California-Los Angeles.

COSTS AND AID

Out-of-state tuition	$12,245
Cost of books	$1,800
Fees	$15,977

Financial Aid

% students receiving aid	86
Average grant	$11,152
Average loan	$19,761
Average debt	$65,672

University of Chicago

The University of Chicago Pritzker School of Medicine

BSLC 104, 924 East 57th Street, Chicago, IL 60637-5416 • Admission: 773-702-1937 • Fax: 773-834-5412 • E-mail: pritzkeradmissions@bsd.uchicago.edu • Website: http://pritzker.bsd.uchicago.edu

STUDENT BODY

Type	Private
Enrollment	416
% male/female	48/52
% underrepresented minorities	15
# applied (total/out)	5,619/4,872
# accepted (total/out)	265/197
# enrolled (total/out)	104/63
Average age	23

ADMISSIONS

Average GPA and MCAT Scores

Overall GPA	3.6
MCAT Bio	10.6
MCAT Phys	10.4
MCAT Verbal	9.8
MCAT Essay	Q

Application Information

Regular application	10/15
Regular notification	rolling
Early application	8/1
Early notification	10/1
Are transfers accepted?	Yes
Admissions may be deferred?	Yes
Interview required?	Yes
Application fee	$75

Academics

Pritzker offers a curriculum best characterized as a modified traditional one. Although most preclinical topics are presented in lecture, case-based methods and clinical exposure supplement lectures. For example, as students study particular parts in anatomy, they view afflictions of that body part in a clinical setting. About 24 percent of the students in each class earn a graduate degree in addition to the MD degree. Students are MSTP participants, are privately funded MS/PhD students, or earn a JD or an MBA along with the MD.

BASIC SCIENCES: Chicago follows a quarter system. Fall quarter, first-year medical students study biochemistry and molecular biology; human morphology I; cell and organ physiology; and clinical skills 1A, which introduces students to the patient interview. During the winter, first-year students study molecular and cell biology; organ physiology and endocrinology; human morphology II; doctor/patient relationship; and clinical skills, which covers social issues related to medicine. Spring curriculum includes neurobiology, medical genetics, development and psychopathology, nutrition and epidemiology, clinical investigation, and an opportunity for elective study. Second-year, fall-quarter curriculum includes immunobiology, microbiology, pharmacology, and cell pathology. Winter quarter includes clinical pathophysiology and clinical skills 2A, called physical diagnosis. The final quarter of preclinical studies includes therapeutics, more clinical skills, review of basic sciences, and electives. First- and second-year students spend their time in the new biological sciences learning center, which is both a center for instruction and research. Classrooms are equipped with audio/video technology, and excellent computer-based learning tools are available. The Knapp Center is a new medical research facility with modern laboratory space. The Crerar Library has one of the largest science collections in the United States and has almost one million volumes. Grades of pass and fail are used to evaluate students, although they receive graded feedback on exams. Tutoring is available for students who are in danger of failing. The USMLE is not a graduation requirement, although most students choose to take Step 1 after year two.

CLINICAL TRAINING

Students are introduced to clinical techniques and experiences during their first quarter in clinical skills 1A. The third year consists of a series of clerkships with short breaks between rotations. Clerkships take place at the University of Chicago Hospitals and Health Systems and at Weiss Memorial Hospital. Recently, a new primary care clerkship was developed and established at MacNeal Hospital. These hospitals serve a broad community, and students learn to treat a diverse patient population. Students rotate through the following departments: internal medicine (three months), obstetrics/gynecology (one-and-a-half months), psychiatry (one-and-a-half months), surgery (three months), pediatrics (two months), and family medicine (one month); family medicine is a new addition to the requirements. During the fourth year, students choose selectives from the following categories: inpatient/subinternship, scientific basis of medical practice, neurology, and anesthesia. The fourth year is also an opportunity for students to pursue individual research projects or to study overseas. The University of Chicago Medical facilities have significantly expanded during the past decade, suggesting a strong patient base and economic situation. Evaluation of clinical performance uses grades of honors, high pass, pass, low pass, and fail. As students do not need to take the USMLE II to graduate, they may substitute it with a comprehensive exam, which is otherwise required.

Students

Typically, Pritzker attracts research-oriented students. Underrepresented minorities have accounted for about 14 percent and women for about 50 percent of the student body. Class size is 104. The unique feature of the Pritzker School of Medicine is its integration—geographically, administratively, and programmatically—into the rest of the University of Chicago. Consequently, it attracts students and faculty who have broader scholarly interests and who see the entire university as a resource for their academic goals. Over 24 percent of Pritzker's graduates earn two degrees. Pritzker is among the top schools in training faculty for academic medicine. Pritzker students obtain additional degrees in business, law, biological sciences, physical sciences, social sciences, humanities, and public health.

STUDENT LIFE

The University of Chicago is located in Hyde Park, a diverse and interesting community; downtown Chicago is a twenty-minute commute by car or by public transportation. Students are also active in curriculum development and have representatives on important administrative councils. Student volunteer organizations are involved in projects such as organizing and implementing health education into public schools. Medical students take part in university-wide activities such as intramural sports.

GRADUATES

During the past five years, the residency programs that attracted the most Pritzker graduates were University of Chicago Hospitals, UCSF, University of Michigan, Mass General, University of Washington, University of Penn, Brigham and Women's Boston, McGaw Medical Center, Beth Israel Boston, Barnes Hospital, Washington University, and UCLA. The following specialties were the most popular within the 2000 graduating class: internal medicine (twenty-four), pediatrics (ten), surgery (five), obstetrics/gynecology (five), dermatology (four), ophthalmology (four), family practice (three), orthopedic surgery (four), internal medicine/pediatrics (two), anesthesiology (four), and emergency medicine (four). About 20 percent of Pritzker graduates ultimately serve as faculty members at universities.

Admissions

REQUIREMENTS

One year of lecture plus lab is required in biology, general chemistry, organic chemistry, and physics. Biochemistry with lab may be substituted with one semester or quarter of organic chemistry. For applicants who graduated from college more than three years prior to applying, recent science course work is important. The MCAT is required and should be no more than three years old. Although Pritzker is private, it seeks to matriculate 35 percent of the student body as Illinois residents.

SUGGESTIONS

Biochemistry is strongly recommended, as is significant course work in social sciences and humanities. The Admissions Committee is interested in what factors motivated applicants to pursue medicine and is also concerned with demonstrated problem solving skills, leadership, experience with persons different from themselves, and experience in research.

PROCESS

Secondary applications are available to all AMCAS applicants and should be completed as soon as possible and no later than December 1. About 18 percent of applicants who return secondaries are interviewed between September and February. Interviewees participate in three one-on-one sessions with faculty members and medical students. About two-fifths of all interviewed candidates are accepted on a rolling basis, and the rest are placed on a wait-list. Wait-listed candidates are encouraged to submit information that will strengthen their applications and will indicate their interest in the school.

Admissions Requirements (Required)

MCAT scores, science GPA, non-science GPA, letters of recommendation, interview, essays/personal statement, extracurricular activities, exposure to medical profession.

Admissions Requirements (Optional)

state residency.

Overlap Schools

Columbia University, Cornell University, Harvard University, Stanford University, University of Illinois at Chicago, Washington University, Yale University.

COSTS AND AID

Tuition	$29,046
Cost of books	$1,009
Fees	$1,949

Financial Aid

% students receiving aid	89
Average grant	$21,161
Average loan	$38,334
Average debt	$110,004

University of Cincinnati
College of Medicine

Office of Admissions, PO Box 670552, Cincinnati, OH 45267-0552 • Admission: 513-558-7314 • Fax: 513-558-1165 • E-mail: comadmis@ucmail.uc.edu • Website: www.med.uc.edu

STUDENT BODY

Type	Public
Enrollment	634
% male/female	60/40
% underrepresented minorities	8
# applied (total/out)	2,090/1,316
# accepted (total/out)	387/135
# enrolled (total/out)	161/39
Average age	22

FACULTY

Total faculty (number)	1,215
% female	29
% minority	17
% part-time	9

ADMISSIONS

Average GPA and MCAT Scores

Overall GPA	3.6
MCAT Bio	10.3
MCAT Phys	10
MCAT Verbal	9.4

Application Information

Regular application	12/15
Regular notification	Rolling
Early application	6/1-8/1
Early notification	10/1
Are transfers accepted?	Yes
Admissions may be deferred?	Yes
Interview required?	Yes
Application fee	$25

Academics

Most students follow a four-year curriculum that leads to the MD degree. There is also a a five-year curriculum that leads to a combined MD/MBA degree. Up to six positions a year are available in an NIH funded Physician Scientist Training Program (PSTP), a seven- to eight-year curriculum that leads to a combined MS/PhD program. The PhD may be earned in one of the following disciplines: cell and molecular biology, molecular and developmental biology, environmental health sciences (includes clinical/genetic epidemiology), molecular, cellular, and biochemical pharmacology, molecular and cellular physiology, molecular genetics, biochemistry, and microbiology, neuroscience, pathobiology and molecular medicine and biomedical engineering. Medical students who are interested in shorter-term research projects may pursue them during the summer or as electives. Grades of honors, high pass, pass, and fail are used to evaluate medical students. Passing the USMLE Step 1 is a requirement for advancing to year three, and passing Step 2 is a requirement for graduation.

BASIC SCIENCES: During the first and second years, courses are integrated around content blocks that foster critical thinking skills and problem solving. In both years, a major effort is made to limit lecture and laboratory time, to use more small group activities, and to ensure sufficient daily free time for active, independent learning. First-year classes are gross anatomy, microscopic anatomy, biochemistry, physiology, and brain and behavior I. The first-year clinical foundations of medical practice course includes interviewing, history-taking, and basic physical examination skills as well as ethics, biopsychosocial issues, human sexuality, and death and loss, and provides each student with a one-on-one clinical experience in a physician's practice. Second-year courses are pathology, microbiology, pharmacology, brain and behavior II, and introduction to clinical practice, which expands physical diagnosis and clinical skills training. An average of twenty contact hours per week and ample study time before each exam allow time for self directed learning, group study, volunteering, and other activities in the basic science years. There continues to be a concerted effort to vertically integrate content blocks between the basic science and clinical science years. OhioLINK, a consortium of Ohio's college and university libraries and the State Library of Ohio, gives AIT&L customers access to more than thirty-nine million library items, 100 research databases, 5,600 full-text electronic journals, and 1,800 electronic books. AIT&L currently ranks fifth in electronic journals and ninth in electronic books among academic health sciences libraries in the United States.

CLINICAL TRAINING

Third-year required clerkships are internal medicine (eight weeks), surgery (eight weeks), pediatrics (eight weeks), obstetrics/gynecology (eight weeks), psychiatry (six weeks), family medicine (four weeks), radiology (two weeks), and two specialty selectives (two weeks each). During the fourth year, students complete an eight-week internal medicine acting internship, a four-week neuroscience selective, and twenty-four weeks of electives, some of which must be in primary care fields.

Students

Among students in the 2003 entering class, 76 percent were Ohio residents, 8 percent were minorities, and 16 percent were over twenty-five years old at the time of application. Eight percent of the class had earned a master's degree. Seventy one percent of students were science majors, and a total of fifty-nine undergraduate institutions were represented. The 2003 entering class size was 161.

STUDENT LIFE

Medical students enjoy a cooperative and supportive environment. There are over thirty student organizations, clubs, and service groups available. Clubs include family practice, cultural diversity, complementary medicine, international health, and medical volunteers. Medical students have access to a UC fitness center and other campus athletic and recreational facilities. Cincinnati offers many attractions, including theaters, restaurants and bars, museums, parks, bookstores, and professional sporting events. University-owned apartments for single and married students are available on a limited basis.

GRADUATES

Of those who graduated in 2003, 35 percent entered residency programs in Cincinnati, 9 percent entered programs elsewhere in Ohio, and the remainder were successful in securing positions throughout the United States. The most prevalent fields for post-graduate study were family medicine (11.1 percent), internal medicine (all types, 37.2 percent), pediatrics (9.2 percent), emergency medicine (6.5 percent), obstetrics/gynecology (5.9 percent) and psychiatry (6.5 percent).

Admissions

REQUIREMENTS

The MCAT is required, and scores should be from within the past three years. Ohio residents are given preference. Although no courses are specified, applicants are expected to have the knowledge usually gained in a one-year lecture and laboratory course in biology, general chemistry, organic chemistry, physics, and math. Applicants are expected to have an undergraduate preparation that provides insight into behavioral, social, and cultural issues. Academically, applicants are evaluated based on the following: GPA, MCAT scores, and undergraduate, graduate, and post-baccalaureate achievement.

PROCESS

All applicants must submit an AMCAS application and complete the UC online application, which is available at www.med.uc.edu. Approximately 700 to 750 applicants are invited to interview. Interviewees attend an informational program, eat lunch, and tour the college. Notification of the committee's decision occurs on a monthly basis, from on October 15 until May 15. After that time, students are accepted from the alternate list as openings occur until the class is filled. Additional programs include the College of Medicine has a dual admissions program for exceptional high school seniors who know they want to pursue a career in medicine. These eight-year programs are in conjunction with John Carroll University, University of Dayton (JAMS), Miami University, Xavier University, and the University of Cincinnati (Connections). There is also a nine-year Medicine and Engineering Dual Admissions Program (Connections E) that involves five years of undergraduate/graduate engineering studies at University of Cincinnati College of Engineering and four years of medical school. High school students who are interested in such programs should contact the admissions or pre-med office at the undergraduate colleges. The University of Cincinnati College of Medicine and College of Business Administration have partnered to develop a joint MD/MBA degree program. Students should apply for the program after their first year of medical school.

Admissions Requirements (Required)

MCAT scores, science GPA, non-science GPA, letters of recommendation, interview.

Admissions Requirements (Optional)

state residency, essays/personal statement, extracurricular activities, exposure to medical profession, Optional experiences are strongly encouraged..

COSTS AND AID

In-state tuition	$18,630
Out-of-state tuition	$33,159
Room and board	$14,081
Cost of books	$2,818
Fees	$1,032

Financial Aid

% students receiving aid	85
Average debt	$90,298

UNIVERSITY OF COLORADO

UNIVERSITY OF COLORADO SCHOOL OF MEDICINE

MEDICAL SCHOOL ADMISSIONS, 4200 EAST 9TH AVENUE, C-297, DENVER, CO 80262 • ADMISSION: 303-315-7361 • FAX: 303-315-1614 • E-MAIL: SOMADMIN@UCHSC.EDU • WEBSITE: WWW.UCHSC.EDU/SM/SM

STUDENT BODY

Type	Public
Enrollment	532
% male/female	54/46
% underrepresented minorities	12
# applied (total/out)	2,357/1,727
# accepted (total/out)	240/98
# enrolled (total/out)	132/26
Average age	24

FACULTY

Total faculty (number)	1,300

ADMISSIONS

Average GPA and MCAT Scores

Overall GPA	3.7
MCAT Bio	10.67
MCAT Phys	10.01
MCAT Verbal	9.81
MCAT Essay	P

Application Information

Regular application	11/1
Regular notification	rolling
Are transfers accepted?	Yes
Admissions may be deferred?	Yes
Interview required?	Yes
Application fee	$80

Academics

The School of Medicine is part of the University of Colorado Health Sciences Center, which includes the schools of dentistry, nursing, pharmacy, and graduate studies. A combined MS/PhD degree through the MSTP is possible in the following fields: biochemistry, biophysics, cell biology, immunology, molecular biology, microbiology, pharmacology, and physiology.

BASIC SCIENCES: The first two years are organized into quarters. Throughout year one, microanatomy, physiology, and foundations of doctoring are studied. Foundations of doctoring, which establishes one-on-one mentoring relationships between students and local practicing physicians, is the first of three segments that together constitute the curricular element of the generalist initiative. In addition, during the fall, students take biochemistry and human anatomy. Year one, winter-quarter courses are genetics and neurobiology. Spring courses are biochemistry and nutrition, embryology, and ethics. Yearlong courses during year two are the following: pathology, pharmacology, human behavior, and foundations of doctoring. Immunology and microbiology are also taken in the fall, and neuroscience, pathophysiology, and epidemiology are taken in the winter. Students spend about twenty-eight hours per week in a structured-learning environment. About 40 percent of this time is devoted to lecture, and another 40 percent is devoted to lab. Small group sessions are also employed as an instructional technique. Academic tutoring and counseling are available to students through a student advocacy program. Grades of honors, pass, and fail are used to evaluate medical students. Students must pass the USMLE Step 1 to begin the clinical years.

CLINICAL TRAINING

Patient contact begins the first year, when students work closely with practicing physicians and and gradually gain independent responsibility. Third-year, required clerkships include medicine (twelve weeks), surgery (six weeks), family medicine (six weeks), obstetrics/gynecology (six weeks), neurology (four weeks), pediatrics (six weeks), and psychiatry (six weeks). One afternoon each week is dedicated to the continuing primary care experience as the third segment of the foundations of doctoring sequence. During year four, students select from surgical specialties (six weeks, including one week each of anesthesiology, ophthalmology, orthopedics, otolaryngology, and urology) and from a wide variety of general electives. Most clerkships take place at University Hospital, VA Medical Center, Denver Health Medical Center, Children's Hospital, and the National Jewish Center for Immunology and Respiratory Medicine. Electives and some required clerkships may be fulfilled at community hospitals and clinics around the state or under the supervision of affiliated private physicians in the area. Denver is a rapidly growing city with a population of over two million. It is an international tourist destination, making the patient population more diverse than that associated with medical schools in other predominantly rural states. Evaluation during the clinical years uses grades of honors, pass, and fail to evaluate medical students; these grades are supplemented by narratives from professors. There are opportunities for clinical experiences outside of traditional rotations, generally through outreach activities and volunteer work. Students may volunteer at clinics that provide care to Denver's homeless population or may spend time working with low-income children in need of care. The Medical Student International Program is popular, granting students credit for up to four months of overseas study or work. Passing the USMLE Step 2 is graduation requirement.

Students

At least 85 percent of students are Colorado residents. Science and nonscience majors are equally represented. Of the 2001 entering class, 15 percent were underrepresented minorities, most of whom were Hispanic Americans. With a mean age of twenty-six for entering students, there is clearly a wide age range within the student body. Class size is 132.

STUDENT LIFE

Denver is a comfortable, affordable, and student-friendly place to live. It is less than an hour from perhaps the best skiing in the United States. During the summer, hiking, swimming, climbing, and mountain biking are all outstanding. Single students live off campus in apartments and shared houses. Married students can find affordable family housing in various Denver neighborhoods. On-campus activities include student-run organizations and events that have either a professional or social focus. The Office of Diversity provides support for minority students.

GRADUATES

The most popular residency programs of the 2001 graduating class were internal medicine (twenty-nine students), family medicine (twenty-one), surgery (nine), pediatrics (thirteen), emergency medicine (four), anesthesiology (fifteen), obstetrics/gynecology (four), and orthopedics (six). More than half of the graduates entered primary care fields. Graduates often stay in Denver for training. Other states that are popular for post-graduate training are Texas, Minnesota, and California.

Admissions

REQUIREMENTS

Required courses are college mathematics (six hours), biology with lab (eight semester hours), chemistry with lab (eight hours), organic chemistry with lab (eight hours), physics with lab (eight hours), English literature and English composition or creative writing (nine hours). Applicants must demonstrate competency in mathematics at least through college level trigonometry, either with college courses or placement test results. The MCAT is required and the best scores are used for students who retake the exam.

SUGGESTIONS

In addition to required courses, a course in biochemistry is recommended. For applicants who have been out of school for a significant period of time, recent course work is suggested. Personal qualities are valued a great deal, as are extracurricular activities that involve medical research or health-related experience. As part of the generalist initiative, applicants from rural backgrounds are encouraged to apply.

PROCESS

All AMCAS applicants receive secondary applications. Seventy-five percent of Colorado residents who complete secondaries are interviewed. Less than 20 percent of out-of-state applicants are interviewed. Interviews take place on campus from September through April and consist of two sessions, each with a member of the Admissions Committee. The Admissions Committee is made up of students, faculty, and community physicians. Notification occurs on a rolling basis. About one-quarter of Colorado residents who interview are accepted, and about one-tenth of out of state interviewees are accepted. A wait-list is established, from which twenty to forty students are usually taken. Wait-listed candidates are not encouraged to send supplementary material.

Admissions Requirements (Required)

MCAT scores, science GPA, nonscience GPA, letters of recommendation, interview, state residency, essays/personal statement, extracurricular activities, exposure to medical profession.

COSTS AND AID

In-state tuition	$15,677
Out-of-state tuition	$67,000
Cost of books	$1,000
Fees	$1,858

Financial Aid

Average grant	$4,000
Average loan	$20,000

UNIVERSITY OF CONNECTICUT
SCHOOL OF MEDICINE

MEDICAL STUDENT AFFAIRS, 263 FARMINGTON AVENUE, ROOM AG-062, FARMINGTON, CT 06030 • ADMISSION: 203-679-3874 • FAX: 860-679-1282 • E-MAIL: SANFORD@NSO1.UCHC.EDU • WEBSITE: WWW.UCHC.EDU

STUDENT BODY

Type	Public
Enrollment	326
% male/female	48/52
% underrepresented minorities	12
# applied (total/out)	2,154/1,816
# accepted (total/out)	182/59
# enrolled (total/out)	80/13
Average age	23

FACULTY

Total faculty (number)	389
% female	34
% part-time	28
# student/faculty ratio	1:1

ADMISSIONS

Average GPA and MCAT Scores

Overall GPA	3.6
MCAT Bio	10.5
MCAT Phys	9.9
MCAT Verbal	9.7
MCAT Essay	Q

Application Information

Regular application	12/15
Regular notification	10/15
Early application	6/1-8/1
Early notification	10/1
Are transfers accepted?	Yes
Admissions may be deferred?	Yes
Interview required?	Yes
Application fee	$75

Academics

In addition to the required courses, about 70 percent of students take part in a research project while they are in school. Grading is strictly pass/fail, based on the notion that all students are at the top of their class. A combined-degree program that leads to both an MD and a PhD is pursued by about four students each year in conjunction with the following graduate programs: cell biology, developmental biology, immunology, genetics, molecular biology and biochemistry, neuroscience, skeletal biology, and cellular and molecular pharmacology. It is also possible for medical students to earn a master's in public health or a master's in business administration from the University of Connecticut's graduate program.

BASIC SCIENCES: The first two years cover the basic sciences, introduce clinical studies, and integrate behavioral and social aspects of medicine and health care. Instruction uses lectures, labs, case conferences, and problem-based learning. First-year courses are human systems, which is composed of: human biology; organ systems I (neuroscience, anatomy of the head and neck); organ systems II (cardiovascular, respiratory and renal systems, anatomy of the thorax and abdomen); and organ system III (gastrointestinal, endocrine and reproductive, genetics, and anatomy of the pelvis); electives; correlated medical problem solving; and principles of clinical medicine, which teaches history-taking, the physical examination, and general concepts related to clinical care. Second-year courses are human development and health, which encompasses ethical, social, and legal issues; mechanisms of disease, which includes concepts related to pathology; pharmacology; infectious disease; homeostasis; oncology; metabolism; nervous system; reproductive system; and skin, connective tissue, and joints; correlated medical problem solving; and clinical medicine. Facilities include modern lecture halls, classrooms for small group discussions, the Lyman Maynard Stowe Library, and computer resources. Passing the USMLE Step 1 is a requirement for promotion to year three.

CLINICAL TRAINING

The third year is organized into two segments: one involves clinical training in ambulatory settings and the other takes place in hospitals. The ambulatory experience consists of the following clerkships: general internal medicine (seven weeks), pediatrics (five weeks), psychiatry (two weeks), family medicine (seven weeks), obstetrics/gynecology (four weeks), and subspecialties (three weeks). The hospital, or inpatient, segment includes rotations in medicine (four weeks); surgery (four weeks); pediatrics (two weeks); psychiatry (two weeks); obstetrics (two weeks); and beginning to end (two weeks), in which students follow patients from their admittance to each diagnosis/service area that they visit in the hospital. The fourth-year includes twenty weeks of electives, which may be taken at local or distant sites. Other fourth-year requirements are advanced inpatient experience (four weeks), critical care experience (four weeks), emergency/urgent experience (four weeks), and selectives (students choose from rotations in research, community health, or education-related fields). All students are paired with a faculty member of their choice to assist in scheduling electives and in selecting postgraduate training programs. Clinical training takes place at the University Hospital (232 beds) and at about ten affiliated hospitals in the area. Some students gain clinical experience overseas, by participating in projects in Latin America, Asia, or Africa. Passing the USMLE Step 2 is a requirement for graduation.

Students

Underrepresented minorities, mostly African American, make up about 15 percent of the student body. The average age of incoming students is typically about twenty-four and range from twenty-one to thirty-nine. About 80 percent of the students are Connecticut residents, and about 10 percent graduated from the University of Connecticut undergraduate college. Approximately 80 percent of students majored in a scientific discipline in college. Class size is about eighty. Dental students participate in the basic sciences classes.

STUDENT LIFE

Life outside the classroom includes theater, concerts, and restaurants in Hartford; organized team sports on campus; and numerous clubs and groups that are related to professional or extracurricular interests. The Department of Health Career Opportunities provides support services throughout the academic year to minority medical students. Community-service activities such as volunteering at homeless shelters bring students together around important projects. Facilities such as golf courses, ski slopes, and public parks are accessible to the campus. On-campus housing is not available. Students live off campus in communities surrounding the university.

GRADUATES

Of the class that graduated in 2002, the most prevalent specialty choices were internal medicine (18 percent), pediatrics (16 percent), emergency medicine (13 percent), obstetrics/gynecology (8 percent). About 20 percent of graduates entered residency programs at the University of Connecticut Health Center. Other popular destinations were Massachusetts, New York, Pennsylvania and Maryland.

Admissions

REQUIREMENTS

Requirements are one year of chemistry, organic chemistry, physics, and biology. The MCAT is required and should be no more than three years old.

SUGGESTIONS

A broad and in-depth liberal arts education, which includes English, math, foreign language, literature, history, art, and political science, is advised. The Admissions Committee looks very seriously at the nonacademic traits of applicants such as their characters and motivation.

PROCESS

All AMCAS applicants are sent secondary applications. About 80 percent of Connecticut applicants and about 10 percent of out-of-state applicants are interviewed. Interviews are held from August through April and consist of two one-hour sessions with faculty, administrators, or students. Candidates have lunch and tour the campus with medical students. Some candidates are accepted shortly after their interviews and others are notified later in the year. A wait-list is established in the spring. Wait-listed candidates may send supplementary information such as transcripts.

Admissions Requirements (Required)

MCAT scores, science GPA, non-science GPA, letters of recommendation, interview, essays/personal statement, extracurricular activities, exposure to medical profession.

Admissions Requirements (Optional)

state residency.

COSTS AND AID

In-state tuition	$10,440
Out-of-state tuition	$23,750
Cost of books	$1,575
Fees	$4,430

Financial Aid

% students receiving aid	90
Average grant	$21,000
Average loan	$21,000
Average debt	$70,000

University of Florida
College of Medicine

Box 100216, 1600 SW Archer Road, Room M-108, Gainesville, FL 32610 • Admission: 352-392-4569 • Fax: 352-846-0622 • E-mail: admissions@mail.med.ufl.edu • Website: www.med.ufl.edu

STUDENT BODY

Type	Public
Enrollment	472
% male/female	54/46
% underrepresented minorities	10
# applied (total/out)	2,003/843
# accepted (total/out)	171/3
# enrolled (total/out)	116/1
Average age	22

FACULTY

Total faculty (number)	1,020
% part-time	2

ADMISSIONS

Average GPA and MCAT Scores

Overall GPA	3.7
MCAT Bio	10.51
MCAT Phys	10.7
MCAT Verbal	9.74
MCAT Essay	P

Application Information

Regular application	12/1
Regular notification	rolling
Are transfers accepted?	No
Admissions may be deferred?	Yes
Interview required?	Yes
Application fee	$30

Academics

Students may pursue their own interests with specialized institutes and centers such as the Health Policy Institute, the Center for Mammalian Genetics, and the Brain and Cancer Institutes. Students who have an interest in public health are encouraged to pursue the MPH degree in conjunction with other academic institutions. Grades of A through F and a ranking system are used to evaluate medical students. Students need both steps of the USMLE to graduate.

BASIC SCIENCES: Instructional methods include lectures, labs, and small group sessions that together occupy twenty-five hours per week or less. First-year basic science courses are biochemistry, anatomy, radiology, genetics, cell and tissue biology, physiology, and neuroscience. Integrated into basic sciences are behavioral sciences, ethical issues, and clinical training. Examples of first-year courses in these areas are essentials of patient care, keeping families healthy, human behavior, and the preceptor program. second-year courses are pathology, oncology, physical diagnosis, clinical diagnosis, pharmacology, clinical radiology, social and ethical issues in medical practice, public health, and microbiology. Classrooms, labs, and the library are in one complex. A satellite library also operates in Jacksonville.

CLINICAL TRAINING

Required third-year rotations are medicine (eight weeks), neurology (two weeks), psychiatry (six weeks), surgery (eight weeks), obstetrics/gynecology (six weeks), pediatrics (eight weeks), and interdisciplinary generalist clerkships (ten weeks). Fourth-year clerkships are advanced surgery (four weeks), advanced medicine, pediatrics, or family medicine (four weeks), clinical pharmacology (four weeks), and electives (twenty-eight weeks). The primary teaching hospitals are Shands Hospital (576 beds), the Gainesville Veterans' Affairs Medical Center (403 beds), and the University Medical Center (528 beds). Training also takes place at outpatient clinics in nearby communities and at clinical research facilities. Educational affiliations have been established in Tallahassee, Pensacola, Jacksonville, Leesburg, Broward County, and Orlando. With approval, up to three months of elective credits may be earned at other institutions around the United States and overseas. Outside of formal rotations, students gain clinical experience through outreach projects such as Camps for Sick Kids and Care for the Homeless.

Students

About 99 percent of the students are Florida residents. Underrepresented minorities account for 11 percent of the student body, and students who have taken time off after college make up at least one-quarter of each entering class. Class size is 120.

STUDENT LIFE

Popular extracurricular activities include viewing intercollegiate sports, taking part in outdoor activities made possible by the year-round temperate climate, and occasionally going out at night to restaurants, clubs, and theaters. The university has an active student union with a theater, pool tables, a bowling alley, and a cafeteria. Athletic facilities, including a student gym, are expansive and are well-used by medical students. Outside of the classroom, students get to know each other through involvement with organizations and projects. A few examples of the numerous medical student organizations are Physicians for Social Responsibility, the Christian Medical and Dental Group, and the

Family Practice Student Organization. Service projects, such as the School of Medicine Outreach to Rural Students (SMORS) and the EqualAccess Clinic improve students' interactive skills and give them the opportunity to contribute to their community. There are numerous groups that devote time each year on medical missions to underserved countries.

GRADUATES

There are about 6,500 graduates of the College of Medicine, a number of whom are renowned for important contributions they have made in their respective fields. At University of Florida-affiliated hospitals there are fifty-six post-graduate programs. Many of the positions in these programs are filled by graduates of the College of Medicine.

Admissions

REQUIREMENTS

Requirements are chemistry (eight hours), organic chemistry (four hours), biochemistry (four hours), biology (eight hours), and physics (eight hours). The MCAT is required, and scores must be no more than three years old from the date of expected matriculation. Generally, the highest scores are considered.

SUGGESTIONS

Early submission, preferably by June, of the AMCAS application is advised. No undergraduate major is preferred, and science and nonscience majors are considered equally. Course work in statistics, biochemistry, genetics, and microbiology is useful. Although there is no math requirement, the school assumes that students have taken math up through calculus as an undergraduate prerequisite for chemistry. Extracurricular activities, nonmedically related community service, health care experience, and research are important.

PROCESS

Typically, the college receives 2,000 AMCAS applications for 120 available spaces. About 1,000 of the AMCAS applicants receive secondary applications, and about three hundred of those returning secondaries are invited to interview. Interviews are held on Fridays from September through March and consist of two sessions with faculty members. On interview day, candidates get to have lunch and take a tour. Interview notification occurs on a rolling basis. After their interviews, applicants are either accepted, rejected, or put on hold. In April, an alternate list is established. Additional material and updates may be submitted by wait-listed candidates. There are two routes of admission to the College of Medicine: junior honors (twelve places) and regular admissions (120 places). To apply for the junior honors program, students apply directly to the College of Medicine during their sophomore year of college. If accepted to the program, they complete a special series of seminars at the University of Florida during their junior year and begin medical school after the completion of their junior year. For more information about junior honors, call 352-392-4569.

Admissions Requirements (Required)

MCAT scores, science GPA, non-science GPA, letters of recommendation, interview, state residency, essays/personal statement, extracurricular activities, exposure to medical profession.

COSTS AND AID

In-state tuition	$13,926
Out-of-state tuition	$40,082
Room and board	$7,292
Cost of books	$2,665
In-state fees	$1,740
Out-of-state fees	$3,119

Financial Aid

% students receiving aid	88
Average grant	$1,400
Average loan	$20,930
Average debt	$55,102

UNIVERSITY OF HAWAII

JOHN A. BURNS SCHOOL OF MEDICINE

JOHN A. BURNS SCHOOL OF MEDICINE, 1960 EAST-WEST ROAD, BIOMED. B-104, HONOLULU, HI 96822 • ADMISSION: 808-956-8300 • FAX: 808-956-9547 • E-MAIL: MNISHIKI@HAWAII.EDU • WEBSITE: HTTP://HAWAIIMED.HAWAII.EDU

STUDENT BODY

Type	Public
Enrollment	264
% male/female	45/55
% underrepresented minorities	17
# applied (total/out)	1,284/1,079
# enrolled (total)	62
Average age	25

FACULTY

Total faculty (number)	458
% female	23
% minority	15
% part-time	51
# student/faculty ratio	1:1

ADMISSIONS

Average GPA and MCAT Scores

Overall GPA	3.6
MCAT Bio	9.98
MCAT Phys	9.39
MCAT Verbal	8.98
MCAT Essay	0

Application Information

Regular application	12/1
Regular notification	10/15
Early application	6/1-8/1
Early notification	10/1
Are transfers accepted?	Yes
Admissions may be deferred?	Yes
Interview required?	Yes
Application fee	$50

Academics

The School of Medicine, the School of Nursing, and the School of Social Work make up the College of Health Sciences and Social Welfare. JABSOM offers an MD/PhD joint degree program designed to train aspiring medical scientists who wish to prepare for careers that combine biomedical or clinical research and clinical practice. The program combines rigorous scientific research preparation for the PhD degree with a full MD curriculum. The PhD degrees offered in this program are cell and molecular biology, public health (biostatistics-epidemiology), and tropical medicine & medical microbiology. A master's degree may also be earned from the Department of Public Health Sciences and Epidemiology or from other selected departments within the school of medicine.

BASIC SCIENCES: Instruction is entirely case-based and emphasizes self directed learning and early clinical training. Throughout the first two years, students take clinical skills, which involves patient contact, and community medicine, which is an interdisciplinary course. Other subjects are organized into units, each one occupying three or four months. Unit 1 courses are health and illness and introduction to problem-based learning. Unit 2 focuses on cardiovascular, respiratory, and renal problems. Unit 3 courses focus on hematology, endocrine, and gastrointestinal problems. During the summer following the first year, students take part in a primary care precept, which entails working with local physicians. Unit 4 courses focus on locomoter, neurologic, and behavioral problems. Unit 5 courses focus on life cycle problems in obstetrics/gynecology, pediatrics, adolescents, and geriatrics. The final three months of the second year are used for a basic science review in preparation for the USMLE Step 1, which is required for promotion to year three. Scheduled classes during the first two years occupy about twenty hours per week and thus provide ample time for independent, self directed study. Grades of pass and fail are used to evaluate students, and they are not ranked.

CLINICAL TRAINING

Preclinical training: Instruction in the various basic science disciplines is integrated into the problem-based learning experience as well as provided through a basic science foundation lecture and laboratory series. The first two years of the curriculum are divided into five units; learning centers around problem-based learning in small group learning sessions. The themes of Unit 1 are health and illness and an introduction to problem-based learning. Unit 2 focuses on cardiovascular, respiratory, and renal problems. Unit 3 focuses on hematology, endocrine, and gastrointestinal problems. During the summer following the first year, students take part in a primary care preceptorship, which entails working for nine weeks with a practicing physician. Students also concurrently participate in a research project during this summer block period. Unit 4 focuses on locomotor, neurologic, and behavioral problems. Unit 5 focuses on life cycle problems in obstetrics/gynecology, pediatrics, adolescents, and geriatrics. In the final three months of the second year, there is basic science review in preparation for the USMLE Step 1. Throughout the first two years, students have weekly clinical skills experiences, during which they participate in patient care under the supervision of medical school faculty.

Students

Hawaii's multi-ethnic population is reflected in the student body, which is made up of men and women of Caucasian, Chinese, Korean, Japanese, Hawaiian, Filipino, Samoan, and Micronesian ancestries. Class size is sixty-two. Graduate residency programs in Hawaii include the following specialties: transitional, internal medicine, obstetrics/gynecology, orthopedics, pathology, pediatrics, psychiatry, surgery, and family practice. Four percent of graduates are in the military service, and 1 percent are in full-time academic positions.

STUDENT LIFE

Although the School of Medicine is relatively small and intimate, the University of Hawaii at Manoa enrolls approximately 17,000 students. Medical students take part in campus activities but are integrated into the greater community of the city of Honolulu and the island of Oahu. Almost all students live off campus. Honolulu is a city with a population of about one million. It is a major tourist center that offers beautiful beaches and many cultural, recreational, and outdoor activities.

GRADUATES

Residency programs in Hawaii are popular with graduates and include the following specialties: transitional, internal medicine, obstetrics/gynecology, orthopedics, pathology, pediatrics, psychiatry, surgery, and family practice. Four percent of graduates are in the military service, and 1 percent are in full-time academic positions.

Admissions

REQUIREMENTS

The initial screening of applicants selects candidates who have close ties to Hawaii and who are most likely to practice in Hawaii and in the Pacific upon completion of postgraduate study. An exception is made for applicants from Wyoming and Montana, states without medical schools that belong to WICHE (Western Interstate Commission on Higher Education). Undergraduate course requirements are biology (twelve semester units, including at least four units of cell and molecular biology), chemistry (four units), biochemistry (three units), and physics (eight units). All courses except biochemistry must include laboratory experience. The MCAT is required and must be no more than three years old. The most recent set of scores is used for candidates who have retaken the exam.

SUGGESTIONS

Additional courses in biological and social science are advised, such as immunology, genetics, microbiology, anatomy, physiology, embryology, psychology, and sociology. Previous medical experience is important, as are personal qualities that suggest the applicant will become a humanistic physician. For candidates who have been out of school for a significant period of time, recent course work is recommended. Each year, a post-baccalaureate program selects ten promising students for medical school. If these students successfully complete the yearlong pre-medical training, they are offered a position in the subsequent incoming class of medical students.

PROCESS

Annually, about 15 to 20 percent of applicants are interviewed. Interviews are conducted from October through March and consist of two sessions with faculty members, practicing physicians, or members of the community. Of those interviewed, about 20 percent of in-state applicants and 5 percent of out-of-state applicants are accepted. Historically, approximately 10 percent of each incoming class are nonresidents. Most applicants are notified of the committee's decision in late April, although a few highly qualified applicants may be contacted earlier. A wait-list is established at this time. Wait-listed candidates are not advised to send supplementary information.

Admissions Requirements (Required)

MCAT scores, science GPA, non-science GPA, letters of recommendation, interview, essays/personal statement.

Admissions Requirements (Optional)

state residency, extracurricular activities, exposure to medical profession.

COSTS AND AID

In-state tuition	$14,808
Out-of-state tuition	$28,512
Cost of books	$2,874

Financial Aid

Average grant	$6,545
Average loan	$12,561

UNIVERSITY OF ILLINOIS AT CHICAGO
UIC COLLEGE OF MEDICINE

808 S. WOOD STREET, ROOM 165 CME, M/C 783, CHICAGO, IL 60612 • ADMISSION: 312-996-5635 • FAX: 312-996-6693 • E-MAIL: MEDADMIT@UIC.EDU • WEBSITE: WWW.MEDICINE.UIC.EDU

STUDENT BODY

Type	Public
Enrollment	1,242
% male/female	59/41
% underrepresented minorities	21
# applied (total/out)	3,925/2,405
# accepted (total/out)	560/39
# enrolled (total/out)	317/20
Average age	22

ADMISSIONS

Average GPA and MCAT Scores

Overall GPA	3.5
MCAT Bio	9.6
MCAT Phys	9.4
MCAT Verbal	9
MCAT Essay	Q

Application Information

Regular application	12/31
Regular notification	6/1
Early application	6/1-8/1
Early notification	10/1
Are transfers accepted?	Yes
Admissions may be deferred?	Yes
Interview required?	Yes
Application fee	$40

Academics

Students participate in one of two educational tracks: 175 students complete all four years in Chicago, while 125 spend their first year at Urbana-Champaign. After the first year at Urbana-Champaign, fifty students complete years two, three, and four in Peoria or Rockford. The remaining twenty-five students at Urbana-Champaign participate in the medical scholars program.

BASIC SCIENCES: The first and second years include the principles of anatomy, behavioral science, biochemistry, genetics, histology, immunology, microbiology, neuroscience, pathology, pathophysiology, pharmacology, and physiology. All students participate in a clinical medicine course. Lectures and labs are the predominant instructional modality.

CLINICAL TRAINING

Patient contact begins in the first year when students are assigned individual physician preceptors. Students sharpen their skills in diagnosis and treatment through problem solving sessions. In the third and fourth years, students focus on patient care with a series of clerkships supplemented by conferences and lectures. The twenty-five affiliated facilities range from rural ambulatory health care centers to major metropolitan hospitals. The diverse clinical experiences prepare UIC graduates to succeed within the nation's ever-changing health care system. Required clerkships include family medicine, internal medicine, obstetrics/gynecology, pediatrics, psychiatry, and surgery. The elective phase provides students with the opportunity to identify special interest areas and to select educational experiences most relevant to their goals. The objective of the MS/PhD program is to train students for careers in academic medicine and research. The Medical Scholars Program (MSP)—located on the Urbana-Champaign campus—permits students to integrate medicine with graduate studies in both science and nonscience fields. The Independent Study Program (ISP) allows students to design their own academic programs with advice from faculty. ISP students complete an in-depth study, usually involving the basic sciences or clinical medicine. The ISP program is offered on the Chicago, Peoria, and Rockford campuses. The Rural Medical Education Program (RMED) and Rural Illinois Medical Student Assistance Program (RIMSAP) recruit students who commit to practice in medically underserved areas of Illinois.

Students

UIC is one of the most ethnically diverse medical schools in the country. Students are assigned to a faculty member who serves as an adviser. The adviser's major role is to be available to students throughout their medical education for academic and personal counseling. Research interests are widely diversified and range from basic molecular biology to patient related clinical research.

STUDENT LIFE

Students in Chicago enjoy living in one of the most exciting cities in the United States. In Urbana-Champaign, students benefit from a large and exciting university community. Rockford and Peoria are midsize cities that offer basic urban amenities. Campus housing in Chicago includes three residence halls near the college. In Urbana-Champaign, university-certified housing includes campus, private residence halls, and university apartments (for family housing). In Peoria and Rockford, housing is easily accessible and reasonable.

GRADUATES

UIC students undertake career specialization and training in all disciplines. Most graduates who participate in the National Residency Matching Program receive one of their top three residency choices.

Admissions

REQUIREMENTS

Only applicants who indicate plans to obtain a baccalaureate degree prior to enrollment will be considered for admission. Major fields may be in humanities, behavioral, biological, or physical sciences. All applicants must complete two semesters of introductory biology or the equivalent with laboratory, two semesters of general inorganic chemistry or the equivalent with laboratory, two semesters of organic chemistry with laboratory (introductory biochemistry may substitute for one semester of organic chemistry), and two semesters of general physics or the equivalent. All applicants are expected to complete three semesters of social science courses with an emphasis in the behavioral sciences. In addition, candidates are expected to take at least one of the following courses: advanced-level biology, biochemistry, physiology, mammalian histology, comparative vertebrate anatomy, or molecular genetics. All applicants must take the MCAT no later than the fall of the year prior to enrollment and no more than three years prior to application. All applicants must complete an application to the AMCAS no later than December 31 of the year prior to enrollment. All applicants must be U.S. citizens or possess a permanent resident immigrant visa at the time of application. Eligible applicants will be sent a UIC Supplemental Application. Materials must be postmarked by February 15 of the year prior to enrollment. A minimum of three academic letters of recommendation or one composite recommendation from a pre-professional committee must be postmarked by February 15 of the year prior to enrollment. If you are currently enrolled in a graduate or professional school, one of your three letters of recommendation must be from a faculty member at your graduate or professional school. It is advisable that letters of recommendation be sent from the institution at which the applicant had been most recently enrolled and must be completed on official university or business letterhead. Personal letters of recommendation are not acceptable.

SUGGESTIONS

At least 90 percent of UIC students are Illinois residents. Although Illinois residents are given preference, positions are open to highly qualified nonresidents. In addition to academic strength, experience, and background are considered important factors in admissions decisions.

PROCESS

About one-third of AMCAS applicants are sent a UIC Supplementary Application. The most highly qualified are invited to interview between September and April. The interview is a requirement and will be arranged by the Office of Medical College Admissions. Interviews are granted by invitation only. Interviews are held on all four campuses, and the interview location does not determine the campus where matriculants may attend. The interview consists of one panel interview session. Candidates have the opportunity to meet faculty members and students, receive financial aid information, tour the campus, and learn more about the College of Medicine. Interviewed candidates are accepted on a batch system. Students not immediately accepted may be put on an alternate list.

Admissions Requirements (Required)

MCAT scores, science GPA, non-science GPA, letters of recommendation, interview, state residency, essays/personal statement.

Admissions Requirements (Optional)

extracurricular activities, exposure to medical profession.

Overlap Schools

Loyola University Chicago, Northwestern University, Rush Medical College of Rush University, Southern Illinois University-Carbondale, University of Chicago.

COSTS AND AID

Cost of books	$1,280

University of Iowa
Roy J. and Lucille A. Carver College of Medicine

100 Medicine Administration Building, Iowa City, IA 52242 • Admission: 319-335-8052 • Fax: 319-335-8049 • E-mail: medical-admission@uiowa.edu • Website: www.medicine.uiowa.edu/osac/admissions/

STUDENT BODY

Type	Public
Enrollment	589
% male/female	56/44
% underrepresented minorities	21
# applied (total)	2,326
# accepted (total)	240
# enrolled (total)	142

ADMISSIONS

Average GPA and MCAT Scores

Overall GPA	3.7
MCAT Bio	10.3
MCAT Phys	10
MCAT Verbal	9.9
MCAT Essay	P

Application Information

Regular application	11/1
Regular notification	rolling
Early application	6/1-8/1
Early notification	10/1
Are transfers accepted?	No
Admissions may be deferred?	Yes
Interview required?	Yes
Application fee	$50

Academics

Most students at Iowa follow a four-year course of study that leads to the MD. About 5 percent of students are MSTP participants and concurrently earn a PhD with the MD. The doctoral degree may be earned in anatomy, biochemistry, microbiology, pharmacology, and physiology, and biophysics. Other joint degree programs such as those leading to a master's degree along with the MD are also possible. Medical students are evaluated with grades of near honors, pass, and fail for all courses except electives, which are graded as pass and fail. Although the first two years are primarily devoted to basic sciences, introductory clinical training is also an important part of the curriculum. The second two years are devoted to clinical rotations.

BASIC SCIENCES: First-year courses are biochemistry, cell biology, medical genetics, gross anatomy, structure and functions of human organ systems, neuroscience, immunology, and foundations of clinical practice, which continues through the second year. This course covers topics that include biomedical ethics, problem-based learning, behavioral medicine, human sexuality, and continuity of care and that covers important clinical techniques such as history-taking, the physical examination, and the doctor-patient relationship. The course structure and functions of human organ systems covers principles of histology and physiology and is organized around body/organ systems. After completing their first years, many students spend the summer working and learning in an Iowa community hospital or conducting medical research projects. Second-year courses are principles of infectious diseases, foundations of clinical practice, pharmacology, pathology. Throughout the first two years, students are in lectures, discussions, labs, or tutorials for about twenty-three hours per week. Basic sciences are taught in the Medical Education and Research Faculty and the Bowen Science Building. The Hardin Library holds over 200,000 volumes and nearly 3,000 periodicals and is used by students, faculty, and the medical community for research and studying. It also has a multimedia computer classroom and computer-based informational resources.

CLINICAL TRAINING

Third- and fourth-year required core clerkships are community-based primary care (six weeks), family practice (three weeks), internal medicine (inpatient, six weeks), internal medicine (ambulatory, 3 weeks), obstetrics/gynecology (six weeks), pediatrics (six weeks), and surgery (six weeks). Subspecialty clerkships are neurology (four weeks), psychiatry (four weeks), and two weeks of each of the following: anesthesia, dermatology, ophthalmology, orthopedics, otolaryngology, radiology, urology, electrocardiography, and laboratory medicine. Two advanced clerkships and at least twelve weeks of electives are also required. Clinical training takes place at the University Hospital (1,100 beds), the Veterans' Affairs Hospital (440 beds), and various sites within the state.

Students

Each entering class has 142 students. About 70 percent of students are Iowa residents. Generally, about thirty undergraduate majors are represented in a class. Approximately 9 percent of students are underrepresented minorities. The majority of students entered medical school one year after college graduation. The Medical Education and Research facility opened for classes in fall 2001. It also houses four learning communities to which each student is assigned.

STUDENT LIFE

Medical students are active in student organizations that include groups that support minorities, professional interest groups, and a medical school band. The learning communities also sponsor activities that encourage peer-to-peer support and mentoring. Each community is staffed by a faculty director, professional, and support staff and leadership is provided by the elected student representatives. As part of the greater University of Iowa, medical students enjoy its facilities, resources, and sponsored events, such as Big Ten athletics. The campus is central to Iowa City and is convenient to restaurants, clubs, theaters, shopping areas, and parks. Although the city has a population of 60,000 people, it is relatively safe and has the feeling of a friendly small town. Just outside of the city are lakes, hiking areas, and other outdoor attractions. Urban centers such as Chicago, St. Louis, Minneapolis, Omaha, and Kansas City are within a five-hour drive. On campus housing options include coed medical fraternities with both single and double rooms and university-owned family housing. Off-campus, reasonably priced apartments are available.

GRADUATES

Graduates are successful in entering the residency programs of their choice. Iowa itself offers post-graduate training programs in about fifteen fields.

Admissions

REQUIREMENTS

Prerequisites are one year each of physics, chemistry, organic chemistry, general biology, one semester of advanced biology, and college-level math. All science courses should include laboratory instruction. The MCAT is required, and scores must be from exams no earlier than April 1998 and no later than August 2003 for the 2004 entering class. All sets of scores are evaluated.

SUGGESTIONS

Although preference is given to Iowa residents, well-qualified nonresidents are also considered. Nonscience majors might benefit from additional science courses beyond requirements. Computer literacy, the ability to write well, strong verbal skills, and general decision-making capabilities are some of the skills sought in applicants. Also important are an applicant's personal characteristics, which are evaluated with the help of letters of reference and interviews. Some medically related experience is important.

PROCESS

Iowa participates in the AMCAS process. Most candidates who apply through AMCAS are sent secondary applications. About one-third of Iowa residents who apply are accepted, and about 6 percent of nonresidents are accepted. Applicants are notified on a rolling basis and are either accepted, rejected, or wait-listed. Wait-listed candidates are not encouraged to send additional information.

Admissions Requirements (Required)

MCAT scores, science GPA, nonscience GPA, letters of recommendation, interview, state residency, essays/personal statement, extracurricular activities.

Admissions Requirements (Optional)

exposure to medical profession.

COSTS AND AID

In-state tuition	$17,838
Out-of-state tuition	$36,306
Cost of books	$3,000
Fees	$1,472

Financial Aid

Average grant	$8,408
Average loan	$31,071

UNIVERSITY OF KANSAS

UNIVERSITY OF KANSAS SCHOOL OF MEDICINE

3901 RAINBOW BOULEVARD, 3040 MURPHY BUILDING, KANSAS CITY, KS 66160 • ADMISSION: 913-588-5245 • FAX: 913-588-5259 • E-MAIL: PREMEDINFO@KUMC.EDU • WEBSITE: WWW.KUMC.EDU/SOM/SOM.HTML

STUDENT BODY

Type	Public
Enrollment	700
% male/female	54/46
% underrepresented minorities	13
# applied (total/out)	1,319/902
# accepted (total/out)	242/61
# enrolled (total/out)	175/22
Average age	25

FACULTY

Total faculty (number)	569
% female	30
% minority	18
% part-time	20
# student/faculty ratio	1:1

ADMISSIONS

Average GPA and MCAT Scores

Overall GPA	3.7
MCAT Bio	9.5
MCAT Phys	9.3
MCAT Verbal	9.3
MCAT Essay	P

Application Information

Regular application	10/15
Regular notification	3/1
Early application	July 1 recommended
Early notification	10/1
Are transfers accepted?	Yes
Admissions may be deferred?	Yes
Interview required?	Yes

Academics

In comparison to many medical schools, clinical training at the University of Kansas emphasizes rural and primary health care. Joint MS/PhD degrees are offered in the following fields: anatomy and cell biology, biochemistry and molecular biology, microbiology, molecular genetics and toxicology, pathology and oncology, pharmacology, and physiology. A joint MD/MPH is also offered.

BASIC SCIENCES: Basic sciences are taught in Kansas City. The facilities are modern and fully equipped with learning tools such as computers and visual-aid equipment. The School of Medicine has recently implemented a systemic methodology for teaching basic sciences. Students take part in individual and small group projects that require them to develop initiative and problem solving skills. First-year students take cell and tissue biology, physiology, biochemistry, gross anatomy, neuroscience, and introduction to clinical medicine. Second-year students take microbiology, pathology, pharmacology, and introduction to clinical medicine. Tutoring is available through the learning resources counseling service. A student-operated note service, in which students share note-taking, covers regularly scheduled lectures. Students are evaluated using the following descriptions: superior, high satisfactory, satisfactory, low satisfactory, and unsatisfactory. These marks are translated into numeric scores to determine class rank. The USMLE is required upon completion of year two. The Dykes Library of the Health Sciences supports the educational and research demands of medical students, faculty, and the public. It contains 150,000 books and offers online informational services. In addition, the Clendening History of Medicine Library has one of the top five collections of rare medical books in the country.

CLINICAL TRAINING

Patient contact begins in year one, when students take part in biweekly sessions with practicing physicians. Required clinical clerkships are ambulatory medicine/geriatrics (six weeks), family medicine (six weeks), obstetrics/gynecology (six weeks), medicine (eight weeks), pediatrics (six weeks), neuropsychiatry (eight weeks), and general surgery (eight weeks). Year four is filled primarily with electives, which include preventive medicine and the history of medicine. Clinical training takes place both at the University of Kansas Hospital (464 beds), which houses nearly all the diagnostic and treatment facilities of the Medical Center, and at hospitals in Wichita. Included at the Medical Center in Kansas City are the Kansas Cancer Institute, the Burnett Burn Center, the Smith Mental Retardation Center, the Center on Aging, and the Center on Environmental and Occupational Health. Patients are drawn from Kansas, Missouri, Oklahoma, Arkansas, and Nebraska. The grading scale is the same for performance in clinical rotations as it for basic science courses. In addition to formal rotations, students gain clinical experience through volunteer activities such as the Mobile Medical Unit, which brings basic prevention and care to communities in need. Many students devote free summers to volunteer work in medically related activities.

Students

About 90 percent of a typical class are Kansas residents, and most students have liberal arts backgrounds. In recent years, about 13 percent of the student body have been underrepresented minorities, mostly African and Hispanic Americans. Usually, almost a quarter of matriculants in a given year are older than twenty-five years. Class size is 175.

STUDENT LIFE

Medical students from all four classes are organized into academic societies which bring students together around academic and extracurricular activities. The Kirmayer Fitness Center is a modern facility that is open to all medical students. Numerous organized activities enrich the lives of medical students. Activities such as Rural Health Weekend provide opportunities for interaction with practicing physicians throughout the state. Organizations such as the Community Outreach Project provide opportunities for community service. All students live off campus.

GRADUATES

About 50 percent of graduates enter primary care fields. Graduates are successful in obtaining residency positions throughout the country. The medical school sponsors events and scholarships that encourage students and residents to consider practicing in Kansas.

Admissions

REQUIREMENTS

Required college courses are one year of biology with lab, chemistry with lab, organic chemistry with lab, physics with lab, one year of English, and one semester of college-level mathematics. A bachelor's degree is required. GPAs are evaluated no matter where course work was completed. The MCAT is required, with the two most recent sets of scores considered. The August MCAT is acceptable.

SUGGESTIONS

Experience in a health care setting is valued, and the breadth of an applicant's undergraduate course work is important. Demonstrated interests in rural and primary care medicine are pluses. Out-of-state residents should have particularly strong qualifications. A few students each year are accepted from the University of Kansas post-baccalaureate program and through the Scholars in Primary Care program.

PROCESS

All Kansas residents are sent secondary applicants, while only about 10 percent of out-of-state applicants receive them. About 75 percent of Kansas residents and about 5 percent of out-of-state applicants are interviewed. Interviews are conducted in Kansas City, from October through March, and consist of one or two sessions each with one or two members of the interview panel. Approximately one-half of those interviewed are offered positions in the class and are notified on a rolling basis after the interview. The wait-list is short, and wait-listed candidates are not encouraged to send supplementary material.

Admissions Requirements (Required)

MCAT scores, science GPA, non-science GPA, letters of recommendation, interview, essays/personal statement, extracurricular activities, exposure to medical profession, secondary application, prerequisite courses, and bachelor degree.

Admissions Requirements (Optional)

state residency.

COSTS AND AID

In-state tuition	$15,078
Out-of-state tuition	$32,336
Cost of books	$3,600
Fees	$370

Financial Aid

% students receiving aid	85
Average grant	$2,500
Average loan	$27,500
Average debt	$70,000

UNIVERSITY OF KENTUCKY
COLLEGE OF MEDICINE

MN102 UKMC, 800 ROSE STREET, LEXINGTON, KY 40536-0298 • ADMISSION: 859-323-6161 • FAX: 859-323-2076 • E-MAIL: KYMEDAP@UKY.EDU • WEBSITE: WWW.COMED.UKY.EDU/MEDICINE

STUDENT BODY

Type	Public
Enrollment	389
% male/female	62/38
% underrepresented minorities	6
# applied (total/out)	941/541
# enrolled (total/out)	95/7
Average age	23

FACULTY

# student/faculty ratio	1:1

ADMISSIONS

Average GPA and MCAT Scores

Overall GPA	3.6
MCAT Bio	9.6
MCAT Phys	9.5
MCAT Verbal	9.5
MCAT Essay	0

Application Information

Regular application	11/1
Regular notification	Rolling
Early application	6/1- 8/1
Early notification	10/1
Are transfers accepted?	Yes
Admissions may be deferred?	Yes
Interview required?	Yes
Application fee	$30

Academics

The curriculum includes early patient contact and teaches lifelong learning skills, ethics, and computer-assisted learning along with traditional basic science and clinical techniques. The goal of the medical education program is to focus on principles and the organization of factual bodies of knowledge rather than on unconnected detail. Although most students complete a four-year curriculum, a few students each year enter a combined MS/PhD program. The doctorate may be earned in anatomy, biochemistry, biophysics, cell biology, genetics, immunology, microbiology, molecular biology, neuroscience, pharmacology, or physiology. Combined MD/MPH and MD/MBA programs are also available. Medical students are evaluated with grades of A through F and with grades of pass and fail in some cases. Passing Step 1 of the USMLE is a requirement for promotion to year three, and passing Step 2 is a graduation requirement.

BASIC SCIENCES: During the first and second years, students are in class or other scheduled sessions for about twenty-four hours per week. Lectures and tutorials are the primary instructional methods. Laboratories, hands-on clinical work, and conferences are also important parts of the curriculum. The first year is devoted to basic sciences and interdisciplinary perspectives. The year is organized into blocks, each of which contains one or two courses. First-year courses are patients, physicians, and society; introduction to the medical profession; human structure/gross anatomy; human structure/histology; healthy human; cellular structure and function/biochemistry; cellular structure and function/genetics; neuroscience; and human function. The second year is focused on the disease process and is also broken into blocks. These are patients, physicians, and society II; introduction to the medical profession II; immunity, infection, and disease; and mechanisms of disease and treatment, which covers pathology and pharmacology. Students spend most of their first two years in the medical science building, which houses classrooms and laboratories. Computers are important educational tools, and all incoming students are required to have their own computers. The College of Medicine has a nationally recognized program of academic computing in medical education, which provides a wide variety of services to enhance student learning. These educational support services are offered in facilities located in the College of Medicine, the Chandler Medical Center, and in the Area Health Education Centers. The library, which contains more than 150,000 volumes, is also an important resource.

CLINICAL TRAINING

Third-year required clerkships are women's maternal and child health (twelve weeks), clinical neuroscience (eight weeks), principles of primary care (twelve weeks), and medical and surgical care (sixteen weeks). The fourth year consists of a one month acting internship selected from medical specialties (family practice, internal medicine, pediatric, neurology, psychiatry, and rehabilitation medicine), a one month acting internship selected from surgical specialties (general, subspecialty, and obstetrics/gynecology), a one month emergency medicine clerkship, a one month clinical pharmacology and anesthesiology clerkship, and a one month primary care or rural medicine selective. In addition, eight weeks of electives are required. Training takes place primarily at the University of Kentucky Hospital (473 beds), although a number of affiliated hospitals and clinics are also used.

Students

Approximately 90 percent of students are Kentucky residents. About 6 percent of students are underrepresented minorities, most of whom are African American. Generally, about 25 percent of students in each class are nontraditional and have pursued other careers or interests in between college and medical school.

STUDENT LIFE

Medical students enjoy extracurricular activities associated with the main university such as attending university basketball games. Student groups provide additional extracurricular activities, including opportunities for involvement in community service projects. They also serve as a means of interacting outside of class. Women in Science and Medicine is a group primarily made up of faculty and administrators that focuses on improving all aspects of life for women in medicine. Lexington is an attractive and safe city where students can find affordable housing.

GRADUATES

Graduates enter residency programs all over the United States in both primary care and specialty fields. The University of Kentucky has post-graduate training programs in over twenty fields.

Admissions

REQUIREMENTS

One year each of biology, general chemistry, organic chemistry, physics, and English are required. All science courses should include associated labs. The MCAT is required, and scores should be from within the past two years. For applicants who have retaken the exam, the most recent set of scores is weighed most heavily.

SUGGESTIONS

In addition to academic qualifications, the school seeks students who have the character, personality, values, and motivation for human service. Individual initiative and good judgment are important traits. Some medically related experience is important.

PROCESS

All AMCAS applicants who are Kentucky residents are sent secondary applications. Highly qualified nonresidents are also sent secondaries. About 50 percent of applicants who return secondary applications are invited to interview between September and March. On interview day, candidates also tour the campus, attend group informational sessions, and have the opportunity to informally meet with current students. About 45 percent of interviewed candidates are accepted on a rolling basis. Other candidates are rejected or wait-listed. Wait-listed candidates may send additional information to update their files. The admissions process is rolling, and the class is typically full by January so early completion of both the primary and the secondary application is strongly recommended.

Admissions Requirements (Required)

MCAT scores, science GPA, non-science GPA, letters of recommendation, interview, exposure to medical profession.

Admissions Requirements (Optional)

state residency, essays/personal statement, extracurricular activities.

Overlap Schools

University of Louisville.

COSTS AND AID

In-state tuition	$13,604
Out-of-state tuition	$31,196
Cost of books	$2,475
Fees	$608

Financial Aid

% students receiving aid	86
Average grant	$6,840
Average loan	$23,617
Average debt	$89,171

UNIVERSITY OF LOUISVILLE
SCHOOL OF MEDICINE

ABELL ADMINISTRATION CENTER, ROOM 413, 323 E. CHESTNUT STREET, LOUISVILLE, KY 40202 • ADMISSION: 502-852-5193 • FAX: 502-852-0302 • E-MAIL: MEDADM@LOUISVILLE.EDU • WEBSITE: WWW.LOUISVILLE.EDU

STUDENT BODY

Type	Public
Enrollment	589
% male/female	50/50
% underrepresented minorities	17
# applied (total/out)	1,291/900
# accepted (total/out)	252/76
# enrolled (total/out)	149/28
Average age	25

FACULTY

Total faculty (number)	680
% female	27
% minority	19
% part-time	11
# student/faculty ratio	1:1

ADMISSIONS

Average GPA and MCAT Scores

Overall GPA	3.6
MCAT Bio	9.2
MCAT Phys	9.2
MCAT Verbal	9.2
MCAT Essay	0

Application Information

Regular application	11/1
Regular notification	rolling
Early application	6/1-8/1
Early notification	10/1
Are transfers accepted?	Yes
Admissions may be deferred?	Yes
Interview required?	Yes
Application fee	$75

Academics

Although most students complete a four-year program that leads to the MD, a few of them earn a combined MS/PhD, which typically demands about seven years. Summer research scholarships allow first- and second-year students to participate in research projects alongside faculty mentors. Throughout all four years, students work closely with faculty advisers who assist them with decisions related to academic and professional goals. Medical students are evaluated with grades of pass and fail in both basic science and clinical courses. Passing Step 1 of the USMLE is a requirement for promotion to year three, and passing Step 2 is a requirement for graduation.

BASIC SCIENCES: The purpose of the core curriculum, which extends over the four-year course of study, is to provide each student with the general education and training considered to be essential to all physicians. It stresses understanding of concepts and general principles instead of superficial knowledge of details. It provides opportunity for correlation among the sciences so that information received in one subject can reinforce ideas and build upon concepts developed in another subject. The incorporation of clinical correlation into the first two years demonstrates how knowledge of the basic sciences applies directly to the solution of problems with human disease. The core curriculum, for the first two academic years, is divided into four quarters (one-half semester intervals) of nine weeks each. Within these smaller subdivisions it is possible to vary the balance of departmental activities to accommodate a better integrated understanding of the subject matter. The purpose of the preclinical elective program is to allow students to extend their education in certain areas of scientific knowledge. The electives make it possible for the school to construct a program of medical education that best meets the needs, abilities, and goals of the individual student. Students also are permitted to take courses as electives in divisions of the University of Louisville other than the School of Medicine, if their class schedules so permit. In addition to the courses listed, students who are interested in research are permitted to participate in an approved research activity for credit. Elective courses constitute an integral part of students' total program in medical school. Second-year students take two credit hours of elective courses.

CLINICAL TRAINING

Third-year required rotations are psychiatry (six weeks), basic surgery (eight weeks), obstetrics/gynecology (eight weeks), and primary care (integrated medicine, pediatrics, and family medicine, twenty-four weeks). Fourth-year requirements are inpatient medicine (four weeks), inpatient surgery (four weeks), neurology (four weeks), AHEC (four weeks), ambulatory primary care (four weeks), ambulatory rotation (four weeks) and perioperative medicine (two weeks). The remaining eleven weeks in the fourth year are reserved for electives.

Students

In the entering class of 2003, 123 of 149 students were Kentucky residents. African Americans represented 9 percent of the class, and students older than twenty-seven years old represented 5 percent of the class.

STUDENT LIFE

Students profit from the school's location in the center of Louisville. Louisville is the largest city in Kentucky and offers cultural and recreational activities such as orchestra, theater, ballet, opera, numerous restaurants and bars, and shopping areas. Just outside of Louisville is the home of the Kentucky Derby. Many medical students take advantage of the university-owned medical-dental dormitory and apartment building, which is two blocks from both the School of Medicine and the University Hospital. In this residential complex, there are apartments of all sizes as well as dorm rooms.

GRADUATES

A large proportion of practicing physicians in Kentucky are Louisville School of Medicine graduates. Louisville offers at least seventeen post-graduate training programs.

Admissions

REQUIREMENTS

Requirements are two semesters each of biology, chemistry, organic chemistry, physics, and calculus or other college-level math. All science courses must include lab work. One semester of English is also required. The MCAT is required, and scores should be no more than two years old. For applicants who have retaken the exam, the most recent set of scores is considered. Thus, there is no advantage in withholding scores.

SUGGESTIONS

Approximately 90 percent of positions in each class are reserved for Kentucky residents, making out-of-state admission very competitive. Pre-medical students should develop a strong background in the humanities, philosophy, and the arts. Communication and reading abilities are also important. The committee values volunteer work, medically related experience, and evidence of strong interpersonal skills. Applicants are advised to take the April MCAT, rather than August one.

PROCESS

All qualified Kentucky residents and highly qualified nonresidents who submit AMCAS applications are sent secondaries. About one-half of Kentucky applicants are invited to interview between September and April. Ten percent of nonresidents are invited to interview. On interview day, candidates receive two thirty-minute interview sessions each with a faculty member, administrator, or medical student. In addition, interviewees go on a guided campus tour, have lunch, and have the opportunity to informally meet with current students. About 40 percent of interviewed candidates are accepted on a rolling basis. Wait-listed candidates may send information to update their files in the spring.

Admissions Requirements (Required)

MCAT scores, science GPA, non-science GPA, letters of recommendation, interview, state residency, essays/personal statement, extracurricular activities, exposure to medical profession.

Overlap Schools

University of Kentucky.

COSTS AND AID

In-state tuition	$14,544
Out-of-state tuition	$36,262
Cost of books	$2,146
Fees	$660

Financial Aid

% students receiving aid	89
Average grant	$3,076
Average loan	$21,969
Average debt	$73,192

University of Manitoba

270-727 McDermot Avenue Winnipeg, MB R3E 0W3 • Admission: 204-789-3499 • Fax: 204-789-3929 • E-mail: registrar_med@umanitoba.ca • Website: www.umanitoba.ca/medicine

STUDENT BODY

Type	Public
Enrollment	339
% male/female	50/50
% underrepresented minorities	5
# applied (total/out)	525/266
# accepted (total/out)	122/34
# enrolled (total/out)	89/9
Average age	24

ADMISSIONS

Average GPA and MCAT Scores

Overall GPA	3.9
MCAT Bio	10.06
MCAT Phys	10.04
MCAT Verbal	9.87
MCAT Essay	0

Application Information

Regular application	10/29
Regular notification	5/31
Are transfers accepted?	Yes
Admissions may be deferred?	Yes
Interview required?	Yes
Application fee	$50

Academics

Medical students complete a four-year curriculum that leads to the MD degree. Classes during the first two years are largely systems-based. Small groups are the predominant format for instruction; lectures, labs, computer-based learning, and early clinical exposure are important educational tools. Students spend the second two years in clinical clerkships.

BASIC SCIENCES: The first academic period begins in September and lasts thirty-five weeks. It is divided into introduction to medicine (population health and medicine, structure and function, and disease mechanisms), human development, systems (cardiovascular, respiratory, dermatology, ENT), clinical/communications skills, problem solving, and medical humanities. The second academic period is organized around anatomical and physiological systems. These are reproduction, endocrine, renal, neuroscience, musculoskeletal, ophthalmology, gastrointestinal, liver, and blood/lymphoid. Students also continue first-year studies in clinical/communication skills and medical humanities.

CLINICAL TRAINING

During their third and fourth years, students complete required clinical clerkships. These are family/community medicine (seven weeks), internal medicine (twelve weeks), obstetrics/gynecology (seven weeks), pediatrics (seven weeks), psychiatry (seven weeks), surgery (nine weeks), anesthesia (two weeks), emergency medicine (four weeks), and ophthalmology/ENT (one week). Fifteen weeks are available for clinical electives. Teaching hospitals include those of the Health Sciences Centre (consisting of the Children's, Adults', Women's, and Respiratory and Rehabilitation Hospitals for a total of over 1,000 beds), St. Boniface General Hospital (900 beds), Deer Lodge Veterans Hospital (500 beds), Grace Hospital (306 beds), Steven Oaks Hospital (336 beds), Victoria Hospital (254 beds), Misericordia Hospital (409 beds), and the Diabetes Research and Treatment Center.

Students

In the entering class of 2002, approximately 46 percent of students were women. The average age of incoming students was slightly over twenty-three years. All students have bachelor's degrees.

STUDENT LIFE

Medical students often choose to live in an apartment complex operated by the Health Sciences Centre. Other options include dormitories and off-campus housing, which is facilitated by listings available through the off-campus housing office. Recreational activities and events are sponsored by the student union. In addition, numerous student groups and organizations offer medical students a wide variety of social and community-based activities.

Admissions

REQUIREMENTS

Applicants must have or be eligible to receive their bachelor's degree by June 30, 2004 from a university recognized by the University of Manitoba. Applicants must have completed a full course of English or French and a full course of biochemistry at the university level and received a grade of C or higher. Two full courses in humanities/social sciences are also required. The MCAT is required and should be taken within the past three years but no later than August of the year of application. Students usually prepare for the MCAT by taking university courses in physics, organic chemistry, physical chemistry, and biology.

SUGGESTIONS

Priority is given to residents of Manitoba who are Canadian citizens or permanent residents. The most successful applicants have grade point averages between 3.8 and 4.2 on a 4.5 scale and at least an 8 on each scored section of the MCAT. In addition to academic and intellectual credentials, the Admissions Committee selects applicants who demonstrate social skills, maturity, and a sense of responsibility. The Admissions Committee selects ninety students for admission from about 550 applicants. Typically, about nine places are offered to applicants from outside Manitoba.

PROCESS

For application material, contact the faculty via E-mail at admissions@umanitoba.ca or via telephone at 204-474-8808. The application deadline is November 16. Applicants who meet scholastic and MCAT requirements will be invited to interview and asked to submit a personal statement. About 250 applicants are interviewed, from which the class is selected in early June. There is a special consideration category for some Manitoba residents who fall into one of the following three groups: candidates who are sponsored by faculty-approved agencies, candidates who are from native populations of Manitoba, and candidates who have been employed for two or more years in the areas of health, social welfare, or health education.

Admissions Requirements (Required)

MCAT scores, science GPA, non-science GPA, letters of recommendation, interview, essays/personal statement, extracurricular activities.

Admissions Requirements (Optional)

state residency, exposure to medical profession.

COSTS AND AID

Tuition	$7,595
Room and board	$6,000
Cost of books	$4,000

Financial Aid

% students receiving aid	35
Average grant	$1,300
Average loan	$10,615
Average debt	$43,000

UNIVERSITY OF MARYLAND
SCHOOL OF MEDICINE

ROOM 1-005, 655 WEST BALTIMORE STREET, BALTIMORE, MD 21201-1559 • ADMISSION: 410-706-7478 • FAX: 410-706-0467 • E-MAIL: MFOXWELL@SOM.UMARYLAND.EDU • WEBSITE: MEDSCHOOL.UMARYLAND.EDU

STUDENT BODY

Type	Public
Enrollment	585
% male/female	43/57
% underrepresented minorities	35
# applied (total/out)	3,258/2,536
# accepted (total/out)	301/113
# enrolled (total/out)	150/38
Average age	23

FACULTY

Total faculty (number)	1,212
% female	34
% minority	7
% part-time	16
# student/faculty ratio	2:1

ADMISSIONS

Average GPA and MCAT Scores

Overall GPA	3.6
MCAT Bio	10.2
MCAT Phys	9.8
MCAT Verbal	9.7
MCAT Essay	P

Application Information

Regular application	11/4
Regular notification	12/4
Early application	8/1-9/30
Early notification	10/1
Are transfers accepted?	Yes
Admissions may be deferred?	Yes
Interview required?	Yes
Application fee	$50

Academics

Maryland changed its curriculum in 1994 to emphasize independent and small group learning, informatics, and the integration of basic and clinical science knowledge. The traditional degree program takes most students four years to complete. However, with permission of the dean, students may spend three years covering the basic sciences and complete the degree requirements in five years. For students who are interested in a research career, the medical school offers a combined MS/PhD program in which the doctoral degree is offered in numerous disciplines such as biochemistry, biomedical engineering, genetics, molecular biology, neuroscience, and pharmacology. Grades of A through F are used to evaluate students, and they must pass Step 1 of the USMLE before beginning clinical training.

BASIC SCIENCES: The basic science curriculum is divided into integrated blocks by using interdisciplinary teaching with both basic and clinical science instructors. Lectures and labs rarely last longer than four hours per day, and small group and independent study are emphasized. Course work during the first year occupies thirty-seven weeks and is organized into the following blocks: structure and development, informatics, principles of human development, cell and molecular biology, neuroscience, and functional systems. Introduction to clinical medicine runs concurrently throughout the year, as does problem based learning. Intimate human behavior is also part of the first-year curriculum. The second year is particularly rigorous. Students learn pathophysiology and therapeutics by organ system, and are trained in conducting a physical diagnosis in the introduction to clinical medicine course. Computers, not microscopes, are the laboratory tool of choice at Maryland. Lap tops are a required purchase, and students spend the first block of medical school in a medical informatics course that discusses medical applications and practical uses for the computer. The multidisciplinary laboratories seat ten students and have the latest in educational technology. The recently renovated library is among the largest medical libraries in the United States, with at least 240,000 volumes, and is fully connected to the information superhighway. The Office of Student Affairs closely monitors students and provides them with tutoring and other support services. In addition, a pre-matriculation summer program allows entrants to review pre-medical course work and preview first-year material.

CLINICAL TRAINING

The third year consists of seven required rotations in family medicine (four weeks), medicine (twelve weeks), surgery (twelve weeks), pediatrics (six weeks), psychiatry (four weeks), obstetrics/gynecology (six weeks), and neurology/rehabilitation (four weeks). The senior year includes a mandatory ambulatory care experience (eight weeks), a subinternship (eight weeks), and sixteen weeks of elective rotations. The majority of training takes place at University Hospital, a 747-bed tertiary care center adjacent to the medical school. Rotations are also spent at the Baltimore VA Medical Center, Mercy Hospital, and other community hospitals. In total, 1,400 patient beds are used for teaching. One of the most popular electives is a rotation through the R. Adams Cowley Shock Trauma. Shock Trauma was the first trauma center in the United States and continues to be a model for the rest of the nation.

Students

The majority of students are Maryland residents, but the medical school attracts and accepts a significant number of out-of-state applicants. In a typical class, approximately thirty-eight of the 150 students are from out-of-state. The student body is highly diverse, with about 20 percent of students from underrepresented minority backgrounds. Increasingly, older students are making up a higher percentage of incoming classes. At least one-third of incoming classes took time off between college and medical school.

STUDENT LIFE

An extensive orientation program in rural Maryland allows entering students to get to know fellow classmates, upperclassmen, and faculty advisers. Almost half of the incoming class attends. Other organized events such as pot-luck suppers, community activities, and meetings of student organizations all serve to bring students together. Baltimore is a lively city with interesting neighborhoods and real character. The harbor, the commercial district (Fells Point), the Orioles baseball stadium, the Ravens football stadium, and other attractions are accessible to the campus. The university has athletic facilities. Most students find affordable, private apartments off campus or live in the dorms. While the surrounding area has undergone a renaissance in recent years, safety remains a concern, as in most large cities.

GRADUATES

Over half of each year's graduates enter one of the primary care fields. Graduates, however, are competitive candidates for the entire range of specialties.

Admissions

REQUIREMENTS

Maryland requires one year each of biology, general chemistry, organic chemistry, physics, and English as prerequisite courses. A grade of C or better is mandatory in each course. While the MCAT is also required, there is no set formula for determining competitive scores. Students with a wide variety of scores are accepted each year. In addition, Maryland considers the best scores for those applicants who retake the exam.

SUGGESTIONS

Maryland gives clinical experience with direct patient exposure considerable weight. Research experience and service activity are also valued.

PROCESS

Maryland uses the AMCAS application. Secondary applications are sent to all applicants. Approximately 25 percent of those applicants are interviewed beginning in October. The interview day consists of a faculty interview, a medical student interview, a casual lunch with students, and a tour of the campus. Interviewed applicants normally receive a decision within a month after the interview. Half of all applicants who are interviewed are accepted, and the other half are either rejected or wait-listed.

Admissions Requirements (Required)

MCAT scores, science GPA, non-science GPA, letters of recommendation, interview, essays/personal statement, extracurricular activities, exposure to medical profession, service.

Admissions Requirements (Optional)

state residency.

Overlap Schools

Jefferson Medical College of Thomas Jefferson University, Johns Hopkins University, The Pennsylvania State University, University of Pennsylvania, University of Pittsburgh, University of Virginia, Virginia Commonwealth University.

COSTS AND AID

In-state tuition	$17,493
Out-of-state tuition	$32,558
Room and board	$15,450
Fees	$765

Financial Aid

% students receiving aid	85
Average grant	$6,300
Average loan	$25,840
Average debt	$97,000

University of Massachusetts

University of Massachusetts Medical School

Associate Dean for Admissions, 55 Lake Avenue North, Worcester, MA 01655 • Admission: 508-856-2323 • Fax: 508-856-3629 • E-mail: admissions@umassmed.edu • Website: www.umassmed.edu/som/admissions/

STUDENT BODY

Type	Public
Enrollment	425
% male/female	49/51
% underrepresented minorities	7
# applied (total)	814
# accepted (total)	10
Average age	25

ADMISSIONS

Application Information

Regular application	11/1
Regular notification	5/15
Early application	6/1-8/1
Early notification	10/1
Are transfers accepted?	Yes
Admissions may be deferred?	Yes
Interview required?	Yes
Application fee	$50

Academics

The four-year program emphasizes varied educational modalities, lifelong learning, communication skills, and a generalist approach that prepares students for all medical career paths. Ethical issues are an important aspect of the education, demonstrated by the existence of an active Office of Ethics. Yearlong and summer research fellowships are available, as is a joint MS/PhD program. The doctoral degree may be earned in biomedical sciences, biochemistry and molecular biology, cell biology, cellular and molecular physiology, immunology and virology, molecular genetics, microbiology, neuroscience, and pharmacology and molecular toxicology. A combined MD/MPH degree program is also offered. For preclinical courses, grades are honors, near honors, satisfactory, marginal, unsatisfactory, or incomplete, with the exception of a few courses that are taken as credit/no credit. During the clinical years, ratings are outstanding, above expected performance, expected performance, below expected performance, and failure.

BASIC SCIENCES: First-year courses are biochemistry/metabolism; the gene; human anatomy; cells and tissues; systems I; physiology; immunology; mind, brain and behavior I; physician, patient and society (PPS); and longitudinal preceptor program (LPP). PPS and LPP together introduce students to medical interviewing, physician-patient relationships, physical diagnosis, medical reasoning and decision analyses, population-based medicine, ethics, epidemiology, medical informatics, and preventive medicine. Systems I covers several body/organ systems, including hematology, cardiovascular, respiratory, renal and acid/base, endocrine regulation, GI/nutrition, and reproduction. Second-year courses focus on the biology of disease and include general pathology; neoplasia; general pharmacology; microbiology; mind, brain and behavior II; systems II; and a continuation of PPS and LPP. In Systems II, dermatology, musculoskeletal/renal, and pumps, wind and water are among the body systems studied. Basic sciences are taught in a wing of the school's central complex. A new learning center houses amphitheaters, flexible classrooms, and a video conference facility. The Lamar Soutter Library holds over 239,000 volumes, subscribes to 1,500 journals, and provides access to online search and database tools. The library computer area contains personal computers and workstations for computer-assisted instruction, interactive programs, and educational databases.

CLINICAL TRAINING

Third-year required rotations are medicine (twelve weeks), surgery (twelve weeks), family and community medicine (six weeks), obstetrics/gynecology (six weeks), pediatrics (six weeks), and psychiatry (six weeks). Fourth-year requirements are neurology (four weeks), a subinternship in medicine (four weeks), and twenty-four weeks of elective study. Clinical training takes place at the UMass hospital (388 beds), a comprehensive facility with general and specialty services. Clinical specialties include the cancer center, level I trauma center, kidney-pancreas transplantation, Children's Medical Center, Center of Stone Disease, advanced laser technology, cardiovascular center, breast center, AIDS programs, burn unit, and public sector psychiatry. UMass benefits from affiliations with the following hospitals in and around the Worcester area: Memorial Health Care (319 beds), Saint Vincent Hospital, and Berkshire Medical Center (330 beds).

Students

All students are Massachusetts residents. The average age of incoming students is twenty-five, and at least half of students took some time off after college. About 60 percent of students were science majors as undergraduates. Approximately 7 percent of students are underrepresented minorities. Class size is 100.

STUDENT LIFE

Recreational and athletic facilities are conveniently located in the lower level of the basic science building. Facilities include a lounge with a television, pool and ping pong tables, study areas, and an exercise and weight room. Students are involved in organizations focused on community service, recreational interests, and professional pursuits. Worcester is a city of nearly 200,000 that offers a full range of services and activities. Students live off campus; most of them choose to live in the local community. Some students rely on public transportation, while others use cars.

GRADUATES

Among 1997 graduates, the most popular fields for post-graduate training were internal medicine (28 percent), family practice (25 percent), pediatrics (15 percent), emergency medicine (7 percent), obstetrics/gynecology (4 percent), and surgery (5 percent). A significant proportion entered residency programs in Massachusetts.

Admissions

REQUIREMENTS

Massachusetts residency is a requirement. Prerequisites are one year each of biology, general chemistry, organic chemistry, physics, and English. All science courses should include associated labs. The MCAT is required, and scores should be from within the past two years. For applicants who have retaken the exam, the best scores are weighed most heavily. Thus, withholding scores is not advantageous.

SUGGESTIONS

Applications should be submitted as early as possible. In addition to requirements, course work in computer science, calculus, statistics, sociology, and psychology is advised. For applicants who have been out of college for a significant period of time, some recent course work is important. Medically related experiences or research may strengthen an application.

PROCESS

All in-state AMCAS applicants are sent secondary applications. About half of those candidates are interviewed between October and March. Interviews consist of two thirty-minute sessions with faculty members and/or medical students. On interview day, candidates also have a group information session and campus tour. Approximately one-third of interviewees are accepted on a rolling basis. Wait-listed candidates may send supplementary information to update their files.

Admissions Requirements (Required)

MCAT scores, science GPA, non-science GPA, letters of recommendation, interview, extracurricular activities, exposure to medical profession.

Admissions Requirements (Optional)

state residency, essays/personal statement.

COSTS AND AID

In-state tuition	$8,352
Cost of books	$460
Fees	$1,835

Financial Aid

% students receiving aid	75
Average debt	$70,068

UMDNJ

New Jersey Medical School

185 South Orange Avenue, Medical Science Building, Room C-653, Newark, NJ 07103 • Admission: 973-972-4631 • Fax: 973-972-7986 • E-mail: njmsadmiss@umdnj.edu • Website: http://njms.umdnj.edu

STUDENT BODY

Type	Public
Enrollment	142
% male/female	46/54
% underrepresented minorities	16
# applied (total/out)	2,498/1,553
# accepted (total/out)	335/40
# enrolled (total/out)	156/19
Average age	23

FACULTY

Total faculty (number)	850
% female	35
% minority	23

ADMISSIONS

Average GPA and MCAT Scores

Overall GPA	3.6
MCAT Bio	10.2
MCAT Phys	10
MCAT Verbal	9
MCAT Essay	P

Application Information

Regular application	12/1
Regular notification	Rolling
Early application	6/1-8/1
Early notification	10/1
Are transfers accepted?	Yes
Admissions may be deferred?	Yes
Interview required?	Yes
Application fee	$75

Academics

BASIC SCIENCES: During the first two years, small group sessions and tutorials account for about one-third of scheduled sessions, with the remainder of class time used for lectures and labs. Students are paired with physicians in the community, working with them one afternoon each week as part of primary care preceptorships. Courses demand about twenty-seven hours per week, in addition to individual study time. First-year courses are biochemistry and molecular biology, cell and tissue biology, genetics, gross and developmental anatomy, neuroscience, physiology, psychiatry, public health, the art of medicine, problem-based learning, and clinical skills, which focuses on the physical examination. During the second year, topics are coordinated among courses and are organized around organ systems. Courses are clinical preventive medicine and nutrition, immunology, microbiology, pathology, pharmacology, introduction to clinical sciences, and psychiatry and the clinical interview. The medical sciences building, where basic sciences are taught, is connected to the University Hospital and the George F. Smith Library, the latter of which houses 70,000 volumes and over 2,000 periodicals. The proximity of clinical facilities to classrooms and labs encourages first- and second-year students' involvement in clinical activities. The Office of Student Affairs provides services ranging from personal counseling to guidance on elective and residency selection.

CLINICAL TRAINING

Required third-year clerkships are internal medicine (twelve weeks), general surgery (eight weeks), pediatrics (eight weeks), obstetrics/gynecology (eight weeks), psychiatry (six weeks), and family medicine (six weeks). During the fourth year, sixteen weeks of electives are required in addition to neurology (four weeks), emergency medicine (four weeks), substance abuse (two weeks), physical medicine and rehabilitation (two weeks), ophthalmology (one week), orthopedics (one week), otolaryngology (one week), and urology (one week). There is also a required acting internship in medicine, pediatrics, family medicine, obstetrics, or surgery (four weeks). Most clinical training takes place at the contiguous 518-bed University Hospital, which serves the needs of the immediate community and attracts patients from around the state with its specialized care units. Other affiliated teaching hospitals are Hackensack University Hospital, Morristown Memorial Hospital, Veterans' Affairs Health Care System, East Orange, and Kessler Institute for Rehabilitation.

Students

Generally, about 90 percent of entering students are New Jersey residents. Underrepresented minorities, most of whom are African American or Puerto Rican, account for about 13 percent of the student body. There is a large age range within each class. Class size is 170. The Health Science Library's homepage (www3.umdnj.edu/stlibweb) provides access to over forty online databases, 185 electronic books, and over 2,000 online journals. The online catalog enables users to identify materials in the print, media, and electronic collections. Students, faculty, and staff may access these resources from on-campus computers or remotely, via the university libraries' proxy service. Online help is available through the homepage or E-mail. The library manages forty-seven public computer workstations, all of which have access to the Web and E-mail. The comuters in the library's microcomputer lab also provide students with access to desktop applications (Microsoft Office Suite), educational software, and tutorials. Scanning and slide production equipment is also available in the microcomputer lab. Staff support and user training is available for all programs.

STUDENT LIFE

Students take advantage of the school's athletic and recreational facilities and are involved in intramural sports and organized student events. Each entering student is assigned to a peer group of first- and second-year students. These groups provide support for students and assist them with academic and personal issues (they wait-list periodically). Students initiate and develop service activities such as Community 2000, which conducts clinical screening and health education with local churches. Students are actively involved in community service projects through the CHARE center. NJMS was recognized in 1994 by the AAMC with the Outstanding Community Service award. Newark is an up-and-coming city with inexpensive ethnic restaurants, performing arts, jazz clubs, and diverse neighborhoods. New York City is just an easy train ride away. All students live off campus, in Newark, or in the surrounding suburbs. The Office of Student Affairs actively assists students in securing housing.

GRADUATES

Each year, graduates are successful in obtaining residencies at prestigious institutions such as Massachusetts General, Columbia Presbyterian, and Children's Hospital in Washington, DC. The alumni association is very enthusiastic, and among its activities is the provision of scholarships and research stipends to medical students.

Admissions

REQUIREMENTS

All applicants are processed and reviewed without regard to state of residence. The minimum course requirements are sixteen semester hours of biology; eight semester hours of physics, chemistry, and organic chemistry, all with associated labs; and six semester hours each of English, math, and social sciences. Applicants should have at least a 3.0 GPA in both sciences and overall, as the average GPA of applicants is about 3.4. The MCAT is required and must be no more than three years old. The average MCAT of successful applicants is in the 8 to 9 range. Just under 10 percent of appoximately 2,200 applicants are interviewed with interviews taking place between August and April. About one-third of interviewees are accepted. Wait-listed candidates may send supplementary information to update their files.

SUGGESTIONS

Research or experience in a health care setting is useful. Personal traits such as compassion, dedication, and interpersonal skills are very important.

PROCESS

In previous years, a secondary application has not been part of the admissions process. About one-quarter of applicants are invited to interview between August and April. Interviews consist of one hour sessions with a faculty member. About 30 percent of interviewees are accepted on a rolling basis. Wait-listed candidates are generally not encouraged to send supplementary material. As an alternative admissions route, New Jersey residents who attend participating undergraduate institutions may apply for the baccalaureate/MD program. This program allows students to earn both degrees within a more compact time frame.

Admissions Requirements (Required)

MCAT scores, science GPA, non-science GPA, letters of recommendation, interview, essays/personal statement.

Admissions Requirements (Optional)

state residency, extracurricular activities, exposure to medical profession.

COSTS AND AID

In-state tuition	$19,776
Out-of-state tuition	$30,947
Cost of books	$1,768
Fees	$2,391

Financial Aid

% students receiving aid	78
Average grant	$5,000
Average loan	$25,000
Average debt	$102,000

UMDNJ

Robert Wood Johnson Medical School

Office of Admissions, 675 Hoes Lane, Piscataway, NJ 08854 • Admission: 732-235-4576 • Fax: 732-235-5078 • E-mail: rwjapadm@umdnj.edu • Website: rwjms.umdnj.edu

STUDENT BODY

Type	Public
Enrollment	699
% male/female	58/42
% underrepresented minorities	18
# applied (total/out)	2,248/1,810
# accepted (total)	170
# enrolled (total)	170

ADMISSIONS

Average GPA and MCAT Scores

Overall GPA	3
MCAT Bio	10.3
MCAT Phys	10.3
MCAT Verbal	9.7
MCAT Essay	Q

Application Information

Regular application	12/1
Regular notification	10/15
Early application	6/1-8/1
Early notification	10/1
Are transfers accepted?	Yes
Admissions may be deferred?	Yes
Interview required?	Yes
Application fee	$75

Academics

Students are encouraged to pursue a variety of educational opportunities. In addition to the traditional four-year medical school curriculum, students may enroll in one of the dual degree options including MD/PhD, MD/JD, MD/MPH, MD/MBA, MS/MS biomedical informatics, and MD/MS Jurisprudence. The flexible curriculum allows the rearranging of certain courses to enable students to pursue the dual degrees, relevant projects, personal interests, research, or employment. Student scholars may take an additional year to pursue the basic science or clinical research or off-campus community health projects. Students who complete a thesis graduate with distinction in research. The grading policy uses grades of honors, high pass, pass, low pass, and fail. Both Steps of the USMLE are required for graduation.

BASIC SCIENCES: Curricular changes in the first two years have been implemented toward fulfilling a two-fold mission: better preparation of clinicians as lifelong learners and a shift toward self directed learning. The changes include more small group learning, problem-based approaches, and a reduction in lecture time, in addition to a systems based approach in the second year. Clinical correlation is emphasized in all first-year disciplines with patient encounters in the case-based learning and the introduction to the patient courses. First-year courses are cell biology and histology, gross and developmental anatomy, neuroscience, epidemiology and biostatistics, biological chemistry, principles of environmental and community medicine, medical ethics, medical genetics, introduction to the patient, case-based learning, medical physiology, medical microbiology and immunology, and based life support I. Second year courses are clinical pathophysiology, behavorial science and psychiatry, human sexuality, pathology and laboratory medicine, physical diagnosis and clinical decision making, physical diagnosis and clinical decision making in psychiatry, pharmacology, clinical prevention and environmental medicine, medicine and the law, biochemical basis of nutrition, basic life support II, and universal precautions/venipuncture. A vast array of noncredit preclinical electives enriches the experience during the first and second years. Courses inlcude issues in women's health, community and child health, humanities in medine, business in medicine elective, emergency room elective, geriatric issues, and alternative and complementary medicine. Renovations at the medical science complex include twenty-six state-of-the-art multipurpose classrooms and anatomy laboratories for the educational programs.

CLINICAL TRAINING

Most clinical training takes place at the teaching hospitals—Robert Wood Johnson University Hospital on the New Brunswick campus and Cooper Hospital University Medical Center on the Camden campus. A Clinical Competency Center with a standardized patient program is used to teach and assess the clinical skills of second, third, and fourth year medical students. During the third year of medical school students rotate through eight-week clerkships in medicine, surgery, pediatrics, family medicine, psychiatry, and obstetrics/gynecology. Additionally, there is the opportunity for elective work during the third year. During the fourth year students are required to take four weeks of medicine, surgery, neurology and a sub-internship, in addition to sixteen to twenty weeks of electives.

Students

Approximately 87 percent of the students are New Jersey residents. There is great diversity among the student body: 51 percent of all students are self-described minorities and 16 percent of them are from underrepresented groups. Typically between 10 to 20 percent of the student body took off some time between undergraduate studies and medical school. The class size is 142. One-third of the class completed their clinical training on the Camden campus.

STUDENT LIFE

New Brunswick offers the many amenities of a university city. Princeton and New York City are short train rides away. Students who complete clinical training on the Camden campus enjoy the proximity of Philadelphia. The medical school does not have on-campus housing; however, the school helps students secure accommodations in the area. Medical students have access to Rutgers University's athletic facilities, which include swimming pools, gyms, golf, squash, racquetball, and volleyball courts. Rutgers also offers social, cultural, and recreational activities for medical students. There are many student organizations and interest groups, including chapters of the major national medical student associations. Many students participate in volunteer organizations including the student-run HIPHOP (Homeless and Indigent Persons Health Outreach Project) and UIP (Urban Health Initiatives). Honor societies include AOA and the Humanism in Medicine Honor Society.

GRADUATES

Graduates have done particularly well in securing outstanding training positions throughout the United States and within our own training programs. About one half of the class chooses internal medicine, pediatrics, or family medicine but all specialties are represented.

Admissions

REQUIREMENTS

Two semesters of biology, general chemistry, organic chemistry, and physics (all with labs), two semesters of English or writing intensive courses, and one semester of college-level mathematics are required. The MCAT is required and must be no more than four years old. For applicants who have retaken the exam, all scores are considered, but the most recent score is given the most weight.

SUGGESTIONS

Course work in the behavioral sciences and humanities is recommended. Medically related experiences, research, and community service are all valued by the Admissions Committee.

PROCESS

As a state institution, preference is given to in-state residents; however, the importance of geographic diversity is recognized and out-of-state residents are encouraged to apply. A new process allows accepted out-of-state residents to become in-state residents and hence be eligible for in-state tuition. Approximately one half of New Jersey applicants and five percent of out-of-state applicants are interviewed on one of the three campuses: Piscataway, New Brunswick, or Camden. Generally, students are interviewed by one faculty member. Some applicants are also interviewed by a student member of the Admissions Committee. All applicants have the opportunity to meet and tour with a current student. About one-third of candidates who are interviewed are accepted. Acceptances are offered on a rolling basis. Several alternative means of accpetance exist. There is a combined BA/MD program with Rutgers University. There is also an Accelerated Acceptance program for post-baccalaureate students completing pre-medical studies at a number of institutions.

Admissions Requirements (Required)

MCAT scores, science GPA, non-science GPA, letters of recommendation, interview, essays/personal statement, extracurricular activities.

Admissions Requirements (Optional)

state residency, exposure to medical profession.

COSTS AND AID

Financial Aid

% students receiving aid	70

UNIVERSITY OF MIAMI

UNIVERSITY OF MIAMI SCHOOL OF MEDICINE

ADMISSIONS R-159, POB 016159, MIAMI, FL 33101 • ADMISSION: 305-243-6791 • FAX: 305-243-6548 •
E-MAIL: MED.ADMISSIONS@MIAMI.EDU • WEBSITE: WWW.MIAMI.EDU/MEDICAL-ADMISSIONS

STUDENT BODY

Type	Private
Enrollment	573
% male/female	49/51
% underrepresented minorities	7
# applied (total/out)	2,621/1,440
# accepted (total/out)	271/83
# enrolled (total/out)	141/35
Average age	22

FACULTY

Total faculty (number)	1,077
% female	12
% minority	4

ADMISSIONS

Average GPA and MCAT Scores

Overall GPA	3.7
MCAT Bio	10
MCAT Phys	9.6
MCAT Verbal	9.4
MCAT Essay	Q

Application Information

Regular application	12/15
Regular notification	10/15
Are transfers accepted?	No
Admissions may be deferred?	No
Interview required?	Yes
Application fee	$65

Academics

Most students follow a four-year curriculum that leads to the MD. A number of students participate in a six-year BS/MD program organized with Miami's undergraduate college. Up to six students each year enter a combined MS/PhD program and earn the doctoral degree in biochemistry and molecular biology; molecular, cell, and developmental biology; microbiology and immunology; molecular and cellular pharmacology; neuroscience; or physiology and biophysics. Opportunities for summer research are also available to medical students. Students are graded with percentile scores during the first two years and with ratings of honors, high pass, pass, and fail during the second two years. Promotion to year three requires a passing score on the USMLE Step 1. Step 2 of the USMLE must be taken to graduate.

BASIC SCIENCES: Although the first two years are devoted primarily to basic sciences, students are introduced to clinical concepts and techniques from day one in the clinical skills course. In this two-year course, students work alongside community physician mentors, learning about the patient interview, the physical examination, and clinical diagnosis. Other first-year courses are gross anatomy, genetics, embryology, immunology, cell and molecular biology, behavioral and life sciences, physiology, histology, neuroanatomy, systemic biochemistry, endocrine module, and ethics/social policy. Second-year courses are microbiology, pharmacology, pathology, mechanisms of disease, introduction to psychiatry, and pathology. During the first two years, students are in class or other scheduled sessions for about twenty-four hours per week. Lectures are the primary instructional modality, but small group discussions are also used and are increasingly important in the second year. Basic sciences are taught in the Rosensteil Medical Sciences Building and the Glaser Medical Research Building, which house newly renovated lecture halls, teaching laboratories, and the brand new Glaser Computer Laboratory. The Louis Calder Memorial Library has almost 200,000 volumes and 2,300 current journals and periodicals. It also offers an electronic classroom with computer instructional aids and a learning resource center with multimedia programs.

CLINICAL TRAINING

Required third-year clerkships are introduction to medicine (one week), radiology (one week), medicine (eight weeks), surgery (eight weeks), primary care (eight weeks), obstetrics/gynecology (six weeks), psychiatry (six weeks), pediatrics (six weeks), and family medicine (four weeks). Fourth-year requirements are geriatrics (two weeks) and neurology (four weeks). The remainder of the fourth year is devoted to selectives, which must include at least eight weeks of direct patient care, and electives which may be clinical or research-based. Clinical training takes place at: Jackson Memorial Hospital (1,567 beds), Veterans' Affairs Medical Center (900 beds), Bascom Palmer/Anne Bates Leach Eye Hospital, Sylvester Comprehensive Cancer Center, Ryder Trauma Center, Diabetes Research Institute, and The Mailman Center for Child Development. Up to three months of the fourth year may be spent in clerkships at other institutions.

Students

A recently entering class had students with ages ranging from eighteen to thirty-seven. Fifty-five percent of that same class were women, 10 percent were underrepresented minorities, 97 percent were Florida residents, and 65 percent were science majors. Thirty-six colleges and universities were represented. Class size is 148.

STUDENT LIFE

Although the medical campus is separate from the main campus, medical students have access to extracurricular programs and events sponsored by the greater university. In addition, the medical campus has athletic and other recreational facilities of its own. Medical students are involved in student organizations and volunteer activities in areas such as AIDS prevention, general health education, and drug abuse counseling. Students enjoy the good weather and multicultural environment of Miami. Medical students live off campus in various parts of Miami and usually drive to school or take Metrorail.

GRADUATES

Graduates are successful in securing residency positions throughout the United States. A significant proportion enter programs at Jackson Memorial Hospital, which features at least fifteen post-graduate training programs.

Admissions

REQUIREMENTS

Prerequisites are one year each of biology, chemistry, organic chemistry, physics, math, and English. Science courses should include associated labs. The MCAT is required, and scores must be from within the past three years. For applicants who have retaken the exam, the best set of scores is weighed most heavily.

SUGGESTIONS

Florida residents are given preference, and only highly qualified out-of-state residents are encouraged to apply. Recommended course work includes biochemistry, cell and molecular biology, microbiology and immunology, genetics, embryology, mammalian physiology, and computer science. Students should display achievement in the humanities and social sciences as well as in the natural sciences. Beyond academic credentials, the Committee on Admissions values interpersonal skills, leadership, maturity, motivation, and compassion. Meaningful patient-contact experience is essential.

PROCESS

About 75 percent of Florida residents and 20 percent of out-of-state residents are sent secondary applications. About 300 applicants are interviewed on campus. Interviews take place on Fridays, between August and April, and consist of one session with a faculty member. About 60 percent of interviewed candidates are accepted, with notification occurring on a rolling basis. Approximately twenty-five positions in each entering class are reserved for participants in the University of Miami Honors Program in Medicine, a six-year BS/MD program.

Admissions Requirements (Required)

MCAT scores, science GPA, non-science GPA, letters of recommendation, interview, essays/personal statement, extracurricular activities, exposure to medical profession.

Admissions Requirements (Optional)

state residency.

COSTS AND AID

Tuition	$28,050
Cost of books	$800
Fees	$130

Financial Aid

Average grant	$10,000
Average loan	$40,000

University of Michigan
Medical School

Admissions Office, M4130 Medical Science I Building, Ann Arbor, MI 48109 • Admission: 313-764-6317 • Fax: 313-936-3510 • E-mail: PIBS@UMICH.EDU • Website: WWW.MED.UMICH.EDU/MEDSCHOOL

STUDENT BODY

Type	Public
Enrollment	660
% male/female	59/41
% underrepresented minorities	15
# applied (total/out)	5,114/4,154
# accepted (total/out)	11/7
# enrolled (total/out)	/24

ADMISSIONS

Average GPA and MCAT Scores

Overall GPA	3.8

Application Information

Regular application	11/15
Regular notification	rolling
Early application	6/1-8/1
Early notification	10/1
Are transfers accepted?	No
Admissions may be deferred?	Yes
Interview required?	No
Application fee	$50

Academics

Most students follow a four-year program that leads to the MD, although a growing number of students opt to pursue combined degrees. A combined MS/PhD curriculum allows students to pursue graduate studies in numerous departments, including anatomy and cell biology, biological chemistry, cellular and molecular biology, human genetics, microbiology and immunology, neuroscience, pharmacology, and physiology. Some MS/PhD students are MSTP participants, while others are funded through institutional sources. For students who are interested in research but not interested in earning an additional degree, summer and yearlong research fellowships are available. In addition, combined programs with public health and business administration are available. Passing Step 1 of the USMLE is a requirement for promotion to year three, and passing Step 2 is a requirement for graduation.

BASIC SCIENCES: During the first year, grading is strictly satisfactory and fail. This promotes student cooperation and allows for variation in the level of scientific knowledge among incoming students. Throughout the first and second years, students take introduction to the patient, which includes interdisciplinary perspectives and the use of simulated patients, and multidisciplinary conferences, which provides clinical correlations for basic science concepts. Other first-year courses are molecular and cell biology, grossanatomy, human genetics, pathology, embryology, histology, host defenses, microbiology, pharmacology, and physiology. Year two is organized around organ and body systems.These are infectious diseases, hematology, oncology, cardiovascular, respiratory, renal, dermatology, gastrointestinal, neuroscience, endocrine, reproduction, and musculoskeletal. The medical school's basic science instructional facilities include recently renovated lecture halls with audiovisual and computer equipment. A Learning Resource Center is open twenty-four hours per day and has over fifty computers for student use. The Taubman Medical Library is one of the largest in the United States in terms of the number of volumes, journals, and electronic resources that it holds. The Office of Academic Enrichment provides academic counseling and organizes study groups and tutoring services.

CLINICAL TRAINING

During the second, third, and fourth years, students are evaluated with grades of honors, high pass, pass, and fail. Third-year required rotations are family practice (four weeks), internal medicine (twelve weeks), neurology (four weeks), obstetrics/gynecology (six weeks), pediatrics (six weeks), psychiatry (four weeks), and surgery (twelve weeks). Students attend weekly conferences and discuss a range of topics including the ethical, social, and economic issues related to practicing medicine. Fourth-year requirements are subinternship (eight weeks), intensive care unit experience (four weeks), advanced basic science experience (four weeks), and electives (twelve to twenty weeks) that are selected from more than 300 subjects. Clinical training takes place at the University Hospital (888 beds), St. Joseph Mercy Hospital (522 beds), the Veterans' Affairs Hospital (486 beds), and at other affiliated institutions. With approval, students may earn elective credits at other academic or clinical sites in the United States and overseas.

Students

About 50 percent of students are Michigan residents; the remainder of the student body comes from all regions of the United States. Typically, at least 10 percent of entering students are older and have taken some time off after college. Approximately 15 percent of students are underrepresented minorities. Class size is 170.

STUDENT LIFE

Incoming medical students benefit from the support and advice of more senior medical students through a peer-counseling program called Big Sib, Little Sib. Students interact outside of the classroom through participation in organizations that focus on issues such as community service, support for minority and gay/lesbian students, and recreational and professional pursuits. The Furstenberg Student Study Center features a well-being room for information and activities related to student health, computer stations, lounges, and quiet study rooms. Expansive sports and recreation centers also enrich student life on campus. Ann Arbor is an academic and cultural center, attracting scholars from around the world. To serve the university community, the area around the campus is filled with coffeeshops, bookstores, restaurants, bars, and shops. In addition to commercial districts, Ann Arbor offers parks, lakes, theaters, farmers' markets, and attractive residential areas. Although some limited campus-owned housing is available to medical students, most of them opt to live in privately owned apartment complexes that are within walking distance of the medical center.

GRADUATES

Medical students consistently score above the national average on both steps of the USMLE, contributing to their success in securing top residency positions. Among 1996 graduates, popular choices for specialty areas were internal medicine (23 percent), pediatrics (12 percent), surgery (11 percent), family practice (10 percent), obstetrics/gynecology (7 percent), and emergency medicine (6 percent).

Admissions

REQUIREMENTS

Prerequisites are chemistry (eight semester hours, to include both organic and inorganic), biochemistry (three semester hours), biology (six semester hours), physics (six semester hours), and English composition and literature (six semester hours). In addition, at least eighteen semester hours must be completed in areas other than the natural sciences or math.

SUGGESTIONS

In addition to the required science courses, genetics and cell biology are considered useful preparation for medical school. Humanities and social sciences course work are also important.

PROCESS

All AMCAS applicants are sent supplementary applications. Of those returning secondaries, about 15 percent are interviewed between September and March. Interviews consist of two thirty-minute sessions each with a faculty member or medical student. Candidates are also given a group informational presentation, a campus tour, and lunch with medical students. About one-third of interviewees are accepted and are notified between November and May. Others are rejected or put on a wait-list. Previously, thirty-five high school students were admitted each year to the Inteflex Program, a combined BS/MD program organized in conjunction with Michigan's undergraduate college, but admissions were suspended as of 1999.

Admissions Requirements (Required)

MCAT scores, science GPA, non-science GPA, letters of recommendation, state residency, extracurricular activities, exposure to medical profession.

Admissions Requirements (Optional)

interview, essays/personal statement.

COSTS AND AID

In-state tuition	$20,524
Out-of-state tuition	$31,524

University of Minnesota
Medical School—Twin Cities

Office of Admissions, Box 293, 420 Delaware Street, Southeast, Minneapolis, MN 55455 • Admission: 612-624-1188 • Fax: 612-625-8228 • E-mail: meded@umn.edu • Website: www.med.umn.edu

STUDENT BODY

Type	Public
Enrollment	112
% male/female	53/47
% underrepresented minorities	16
# applied (total/out)	458/64
# accepted (total/out)	77/5
# enrolled (total/out)	53/1
Average age	24

FACULTY

Total faculty (number)	44
% female	27
% minority	6
% part-time	5
# student/faculty ratio	2:1

ADMISSIONS

Average GPA and MCAT Scores

Overall GPA	3.6
MCAT Bio	9.64
MCAT Phys	9.4
MCAT Verbal	8.92
MCAT Essay	Q

Application Information

Regular application	11/15
Regular notification	Rolling
Early application	8/1
Early notification	10/1
Are transfers accepted?	No
Admissions may be deferred?	Yes
Interview required?	Yes
Application fee	$75

Academics

In addition to a four-year curriculum that leads to the MD degree, Minnesota offers joint MS/PhD programs, generally MSTP-sponsored, that lead to the doctoral degree in biochemistry, biomedical engineering, biophysics, cell biology, genetics, immunology, microbiology, molecular biology, neuroscience, pharmacology, and physiology. Evaluation of medical student performance uses grades of outstanding, excellent, satisfactory, incomplete, and no credit. Students must pass both steps of the USMLE to graduate. Faculty members serve as informal advisers to medical students throughout the four years.

BASIC SCIENCES: Basic sciences are taught as part of an interdisciplinary curriculum that also includes behavioral, social, and ethical aspects of medicine, in addition to introductory clinical instruction. On average, students are in class or other scheduled sessions for twenty-four hours per week. First-year courses are gross anatomy, human histology, biochemistry, molecular and cellular biology, human nutrition, medical physiology, neuroscience, microbiology, human behavior, human sexuality, human genetics, foundations of preventive medicine, pathology, pharmacology, and clinical medicine, the last of which focuses on history-taking and the physical examination. Second-year courses are pharmacology, organ system pathology, pathophysiology, laboratory medicine, and clinical medicine. In addition, second-year students participate in four six-week tutorials in internal medicine, family practice, pediatrics, and neurology. First- and second-year instruction takes place in the Moos Health Tower and other buildings in the basic science complex. The Bio-Medical Library contains more than 428,000 volumes, 4,393 journals, 1,194 audiovisual programs, and 223 computer programs. The reference department has over fifty computers and has access to several online databases.

CLINICAL TRAINING

Students rotate through the following required clerkships during their third and fourth years: medicine (twelve weeks), obstetrics/gynecology (six weeks), surgery (six weeks), pediatrics (six weeks), psychiatry (six weeks), neurology (four weeks), surgical specialty (four weeks), and ambulatory care (eight weeks). The remaining time is reserved for elective study. Clinical facilities include the Fairview-University Medical Center, Variety Club Heart and Research Center, Masonic Cancer Center, Veterans of Foreign Wars Cancer Research Center, Children's Rehabilitation Center, Paul F. Dwan Cardiovascular Research Center. Each year, through the Rural Physician Associate Program, up to forty third-year medical students study primary health care in Minnesota communities under the supervision of local physicians. One-quarter of clinical electives may be fulfilled at nonaffiliated institutions in other parts of the country or abroad.

Students

Of the 165 students in last year's entering class, 89 percent were Minnesota residents, and 62 percent attended college in Minnesota. About 5 percent were from underrepresented minority groups. Typically, the average age of incoming students is twenty-four or twenty-five.

STUDENT LIFE

Some students work part-time as graduate research or teaching assistants while they are in medical school. These positions provide academic opportunities and a source of income or tuition reduction. The Medical Student Adytum (adytum is Greek for "innermost sanctuary") is a spacious, comfortable area reserved solely for medical students and their guests. Students use the facility for studying, socializing, eating, and relaxing. Medical students also have the opportunity to interact with other health sciences students at an alternate student center. Organizations bring students together around common interests, allow them to contribute to the community, and organize extracurricular activities. Examples of student organizations are the Marathon Training Club, which in a recent year motivated 10 percent of the student body to complete a marathon; the Student Committee on Bioethics; and the Medical Students in Community Service, which operates a health clinic. The medical school is part of the greater university, and medical students have access to its athletic and recreational facilities. Beyond the campus, the city of Minneapolis has restaurants, shopping, cultural activities, and entertainment. Housing options include residence halls, medical fraternities, and privately owned apartments that are adjacent to the medical center.

GRADUATES

In the 1999 graduating class, the most popular fields for residencies were family practice (33 percent), internal medicine (18 percent), surgery (8 percent), pediatrics (7 percent), emergency medicine (5 percent), obstetrics/gynecology (4 percent), and radiology (3 percent). Generally, at least half of graduates enter post-graduate programs in Minnesota.

Admissions

REQUIREMENTS

Prerequisites are biology (seven semester hours), general chemistry (eight hours), organic chemistry (eight hours), physics (eight hours), English (eight hours), math (one college-level course), and biochemistry (three hours). In addition, at least eighteen hours of social and behavioral sciences and humanities are required. This requirement is fulfilled with courses such as history, economics, anthropology, psychology, sociology, philosophy, and foreign languages. The MCAT is required, and scores must be no more than three years old. For applicants who have retaken, the highest set of scores is considered.

SUGGESTIONS

Minnesota residents are given preference. As indicated by the social science/humanities requirement, breadth in undergraduate preparation is important. In addition to academic strength, applicants should demonstrate extensive volunteer/community service activity, personal integrity, high ethical standards, motivation, intellectual curiosity, enthusiasm, dedication to lifelong learning, and the ability to work well with others. Computer literacy is recommended.

PROCESS

Qualified applicants who submit AMCAS applications are sent secondaries. Of those returning secondaries, about 80 percent of Minnesota residents and 30 percent of out-of-state applicants are invited to interview. Interviews take place on campus from September through March and consist of one session with a faculty member. Of interviewed candidates, about 25 percent of Minnesota residents and 15 percent of out-of-state residents are offered a place in the class. Applicants are accepted on a rolling admission basis from October to April. Additional materials from wait-listed candidates are not accepted.

Admissions Requirements (Required)

MCAT scores, science GPA, non-science GPA, letters of recommendation, interview, state residency, essays/personal statement.

Admissions Requirements (Optional)

extracurricular activities, exposure to medical profession.

Overlap Schools

University of Minnesota.

COSTS AND AID

In-state tuition	$25,074
Out-of-state tuition	$46,590
Cost of books	$2,332
Fees	$2,030

Financial Aid

% students receiving aid	97
Average grant	$2,000
Average loan	$40,000

University of Minnesota
School of Medicine Duluth

180 Medicine, 1035 University Drive, Duluth, MN 55812 • Admission: 218-726-8511 • Fax: 218-726-7057 • E-mail: medadmis@d.umn.edu • Website: http://penguin.d.umn.edu/

STUDENT BODY

Type	Public
Enrollment	868
% male/female	55/45
% underrepresented minorities	18
# applied (total/out)	1,987/1,406
# accepted (total)	299
# enrolled (total)	165

FACULTY

ADMISSIONS

Average GPA and MCAT Scores

Overall GPA	3.7
MCAT Bio	10.8
MCAT Phys	10.3
MCAT Verbal	10
MCAT Essay	P

Application Information

Regular application	11/15
Regular notification	rolling
Early application	6/1-8/1
Early notification	10/1
Are transfers accepted?	Yes
Admissions may be deferred?	Yes
Interview required?	Yes
Application fee	$75

Academics

Although formal clinical rotations are not included in the two-year UMD curriculum, early patient contact and clinical correlations are important aspects of the program. Successful completion of UMD requirements guarantees transfer after year two to the Minneapolis campus. Evaluation of medical student performance uses grades of outstanding, excellent, satisfactory, incomplete, and no pass. Passing Step 1 of the USMLE is a requirement for promotion to the Minneapolis program.

BASIC SCIENCES: The two-year curriculum is a unique blend of basic medical and behavioral sciences and clinical hands-on experience. The basic sciences, presented using an organ systems approach that begins with principles of basic science, extends to various aspects of the prevention and pathophysiology of organ system disease and concludes with discussions of several presenting clinical symptoms and multisystems diseases. The behavioral sciences portion of the curriculum emphasizes knowledge about the psycho-social aspects of health and illness that are relevant to the clinical setting and is interwoven with the organ systems component. The clinical experience is directed by community specialists and is augmented by UMD's nationally recognized family practice preceptorship program. In addition to classrooms and labs, the Learning Resource Center serves as a computer and multimedia instructional facility. It is open twenty-four hours per day. The Health Science Library houses 95,000 volumes, 600 current journals, and several online databases.

CLINICAL TRAINING

In Duluth, clinical affiliates are St. Luke's Hospital and St. Mary's Medical Centers. After successfully completing year two, students transfer to Minneapolis, where they rotate through required clerkships during their third and fourth years. These are medicine (twelve weeks), obstetrics/gynecology (six weeks), surgery (six weeks), pediatrics (six weeks), psychiatry (six weeks), neurology (four weeks), surgical specialty (four weeks), and ambulatory care (eight weeks). The remaining time is reserved for elective study. Clinical facilities include Abbott Northwestern Hospital, Children's Health Care, Fairview-University Medical Center, Hennepin County Medical Center, Regions Hospital, St. Luke's Hospital, St. Mary's Medical Center, and other sites. Each year, through the Rural Physician Associate Program, up to forty third-year medical students study primary health care in Minnesota communities under the supervision of local physicians. Up to twelve weeks of clinical electives may be fulfilled at nonaffiliated institutions in other parts of the country or abroad.

Students

STUDENT LIFE

Small class size, and students' shared interest in family medicine promotes a supportive and cohesive atmosphere. University recreational events, facilities, and activities are open to medical students, including the student center, the gym, intramural sports, and student organizations. Students also take advantage of the extracurricular opportunities afforded by the school's location. Activities such as cycling, running, skiing, hiking, and camping are easily accessible within or around Duluth. Duluth functions as a cultural center for Northern Minnesota and has a symphony, a ballet, theaters, and art museums. Affordable off-campus housing options in the immediate area are available.

GRADUATES

About 98 percent of students are Minnesota residents. About 16 percent of students are underrepresented minorities, most of whom are Native American. Class size is fifty-three. At least 70 percent of graduates enter primary care fields, and most go on to practice in rural areas.

Admissions

REQUIREMENTS

Priority consideration is given to Minnesota residents who wish to pursue a family practice or other primary care physicians in a rural setting. Applicants from other states who demonstrate a high potential and motivation for practicing medicine in Minnesota will also be considered. Applicants must be U.S. citizens or permanent residents and must have completed all requirements for a baccalaureate degree by the time of possible matriculation. Prerequisites are one year each of biology, general chemistry, physics, English, behavioral sciences, and humanities/social sciences. One math course in calculus or upper-level statistics and one biochemistry course are also required. The MCAT is required, and scores must be no more than three years old.

SUGGESTIONS

UMD looks for applicants who demonstrate interest in entering family practice and other primary care specialties and working with underserved rural or small town communities in Minnesota or American Indian communities.

PROCESS

Applicants are sent secondary applications after preliminary screening of academics and MCAT scores. Of those returning secondaries, about 45 percent are invited to interview between October and April. Interviews consist of two one-hour sessions, each with a member of the Admissions Committee. Notification occurs on a rolling basis, and about 30 percent of interviewees are offered a place in the class.

Admissions Requirements (Required)

MCAT scores, science GPA, non-science GPA, letters of recommendation, interview, essays/personal statement, extracurricular activities, exposure to medical profession.

COSTS AND AID

In-state tuition	$16,060
Out-of-state tuition	$29,840
Cost of books	$1,650
Fees	$642

Financial Aid

% students receiving aid	90
Average grant	$2,500
Average loan	$26,000

UNIVERSITY OF MISSISSIPPI
UNIVERSITY OF MISSISSIPPI MEDICAL CENTER

2500 NORTH STATE STREET, JACKSON, MS 39216 • ADMISSION: 601-984-5010 • FAX: 601-984-5008 •
E-MAIL: ADMITMD@SOM.UMSMED.EDU • WEBSITE: SOM.UMC.EDU

STUDENT BODY

Type	Public
Enrollment	394
% male/female	61/39
% underrepresented minorities	7
# applied (total)	239
# accepted (total)	120
# enrolled (total)	100
Average age	24

FACULTY

Total faculty (number)	582
% female	23
% minority	14
% part-time	15
# student/faculty ratio	1:1

ADMISSIONS

Average GPA and MCAT Scores

Overall GPA	3.7
MCAT Bio	9.6
MCAT Phys	9
MCAT Verbal	9.68
MCAT Essay	0

Application Information

Regular application	10/15
Regular notification	3/15
Early application	8/1
Early notification	10/1
Are transfers accepted?	Yes
Admissions may be deferred?	Yes
Interview required?	Yes

Academics

While most medical students follow a four-year curriculum that leads to the MD, some take advantage of other schools within the medical center and pursue joint degree programs such as the combined MS/PhD curriculum, which leads to the doctorate in anatomy, biochemistry, microbiology, neuroscience, pathology, and pharmacology. Medical students receive percent scores and a class rank and may be awarded honors at graduation. To be eligible for promotion, a student must achieve at least a seventy in each course, have a weighted average of seventy-five or higher, and attend 80 percent of the lectures and classes. Passing the USMLE Step 1 is a requirement for promotion to year three, and passing Step 2 is a requirement for graduation.

BASIC SCIENCES: The basic sciences are integrated with clinical science courses and are taught through a combination of lectures, small groups, labs, and hands-on clinical experiences. Students are in class or other scheduled activity for about twenty-two hours per week. First-year courses are gross anatomy, histology, neurobiology, biochemistry, medical physiology, behavioral science and psychiatry, and cardiopulmonary resuscitation. Second-year courses are medical microbiology, general and systemic pathology, pharmacology, biostatistics, preventive medicine and public health, medical genetics, clinical psychiatry, and introduction to clinical medicine (ICM). In the ICM course students learn history-taking, examination, and diagnosis skills through classroom presentations and small group sessions. The ICM experience helps prepare students for the clinical phase of the curriculum. Basic science instruction facilities are central to the campus and include the Holmes Learning Resources Center, which houses the Rowland Medical Library. The library is impressive, with more than 160,000 volumes and 2,500 periodicals.

CLINICAL TRAINING

Required third-year rotations are family medicine (six weeks), medicine/neurology (twelve weeks), obstetrics/gynecology (six weeks), psychiatry (six weeks), pediatrics (six weeks), and surgery (twelve weeks). The fourth year is organized into eight-month blocks of selectives. Students choose specialty areas from within internal medicine, obstetrics/gynecology, pediatrics, and surgery. In addition, three blocks of selectives in an ambulatory setting and two blocks in inpatient settings are required. Throughout the fourth year, students participate in a senior seminar, which provides a forum for interdisciplinary instruction and discussion of issues relevant to modern medical practice. Clinical training takes place at the University Hospital (593 beds), Blair E. Batson Hospital for Children, the Veterans' Administration Hospital, McBryde Rehabilitation Center for the Blind, Jackson Medical Mall Ambulatory Clinic, and State Health Department offices.

Students

In recent years all students have been Mississippi residents. Approximately 10 percent of students are underrepresented minorities, most of whom are African Americans. The average age of incoming students is generally around twenty-four. Class size is 100.

STUDENT LIFE

Medical students use the resources and facilities of the university, in addition to those of the greater community. As the state capital of Mississippi, Jackson offers numerous cultural and recreational attractions. Beyond clinical-care provision, the medical school contributes directly to the community through activities such as the Base-Pair Mentorship Program, which pairs medical school researchers and high school students and encourages them to jointly pursue academic projects. On-campus housing options include a residence hall for female students and an apartment complex with one-, two-, and three-bedroom units.

GRADUATES

Graduates are successful in securing positions in a range of specialty areas. At the University Hospital in Jackson there are more then twenty residency programs into which a number of graduates enter each year.

Admissions

REQUIREMENTS

Due to high competition in the admissions process, state residency is virtually a requirement. Required science courses are eight semester hours each of biology, chemistry, organic chemistry, and physics, all with associated labs. Three semester hours of college-level algebra and three of college-level trigonometry, or three semester hours of calculus, satisfies the math requirement. Six semester hours of English are an additional prerequisite. The MCAT is required, and scores for the class entering in 2002 must be from after 1997.

SUGGESTIONS

The April MCAT is preferred over the August one. Beyond requirements, some advanced science course work in areas such as biochemistry, anatomy, embryology, genetics, physical chemistry, histology, or advanced physics is recommended. Other suggested courses are advanced English, sociology, psychology, philosophy, history, geography, foreign language, computer science, and fine arts. Math and science courses designed for non-science majors are not counted toward minimum requirements.

PROCESS

All Mississippi residents who submit AMCAS applications are sent secondaries. About half of those returning secondary applications are interviewed between August and January. Candidates have three interview sessions, each with a faculty member or administrator. In addition, a tour of the campus and the opportunity to have lunch with a current medical student is provided. Among interviewees, about half are accepted and are notified throughout the application cycle. Wait-listed candidates may send additional information to update their files.

Admissions Requirements (Required)

MCAT scores, science GPA, non-science GPA, letters of recommendation, interview, state residency, essays/personal statement, extracurricular activities, exposure to medical profession.

COSTS AND AID

In-state tuition	$6,938
Out-of-state tuition	$13,298
Cost of books	$4,000

Financial Aid

% students receiving aid	94
Average grant	$7,000
Average loan	$18,500
Average debt	$66,000

UNIVERSITY OF MISSOURI—COLUMBIA

SCHOOL OF MEDICINE

MA215 MEDICAL SCIENCES BUILDING, COLUMBIA, MO 65212 • ADMISSION: 573-882-9219 • FAX: 573-884-2988 • E-MAIL: NOLKEJ@HEALTH.MISSOURI.EDU • WEBSITE: WWW.MUHEALTH.ORG/~MEDICINE

STUDENT BODY

Type	Public
Enrollment	375
% male/female	51/49
% underrepresented minorities	5
# applied (total/out)	822/433
# accepted (total/out)	137/15
# enrolled (total/out)	96/5

FACULTY

Total faculty (number)	559
% female	30
% minority	14
% part-time	16
# student/faculty ratio	1:1

ADMISSIONS

Average GPA and MCAT Scores

Overall GPA	3.7
MCAT Bio	9.9
MCAT Phys	9.5
MCAT Verbal	9.4
MCAT Essay	0

Application Information

Regular application	11/1
Regular notification	3/15
Early application	8/1
Early notification	10/1
Are transfers accepted?	Yes
Admissions may be deferred?	Yes
Interview required?	Yes
Application fee	$50

Academics

Although most students complete the MD curriculum in four years, some follow an extended program that leads to the MS or PhD along with the MD. Doctoral programs are available in diverse areas.

BASIC SCIENCES: Missouri is one of the leaders in the movement toward problem-based learning. Students learn in small groups and, because they spend less than twenty hours per week in scheduled sessions, have ample time for self-study or individualized projects. The first two years are organized into eight ten-week blocks, each of which consists of eight weeks of instruction followed by one week of evaluation and one week of vacation. Each block is divided into two general instructional components: problem-based learning and introduction to patient care. Block one is devoted to the structure and function of the human body, covering biochemistry, anatomy, histology, embryology, and molecular biology and genetics. Blocks two, three, and four each focus on a set of body/organ systems, which include the following: cardiovascular, respiratory, renal, gastrointestinal, metabolism, endocrine, neuroscience, liver, pulmonary, hematology, reproductive, immune response, and pharmacokinetics. Year two is made up of blocks five through eight, which concentrate on pathophysiology and clinical management. One of the main objectives of the second year is to prepare students for clinical rotations. Grading for the first year is satisfactory and unsatisfactory and grading for the second year is honors, satisfactory, and unsatisfactory. The medical library and computer facilities are comprehensive and serve as educational resources for faculty, students, and the medical community.

CLINICAL TRAINING

The third year is divided into six eight-week blocks of required clerkships, which are child health, family medicine, internal medicine, obstetrics/gynecology, psychiatry/neurology, and surgery. A separate rural track offers up to six months of clinical experience in a rural community during the third year in lieu of some of the required rotations. The fourth year consists of twelve weeks of general electives and three four-week advanced clinical selectives—one must be in a core medical specialty and another must be in a core surgical specialty. Finally, fourth-year students must complete eight weeks of advanced basic science selectives. The majority of clinical training is conducted at University Hospital and Clinics, a 288-bed tertiary care facility that draws patients from throughout central Missouri. Other training sites include Children's Hospital, Ellis Fischel Cancer Center, Columbia Regional Hospital, Truman VA Hospital, and the Missouri Rehabilitation Center. In total, clinical training sites encompass over 1,000 patient beds. Grades of honors, letters of commendation, satisfactory, and unsatisfactory are used to evaluate the clinical years. Students must pass Step 1 of the USMLE to be promoted to year four and Step 2 to graduate.

Students

The University of Missouri—Columbia is a state school, and the vast majority of the ninety-six entering students are Missouri residents. A large percentage attended the various public undergraduate colleges and universities throughout the state. Among students in the 2003 entering class, 81 percent were science majors as undergraduates. Approximately 4 percent of medical students are underrepresented minorities. The average age of incoming students is usually twenty-four.

STUDENT LIFE

The School of Medicine is located in the heart of the University of Missouri's main campus, which allows students to take advantage of its recreational, athletic, and entertainment facilities. The new curriculum gives students flexibility within their schedules, allowing them to explore both their academic and nonacademic interests. Student organizations are active, particularly the local chapter of the American Student Medical Association, which coordinates academic, social, and cultural events and sponsors community-service projects. Columbia is located within a few hours of both Kansas City and St. Louis. Most medical students live in privately owned apartments, generally a short distance from campus.

GRADUATES

About half of the graduates enter residencies in one of the primary care fields. A limited number of students who seek primary care careers are selected for a program that integrates the senior year of medical school with residency training in family medicine, internal medicine, pediatrics, or psychiatry.

Admissions

REQUIREMENTS

The School of Medicine requires eight credit hours each of the following courses, all of which must be taken with associated labs: biology, general chemistry, organic chemistry, and general physics. In addition to the traditional pre-medical courses, one semester of math and two semesters of English composition are also prerequisites. The MCAT is required; scores must be from after 1998. If a student has retaken the MCAT, the highest total set of MCAT scores is considered.

SUGGESTIONS

Course work in biology and chemistry beyond requirements and biochemistry are strongly recommended. In addition, applicants are encouraged to study humanities and social sciences while in college.

PROCESS

All Missouri residents (and some residents of continguous states) who submit an AMCAS application receive a secondary, which should be submitted as soon as possible. Almost 50 percent of the Missouri-resident applicants are invited to interview between October and April. Students are interviewed one-on-one by two members of the Admissions Committee. A current medical student gives a short tour of the facilities and answers questions. About a month after interviewing, applicants may be notified of the Committee's decision. Approximately 40 percent of interviewed candidates are accepted. Wait-listed candidates are not encouraged to send supplementary information.

Admissions Requirements (Required)

MCAT scores, science GPA, non-science GPA, letters of recommendation, interview, essays/personal statement, extracurricular activities, exposure to medical profession.

Admissions Requirements (Optional)

state residency, required coursework from an accredited college.

COSTS AND AID

In-state tuition	$18,792
Out-of-state tuition	$37,418
Room and board	$8,027
Cost of books	$2,117
Fees	$780

Financial Aid

% students receiving aid	94
Average grant	$3,577
Average loan	$31,583
Average debt	$96,200

UNIVERSITY OF MISSOURI—KANSAS CITY
SCHOOL OF MEDICINE

COUNCIL ON SELECTION, 2411 HOLMES, KANSAS CITY, MO 64108-2792 • ADMISSION: 816-235-1870 • FAX: 816-235-6579 • E-MAIL: MORGENEGGM@UMKC.EDU • WEBSITE: WWW.UMKC.EDU/MED

STUDENT BODY

Type	Public
Enrollment	630
% male/female	40/60
% underrepresented minorities	9
# applied (total/out)	476/199
# accepted (total/out)	176/44
# enrolled (total/out)	118/21
Average age	18

FACULTY

Total faculty (number)	484
% female	32
% minority	14

ADMISSIONS

Average GPA and MCAT Scores

MCAT Essay	M

Application Information

Regular application	11/15
Regular notification	4/1
Are transfers accepted?	No
Admissions may be deferred?	No
Interview required?	Yes
Application fee	$25

Academics

Rather than distinguishing pre-medical course work, preclinical medical course work, and clinical instruction, the curriculum integrates liberal arts, didactic medical sciences, and clinical training. Grades of A through F, honors, credit, no credit, and narratives are used to evaluate students. They must pass both steps of the USMLE to graduate.

BASIC SCIENCES: During the first two years, students focus most of their efforts on working toward a baccalaureate degree through arts and science course work. Seventy-five percent of classroom hours are devoted to liberal arts studies and 25 percent to introductory medical course work. The first year (thirty-five weeks) consists of undergraduate level courses in general chemistry, biology, sociology, psychology, and introduction to medicine. The introduction to medicine course gives special attention to the effects of illness on patients, families, and communities. Students become acclimated to the hospital environment and are introduced to the medical vocabulary and to basic clinical skills such as patient interviews and simple data gathering. The second year (twenty-four weeks) includes organic chemistry, human biochemistry, life cycles, medical physiology, biostatistics, and ongoing introductory clinical experiences. In the third and fourth years (both forty-eight weeks) students take courses in anatomy, microbiology, pathology, and pharmacology and participate in clinical rotations, including a weekly continuing care clinic and family medicine preceptorship. Throughout the first four years, additional liberal arts courses are included in the curriculum that are considered part of the BA. To assist with clinical training, a physician-scholar (or docent) instructs and advises groups of eleven or twelve students. The docent acts as a mentor, guide, and preceptor throughout the entire six years.

CLINICAL TRAINING

Students enter fifth- and sixth-year clerkships having already had significant clinical exposure. They continue their weekly continuing care clinic experience. The fifth year (forty-eight weeks) is made up of rotations in community medicine/family practice (one month), psychiatry (one month), obstetrics/gynecology (two months), pediatrics (two months), surgery (two months), and internal medicine (two months). One month is reserved for electives. The sixth year (forty-eight weeks) gives students ample opportunity to explore their specific areas of interest with six months of elective rotations. Required rotations include internal medicine (two months) and emergency medicine (one month). During the fifth or sixth year, students also take one month of liberal arts courses. Most training takes place at Truman Medical Center, one of the clinical facilities associated with UMKC.

Students

At least 85 percent of students are Missouri residents. Others come from high schools in neighboring states and other regions of the United States. Underrepresented minorities account for about 6 percent of the student body. As a result of the structure of the program, students within a class are all approximately the same age.

STUDENT LIFE

For the most part, classes run year-round. Although the atmosphere is intense, students are committed and supportive of one another particularly because of the junior-senior partnership program. Students enjoy the resources of both the undergraduate campus and Kansas City. All students live on campus during the first year, but most choose to live off campus for the remainder of their studies.

GRADUATES

Graduates are successful in securing residency positions in all fields. Approximately 25 percent enter programs affiliated with UMKC.

Admissions

REQUIREMENTS

Applicants for admission at the freshman level must take the ACT or the SAT (out-of-state applicants only). Applicants should have completed four years of high school English, four years of math, three years of science (including one year each of biology and chemistry), three years of social studies, one year of foreign language, and one year in the fine arts. In addition, one year of physics and one semester of computer science are highly recommended by the school. Furthermore, the school recommends that candidates take Advanced Placement (AP) courses if they are available. A limited number of positions are available at the third-year level. Applicants to the third must be Missouri residents and must have completed the standard pre-medical requirements of one year each of biology, chemistry, organic chemistry, and other requirements. The MCAT is required of these applicants, and scores must be from within the past three years.

SUGGESTIONS

For applicants to the BA/MD program and for those who apply after taking time off after college, some medically related experience is considered useful. High school students are encouraged to volunteer or work in a hospital or other health care environment.

PROCESS

UMKC does not participate in AMCAS. Applications may be obtained from the address above and are due by December 1. Interviews take place between December and mid-March and consist of two sessions, each of which is one-on-one. In addition to the interview, students and their parents attend group orientation sessions that cover a range of topics, including financial aid. Applicants tour the campus and have the opportunity to meet with current students. All candidates are notified of the Admissions Committee's decision on April 1. Some are accepted from a wait-list later in the spring.

Admissions Requirements (Required)

letters of recommendation, interview, essays/personal statement, Performance on the Toledo chemistry assessment.

Admissions Requirements (Optional)

MCAT scores, science GPA, non-science GPA, state residency, extracurricular activities, exposure to medical profession.

COSTS AND AID

In-state tuition	$24,986
Out-of-state tuition	$50,297
Room and board	$6,165
Cost of books	$800
Fees	$977

Financial Aid

Average loan	$27,000

UNIVERSITY OF MONTREAL

FACULTÉ DE MÉDECINE, CP 6128, SUCCURSALE CENTRE-VILLE, MONTRÉAL, QC, CANADA H3C 3J7 • ADMISSION: 514-343-6265 • E-MAIL: FACMED@MEDDIR.UMONTREAL.CA • WEBSITE: WWW.MED.UMONTREAL.CA/

Student Body

Type	Public
# applied (total/out)	1,859/270

ADMISSIONS

Application Information

Regular application	3/1
Regular notification	3/31
Admissions may be deferred?	No
Interview required?	Yes
Application fee	$45

Academics

Instruction is solely in French. Some students enter a one-year pre-medical program that leads to the four-year MD curriculum, while other students who qualify enter the medical curriculum directly. Although clinical exposure begins during the first year of premedical or medical training, intensive clinical training begins in the third year. The premedical program is taught through lectures. The majority of instruction for medical students, however, takes place in a small group setting. In addition to the four-year MD curriculum, graduate degree programs are offered in all major medical science fields. Affiliated with the School of Medicine are other health science programs in areas such as health administration, public health, social and preventive medicine, nutrition, rehabilitation, and speech language therapy.

BASIC SCIENCES: Students who enter the pre-medical program take courses in genetics and embryology, biostatistics, cell biology and general histology, general microbiology and virology, clinical immersion, introduction to clinical anatomy, cell and molecular biology, nutrition and metabolism, cell physiology and pharmacology, introduction to physiology, psychology and human behavior, introduction to sociology, basic concepts in ethics, and an elective. First-year medical school courses are introduction to medical studies; growth, development and aging, general pathology and immunology; infectious diseases; hematology; neurological sciences; mind; musculoskeletal system; introduction to clinical medicine; history of medicine; epidemiology; and an elective. Second-year studies are largely organized by anatomical systems. These are cardiovascular, respiratory, kidney, digestion, endocrinology, and multisystem. Second-year students also take an elective and continue with Introduction to Clinical Medicine.

CLINICAL TRAINING

For clinical training, students complete a series of required clerkships that provide hands-on experience in the major medical disciplines. During the third year, required clerkships are medicine (eight weeks), surgery (eight weeks), pediatrics (eight weeks), psychiatry (eight weeks), obstetrics/gynecology (eight weeks), and family medicine (four weeks). Third-year students also have the opportunity to take a four-week clinical elective. Fourth-year clerkships are anesthesiology (two weeks), ophthalmology (two weeks), radiology (four weeks), geriatrics (four weeks), community medicine (four weeks), and an elective (four weeks). Selectives are chosen from medical or pediatric subspecialties (eight weeks) and from surgical subspecialties (four weeks). Clinical training takes place at over fifteen affiliated hospitals including Hopital Maisonneuve-Rosemont, Hopital Notre-Dame, Hopital Riviere-des-Prairies, Hopital du Sacre-Coeur de Montreal, Hopital Louis-H Lafontaine, Hopital Sainte-Justine, Hopital Saint-Luc, Hotel-Dieu de Montreal, Institute de Cardiologie de Montreal, Institut de Readaptation de Montreal, Centre Hospitalier de Verdun, Cite de la Sante de Laval, Institue de Recherches Clinique de Montreal, Institut Philpe-Pinelde Montreal, and Centre Hospitalier Cote-des-Nieges.

Students

Entering class size is 143. In a recent class, all but four students were from the province of Quebec. About 60 percent of the students are women.

STUDENT LIFE

The School of Medicine is committed to its students and provides them with academic and nonacademic support services. Outside of the classroom, medical students interact through student groups and organized social activities. The resources of the greater university, including athletic and recreational facilities, are available to medical students as well. Finally, the city of Montreal is an internationally recognized cultural center with a wealth of activities that are accessible to students.

GRADUATES

Graduates enter both academic and clinical medicine. There are many post-graduate programs available at hospitals affiliated with the University of Montreal, including anesthesiology, family medicine, medicine, obstetrics/gynecology, ophthalmology, pediatrics, psychiatry, radiology, and surgery.

Admissions

REQUIREMENTS

Only Canadian citizens, landed immigrants, and highly qualified French-speaking applicants from the United States are considered for admission. Fluency in French is a requirement. Two years of college is the minimum requirement for admission to the School of Medicine. Prerequisites are philosophy, behavioral sciences, social sciences, French, English, mathematics (through trigonometry), biology, organic chemistry, general chemistry, and physics.

SUGGESTIONS

Strong preference is given to applicants from the province of Quebec. Selection is based on both academic records and interviews.

PROCESS

The absolute deadline for applications is March 1. About one-third of all applicants are asked to interview based on their academic records. The strongest candidates are then selected from those who are interviewed. Admissions decisions are made in the spring, and the first acceptance notices are sent out in May. Accepted applicants have two weeks to confirm their place in the entering class.

COSTS AND AID

Tuition & Fees

Tuition (in/out)	$2,575/$12,836
Fees	$30

University of Nebraska Medical Center

University of Nebraska College of Medicine

986585 Nebraska Medical Center, Omaha, NE 68198-6585 • Admission: 402-559-6140 • Fax: 402-559-6840 • E-mail: grrogers@unmc.edu • Website: www.unmc.edu/UNCOM/

STUDENT BODY

Type	Public
Enrollment	483
% male/female	61/39
% underrepresented minorities	11
# applied (total/out)	777/521
# accepted (total/out)	152/37
# enrolled (total/out)	117/14

FACULTY

Total faculty (number)	599
% part-time	19

ADMISSIONS

Average GPA and MCAT Scores

Overall GPA	3.7
MCAT Bio	9.8
MCAT Phys	9.5
MCAT Verbal	9.5
MCAT Essay	0

Application Information

Regular application	11/1
Regular notification	rolling
Early application	8/1
Early notification	10/1
Are transfers accepted?	Yes
Admissions may be deferred?	No
Interview required?	Yes
Application fee	$40

Academics

Most medical students complete the MD curriculum in four years, although some students may remain for an additional year to work on research projects or other activities. A combined MS/PhD program is offered to qualified students that leads to the doctoral degree in a number of fields, including cell biology and anatomy, biochemistry and molecular biology, physiology and biophysics, pathology and microbiology, and pharmacology. Medical students who are interested in discrete research projects should look into summer research stipends, which are available on a competitive basis. Students must pass the USMLE Step 1 to be promoted to year three, and all students must record a score on Step 2 to graduate.

BASIC SCIENCES: Throughout the first two years, basic sciences are integrated with introductory clinical instruction; topics are organized into blocks, which are referred to as cores. Students are in class for about thirty-two hours per week, most of which is spent in lectures, small groups, or labs. First-year courses are structure and development of the human body, cellular processes, neuroscience, and function of the human body. Throughout the first and second years, integrated clinical experience (ICE) covers the history and physical examination, interviewing skills, behavioral sciences, ethics, preventive medicine, health care policy, and health care services research. Through ICE, students have the opportunity to work alongside primary care physicians in a longitudinal clinical experience and a summer preceptorship. Also spanning both years is problem-based learning, in which students work in small groups and apply basic science concepts to clinical case studies. Second year cores are introduction to disease processes; cardiology/pulmonary/endocrinology/ear, nose, and throat; neurology, ophthalmology and psychiatry; hematology/oncology/musculoskeletal; dermatology and infectious disease; and genitourinary/gastroenterology. Instruction takes place in the Eppley Institute and in Wittson Hall, which also houses administrative offices, laboratories, and audiovisual resources. The Leon S. McGoogan Library of Medicine holds over 200,000 volumes and 2,100 current journals. Multimedia materials for computer-assisted and self-instruction are available, as are online informational systems.

CLINICAL TRAINING

Required third-year clerkships are internal medicine (twelve weeks), obstetrics/gynecology (six weeks), pediatrics (eight weeks), surgery (ten weeks), psychiatry (six weeks), community preceptorship (eight weeks), basic science selective (four weeks), and a mini-clerkship in an area of choice (two weeks). During the fourth year, a basic science selective in addition to twenty-eight weeks of electives are required. Clinical facilities at UNMC are Nebraska Health System (650 beds); University Medical Associates, which operates over sixty primary care and subspecialty clinics throughout the greater Omaha metropolitan area; Meyer Rehabilitation Institute; Omaha Veterans' Affairs Medical Center; Children's Hospital; Immanuel Hospital; and Methodist Hospital.

Students

Most students in each class are Nebraska residents. Class size is 120.

STUDENT LIFE

Medical students are active in student organizations that include the Student Alliance for Global Health, the Family Practice Club, and a group that focuses on alternative medicine. The local chapter of the American Medical Student Association is particularly active, organizing volunteer projects, film series, and opportunities for enhanced clinical exposure. Omaha is a city of 700,000, offering a symphony, theaters, art museums, shopping, restaurants, and parks, among other attractions. Students live off campus in the surrounding communities, where, for an urban area, housing is relatively inexpensive.

GRADUATES

Students are successful at securing residencies in both primary care and specialty areas. A significant percentage of graduates enter post-graduate programs at UNMC, which oversees eighteen residency programs. In recent years, at least 60 percent of graduates have gone on to practice in the state of Nebraska. Among students who graduated between 1981 and 1990, 130 joined the faculty at UNMC.

Admissions

REQUIREMENTS

Prerequisites are biology (eight semester hours), general chemistry (eight hours), organic chemistry (eight hours), physics (eight hours), humanities and/or social sciences (twelve hours), English composition (three hours), calculus or statistics (three credits), biochemistry (three hours), and genetics (three hours). All science courses must include associated labs. The MCAT is required and scores must be from an exam taken no earlier than 2001.

SUGGESTIONS

State residents are given preference, but other highly qualified candidates are considered, particularly if they have ties to Nebraska and are interested in practicing in underserved communities in the state. Beyond required courses, the following are recommended: molecular biology, immunology and microbiology, communications, ethics, and personnel management.

PROCESS

All Nebraska residents who apply through AMCAS and a small percentage of out-of-state applicants are asked to submit supplementary materials and are interviewed. Interviews are conducted between October and February and consist of a thirty-minute session with a faculty member. On interview day, there is also a group information session and a campus tour. Typically, about 50 percent of Nebraska residents are accepted and are notified beginning in December. Wait-listed candidates may send additional information to update their files.

Admissions Requirements (Required)

MCAT scores, science GPA, non-science GPA, letters of recommendation, interview, state residency, essays/personal statement, extracurricular activities, exposure to medical profession.

COSTS AND AID

In-state tuition	$14,469
Out-of-state tuition	$33,930
Cost of books	$1,800
Fees	$1,672

Financial Aid

% students receiving aid	92
Average debt	$92,317

UNIVERSITY OF NEVADA
SCHOOL OF MEDICINE

OFFICE OF ADMISSIONS, RENO, NV 89557 • ADMISSION: 702-784-6063 • FAX: 702-784-6194 •
E-MAIL: ASA@SCS.UNR.EDU • WEBSITE: WWW.UNR.EDU/UNR/MED.HTML

STUDENT BODY

Type	Public
Enrollment	211
% male/female	61/39
% underrepresented minorities	5
# applied (total/out)	925/749
# accepted (total/out)	71/3
# enrolled (out)	18

ADMISSIONS

Application Information

Regular application	11/1
Regular notification	1/15, varies
Early application	6/1-8/1
Early notification	10/1
Are transfers accepted?	No
Admissions may be deferred?	Yes
Interview required?	No
Application fee	$45

Academics

The first two years provide a foundation in basic clinical sciences, significant preclinical training, and clerkships that take place statewide in community clinics as well as hospital settings. The School of Medicine applicants or current medical students may apply to jointly pursue a MS/PhD program in several areas including biomedical engineering and cell and molecular biology, pharmacology, and physiology. Students who are interested in research but not in pursuing a PhD can make arrangements with faculty members to work on projects.

BASIC SCIENCES: The first two years at Nevada focus on the basic sciences but also give considerable attention to community health and social issues. Additional scientific material is presented through lectures, labs, and small group formats at the Reno campus. Students apply scientific principles to clinical challenges through problem solving courses using case study methods. This approach promotes the development of problem solving skills in medical students. Concurrent with basic and behavioral science courses, students learn fundamental skills in doctor-patient relationship and physical exams through weekly sessions that are supervised by physicians and senior medical students. In this way, students learn not only from full-time faculty but also from knowledgeable and experienced clinical faculty physicians throughout the state. First-year course work includes human biochemistry, human anatomy, embryology, histology, neuroanatomy, human behavior, medical cell biology, neurosciences, systems physiology, clinical problem solving, nutrition, and introduction to patient care. Year two courses include human genetics, medical mircobiology, medical pharmacology, pathology, laboratory medicine, psychiatric medicine, medical ethics, community medicine, introduction to patient care II, and clinical problem solving II. Students receive grades of A through F for most courses and must receive at least a C to be promoted. Students are evaluated on both cognitive and noncognitive factors. Two major medical libraries serve the medical students: the Savitt Medical Library on the Reno campus, which contains more than 40,000 volumes, and the University Medical Center Library in Las Vegas. Both libraries maintain computer labs that feature an assortment of general and curriculum-based software. Additional learning resource labs are available in Las Vegas in the ambulatory care centers. Students have electronic access to all of Nevada's university and community college collections through terminals located throughout the teaching sites in the state. Students are issued computer accounts for E-mail and Internet access. In addition, the USMLE Step 1 is required for promotion to year three.

CLINICAL TRAINING

Training takes place at affiliated hospitals, clinics, and ambulatory care centers throughout the state. Most students have required rotations including the practice of medicine, which is a twenty-four-week integrated clerkship experience that includes family medicine (six weeks), internal medicine (twelve weeks), and pediatrics (six weeks). The practice of medicine also includes a core curriculum that runs throughout the state via distance education facilities. Medical students also complete required specialty rotations of obstetrics/gynecology (six weeks), psychiatry (six weeks), and surgery (twelve weeks). There is an increased emphasis in all of the rotations to blend ambulatory and hospital-based practice to give the students a balanced educational experience. During the fourth year, students rotate through thirty-two weeks of elective clerkships and four weeks of a required rural clerkship. Elective study can take place in Reno, Las Vegas, rural Nevada, other states, or abroad. Although the obvious emphasis and strength of the program is primary care and rural medicine, hospitals in Reno and Las Vegas treat urban and often international populations. Evaluation of clinical performance uses grades of honors, pass, and fail. In addition, special awards and honors are granted to students who have made unique and outstanding achievements in clinical areas. Passing the USMLE Step 2 is required for graduation.

Students

Eighty-five percent of students majored in a science-related discipline in college. About 5 percent are underrepresented minorities, most of whom are Mexican American or Native American. Almost all students are Nevada residents, although many attended college in other states. About one-quarter of each class took some time off between college and medical school.

STUDENT LIFE

Small class sizes promote cohesion among students. A designated lounge on campus gives medical students a place to relax and interact. Athletic facilities are available: Students in the Reno area use the Lombardi Recreational Facility, and students in Las Vegas use the McDermott Physical Education Facility. Student organizations include AMWA & OSR medical specialty interest groups, the Significant Others Group for partners of medical students, and the University of Nevada Student Outreach Clinic, through which medical students, with supervision, volunteer to treat patients from underserved areas. Most students have cars, and on-campus parking is free for students with registered vehicles. Lake Tahoe is just an hour away from Reno where students can enjoy outstanding outdoor activities year-round. Virtually all medical students live off campus since housing is affordable and comfortable.

GRADUATES

The majority of graduates enter residency programs outside the state. Almost all graduates ultimately become practicing clinical physicians.

Admissions

REQUIREMENTS

Required course work includes biology (twelve semester hours), chemistry (eight hours), organic chemistry (eight hours), physics (eight hours), and behavioral science (six hours). The biology and behavioral science requirements specify that at least three semester hours be upper-division credits. GPAs and MCAT scores are used to screen for interview invitations. The most recent MCAT scores are used, and the exam must have been taken within the past three years.

SUGGESTIONS

Only applicants from Nevada, neighboring states, Wyoming, Alaska, Montana, and Idaho, and applicants who have close ties to Nevada are considered for admission. Nevada residents are given preference. Community-focused work and health care experience are considered important.

PROCESS

Interviews are held from September through January. The interview consists of two fifty-minute sessions, which may be with faculty or medical students. About 25 percent of Nevada residents who are interviewed are offered a place in the class; about 10 percent of out-of-state applicants are accepted. The first acceptance notices are sent in January. Wait-listed candidates are ranked, and candidates in the top third are likely to be admitted.

Admissions Requirements (Required)

MCAT scores, science GPA, non-science GPA, letters of recommendation, state residency, extracurricular activities, exposure to medical profession.

Admissions Requirements (Optional)

interview, essays/personal statement.

COSTS AND AID

In-state tuition	$7,265
Out-of-state tuition	$21,292
Fees	$1,894
Financial Aid	
% students receiving aid	80

UNIVERSITY OF NEW MEXICO
SCHOOL OF MEDICINE

OFFICE OF ADMISSIONS, ALBUQUERQUE, NM 87131 • ADMISSION: 505-272-4766 • FAX: 505-272-8239 • E-MAIL: MBALLEJOS@SALUD.UNM.EDU • WEBSITE: HTTP://HSC.UNM.EDU/SOM/

STUDENT BODY

Type	Public
Enrollment	303
% male/female	44/56
% underrepresented minorities	37
# applied (total/out)	828/569
# accepted (total/out)	92/3
# enrolled (total/out)	75/3
Average age	25

FACULTY

Total faculty (number)	715
% part-time	14
# student/faculty ratio	2:1

ADMISSIONS

Average GPA and MCAT Scores

Overall GPA	3.5
MCAT Bio	9.5
MCAT Phys	8.8
MCAT Verbal	8.8

Application Information

Regular application	11/15
Regular notification	3/15
Early application	8/1
Early notification	10/1
Are transfers accepted?	Yes
Admissions may be deferred?	Yes
Interview required?	Yes
Application fee	$50

Academics

The four-year curriculum is organized into three phases, all of which involve at least some basic science instruction and clinical training. In addition, all students conduct research projects under the guidance of a faculty mentor. The complete project consists of research, presentation, and a written paper. Applicants who are interested in pursuing a combined MS/PhD may apply to the graduate committee at the School of Medicine in addition to completing medical school admissions requirements. Medical students are evaluated with grades of outstanding, good, satisfactory, marginal, and unsatisfactory. The USMLE Step 1 must be passed prior to graduation, and Step 2 must be taken to graduate.

BASIC SCIENCES: The first year-and-a-half (Phase I) is organized into discrete segments, most of which focus on an organ system. First-year subjects are foundations, musculoskeletal, GI/nutrition/metabolism, renal/endocrine, neuroscience, and cardiovascular/pulmonary. During the summer following year one, students take part in a three-month practical immersion experience that involves hands-on clinical work in either a rural or urban setting. Phase I continues in the first semester of year two with molecular genetics, human sex and reproduction, infectious disease, and neoplasma. A range of learning methodologies are used, including lectures, labs, discussions, tutorials, and seminars. Concurrent to basic science instruction are weekly clinical experiences in both inpatient and ambulatory settings. Students learn interviewing and examination techniques and are able to improve communication and personal interaction skills. Much of Phases I and II take place in the basic medical sciences building. The nearby Health Sciences Center Library supports educational, research, and clinical activities. It houses 150,000 volumes in addition to audiovisuals, online search services, and computer software.

CLINICAL TRAINING

Phase II begins midway through year two with a three-week pharmacology block and orientation to the hospital. Clinical rotations are accompanied by ongoing small group sessions that focus on problem solving and integrating information. Students rotate through required clerkships throughout the spring and summer of the second year and the fall and winter of the third year. Requirements are internal medicine (eight weeks), surgery (eight weeks), neurology/psychiatry (eight weeks), family medicine ambulatory (eight weeks), pediatrics ambulatory/inpatient (eight weeks), and obstetrics/gynecology and ambulatory/inpatient (eight weeks). Phase III begins in the spring of year three and consists entirely of selectives and electives. A monthlong, community-based preceptorship, in which students work alongside a primary care physician who serves as a mentor, is also required. Clinical training takes place at the University Hospital (370 beds) and at several affiliated sites, namely Regional Federal Medical Center (429 beds), UNM Cancer Center, UNM Mental Health Center, UNM Children's Psychiatric Hospital (73 beds), and the Carrie Tingley Hospital for Children.

Students

About 25 percent of students are underrepresented minorities, most of whom are Mexican Americans. At least 90 percent of students are New Mexico residents, and about half of each class graduated from UNM's undergraduate college. In a recent class, the average age of entering students was twenty-five. Approximately one-third of students took time off after college. Class size is seventy-three.

STUDENT LIFE

The medical school is located on the north campus of UNM, which gives students access to the resources and facilities of the university. The city also provides an outlet for students who need a break from studying. The greater Albuquerque metropolitan area is home to nearly one-third of the state's population and offers numerous cultural and recreational opportunities. Although no on-campus housing is available, off-campus options are convenient and comfortable.

GRADUATES

About 35 percent of graduates enter residencies at UNM, which offers programs in twelve different departments. The majority of graduates enter primary care fields.

Admissions

REQUIREMENTS

Prerequisites are general biology (eight semester hours), general chemistry (eight semester hours), organic chemistry (eight semester hours), physics (six semester hours), and biochemistry (three semester hours). Competency in English and the MCAT are additional requirements.

SUGGESTIONS

Knowledge of Spanish or a Native American language is beneficial. Course work in the humanities and social sciences is important. The April MCAT is preferred over the August one. Students are selected on the basis of academic achievement, motivation for the study of medicine, problem solving ability, self-appraisal, ability to relate to people, maturity, breadth of interest and achievements, professional goals, and the likelihood of serving the health care needs of the state following post-graduate training.

PROCESS

All New Mexico AMCAS applicants receive secondary applications and are invited to interview. Qualified WICHE and other out-of-state applicants who apply for early decision are also sent secondary materials and invited to interview. Interviews are conducted from June through March and consist of two sessions with members of the Admissions Committee, who are either full-time faculty members or community physicians. On interview day, students have lunch and tour the facilities. About 20 to 25 percent of interviewed candidates are accepted. Wait-listed candidates are ranked and notified of their position on the list.

Admissions Requirements (Required)

MCAT scores, letters of recommendation, interview, state residency, essays/personal statement, extracurricular activities, exposure to medical profession.

Admissions Requirements (Optional)

science GPA, nonscience GPA.

COSTS AND AID

In-state tuition	$9,466
Out-of-state tuition	$27,135
Cost of books	$1,431
Fees	$1,709

Financial Aid

% students receiving aid	82
Average grant	$1,000
Average loan	$18,000
Average debt	$70,780

UNIVERSITY OF NORTH CAROLINA—CHAPEL HILL
SCHOOL OF MEDICINE

CB #7000 130 MACNIDER HALL, CHAPEL HILL, NC 27599-7000 • ADMISSION: 919-962-8331 •
E-MAIL: ADMISSIONS@MED.UNC.EDU • WEBSITE: WWW.MED.UNC.EDU

STUDENT BODY

Type	Public
Enrollment	624
% male/female	51/49
% underrepresented minorities	17
# applied (total/out)	5,859/5,153

ADMISSIONS

Overall GPA	3.7
MCAT Bio	10.57
MCAT Phys	10.48
MCAT Verbal	10.25

Application Information

Regular application	11/15
Regular notification	10/15 until filled

Academics

The core curriculum gives students the required comprehensive education needed before they embark on the next stage of their careers. In addition, many students pursue focused research training in the clinic or at the bench. Research stipends are available through training grants or individual research grants. Students with a particular interest in research may apply for the MSTP-supported MD/PhD program at UNC. Other students take the opportunity to combine an advanced degree in public health, law, or business with their medical studies. Grades of honors, pass, and fail are used to evaluate medical students in the first two years. Students must pass the USMLE Step 1 examination before promotion to the third year and pass Step 2 before graduation.

BASIC SCIENCES: The first two years are devoted primarily to studying the scientific basis of clinical practice, with emphasis on demonstrating clinical implications and correlation. Clinical instruction begins early in the first year with the two-year course introduction to clinical medicine (ICM), in which students have the opportunity to develop the clinical skills (such as history-taking, physical examination) and problem-solving abilities needed for the clinical years. ICM also serves as a forum for discussion of a wide range of crosscutting topics such as substance abuse, domestic violence, and computing in medicine. Three months of both the first and second years are spent in a community working with a physician tutor. Other first-year courses are biochemistry, cell biology, gross anatomy, histology, immunology, introduction to pathology, medical embryology, medical physiology, medicine and society, microbiology, and neurobiology. Many of the courses in the second year are organized around the pathophysiology of particular organ systems such as cardiovascular, endocrine, gastrointestinal, hematology/oncology, neurology and special senses, reproductive biology, respiratory, skin, musculoskeletal, and urinary. Closely integrated with the study of particular organ systems are courses in pathology, genetics, humanities and social sciences, and psychiatry. Throughout the first and second years, students participate in small group discussions, lectures, labs, clinical practice sessions, and real clinical experiences. The needs of the curriculum are well served by continuous training in information technology coupled with the requirement that each student have a laptop computer. The Health Sciences Library serves the Schools of Dentistry, Medicine, Nursing, Pharmacy, and Public Health and the UNC Hospitals. The library has approximately 300,000 volumes, 4,000 serial titles, and 9,000 audiovisual and microcomputer software programs.

CLINICAL TRAINING

Students rotate through six major clinical disciplines during their third year. These are medicine (twelve weeks), obstetrics/gynecology (six weeks), pediatrics (eight weeks), family medicine (six weeks), psychiatry (six weeks), and surgery (eight weeks). An additional requirement is life support skills (one week). The purpose of the fourth-year program is to offer a flexible educational experience that can be tailored to the career goals and intellectual interests of each student. Requirements are an ambulatory care selective (four weeks), an acting internship (four weeks), a neuroscience selective (four weeks), and a critical care/surgery selective. A total of twenty-eight weeks of electives is required, some of which may be completed at other universities or clinical settings, either in the United States or overseas.

Students

Approximately 90 percent of students are North Carolina residents. The School of Medicine is committed to admitting students who are representative of the diversity of the population of North Carolina. About one-third of entering students have pursued other interests or careers before applying to medical school.

STUDENT LIFE

The School of Medicine is responsive to students' needs and provides a range of support services. Faculty advisors are assigned to entering students and serve as mentors and academic counselors throughout all four years. The School of Medicine has twenty-six student organizations, including the student body government, student chapters of national medical professional organizations, community service groups, and special interest groups. Students are particularly active in outreach efforts such as Habitat for Humanity, the Domestic Violence Coalition, and Physicians for Social Responsibility and manage two community clinics. During the academic year, scheduled events bring faculty, students, families, and the community together. The university offers single room accommodations for some graduate students in a building near the medical center. Other students live off campus in surrounding neighborhoods.

GRADUATES

Among 2,000 graduates, 53 percent entered primary care fields, and 30.6 percent chose post-graduate training programs within North Carolina. Eighty-four percent of the class of 2000 matched with one of their top three choices for residency training.

Admissions

REQUIREMENTS

Prerequisites are under review and may be changed. Current prerequisites are eight semester hours of biology, at least four hours of which must be accompanied by a lab. Students are strongly encouraged to have taken at least one course in molecular and cell biology. Eight semester hours of general chemistry, organic chemistry, and physics, all with lab, are also required in addition to six semester hours of English. The MCAT is required.

SUGGESTIONS

Preference is given to residents of North Carolina. Thus, successful applicants who are not residents of North Carolina typically have outstanding qualifications.

PROCESS

Approximately 50 percent of AMCAS applicants who are North Carolina residents, and fewer than 10 percent of nonresidents, are sent secondary applications and are invited to interview. Interviews take place between August and March and consist of two sessions with faculty members, one a member of the admissions committee. On interview day, candidates also have lunch with currently enrolled medical students and go on tours of the campus.

Early application	6/1–8/1
Early notification	10/1
Admissions may be deferred?	Yes
Interview required?	Yes
Application fee	$55

COSTS AND AID

In-state tuition	$8,188
Out-of-statetuition	$33,656
Cost of books	$1,050

University of North Dakota
School of Medicine and Health Sciences

501 North Columbia Road, Box 9037, Grand Forks, ND 58202-9037 • Admission: 701-777-4221 • Fax: 701-777-4942 • E-mail: jdheit@medicine.nodak.edu • Website: www.med.und.nodak.edu

STUDENT BODY

Type	Public
Enrollment	226
% male/female	49/51
% underrepresented minorities	9
# applied (total/out)	249/104
# accepted (total/out)	101/28
# enrolled (total/out)	56/11
Average age	24

FACULTY

Total faculty (number)	1,196
% part-time	90
# student/faculty ratio	2:1

ADMISSIONS

Average GPA and MCAT Scores

Overall GPA	3.7
MCAT Bio	9.03
MCAT Phys	8.44
MCAT Verbal	8.62
MCAT Essay	0

Application Information

Regular application	11/1
Regular notification	1/15
Are transfers accepted?	No
Admissions may be deferred?	Yes
Interview required?	Yes
Application fee	$50

Academics

Preclinical instruction takes place at the University of North Dakota campus in Grand Forks, and clinical training takes place throughout the state. After students have been admitted to the MD program, they may apply to pursue a joint MD/PhD program in anatomy, biochemistry, cell biology, immunology, microbiology, molecular biology, physiology and therapeutics, and pharmacology. Evaluation of students uses ratings of satisfactory or unsatisfactory during the first year and honors, satisfactory, unsatisfactory for the final three years. Step 1 and 2 of the USMLE must be passed to graduate.

BASIC SCIENCES: The basic sciences are taught through a combination of lectures, labs, and small group sessions. The new curriculum puts significant emphasis on active student participation and early clinical experience. Social science courses that address topics such as statistics, human behavorial patterns, and social issues that are relevant in North Dakota and other rural areas are integrated into the basic science and clinical curriculum throughout the first and second years. The first-year courses are organized into the following blocks: functional biology of cells and tissues, biology of organ systems I, biology of organ systems II, and biology of the nervous system. These blocks are offered in the morning. The afternoons are reserved for self-study or for introduction to patient care (IPC), which is the clinical component and is also organized into blocks such as IPC block I (interviewing and professionalism). The same format continues into the second year. Second-year blocks include introduction to pathobiology and pathobiology I, II, and III. The IPC component again is covered during afternoon sessions. Students also complete their first clinical rotation, introduction to inpatient and ambulatory practice of medicine (three weeks). Most instruction takes place in the medical sciences building, which houses administrative offices, classrooms, labs, and the library. The Harley E. French Library of the Health Sciences has over 80,000 books, periodicals, and audiovisual programs. It is fully automated and has computers for informational and research purposes. The proximity of basic science instructional facilities to the clinical and research facilities promotes an integrated learning experience during the first two years.

CLINICAL TRAINING

Third-year, required clerkships are medicine (eight weeks), surgery (eight weeks), pediatrics (eight weeks), obstetrics/gynecology (eight weeks), psychiatry (eight weeks), family medicine (eight weeks), and clinical epidemiology (taken throughout the year). Students are assigned to the Bismarck, Fargo, or Grand Forks campuses for the third year or they may participate in the ROME (Rural Opportunities in Medical Education) program. ROME students are assigned to a rural practice site for seven months of the third year and to their home campus for the remainder of the year. During the fourth year, students train at regional sites in Bismarck, Fargo, Minot, and Grand Forks. Each campus is affiliated with from ten to twenty-two hospitals and provides health care services to anywhere from nine to eighteen counties. The fourth year includes acting internships and electives. Clinical students train at sites throughout the state, including community hospitals, clinics that are part of the Indian Health Service, and physicians' offices. The University of North Dakota's Center for Rural Health focuses on policy analysis and research on rural health care delivery at the state, regional, and national level.

Students

Most students are North Dakota residents, although up to eleven students in each class may be from Minnesota, Montana, and Wyoming. Up to seven students in each class (admitted as part of INMED) are Native American. In total, underrepresented minorities account for about 17 percent of the student body. About 20 to 25 percent of an entering class is made up of older students who took time off between college and medical school. Class size is sixty-two.

STUDENT LIFE

Grand Forks is a community of 50,000 people, located in the Red River Valley on the border between North Dakota and Minnesota. The city is affordable and safe, and offers the services that students need. Students have access to the facilities of the greater University, and are encouraged to participate in student organizations, including the local chapters of national medical student organizations. On-campus housing is available, although many students opt to live off campus. Since clinical training takes place around the state, students will experience a variety of living situations throughout their four years.

GRADUATES

About one-half of the graduates enter residency programs in primary care fields, and a significant number go on to practice in North Dakota. Post-graduate training programs are offered at all the regional training sites.

Admissions

REQUIREMENTS

State residency is a requirement, unless applicants are certified by the Western Interstate Commission for Higher Education (WICHE) or are Native Americans who are enrolled members of a federally recognized tribe and admitted through the INMED program. Minnesota residents also are given some consideration. Prerequisite course work is general chemistry (eight hours), organic/biochemistry (eight hours), biology (eight hours), physics (eight hours), psychology/sociology (three hours), language arts (six hours), and college algebra (three hours). All science course work must be completed with the appropriate laboratory sessions. A minimum GPA of 3.0 is expected. The MCAT is required, and scores must be no more than three years old. For applicants who have retaken the test, the most recent set of scores is considered.

SUGGESTIONS

Preference is given to students who are broadly educated in the sciencs and humanities. For students who have been out of college for a period of time, some recent course work is suggested. Computer literacy also is advised.

PROCESS

North Dakota does not participate in AMCAS. Applicants may apply either online or using the traditional paper application. Applications should be requested from the address listed above or at www.med.und.nodak.edu. About 40 percent of applicants are invited to interview in December or January. The committee consists of faculty, administrators, practicing physicians, and medical students. After interviewing, candidates are notified of the committee's decision within four and six weeks. About 40 percent of interviewees are accepted. Wait-listed candidates are not encouraged to send supplementary information.

Admissions Requirements (Required)

MCAT scores, science GPA, non-science GPA, letters of recommendation, interview, state residency, essays/personal statement, extracurricular activities, exposure to medical profession.

COSTS AND AID

In-state tuition	$15,343
Out-of-state tuition	$40,963
Room and board	$8,704
Cost of books	$2,250
Fees	$1,040

Financial Aid

% students receiving aid	99
Average grant	$1,500
Average loan	$33,500
Average debt	$95,287

University of Oklahoma
College of Medicine

PO Box 26901, Oklahoma City, OK 73190 • Admission: 405-271-2331 • Fax: 405-271-3032 •
E-mail: AdminMed@ouhsc.edu • Website: www.ouhsc.edu

STUDENT BODY

Type	Public
Enrollment	585
% male/female	61/39
% underrepresented minorities	27
# applied (total/out)	848/539
# accepted (total/out)	188/24
# enrolled (total/out)	142/7
Average age	23

FACULTY

Total faculty (number)	688
% female	31
% part-time	15
# student/faculty ratio	1:1

ADMISSIONS

Average GPA and MCAT Scores

Overall GPA	3.7
MCAT Bio	9.6
MCAT Phys	9.06
MCAT Verbal	9.16
MCAT Essay	0

Application Information

Regular application	10/15
Regular notification	rolling
Are transfers accepted?	Yes
Admissions may be deferred?	No
Interview required?	Yes
Application fee	$50

Academics

All students spend their first two years on the Oklahoma City campus. On completion of year two, about 25 percent of the class enter clinical rotations at sites affiliated with the University of Oklahoma's Tulsa campus. Tulsa is particularly well-equipped for primary care and community-based medical instruction. Qualified students may pursue the joint MS/PhD degree from any graduate department. OUHSC also offers a joint MD/master's in public health degree. Medical students are evaluated with grades of A through F. They must pass Step 1 of the USMLE to be promoted to year three; graduates must take, but not necessarily pass, Step 2 of the USMLE to earn their diploma.

BASIC SCIENCES: Basic sciences are taught through lectures, labs, computer-assisted instruction, problem based learning, and small group discussions. During the first two years, students are in class or other scheduled sessions for twenty to twenty-five hours per week, which gives students ample time for self directed study. First-year courses are gross anatomy, embryology, histology, biochemistry/molecular biology, physiology, neuroscience, human behavior I, medical statistics, and principles of clinical medicine I. Second-year courses are microbiology and immunology, principles of clinical medicine II, human behavior II, pharmacology, introduction to human illness, and professional ethics and professionalism. Basic sciences are taught in the basic sciences education building, which has classrooms, labs, and a study area. The Robert Bird Library contains more than 250,000 books, journals, and audiovisuals and has two special collections—the Indian Health Collection and the Rare Book Collection. Students can access a number of online catalogs and databases from the library.

CLINICAL TRAINING

Third-year rotations are medicine (eight weeks), surgery (eight weeks), obstetrics/gynecology (six weeks), psychiatry (six weeks), pediatrics (six weeks), family medicine (four weeks), specialty selectives (six weeks) and clinical electives (twenty-eight weeks), and neuroscience (two weeks). Fourth-year clerkships are adult ambulatory medicine (four weeks), and a rural preceptorship (four weeks) and specialty selectives (six weeks) and clinical electives (twenty-eight weeks). Clinical affiliates and training sites are OU Medical Center, Department of Veterans' Affairs Medical Center, Oklahoma Medical Research Foundation, Oklahoma City Clinic, Oklahoma Allergy Clinic, Dean A. McGee Eye Institute, Oklahoma Blood Institute, State Medical Examiner's Office, Department of Mental Health, and Oklahoma State Department of Health. Students also may do training at the Baptist Medical Center, St. Anthony Hospital, and Mercy Health Center in Oklahoma City. At the Tulsa campus, clinical facilities contain more than 2,000 patient beds, and additional rural training sites are currently being developed. The Oklahoma Telemedicine Network is among the largest medical communications systems in the world, successfully bringing information and expertise to rural physicians, clinics, and hospitals.

Students

At least 85 percent of students must be Oklahoma residents, but generally only five or ten students are from out of state. There is a wide age range among incoming students; therefore, it is not unusual to find students older than thirty-five. About 26 percent of students are underrepresented minorities, most of whom are Native Americans. Class size is 150.

STUDENT LIFE

Students are cohesive both inside and outside the classroom. A student-run note service is one example of cooperation among students. The OUHSC student center facilitates both social and academic interaction. It features an exercise room, study areas, computers, a food service court, and common rooms. Medical students also have access to the recreational center at the nearby Healthy Living Center for a fee. Medical students are active in student organizations that offer support and focus on recreational pursuits, professional goals, and community service. Medical students are also involved in coed intramural football, basketball, and soccer. Students are eligible for intercollegiate athletic tickets and other university-wide events. OUHSC has no on-campus housing, but off-campus housing is affordable and comfortable. University-owned housing for married and single students is available at the Norman campus. Downtown Oklahoma City is one mile from the OUHSC campus and offers a range of activities and attractions.

GRADUATES

Typically, about half of all graduates enter residencies in Oklahoma. Other graduates are successful in securing positions throughout the United States. There are seven OUHSC-affiliated post-graduate programs in Tulsa, and over twenty-five in Oklahoma City.

Admissions

REQUIREMENTS

Prerequisites include general zoology/biology with lab (one semester), embryology, genetics, anatomy, cellular biology, or histology (one semester), inorganic chemistry (one year), organic chemistry (one year), general physics (one year), and English (three semesters). Students should also take three semesters of any combination of sociology, psychology, anthropology, humanities, philosophy, or foreign language. The MCAT is required, and scores must be from after 1991. For applicants who have retaken the exam, the most recent set of scores is considered. Basic computer skills are required.

SUGGESTIONS

Strong preference is given to Oklahoma residents, making competition intense for out-of-state residents. Applicants are encouraged to take additional courses in social sciences, humanities, fine arts, computer sciences, and English. In addition to academic achievement, a candidate's personality, maturity, and character are evaluated. Admissions decisions also take into account the importance of social and cultural diversity.

PROCESS

All AMCAS applicants receive secondary applications, of which about 20 percent are interviewed. Interviews are conducted between November and January, and consist of one session with a panel of three members of the Admissions Committee. On interview day, applicants tour the campus and have the opportunity to informally meet with current students. About 80 percent of interviewed candidates (not including wait-listed candidates), are accepted on a rolling basis. Wait-listed candidates may send updated transcripts.

Admissions Requirements (Required)

MCAT scores, science GPA, non-science GPA, letters of recommendation, interview, essays/personal statement, extracurricular activities, exposure to medical profession.

Admissions Requirements (Optional)

state residency.

COSTS AND AID

In-state tuition	$13,299
Out-of-state tuition	$33,677
Cost of books	$7,215
Fees	$985

Financial Aid

Average grant	$5,500
Average loan	$32,800

University of Ottawa

451 Smyth Road, Room 2046, Ottawa, ON K1H 8M5 • Admission: 613-562-5409 • Fax: 613-562-5420 •
E-mail: admissmd@uottawa.ca • Website: www.medecine.uottawa.ca/eng/undergraduate.html

STUDENT BODY

Type	Public
# applied (total/out)	1,851/482

ADMISSIONS

Application Information

Regular application	10/15
Regular notification	5/1
Admissions may be deferred?	Yes
Interview required?	Yes
Application fee	$175 OMSAS, plus $75 for each additional school (subject to change)

Academics

During the four-year MD program, students acquire the knowledge, skills, and attitudes they need to apply effective, efficient strategies for the prevention and management of health problems ranging from the most common to the most severe. The program integrates the basic and clinical sciences throughout all four years. It also emphasizes health promotion and disease prevention and is responsive to individual needs and abilities and to the changes occurring in society and the health care system. Instruction is available in both French and English. In addition to the MD, master's, and PhD programs are offered in biochemistry, cell and developmental biology, epidemiology and community medicine, microbiology and immunology, pharmacology, and physiology.

BASIC SCIENCES: The basic science curriculum spans seventy weeks and emphasizes self-learning and multidisciplinary teaching. Lecture, seminars, computer applications, problem-based learning, and labs are all important teaching methodologies. During the first academic period, students complete blocks focused on development and homeostasis, infection and neoplasia, hematology, and immune, cardiovascular, respiratory, and renal systems. The second academic period teaches endocrinology, human reproduction and sexuality, musculoskeletal, nervous system, mind, special senses, and gastrointestinal. Throughout the first and second years, students also take physicians skills development. In addition to the Health Sciences Library, the other libraries and learning resources of the university are available to students.

CLINICAL TRAINING

During the third year, required rotations are medicine (three weeks), surgery (eight weeks), ambulatory medicine (eight weeks), obstetrics/gynecology (eight weeks), pediatrics (eight weeks), and psychiatry (eight weeks). The fourth year is comprised of fourteen weeks of electives and selectives in medicine, surgery, and ambulatory medicine. Training takes place at Ottawa General Hospital, Ottawa Civic Hospital, Children's Hospital of Eastern Ontario, Royal Ottawa Hospital, National Defense Medical Center, Brockville Psychiatric Hospital, Elisabeth Bruyere Health Center, Monfort Hospital, Pierre Janet Hospital, North Bay Psychiatric Hospital, Saint Vincent Hospital, Riverside Hospital, Sudbury Algoma Hospital, Sudbury Memorial Hospital, Grace General Hospital, and Queensway-Carleton Hospital. Affiliated research institutions include the Institute of Mental Health Research, The Institute for Rehabilitation Research and Development, The Loeb Medical Research Institute, The University of Ottawa Heart Institute Research Center, and the University of Ottawa Eye Institute.

Students

There are eighty-four students in each class. Typically, all but a few are residents of the province of Ontario. About 50 percent of members of the student body are women.

STUDENT LIFE

Medical students benefit from the resources and activities of a large university and an urban environment. Student clubs and organizations exist within the medical school and the greater university. Support services such as counseling, child care, health care, and academic assistance are available to medical students. On-campus housing is offered.

GRADUATES

Graduates enter both clinical medicine and research-oriented careers. Graduate-level medical training is offered at Ottawa in most clinical fields.

Admissions

REQUIREMENTS

To be eligible for admissions, applicants must have successfully completed three years of full-time university studies in any undergraduate program that leads to a bachelor's degree, including one year of general biology, one year of humanities or social sciences, and two years of some combination of biochemistry, general chemistry, and organic chemistry. The MCAT is no longer required. Only Canadian citizens or permanent residents are accepted, with the exception of eligible children of alumni.

SUGGESTIONS

The Admissions Committee primarily considers eligible candidates who have maintained a weighted average of at least a B+ in the last three years of their undergraduate university studies. Priority is given to Franco-Ontarians, Aboriginal applicants, residents of under serviced areas, bona fide residents of the Ottawa-Outaouais region, Ontario residents, and residents of other provinces. In recent entering classes, about 20 percent of all applicants were accepted.

PROCESS

After a written application is submitted, supporting materials and an interview will be requested of applicants with acceptable academic records. The interview is used to further screen applicants. Documents for application to the first year of medicine are available through the faculty or through OMSAS (Ontario Medical School Application Service). Kits are available in July of the preceding year from: OMSAS, PO Box 1328, 650 Woodlawn Road West, Block C, Guelph, Ontario N1H 7P4. Applications must be completed and returned by October 15.

COSTS AND AID

Tuition & Fees

Tuition (in/out)	$4,266/$8,700
Fees	$373

University of Pennsylvania
School of Medicine

Director of Admissions, Edward J. Stemmler Hall, Suite 100, Philadelphia, PA 19104 • Admission: 215-898-8001 • Fax: 215-573-6645 • E-mail: admiss@mail.med.upenn.edu • Website: www.med.upenn.edu

STUDENT BODY

Type	Private
Enrollment	698
% male/female	57/43
% underrepresented minorities	16
# applied (total/out)	7,465/6,614
# accepted (total/out)	4/4
Average age	24

ADMISSIONS

Application Information

Regular application	11/15
Regular notification	3/1
Are transfers accepted?	Yes
Admissions may be deferred?	Yes
Interview required?	No
Application fee	$55

Academics

The four-year curriculum is organized into five modules, some of which overlap. Patient contact begins on day one, and clinical rotations begin midway through the second year. Research and scholarly projects are encouraged and may be pursued in a wide variety of areas, including biomedical science, clinical medicine, behavioral science, and public health related fields. For qualified students, combined MS/PhD and MD/master's degree programs are available. Among other disciplines, graduate degrees may be earned in cell and molecular biology, neuroscience, chemical/structural biology and biophysics, immunology, pharmacological sciences, psychology, bioengineering, epidemiology, health care systems, public policy and management, history and sociology of science, and philosophy. Another option is a joint MD/MBA in conjunction with the Wharton School of Business. Grades of pass and fail are used to evaluate students during module one, and grades of honors, high pass, pass, and fail are used during the remaining modules.

BASIC SCIENCES: Basic sciences are taught primarily through an integrated organ/disease system model, which is correlated with clinical examples and hands-on experiences. Module one occupies the first semester and is devoted to core principles. courses are developmental and molecular biology; cellular physiology, metabolism, and pharmacological processes; human body structure and function; host defenses; and pharmacological responses. Module two is called integrative systems and disease and is organized around body or organ systems; it spans the second semester of the first year and the first semester of the second year. Body and organ systems are cardiology/pulmonary, skin/connective tissue/musculoskeletal/hematology/oncology, gastrointestinal and nutrition, brain and behavior, and endocrinology and reproduction. Throughout the entire first-year-and-a-half, students are introduced to clinical medicine in module three, the technology, art, and practice of medicine. In addition to providing training in basic clinical techniques, module three addresses ethics, technological issues, population-based medicine, public health, and humanistic perspectives. Classroom instruction is enhanced by various academic resources, including multimedia, video, and computerized instructional programs. The Biomedical Science Library houses over 100,000 volumes and receives more than 2,000 periodicals.

CLINICAL TRAINING

Students rotate through required clerkships during module four, which covers the second semester of year two and the first semester of year three. These are internal medicine (nine weeks), family medicine (three weeks), obstetrics/gynecology (six weeks), pediatrics (six weeks), surgery/anesthesia (nine weeks), emergency medicine (three weeks), and psychiatry/substance abuse (six weeks), neurology (three weeks), and clinical specialists (three weeks). Module five begins in the second semester of year three and continues until graduation at the end of year four. It includes a subinternship, advanced electives, and a required three-month scholarly or research experience. A large portion of clinical training takes place at the Hospital of the University of Pennsylvania, also the site of research institutions and labs. Other training sites are Children's Hospital of Philadelphia, Veterans' Affairs of Philadelphia Hospitals, Phoenixville Hospital, Penn Medicine at Radnor, Chestnut Hill Health Care, Chester County Hospital, Friends Hospital, Holy Redeemer Health System, and the Presbyterian-University of Pennsylvania Medical Center.

Students

The student body at U. Penn is nationally represented. About 16 percent of students are underrepresented minorities, and about 20 percent of students took significant time off after college. Class size is 150.

STUDENT LIFE

Grades of pass and fail in the first semester contribute to the high degree of cooperation among students. U. Penn, a comprehensive private university, offers a wide variety of extracurricular activities on and around campus, and students are involved both in school and community organizations. Medical students have access to all recreational facilities, including athletic centers. Philadelphia is an important urban center and is also the home of a very large number of universities. The student community is vast, and the city serves the student community well. Other metropolitan areas such as New York, Baltimore, and Washington, DC, are easily accessible by train, and mountains and beaches are a short drive away. The Graduate Towers and High Rise North is a university-owned graduate student apartment complex available to medical students. However, most students choose to live off campus.

GRADUATES

During a recent three-year period, the most prevalent residency programs selected were medicine (19 percent of graduates), surgical specialties (19 percent), general surgery (6 percent), pediatrics (12 percent), family practice (3 percent), obstetrics/gynecology (3 percent), orthopedics (5 percent), radiology (6 percent), emergency medicine (7 percent), and psychiatry (4 percent).

Admissions

REQUIREMENTS

Applicants must complete a course of study that leads to a baccalaureate degree at an accredited college or university. No prerequisites are specified, although the MCAT is required, which suggests that students should have preparation in science courses. Penn recommends that applicants submit MCAT scores from the spring, but no later than the summer, of the calendar year prior to entrance.

SUGGESTIONS

Recommended undergraduate preparation includes courses in biology, chemistry, organic chemistry, physics, math, history, philosophy, ethics, anthropology, political science, and economics. Students who have taken time off after college are advised to demonstrate recent course work. Experience in hospitals, clinics, or community service projects is important.

PROCESS

All AMCAS applicants receive secondary applications, of which about 20 percent are interviewed between October and February. Interviews consist of two sessions: one with a student and one with a faculty member. On interview day, candidates tour the campus, attend group informational sessions, and have the opportunity to informally meet with students. About 20 percent of interviewed candidates are accepted. Wait-listed candidates may send additional information to update their files.

Admissions Requirements (Required)

MCAT scores, science GPA, non-science GPA, letters of recommendation, state residency, extracurricular activities, exposure to medical profession.

Admissions Requirements (Optional)

interview, essays/personal statement.

COSTS AND AID

Tuition	$34,482
Room and board	$7,975
Cost of books	$1,040
Fees	$2,032

Financial Aid

% students receiving aid	80
Average debt	$80,000

UNIVERSITY OF PITTSBURGH
SCHOOL OF MEDICINE

OFFICE OF ADMISSIONS, 518 SCAIFE HALL, PITTSBURGH, PA 15261 • ADMISSION: 412-648-9891 • FAX: 412-648-8768 • E-MAIL: ADMISSIONS@MEDSCHOOL.PITT.EDU • WEBSITE: WWW.MEDSCHOOL.PITT.EDU

STUDENT BODY

Type	Public
Enrollment	592
% male/female	52/48
% underrepresented minorities	9
# applied (total/out)	4,722/3,745
# accepted (total/out)	8/6
# enrolled (out)	24

FACULTY

Total faculty (number)	1,400
# student/faculty ratio	3:1

ADMISSIONS

Application Information

Regular application	11/1
Regular notification	10/15 until filled
Early application	6/1-8/1
Early notification	10/1
Are transfers accepted?	Yes
Admissions may be deferred?	Yes
Interview required?	No
Application fee	$60

Academics

The four-year curriculum encourages personal interaction among students, between faculty and students, and between patients and students. Students can obtain joint master's degrees in medical ethics and public health with nearby Carnegie-Mellon University. The MSTP-funded MS/PhD is offered in conjunction with Carnegie-Mellon Uniersity.

BASIC SCIENCES: During the first two years, students take classes that are grouped into blocks. Year one has four blocks: the patient-doctor block, which covers ethical, behavioral, and sociological issues related to medicine; the basic science block, which covers the biological elements of medicine; the organ systems block, which includes host defenses and the musculoskeletal system; and the introduction to patient care block, which encompasses physical diagnosis. The blocks are synchronized so that single topics are approached in an interdisciplinary way. The blocks in year two are patient-doctor relationship, patient care, and organ systems, which includes the following systems: homeostasis, digestion, endocrine, dermatology, reproductive, and neuroscience. As in year one, the blocks are planned to complement each other. The final segment of year two integrates all the organ systems and, while doing so, reviews important points of the previous two years. Lectures, small group sessions, conferences, labs, and tutorials are the instructional methods used during the first two years, and students are in a structured learning environment for about twenty-eight hours per week. Problem-based learning is used with most instructional methods. With the exception of clinical work, instruction is given in Scaife Hall, a renovated building with classrooms, labs, and a library, which has 220,000 volumes and subscribes to the major online medical informational services. Grades during the first two years are honors, pass, and fail. The USMLE Steps 1 and 2 are required for graduation.

CLINICAL TRAINING

Patient contact begins in year one during the patient care block. Third-year rotations begin in July immediately following year two. These are ambulatory subspecialties (six weeks, includes dermatology, neurosurgery, ophthalmology, orthopedics, otolaryngology, pediatric surgery, plastic surgery, and urology), family medicine (four weeks), obstetrics/gynecology (six weeks), pediatrics (eight weeks), psychiatry (six weeks), surgery (six weeks), and elective (four weeks). The fourth year is made up solely of selectives and electives. Clinical training takes place at the University Health Center, which is composed of five major hospitals: the Presbyterian University Hospital, Montefiore Hospital, the Eye and Ear Institute, the Western Psychiatric Institute, and the University of Pittsburgh Cancer Institute. The passing rate for students at the University of Pittsburgh on both parts of the USMLE is higher than that for medical schools nationally, and for the past two years 100 percent of all students passed both Step 1 and 2.

Students

About 9 percent of students are underrepresented minorities, most of whom are African Americans. Approximately half of the students in each class are Pennsylvania residents. There is a large age range within the student body, and many students took some time off before entering medical school. Class size is 148.

STUDENT LIFE

The structure of the curriculum promotes student interaction and collegiality. In addition, medical students get to know each other through involvement in organizations and extracurricular activities. Some of the many student groups on campus are Pitt Women in Medicine, the Christian Medical Society, and the History of Medicine Society. Medical students have access to all facilities of the University of Pittsburgh, including athletic facilities. Pittsburgh is an accessible and exciting city, and, although on-campus housing is available, most medical students choose to live off campus.

GRADUATES

Graduates are successful in gaining admittance to some of most prestigious residency programs in the country. In 1999, 78 percent of the graduating class obtained one of their top three choices in the National Residency Matching Program. About 50 percent of graduates enter primary care fields.

Admissions

REQUIREMENTS

Requirements are one year each of biology, physics, chemistry, and organic chemistry, all with associated labs, and English. In assessing grades, consideration is given to the candidate's undergraduate institution and the course load they took. The MCAT is required and must be no more than three years old.

SUGGESTIONS

Competence in math is valued as is evidence of success in social science and humanities courses. The University of Pittsburgh looks for interpersonal skills and commitment to community service in applicants. For applicants who graduated college several years ago, some recent course work is advised.

PROCESS

Secondary applications are sent selectively to AMCAS applicants. About 20 percent of Pennsylvania residents, and 10 percent of out-of-state residents, are interviewed. Interviews are conducted from September through April and consist of two sessions: one with a faculty member and one with a medical student. Notification occurs toward the end of February. Wait-listed candidates may send additional information to strengthen their applications and to indicate interest in the school.

Admissions Requirements (Required)

MCAT scores, state residency, essays/personal statement, exposure to medical profession.

Admissions Requirements (Optional)

science GPA, nonscience GPA, letters of recommendation, interview, extracurricular activities.

COSTS AND AID

In-state tuition	$30,084
Out-of-state tuition	$35,876
Cost of books	$2,000
Fees	$600

Financial Aid

% students receiving aid	26
Average grant	$6,626
Average loan	$3,000
Average debt	$74,952

University of Puerto Rico
College of Health Related Professions

College of Health Related Professions, PO Box 365067, San Juan, PR, 00936-5067 •
Admissions: 787-758-2525, ext. 5211• Fax: 787-282-7117

STUDENT BODY

Type	Public
# applied (total/out)	970/624

ADMISSIONS

Application Information

Regular application	12/1
Regular notification	3/31
Admissions may be deferred?	Yes
Interview required?	Yes
Application fee	$15

Academics

Medical training is accomplished through a variety of educational experiences, both in the classroom and at multiple service settings in the public and private sectors of Puerto Rico. Medical students benefit from the resources of other health professional schools and from interaction with students at other schools. Through the Center for International Health, medical students gain exposure to the research and policy issues surrounding global health. Grades of A through F are used to evaluate medical students in all courses.

BASIC SCIENCES: Basic sciences are taught using a combination of lectures, small group discussions, labs, and exposure to clinical correlates. Required first year course are medical gross anatomy, medical histology, medical embryology, medical neuroscience, introduction to biochemistry, human physiology, human development I, public health and preventive medicine I, integration seminar I, behavioral sciences, and introduction to clinical diagnosis. Second year courses consist of pathobiology-introduction to laboratory medicine, infectious diseases, medical pharmacology, fundamentals of clinical diagnosis, human development II, public health and preventive medicine II, basic clinical clerkship, mechanisms of disease, psychopathology, and integration seminar II. Outside of the classroom, students learn in the Learning Resources Center, the Standardized Patient Laboratory, and the Clinical Learning Laboratory.

CLINICAL TRAINING

The third year consists of clinical rotations. These are radiology (two weeks), psychiatry (four weeks), medicine (twelve weeks), family medicine (four weeks), pediatrics (ten weeks), surgery (ten weeks), and obstetrics/gynecology (six weeks). During year four, clerkships are dermatology (one week), physical medicine and rehabilitation (one week), public health (three weeks), legal, ethical, and administrative aspects in medicine (one week), and selective clerkships (eight weeks). In addition, eighteen weeks are open for clinical and research electives. Clinical education uses a variety of settings including University Hospital, University Pediatric Hospital, San Juan City Hospital, Veterans' Administration Hospital, and the Oncology Hospital. In addition, the school uses certain private hospitals, clinics, and public health facilities. Some electives may be taken at institutions other than those affiliated with the University of Puerto Rico, such as hospitals in other regions of Puerto Rico and in other countries.

Students

Each entering class has about 100 students. Students come from foreign countries and the mainland United States as well as Puerto Rico. Fifty percent of students are women.

STUDENT LIFE

Recreational facilities on campus include the sports and gym center. The medical school promotes student health through its exercise/wellness program and by sponsoring a range of student activities and events. When they have free time, medical students enjoy the city of San Juan and its surroundings.

GRADUATES

The University of Puerto Rico and its affiliated hospitals offer residency programs in most major medical fields.

Admissions

REQUIREMENTS

With few exceptions, entering students must have completed their bachelor's degree. Prerequisite courses are one year each of biology, general chemistry, physics, and organic chemistry. The MCAT is required, and August in the year prior to admission is the latest acceptable test date.

SUGGESTIONS

Both residents of Puerto Rico and nonresidents are considered for admission. Grade point average and MCAT scores are important in admissions decisions. In addition to academic credentials, the University of Puerto Rico looks for integrity and motivation in its students.

PROCESS

All applicants are encouraged to visit the campus. Candidates for the MD program must submit an application by December 1. Candidates who qualify are invited to interview after their applications are reviewed. Final decisions and notifications are made throughout the year and are completed in the spring.

COSTS AND AID

Tuition & Fees

Tuition (in/out)	$5,000/$10,500
Fees	$844

University of Rochester
School of Medicine and Dentistry

Medical Center Box 601A, Rochester, NY 14642 • Admission: 585-275-4539 • Fax: 585-756-5479 •
E-mail: mdadmish@urmc.rochester.edu • Website: www.urmc.rochester.edu/smd/admiss

STUDENT BODY

Type	Private
Enrollment	433
% male/female	46/54
% underrepresented minorities	14
# applied (total/out)	3,434/2,514
# accepted (total/out)	275/191
# enrolled (total/out)	100/58
Average age	24

FACULTY

Total faculty (number)	1,317
% female	33
% minority	3
% part-time	10
# student/faculty ratio	3:1

ADMISSIONS

Average GPA and MCAT Scores

Overall GPA	3.6
MCAT Bio	10.64
MCAT Phys	10.5
MCAT Verbal	10.05
MCAT Essay	P

Application Information

Regular application	10/15
Regular notification	11/1
Are transfers accepted?	No
Admissions may be deferred?	Yes
Interview required?	Yes
Application fee	$75

Academics

Special emphasis is placed on skills acquisition and use, with a commitment to lifelong learning. Sensitivity to the world of the patient is encompassed in the biopsychosocial integration of the curriculum and the learning experience, with mechanisms in place for continuous curricular improvement through the collaboration of students and faculty. The curriculum ensures adequate and early electivity for students to enhance their special interests and provides students with rigorous training and assessment of all of the competencies demanded by modern medical practice; thus, it generates a knowledge base characterized by depth, breadth, rigor, and flexibility. Students who are interested in careers in medical science may participate in the fully-funded medical scientist training program (MS/PhD) or in joint degree programs, including the MPH/MD and M.BA/MD program in health care management in conjunction with the William E. Simon Graduate School of Business Administration. Vacation and full-year fellowships facilitate student research or international medicine experiences. Evaluation of student performance uses grades of satisfactory or fail, except in the required clerkships, where grades of honors, high pass, pass, and fail are used. Passing the USMLE is not required for promotion to the third year.

BASIC SCIENCES: An introductory module at the beginning of the first year prepares students in the acquisition, management, and presentation of medical information. Students learn how to meet the challenges of active and independent learning by becoming competent in data management, information technology, and critical evaluation of the medical literature. Every course is interdisciplinary; basic sciences are integrated with one another and basic and clinical sciences are woven together as the strands of the double helix curriculum throughout the four years. Clinical skills training from day one leads not to shadowing or preceptor experiences in clinics, but rather to real clinical work as part of the health care team. Not only paper cases but also students' actual clinical cases drive the learning of science through the school-wide use of multidisciplinary problem-based learning (PBL) cases. Three two-hour PBL tutorials per week and an average of no more than ten hours of lecture per week, with adequate time for self-study, and the use of labs, conferences, seminars, and computer-assisted learning all characterize the classroom setting of the curriculum. Electives are available during all four years, including electives in medical humanities, international medicine, and community outreach programs. The Edward G. Miner Library holds over 225,000 volumes and a modern, computer-based learning resource center.

CLINICAL TRAINING

Beginning in year one, students complete their introduction to clinical medicine in the fall and then participate in an ambulatory clerkship experience beginning in the spring. This experience, unlike any other in the country, includes all the ambulatory components of family medicine, pediatrics, internal medicine, women's health, psychiatry, and ambulatory surgery, and is completed by the end of the second year. Inpatient clerkships are completed by December of the fourth year and focus on acute illness experiences in adult medicine, women's and children's health, mind/brain/behavior, and urgent/emergent care. Strong Memorial Hospital (700 beds) is the principal site for clinical teaching, along with a newly completed Ambulatory Care Center and five affiliated hospitals (2,000 beds), which cover acute and chronic care.

Students

Students come from all regions of the country. About 13 percent are underrepresented minorities. The average age of incoming students is twenty-four; one-third have majored in areas outside the sciences, and 100 students are accepted each year.

STUDENT LIFE

Most medical students lead active lives outside of the classroom. Many of them participate in community outreach programs, international medicine electives, and student organizations and events. Students have access to resources of the university campus and athletic facilities in the medical center. Located on the southern shore of Lake Ontario, in the Finger Lakes wine-producing region of upstate New York, Rochester is a progressive, metropolitan community of more than one million people. Rochester has a rich cultural life, is an affordable and friendly city, and is a haven for boaters and other outdoor enthusiasts.

GRADUATES

Among the 2001 graduates, the most popular residencies were internal medicine (34 percent), pediatrics (18 percent), surgery (4 percent), emergency medicine (4 percent), obstetrics/gynecology (4 percent), family medicine (4 percent), anesthesiology (4 percent), orthopaedics (4 percent), ENT (4 percent) and ophthamaology (4 percent). About 15 percent stayed in the Rochester area, while an additional 27 percent remained in New York State. The remainder went to twenty-five other states.

Admissions

REQUIREMENTS

Prerequisite science courses are one year of biology, physics, general chemistry, and organic chemistry, all associated with labs. One semester of biochemistry may be substituted for one semester of organic chemistry. One year of English or expository writing is also required. Rochester belongs to AMCAS, and the MCAT exam is required; scores should be from the past three years. The best set of scores is considered.

SUGGESTIONS

In addition to required science courses, 12 to 16 credit hours in the humanities and/or social sciences are required. Experiences in research, clinical settings, and the community are strongly recommended. Rochester looks for evidence of leadership, excellent interpersonal skills, a love of learning, appreciation of diversity, and outstanding scholarship.

PROCESS

Rochester is an AMCAS school. About 10 percent of applicants are interviewed between September and February. Interviews consist of two sessions with faculty, and applicants have a tour, lunch with current students, and a financial aid presentation. About 35 percent of the interviewed applicants are offered acceptance and are notified between November and the end of May. About fifteen positions in each class are reserved for students from several programs such as the Rochester Early Medical Scholar program and the Bryn Mawr post-baccalaureate program.

Admissions Requirements (Required)

MCAT scores, science GPA, non-science GPA, letters of recommendation, interview, essays/personal statement, extracurricular activities, exposure to medical profession.

Admissions Requirements (Optional)

state residency.

Overlap Schools

Cornell University, Harvard University, SUNY at Stony Brook University, SUNY Upstate Medical University, SUNY at Buffalo, University of California, Hastings.

COSTS AND AID

Tuition	$31,500
Cost of books	$1,500
Fees	$2,817

Financial Aid

% students receiving aid	92
Average grant	$1,206
Average loan	$28,436
Average debt	$124,816

UNIVERSITY OF SASKATCHEWAN
COLLEGE OF MEDICINE

B103 HEALTH SCIENCE BUILDING, 107 WIGGINS ROAD, SASKATOON, SK, CANADA • ADMISSION: 306-966-8554 • FAX: 306-966-6164 • E-MAIL: MED.ADMISSIONS@USASK.CA • WEBSITE: WWW.USASK.CA/MEDICINE

STUDENT BODY

Type	Public
Enrollment	60
% male/female	42/58
# applied (total)	27
# accepted (total/out)	60/7
# enrolled (total/out)	60/7
Average age	23

FACULTY

Total faculty (number)	228
% female	28
# student/faculty ratio	1:1

ADMISSIONS

Average GPA and MCAT Scores

MCAT Bio	9.7
MCAT Phys	9.6
MCAT Verbal	9.7
MCAT Essay	P

Application Information

Regular application	1/15
Regular notification	6/1
Are transfers accepted?	No
Admissions may be deferred?	Yes
Interview required?	Yes
Application fee	$40

Academics

The goal of the College of Medicine is to enable medical students to develop the knowledge, skills, values, and attitudes that will serve as a foundation for subsequent education in primary and specialty patient care and research. In its curriculum, the college promotes the integration of basic and clinical sciences. Independent learning, problem solving, and early patient interaction are emphasized. The curriculum is divided into four phases. For the most part, basic science instruction occurs during the first three phases. However, basic science and clinical training are integrated throughout the four-year curriculum.

BASIC SCIENCES: Phase A (one year) consists of thirty-three weeks and includes the introductory study of basic sciences, the history of medicine, professional skills (includes two-week community experience), and life cycle and humanities. Instruction in basic sciences is interdisciplinary, covering fundamental principles of anatomy, physiology, biochemistry, and microbiology. Instruction in the basic sciences continues into phase B (one year) which lasts thirty-three weeks. Subjects include pathology, microbiology, and pharmacology. Also included in phase B is clinical sciences, systems, and genetics. Phase C consists of only fifteen weeks and is a continuation of clinical sciences and systems, but also includes the linking courses, microbiology, and community health and epidemiology.

CLINICAL TRAINING

Phase D (sixteen months) is a discipline-based rotation clerkship that builds on the clinical training and offers students the opportunity to study clinical electives (twelve weeks) and specialty fields. Teaching hospitals are Royal University Hospital, St. Paul's Hospital, Saskatoon City Hospital, Regina General Hospital, and Pasqua Hospital.

Students

The maximum size of entering classes is sixty students. Typically, 90 percent of students are from the province of Saskatchewan. In general, about 50 percent of students are women.

STUDENT LIFE

With a relatively small student body and a curriculum that encourages interaction, students are generally cohesive. Between the medical school and the greater university, a wide variety of extracurricular activities and events are offered. Medical students live both on and off campus.

GRADUATES

Although research is an increasingly important activity for the College of Medicine, a large number of graduates become practicing clinical physicians in the province of Saskatchewan.

Admissions

REQUIREMENTS

A minimum of two years of undergraduate work is required. In general, prerequisites are biochemistry, biology, chemistry, organic chemistry, physics, English, social sciences, and humanities. Incoming students should also have an academic average of 70 percent in prerequisite courses to be considered for admission. Overall academic averages must be at least 78 percent. The MCAT must be taken and a minimum score of 8 in all sections is required.

SUGGESTIONS

Criteria for selection are academic performance and personal qualities. Academic performance is based on applicants' two best full undergraduate years of study. Personal qualities are assessed primarily in the interview. To be competitive academically, an overall two year average of over 80 percent is required.

PROCESS

Application forms may be obtained from the admissions secretary after July 1 or from the Internet at the address above. Applications from Saskatchewan residents must be postmarked no later than January 15. Applications from out-of-province residents must be post-marked no later than December 1. Interviews are approximately forty-five minutes and occur during a weekend in March. The applicant is interviewed by a team of four, including a medical doctor, a faculty member, a medical student, and a community member. Three letters of reference are also considered. All candidates are notified of their acceptance by the end of June.

Admissions Requirements (Required)

MCAT scores, science GPA, non-science GPA, letters of recommendation, interview, state residency.

Admissions Requirements (Optional)

essays/personal statement, extracurricular activities, exposure to medical profession.

Overlap Schools

University of Alberta, University of Calgary.

COSTS AND AID

Tuition	$7,930
Room and board	$4,832
Cost of books	$1,700

UNIVERSITY OF SHERBROOKE

2500 BOULEVARD UNIVERSITÉ SHERBROOKE, QC, J1K 2R1 • ADMISSION: 819-821-7000 •
WEBSITE: WWW.USHERB.CA/

STUDENT BODY

Type	Public
# applied (total/out)	1,401/199

ADMISSIONS

Application Information

Regular application	3/1
Regular notification	5/1–8/1
Admissions may be deferred?	No
Interview required?	No
Application fee	$30

Academics

Sherbrooke offers a four-year curriculum that leads to the MD degree. Educational methodology is based on small group discussions, case studies, audiovisual and computer assisted learning, and hands-on clinical experiences. Combined degree programs such as the MD/MSc program are open to highly qualified students who have an interest in research.

BASIC SCIENCES: The first academic period begins in late August and spans thirty-nine weeks. In general, students are in class or other scheduled session for approximately thirty hours per week. Courses are introduction to MD program, biological medicine I and II, clinical immersion, growth development and aging, nervous system, locomoter system, pscyhosocial sciences, preventive medicine and community health, integration, and clinical skills. The second year is organized into blocks based on anatomical/physiological systems. These are cardiovascular system, respiratory system, urinary system, gastrointestinal system, hemato-immunologic system, infectious disease, endocrine system, reproductive system, and human sexuality. In addition, students take part in a rotation in community hospitals and a course in clinical skills.

CLINICAL TRAINING

The third and fourth years are organized into several components. These are required courses, required primary clerkships, rotations in community, elective programs, integration period, and final exam. Required courses are interdisciplinary concepts, clinical skills, and introduction to clerkships. The required primary clerkships are medicine (ten-and-a-half weeks), surgery (seven weeks), pediatrics (seven weeks), psychiatry (seven weeks), obstetrics/gynecology (seven weeks), and multidisciplinary (anesthesia, ophthalmology, dermatology, ORL, three-and-a-half weeks). Rotations in community consist of family medicine and emergency (seven weeks) and community health (four weeks). The elective program lasts twelve weeks, followed by the integration period (six weeks) and the final exam period (one week). Teaching hospitals are Cuse Fleurimont, Cuse Bowen, Hopital Charles Le Moyne, and Hopital Sainte-Croix.

Students

Each entering class has approximately 105 students. About 80 percent of students are from the Province of Quebec. Women account for 60 percent of students.

STUDENT LIFE

The University of Sherbrooke is a large university with many social, recreational, and other extracurricular activities for medical students. Medical students have both on-campus and off-campus housing options.

GRADUATES

Many graduates enter one of the residency programs offered at hospitals affiliated with Sherbrooke.

Admissions

REQUIREMENTS

Fluency in French is required. The minimum requirement for admissions is two years of university or a BA degree. Prerequisites are general biology (one year), general chemistry (one year), organic chemistry (one year), physics (three semesters), and mathematics through calculus. The MCAT is not required.

SUGGESTIONS

In addition to prerequisite courses, students should complete course work in the humanities and in the social sciences. Priority is given to residents of Quebec, and eighty-six positions in each entering class are reserved for this group of applicants. Fifteen additional places are reserved for applicants from New Brunswick, one place is reserved for an applicant from Prince Edward Island, one for an applicant from Nova Scotia, and two places are available for qualified foreign applicants. Overall, about 5 percent of applicants are admitted each year.

PROCESS

Applications are available from the Admissions Office at the address above. Following review of applications, qualified candidates are invited to a learning skills test (THAMUS).

COSTS AND AID

Tuition & Fees

Tuition and fees (in/out)
$3,127/$15,127

UNIVERSITY OF SOUTH ALABAMA

UNIVERSITY OF SOUTH ALABAMA COLLEGE OF MEDICINE

OFFICE OF ADMISSIONS, 241 CSAB, MOBILE, AL 36688 • ADMISSION: 251-460-7176 • FAX: 251-460-6278 • E-MAIL: MSCOTT@USOUTHAL.EDU • WEBSITE: WWW.USOUTHAL.EDU/USA/DEPS-GRD.HTML

STUDENT BODY

Type	Public
Enrollment	256
% male/female	54/46
% underrepresented minorities	14
# applied (total/out)	766/378
# accepted (total/out)	112/11
# enrolled (total/out)	64/9
Average age	24

FACULTY

Total faculty (number)	300
% female	30
% minority	10
% part-time	9
# student/faculty ratio	1:1

ADMISSIONS

Average GPA and MCAT Scores

Overall GPA	3.7
MCAT Bio	10
MCAT Phys	9.5
MCAT Verbal	10
MCAT Essay	0

Application Information

Regular application	11/15
Regular notification	rolling
Early application	6/1-8/1
Early notification	10/1
Are transfers accepted?	Yes
Admissions may be deferred?	Yes
Interview required?	Yes
Application fee	$50

Academics

The curriculum is semitraditional and uses a lecture format for most of the preclinical instruction. Although some early clinical exposure is offered, during the first two years, the program focuses on ensuring a solid understanding of the basic sciences. Students can combine medical and doctorate studies if they pursue a PhD degree in a medically related discipline. About one-quarter of the class enters the School of Medicine via a combined undergraduate/medical school program that is open to both Alabama and out-of-state high school seniors.

BASIC SCIENCES: The school operates on a quarter system. During the first year, lecture courses are gross anatomy, histology, developmental anatomy, physiology, neuroanatomy, and biochemistry. Generally, students are in lecture for about twenty-five hours per week. The course medical ethics is taught by using both lecture and small group format. Medical practice and society and physical diagnosis use lectures and a case-based approach. During the second year, traditional lecture/lab courses include microbiology, pharmacology, pathology, and genetics. Introduction to behavioral sciences and a course covering principles of public health are also part of the curriculum. In addition, students take part in weekly sessions in clinical settings, as part of an introductory course in clinical medicine. Basic sciences are taught in the medical sciences building, which contains administrative offices, classrooms, and laboratories. The Biomedical Library houses 65,000 volumes and offers computer and online services. Grades of A through F are used to evaluate medical students in most of their courses, and promotions are based not only on grades but also on faculty evaluation of students' ethical and personal maturity. Medical students are involved in the schools' administrative affairs through an elected student governing body, which also participates in issues relating to the greater university. The schedule for the first two years is relatively firm, and students are encouraged to focus on their studies, rather than on pursuing employment or other activities during this period. The USMLE Step 1 is required following the basic science portion of study.

CLINICAL TRAINING

Year three is composed entirely of the following required clerkships: medicine (twelve weeks), surgery (eight weeks), obstetrics/gynecology (eight weeks), psychiatry (six weeks), pediatrics (eight weeks), and family practice (six weeks). The fourth year is also forty-eight weeks but is composed of elective rather than required rotations. Students must select a one-month rotation from each broad field from the following: neuroscience, surgical subspecialties, ambulatory care, primary care, and in-house elective. Students train at university-affiliated hospitals that together constitute the largest medical complex along the Gulf Coast and that contain a total of 880 beds. All levels of trauma care and surgery are available, and patients come not only from around the state but also from neighboring states. In downtown Mobile, the Children's and Women's Hospital offers clinical rotations in pediatric services and neonatal care. The hospital system serves managed care clients, among others, thus ensuring a client base. Cancer research and treatment, organic transplant, aeromedical transport, and preventative care are a few of the noteworthy services available through the university network. Students receive grades of A through F for clinical performance during required rotations and grades of honors, pass, and fail during elective rotations. The USMLE Step 2 is required for graduation. Few students take part in rotations at out-of-state institutions or overseas.

Students

At least 90 percent of medical students must be Alabama residents. Reflecting the state's demographics, about 9 percent are underrepresented minorities, most of whom are African American. Each year, about fifteen students enter who have taken time off after college. The student body is diverse in terms of undergraduate majors and class size is relatively small, at sixty-five-seventy students.

STUDENT LIFE

Students take advantage of the university campus with its recreational facilities and activities. Students also use nearby municipal recreational facilities, which include a golf course. The School of Medicine provides opportunities for students to participate in medically related projects and events such as volunteer activities and special seminars. University housing consists of more than 700 two- and three-bedroom houses, appropriate for married students, in an area adjacent to the campus. Furnished dormitories provide living accommodations that are within walking distance of the medical school. In addition to the typical medical student associations, the Military Medical Students Society operates a chapter on campus.

GRADUATES

Of the graduating class of 1997, 66 percent chose primary care specialties, 18 percent went into internal medicine, 35 percent into family medicine, 11 percent into pediatrics, and 2 percent chose medicine/pediatrics. Obstetrics/gynecology, pathology, and surgery were also popular choices.

Admissions

REQUIREMENTS

Requirements are one year each of general chemistry, organic chemistry, biology, and physics, all with associated labs, and one year each of math, humanities, and English. In total, ninety semester hours of undergraduate course work are required. The quality of the undergraduate institution is considered in evaluating GPA. Generally, courses taken abroad are not counted. The MCAT is required and should be no more than three years old. The most recent score is considered, and there is no preference between the April and August MCAT.

SUGGESTIONS

Preferably, the math requirement should be fulfilled with calculus. Nontraditional students who have taken time off after college are advised to demonstrate recent course work, particularly in the sciences. The goal of the Admissions Committee is to select candidates who have the potential to address the wide spectrum of needs faced by the medical profession, which suggests that diverse backgrounds are valued in addition to medically related experience. Because spots are few, out-of-state candidates should be competitive on a national level.

PROCESS

All Alabama residents receive a secondary application, which is sent upon receipt of the AMCAS application. About one-quarter of out-of-state residents receive a secondary. The secondary application is due on November 15, but the School of Medicine advises applicants to submit it as soon as possible. Fifty percent of Alabama residents and about 10 percent of out-of-state residents are interviewed. Interviews are held on campus from September through March. Students receive three thirty-minute interviews, which may vary in format. The interview day provides applicants and faculty an opportunity to become acquainted and is considered a two-way process. Of those interviewed, about 30 percent are accepted and 20 percent are placed on a ranked wait-list. Candidates are accepted on a weekly basis, beginning in December.

Admissions Requirements (Required)

MCAT scores, science GPA, non-science GPA, letters of recommendation, interview, essays/personal statement, extracurricular activities, exposure to medical profession.

Admissions Requirements (Optional)

state residency.

COSTS AND AID

In-state tuition	$10,500
Out-of-state tuition	$21,000
Cost of books	$2,500
Fees	$1,400

Financial Aid

% students receiving aid	90
Average grant	$5,000
Average loan	$25,000
Average debt	$89,000

University of South Carolina
School of Medicine

Admissions Office, Columbia, SC 29208 • Admission: 803-733-3325 • Fax: 803-733-3328 •
E-mail: mills@gw.med.sc.edu • Website: www.med.sc.edu

STUDENT BODY

Type	Public
Enrollment	297
% male/female	53/47
% underrepresented minorities	20
# applied (total/out)	1,047/715
# accepted (total/out)	133/19
# enrolled (total/out)	80/10
Average age	23

FACULTY

# student/faculty ratio	1:1

ADMISSIONS

Average GPA and MCAT Scores

Overall GPA	3.5
MCAT Bio	9
MCAT Phys	8
MCAT Verbal	9
MCAT Essay	0

Application Information

Regular application	12/1
Regular notification	10/15
Early application	6/1-8/1
Early notification	10/1
Are transfers accepted?	Yes
Admissions may be deferred?	Yes
Interview required?	Yes
Application fee	$45

Academics

In addition to the MD, the School of Medicine offers the MS and PhD degrees in biomedical science with specialization in anatomy, cell biology, experimental pathology, microbiology and immunology, pharmacology, and physiology. For qualified students, a combined MS/PhD program is possible. A combined MD/MPH program, offered in conjunction with the School of Public Health at USC, is available. Also offered is the MS in genetics counseling, biomedical science with specialization in nurse anesthesia, and rehabilitation counseling. The MD curriculum stresses psychological and social perspectives along with biological principles. Elective opportunities are available throughout all four years to assist students pursue individual interests and career goals. Medical students are evaluated with grades of A through F. Passing Step 1 of the USMLE is a requirement for promotion to year three, and passing Step 2 is a graduation requirement.

BASIC SCIENCES: Throughout the first two years, clinical case studies are correlated with basic science material. The two-year introduction to clinical practice course emphasizes active, independent, and cooperative learning and uses a small group format. Other first-year courses are gross anatomy, microscopic anatomy, biochemistry, neuroanatomy, and physiology. Second-year courses are microbiology, pathology/pathophysiology, and pharmacology. An important resource is the USCSM Library, which has a collection of more than 90,0000 volumes. Medical students also use the USC Thomas Cooper Library, which has more than two-and-a-half million bound volumes.

CLINICAL TRAINING

Clerkship experiences in the third year include eight week rotations in medicine, surgery, obstetrics/gynecology, psychiatry, family medicine, and pediatrics. During the fourth year, required clerkships are four weeks each in neurology and surgery and medicine and a four-week acting internship. A four-week, multidisciplinary rotation concludes undergraduate clinical training and prepares students for the transition to residency and clinical practice. The remainder of the year is reserved for electives and selectives, many of which may be completed at locations around the state, at other medical schools, with federal and state agencies, and through an international elective program. While the majority of students complete core clinical training at the five affiliated hospitals in Columbia, about fifteen students in each class train at the Greenville Hospital System in Greenville, South Carolina. In the Columbia area, teaching hospitals include Palmetto Richland Memorial Hospital (649 beds), Dorn Veterans Hospital (447 beds), and the William S. Hall Psychiatric Institute (270 beds).

Students

Approximately 98 percent of students are South Carolina residents. About 10 percent of students are underrepresented minorities, most of whom are African American. Typically, about 20 percent of students in each entering class are nontraditional, having taken time off or pursued other careers or interests after college.

STUDENT LIFE

Because the School of Medicine is an important component of a comprehensive research university, medical students have many opportunities for interaction with students in other disciplines and can take advantage of the numerous student organizations, intramural sporting events, and social opportunities of the main university. Medical student organizations include chapters of the AMSA and the American Medical Women's Association, in addition to professionally focused groups such as the internal medicine, family practice, emergency medicine, and pediatrics clubs and the psychiatry/behavioral science society. Medical students have initiated a number of community service activities, including participation in the Columbia Free Medical Clinic, tutoring and social events at area children's homes, and the Health Education Leadership Program for primary school students. The School of Medicine has its own fitness center, but medical students also have access to all athletic facilities of the main campus. Columbia is a city with a population of almost 500,000 that provide a wide variety of recreational and cultural activities. Both the ocean and the Great Smoky Mountains are within a few hours drive. On-campus housing is available for married couples, although most students live off campus in the area adjacent to the USC campus.

GRADUATES

Two-thirds of USCSM graduates go on to practice in primary care fields, making the School of Medicine a leader among U.S. medical schools in the percentage of graduates who enter primary care. Although many graduates do enter primary care, USCSM grads match in all specialties all over the United States.

Admissions

REQUIREMENTS

Prerequisites are eight semester hours each of general biology or zoology, inorganic chemistry, organic chemistry, and general physics, all with associated labs. In addition, six semester hours of college-level math and English are required. The MCAT is required, and scores must be no more than five years old. For applicants who have taken the exam more than once, the most recent set of scores is weighed most heavily.

SUGGESTIONS

A maximum of six to eight positions in each class are open to residents of states other than South Carolina. Thus, nonresident applicants should be highly qualified. USCSM looks for applicants who are interested in primary care and who are likely to serve within the state.

PROCESS

All competitive AMCAS applicants who are South Carolina residents are sent secondary applications. About 40 percent of nonresident AMCAS applicants are sent secondaries, of which about 25 percent are interviewed between August and April. Interviews consist of two sessions, each with a member of the Admissions Committee. Candidates also have lunch with medical students and attend informational presentations. Notification of the committee's decision occurs on a rolling basis, beginning in October. Approximately one-third of interviewed candidates are accepted. Other candidates are rejected or put on hold and possibly accepted later in the year.

Admissions Requirements (Required)

MCAT scores, science GPA, non-science GPA, letters of recommendation, interview, essays/personal statement, extracurricular activities, exposure to medical profession.

Admissions Requirements (Optional)

state residency.

Overlap Schools

Medical University of South Carolina.

COSTS AND AID

In-state tuition	$16,900
Out-of-state tuition	$48,870
Room and board	$10,050
Cost of books	$7,000
Fees	$50

Financial Aid

% students receiving aid	95
Average grant	$3,000
Average loan	$25,000
Average debt	$71,352

University of South Dakota

University of South Dakota School of Medicine

Office of Medical Student Affairs, 414 East Clark Street, Vermillion, SD 57069 • Admission: 605-677-6886 • Fax: 605-677-5109 • E-mail: usdsmsa@.usd.edu • Website: http://med.usd.edu

STUDENT BODY

Type	Public
Enrollment	206
% male/female	57/43
% underrepresented minorities	3
# applied (total/out)	421/315
# accepted (total/out)	71/13
# enrolled (total/out)	50/9
Average age	24

FACULTY

Total faculty (number)	809
% part-time	75

ADMISSIONS

Average GPA and MCAT Scores

Overall GPA	3.6
MCAT Bio	8.83
MCAT Phys	8.57
MCAT Verbal	9.17
MCAT Essay	0

Application Information

Regular application	11/15
Regular notification	rolling
Are transfers accepted?	Yes
Admissions may be deferred?	Yes
Interview required?	Yes
Application fee	$35

Academics

Students complete 168 credits during their four-year MD program. They are evaluated with letter and numerical grades. Students must pass USMLE Steps 1 and 2, a school administered OSLE, and must take USMLE Step 2-CS to graduate. During the break between years one and two, medical students have the opportunity to undertake clinical or basic science research projects, arranged through the Summer Research Program. This program teams qualified students with physician/faculty mentors and offers fellowship support.

BASIC SCIENCES: Basic biomedical sciences are taught in the Lee Memorial Medical Science Building on the USD campus in Vermillion. The Lommen Health Sciences Library is also on the Vermillion campus. The basic biomedical sciences are taught by lecture, lab, small group discussions, and case-based presentations, all with an emphasis on clinical correlation. Students are in class or other scheduled sessions for about thirty hours per week. First-year courses are biochemistry, gross anatomy with embryology, histology, neuroscience, physiology, and introduction to clinical medicine (ICM). The ICM course is an interdisciplinary sequence that continues into the second year. During the first year, the Introduction to the Patient: Personal and Professional Issues course focuses on integrating biological, social, and psychological models and introducing the patient in all stages of the life cycle. Students also learn doctor/patient communication skills. Second-year courses are advanced behavorial science, ICM, laboratory medicine, microbiology, and pharmacology. During year two, ICM provides students with experiences in performing comprehensive history and physical examinations on patients in a clinical setting. At the end of year two, students travel to a rural community within the state to take a four-week preceptorship with a family practice physician.

CLINICAL TRAINING

During the third and fourth years, students rotate through hospitals and clinics in Sioux Falls, Rapid City, or Yankton. All students participate in three weeks of clinical colloquium. For the Sioux Falls and Rapid City campuses, the third year consists of six clerkships taken two at a time during three blocks of sixteen weeks. The clerkships may be family medicine paired with general internal medicine, pediatrics and adolescent medicine paired with obstetrics and gynecology, and general surgery paired with psychiatry and neurology. In addition, students take radiology and participate in a weekly primary care ambulatory clinic throughout the year. Alternatively, third-year students may enter a unique, primary care curriculum at the Yankton campus that emphasizes community involvement and self directed learning. The entire twelve months is based in a multidisciplinary clinic, and students follow patients in each of the six specialties throughout the year. Fourth-year required clerkships for all students are family medicine (four weeks), emergency room (four weeks), and surgical specialties (seven weeks). An additional twenty-one weeks are reserved for electives. As a community-based medical school, the School of Medicine neither owns nor operates the clinical facilities utilized by USD for teaching. Rather, the school maintains strong affiliations with a range of health care providers throughout the state, including Rapid City Regional Hospital; Sioux Valley Hospital-University of South Dakota Medical Center and Avera McKennan Hospital (both in Sioux Falls); Avera Sacred Heart Hospital and the Yankton Medical Clinic in Yankton; and Veterans' Affairs Hospitals in Sioux Falls, Fort Meade, and Hot Springs.

Students

All admitted students are either South Dakota residents or have significant personal ties to South Dakota. About 3 percent of students are underrepresented minorities, most of whom are Native Americans. The average age of incoming students is about twenty-four. Class size is fifty.

STUDENT LIFE

The small class size encourages cohesion and interaction among students, as well as between faculty and students. Several student organizations give the students an opportunity to become involved in a variety of service and support activities. During years one and two, students have access to the recreational and athletic facilities of the University of South Dakota as well as on-campus residence halls. During years three and four, students have varied options, depending on where their clinical training takes place.

GRADUATES

Graduates are successful in securing residencies nationwide and typically choosing ten to fourteen different specialties. Approximately 25 percent of graduates enter family practice, while an additional 25 percent enter other primary care fields.

Admissions

REQUIREMENTS

Prerequisites are one year each of biology, chemistry, organic chemistry, physics, and college-level math. Advanced Placement and CLEP courses may count for meeting prerequisites if granted on pre-medical transcript. The MCAT is required, and scores must be no more than three years old. For applicants who have retaken the exam, the most recent set of scores is compared to previous scores.

SUGGESTIONS

Residents of South Dakota, nonresidents with strong personal ties to the state (for example, they graduated from high school in South Dakota or their parents live in-state) and applicants of Native American descent who can demonstrate enrollment in federally recognized tribes in South Dakota or in border states are invited to submit secondary applications. Beyond academic credentials, exposure to the medical profession, volunteer activities, interest in practicing primary care medicine, and working with underserved communities are all valued.

PROCESS

All qualified AMCAS applicants who meet residency criteria are sent secondary applications. These applicants are invited to interview with the admissions committee between October and March. Interviews consist of two one-to-one interviews with a faculty member who serves on the admissions committee. Of interviewed candidates, about 30 percent are accepted, with notification beginning in December. Several students are placed on an alternate list and are given a rank order for admission if vacancies occur. USDSM does not consider applications for transfer with advanced standing from students at non-LCME accredited medical schools.

Admissions Requirements (Required)

MCAT scores, science GPA, non-science GPA, letters of recommendation, interview, supplemental application.

Admissions Requirements (Optional)

state residency, essays/personal statement, extracurricular activities, exposure to medical profession.

COSTS AND AID

In-state tuition	$12,498
Out-of-state tuition	$29,937
Room and board	$14,650
Cost of books	$1,750
Fees	$5,119

Financial Aid

% students receiving aid	98
Average grant	$3,691
Average loan	$26,510
Average debt	$97,596

UNIVERSITY OF SOUTH FLORIDA

COLLEGE OF MEDICINE

12901 BRUCE B DOWNS BOULEVARD, MDC-3, TAMPA, FL 33612 • ADMISSION: 813-974-2229 • FAX: 813-974-4990 •
E-MAIL: MD-ADMISSIONS@LYRIS.HSC.USF.EDU • WEBSITE: WWW.MED.USF.EDU/MD/START.HTM

STUDENT BODY

Type	Public
Enrollment	399
% male/female	56/44
% underrepresented minorities	39
# applied (total/out)	1,492/355
# accepted (total)	170
# enrolled (total)	100
Average age	23

ADMISSIONS

Average GPA and MCAT Scores

Overall GPA	4
MCAT Bio	10
MCAT Phys	9.7
MCAT Verbal	9.7
MCAT Essay	0

Application Information

Regular application	12/1
Regular notification	10/15
Early application	8/15
Early notification	10/1
Are transfers accepted?	Yes
Admissions may be deferred?	Yes
Interview required?	Yes
Application fee	$30

Academics

The four-year curriculum is designed to permit the student to learn the fundamental principles of medicine, to acquire skills of critical judgment based on evidence and experience, and to develop an ability to wisely use principles and skills in solving problems of health and disease. Medical students who are interested in careers in research may pursue a combined MS/PhD program, earning the doctorate in a number of biomedical fields. For students who are interested in public and community health issues, a combined MD/MPH program is offered in conjunction with the College of Public Health. Medical students are evaluated with grades of honors, pass with commendation, pass, and fail. Passing Step 1 of the USMLE is a requirement for promotion to year three, and passing Step 2 is a graduation requirement.

BASIC SCIENCES: First-year students focus mainly on basic sciences and are instructed in a variety of ways, including lectures, labs, small group conferences, and interdisciplinary methods. Computers are also an important educational resource. In addition to science courses, first-year students investigate ethical and behavioral aspects of medicine in the courses behavioral medicine and medical ethics. In the second semester, they begin to learn patient-interaction skills through a physical diagnosis course that extends into the second year. Other first-year courses are gross anatomy, biochemistry, microscopic anatomy, human embryology, molecular biology and human genetics, medical neuroscience, and physiology. The second year is a continuation of basic sciences with increased emphasis on clinical correlation. The remainder of physical diagnosis and introduction to clinical medicine further develop patient examination and evaluation skills and prepare students for the clinical phase of the curriculum. Other second-year courses are medical microbiology and immunology, pathology and laboratory medicine, clinical correlation, and pharmacology. Students are in class or other scheduled sessions for about twenty-five hours per week. There are opportunities for involvement in research in between the first and second year.

CLINICAL TRAINING

Third-year required clinical rotations are eight weeks each of the following: internal medicine, surgery, pediatrics, psychiatry, obstetrics/gynecology, and family medicine. The fourth year is devoted primarily to electives, a portion of which may be taken at other academic or clinical institutions at locations around the state, country, or overseas. Most clinical training takes place at Tampa General Hospital (1000 beds), H. Lee Moffitt Cancer Center and Research Institute (162 beds), James A. Haley Veterans Hospital (577 beds), the USF Psychiatry Center, USF Medical Clinic, All Children's Hospital (168 beds), USF Eye Institute, University Diagnostic Institute, Shriners Hospital for Crippled Children, Bayfront Medical Center (518 beds); and Bay Pines Veterans Medical Center (520 beds). A number of community-based clinics are also used as clinical training facilities.

Students

All students are Florida residents. About 7 percent of students are underrepresented minorities. Although most students enter shortly after college graduation, there is a wide age range in each class. Class size is ninety-six.

STUDENT LIFE

Students are cooperative, often studying together and interacting outside of the academic setting. The medical school sponsors student events and organizations, and places a strong emphasis on student involvement in school and community activities. The medical school is located on the main USF campus, giving students access to the amenities of a large university. Tampa has many cultural and recreational opportunities and is generally a popular city among students. Most students live off campus, where housing is relatively affordable and comfortable.

GRADUATES

Graduates are successful in securing residency positions in all specialty areas. At USF, post-graduate training programs are offered in more than ten fields.

Admissions

REQUIREMENTS

Science requirements include one year each of basic introductory courses and laboratories in biological science, general chemistry, organic chemistry, and physics. One year of both English and mathematics is also required. The MCAT is required, and scores should be from within the past three years. For applicants who have retaken the exam, the best set of scores is weighed most heavily. Thus, there is no advantage in withholding scores.

SUGGESTIONS

State residency is a requirement. Courses that are recommended, but not required, include physical or biological chemistry, biochemistry, embryology, cell biology, comparative anatomy, genetics, statistics, logic, and rhetoric. Knowledge of calculus, computer science, and statistics is useful. Consideration is given to a student's participation in honors courses, independent study, and scientific research. All applicants are advised to apply as early as possible because the application process is rolling.

PROCESS

All AMCAS applicants who are residents of Florida and who meet minimum standards are sent secondary applications. About 15 percent of those who return secondaries are invited to interview between September and April. Interviews are one-on-one with a faculty member. On interview day, candidates have the opportunity to tour the campus and to informally meet with current medical students. About 50 percent of interviewees are accepted and are notified on a rolling basis. Other candidates are rejected or wait-listed. Wait-listed candidates may send additional information to update their files.

Admissions Requirements (Required)

MCAT scores, science GPA, non-science GPA, letters of recommendation, interview, state residency, essays/personal statement, extracurricular activities, exposure to medical profession.

Overlap Schools

University of Florida, University of Miami.

COSTS AND AID

In-state tuition	$12,051
Out-of-state tuition	$36,159
Cost of books	$7,764
In-state fees	$1,592
Out-of-state fees	$2,797

Financial Aid

% students receiving aid	85
Average grant	$5,000
Average loan	$20,500
Average debt	$82,500

University of Southern California
Keck School of Medicine

1975 Zonal Avenue (KAM 100-C), Los Angeles, CA 90089-9021 • Admission: 323-442-2552 • Fax: 323-442-2433 • E-mail: medadmit@hsc.usc.edu • Website: www.usc.edu/medicine/

STUDENT BODY

Type	Private
Enrollment	659
% male/female	52/48
% underrepresented minorities	17
# applied (total/out)	5,445/2,087
# accepted (total/out)	334/54
# enrolled (total/out)	161/26
Average age	24

FACULTY

Total faculty (number)	206
% female	26
% minority	19
% part-time	3

ADMISSIONS

Average GPA and MCAT Scores

Overall GPA	3.6
MCAT Bio	10.56
MCAT Phys	10.48
MCAT Verbal	9.66
MCAT Essay	R

Application Information

Regular application	10/1
Regular notification	4/2
Early application	8/1
Early notification	10/1
Are transfers accepted?	Yes
Admissions may be deferred?	Yes
Interview required?	Yes
Application fee	$90

Academics

While the majority of students earn their MD in four years, USC offers a variety of joint degree programs. The MS/PhD program is administered by the USC Graduate School and the School of Medicine, allowing students to earn the doctorate in anatomy, biochemistry, biomedical engineering, biophysics, cell biology, genetics, immunology, microbiology, molecular biology, neuroscience, pathology, pharmacology, and physiology. For students who are interested in more discrete research projects, the Research Scholar Program allows them to spend one year involved in research at USC or another approved institution. Students also have the option of entering a combined MD/MPH program.

BASIC SCIENCES: Lectures, labs, and periodic small group discussions are the instructional modalities used during the first two years. Currently, the faculty and students are working together to design a revised curriculum that may depend more on small group sessions and problem-based learning. The first year (thirty-eight weeks) begins with an introductory review course entitled human biology, which is followed by a sequence of courses based on organ systems. They are cardiovascular, endocrine/reproduction, gastrointestinal/liver, renal/respiratory/skin, neuroscience, and blood. Students benefit from patient contact from the very beginning in introduction to clinical medicine. The second year (thirty-seven weeks) is also organized around body/organ systems and is dedicated to studying the mechanisms of disease. USC's library is comprehensive and has an ample supply of computers. Computers with course material, online resources, and other study aids are also available in individually assigned laboratory spaces, which serve as student study areas. Grades of honors, satisfactory, and unsatisfactory are used to evaluate medical students during the first two years. Students must pass Step 1 of the USMLE to be promoted to year three.

CLINICAL TRAINING

The clinical years are the hallmark of USC's education. The majority of teaching takes place in L.A. County and USC Medical Center. It is among the major public hospitals for Los Angeles and receives patients with every imaginable illness and injury. Students are allowed extensive patient contact. The curriculum of required courses and electives is continuous over the third and fourth years and is individually designed. Required clerkships are internal medicine (two of six weeks each), family medicine (six weeks), pediatrics (six weeks), obstetrics/gynecology (six weeks), general surgery (six weeks), psychiatry (six weeks), neurology (four weeks), specialized surgery (two to three weeks), and a basic or clinical sciences clerkship (four weeks). An additional twelve weeks of selectives are required. Students may take up to sixteen weeks of electives at approved institutions throughout the nation. In addition to L.A. County and USC Medical Center, clinical facilities include Children's Hospital Los Angeles, USC University Hospital, and USC/Norris Comprehensive Cancer Center. During the clinical years grades of honors, near honors, satisfactory, and unsatisfactory are used to evaluate medical students. To graduate, students must record a score on the USMLE Step 2.

Students

Of the 150 students in each class, almost 80 percent are California residents. About 16 percent of students are underrepresented minorities. The average age of incoming students is about twenty-four, with a wide age range including significant numbers of students in their thirties.

STUDENT LIFE

The Medical School campus is not situated in an ideal residential area, and the majority of students commute to school from surrounding communities. Nonetheless, USC has a cohesive and cooperative student body. Many first-year students attend a camping retreat prior to the beginning of classes, during which they are introduced to each other and to returning students. During the academic year, students typically study in groups and spend time together outside of school. The School of Medicine offers a wide variety of extracurricular activities, including volunteer programs, intramural sports, and student clubs and organizations. USC's main campus is easily accessible by car, and medical students regularly use its extensive recreational facilities. University-sponsored activities such as intercollegiate sporting events, films, and parties are also popular with medical students.

GRADUATES

Graduates are successful in securing positions throughout the United States, in both specialty and primary care fields. Most enter residency programs in California.

Admissions

REQUIREMENTS

Prerequisites are two semesters each, with associated labs, in biology, general chemistry, organic chemistry, and physics. In addition, applicants must have completed a course in basic molecular biology and an additional thirty semester hours in a combination of social sciences, humanities, and English composition. The MCAT is required, and scores must be from within the previous two years.

SUGGESTIONS

The Admissions Committee looks very favorably upon hospital or other medical experience that involves patient care and demonstrates a commitment to service. Research experience is also helpful. USC strongly recommends additional course work in statistics and higher mathematics.

PROCESS

All AMCAS applicants are asked to submit a supplemental application. Of those students who return supplemental applications, approximately 800 are invited for interviews. The interview day consists of a tour, lunch with medical students, and one- or two-hour interviews with faculty and/or medical students. Initial acceptances are sent at the beginning of January, but most students are placed in a hold category, with the majority of acceptances offered in May. About 40 percent of interviewed candidates are accepted. Wait-listed candidates may send additional information to update their files.

Admissions Requirements (Required)

MCAT scores, science GPA, non-science GPA, letters of recommendation, interview, essays/personal statement, extracurricular activities, exposure to medical profession.

Admissions Requirements (Optional)

state residency.

COSTS AND AID

Tuition	$35,052
Room and board	$9,802
Cost of books	$2,200
Fees	$1,013

Financial Aid

% students receiving aid	75
Average grant	$10,000
Average loan	$29,800
Average debt	$93,000

UNIVERSITY OF TENNESSEE—MEMPHIS

COLLEGE OF MEDICINE

ADMISSIONS OFFICE, 790 MADISON AVENUE, ROOM 307, MEMPHIS, TN 38163 • ADMISSION: 901-448-5559 •
FAX: 901-448-1740 • WEBSITE: WWW.UTMEM.EDU/MEDICINE

STUDENT BODY

Type	Public
Enrollment	686
% male/female	61/39
% underrepresented minorities	15
# applied (total/out)	1,700/1,054
# accepted (total/out)	15/4
# enrolled (out)	39
Average age	24

FACULTY

Total faculty (number)	1,711
% female	17
% minority	10
% part-time	3
# student/faculty ratio	2:1

ADMISSIONS

Application Information

Regular application	11/15
Regular notification	10/15-4/1
Are transfers accepted?	Yes
Admissions may be deferred?	Yes
Interview required?	No
Application fee	$50

Academics

Most students follow a four-year curriculum that leads to the MD. The optional expanded academic program allows students to expand the first two years into three. The clinical scholars program provides special educational and financial assistance to entering students who are interested in careers in family medicine, general internal medicine, general pediatrics, medicine and pediatrics (med-peds), or obstetrics/gynecology. Students are encouraged to pursue research, either during the summer following year one or as ongoing projects. An MS/PhD program is available for students who are interested in intensive research. Medical students generally receive percentage scores on exams and are evaluated with grades of A through F. Examinations in some courses are administered by computer. Students must pass both steps of the USMLE to graduate.

BASIC SCIENCES: The basic sciences are taught during the first two years primarily through lectures and lab work. Students are in class or other scheduled sessions for about twenty-three hours per week. First-year science courses are the following: biochemistry, fundamentals of cellular and molecular biology, medical genetics, gross anatomy, histology, neuroanatomy, and physiology. Other first-year courses are behavioral sciences and preventive medicine, both of which involve small group discussions. Throughout the first and second years, students take introduction to clinical skills, which correlates basic science concepts with actual medical cases and teaches students introductory clinical techniques. Students also participate in a longitudinal, community-based clinical program. Second-year courses are microbiology, neuroscience, nutrition, pathology, pathophysiology, and pharmacology. Most of the first two years is spent in the Cecil C. Humphreys General Education Building that houses classrooms, labs, and a computer center. A three-year longitudinal community program incorporates content of behavioral science, preventive medicine, nutrition, ICS, and longitudinal community-based clinical program. An important educational resource is the Plane Tree Center with multimedia software technologies for learning anatomy, embryology, histology, EKG readings, and lung and heart sounds. Plane Tree also provides health oriented books, audiovisuals, and Internet connections. The Health Sciences Library is used by students both for research purposes and for studying. It is fully computerized, subscribes to approximately 1,550 current periodicals, and contains a total volume count of over 170,000.

CLINICAL TRAINING

Third-year required clerkships are two months each of the following: family medicine, medicine, obstetrics/gynecology, pediatrics, psychiatry, and surgery. The fourth year consists of five one-month clerkships and three months of electives that provide students the opportunity to select the clinical or basic science experiences to best meet their particular career goals. Electives allow for increased responsibility in patient care as well as the opportunity to pursue areas of individual interest. Fourth-year required clerkships are ambulatory care medicine, neurology, and a senior clerkship in medicine and surgical subspecialties. As part of a selective requirement, one month of either family medicine, medicine, pediatrics, obstetrics/gynecology, psychiatry, or surgery is also required. All students must spend a minimum of ten months of clerkship and elective time on the Memphis campus. This requirement allows a maximum of ten months (excluding option months) to be spent at Knoxville, Chattanooga, and/or Nashville. Two of the ten months away from the Memphis campus may be taken at another institution, either in the United States or overseas.

Students

At least 90 percent of students are Tennessee residents. Others are usually from the eight states contiguous to Tennessee. These are Mississippi, Arkansas, Missouri, Kentucky, Virginia, North Carolina, Georgia, and Alabama. The average age of incoming students is typically about twenty-four, with a wide age range among students. Underrepresented minorities account for about 12 percent of students. Class size is 165.

STUDENT LIFE

Medical students are cohesive and supportive of one another. As part of the Big Sib program, incoming medical students are assigned to senior students as mentors. Typically, the Big Sibs will pass along their class notes to the new students to use as a guide during basic science lectures. Medical students are part of a larger community that includes students from all professional schools and programs. The Student Alumni Center (SAC) is the focal point of campus life, providing meeting areas, a restaurant, lounges, a television room, shopping areas, and other services. More than thirty-five campus-wide organizations are open to medical students. Students enjoy a fitness center that houses a multipurpose gym, a swimming pool, spa, racketball courts, and a weight room. An outdoor complex has playing fields, volleyball courts, tennis courts, golf-practice facilities, and a track. Intramural sports are popular, as is the Outdoor Adventures Program, which leads canoeing, hiking, rafting, and camping trips. Memphis is a festive city, renowned for its music scene. Other attractions include riverside areas, parks, restaurants, a lively arts community, and quiet residential neighborhoods. UT Memphis offers both residence halls and apartment-style facilities for single students. The university assists married students who are looking for housing in the city.

GRADUATES

Among 1999 graduates, the most popular fields for residencies were the following: internal medicine (31 percent), pediatrics (10 percent), family practice (21 percent), obstetrics/gynecology (21 percent), surgery (12 percent), radiology (6 percent), and medicine/pediatrics (8 percent). A significant proportion of graduates remains in Tennessee for post-graduate training.

Admissions

REQUIREMENTS

Prerequisite course work is eight semester hours each of biology, general chemistry, organic chemistry, and general physics, all taken with associated labs. In addition, six hours of English is required. The MCAT is required and scores must be no more than five years old. For applicants who have retaken the exam, all sets of scores are considered.

SUGGESTIONS

Residents of Tennessee are given preference. Children of UT alumni are also considered, regardless of their state of residence. As a state-supported institution, no more than 10 percent of students may be nonresidents. Thus, nonresident applicants should be highly qualified. Students are encouraged to take courses in the humanities, fine arts, and social sciences. Demonstration of analytic ability and independent thinking is important.

PROCESS

All AMCAS applicants who are considered competitive are sent supplemental applications, of which approximately 400 applicants are invited to interview between October and March. The interview gives insights into applicants' character and how well they have formulated plans for the study of medicine. Interviews consist of two sessions, each with a faculty member or current medical student. On interview day, applicants have lunch, attend group informational sessions, sit in on classes, and tour the campus. Of interviewed candidates, about 60 percent are accepted on a rolling basis. Other candidates are either rejected or placed on a wait-list.

Admissions Requirements (Required)

MCAT scores, state residency, extracurricular activities, exposure to medical profession.

Admissions Requirements (Optional)

science GPA, nonscience GPA, letters of recommendation, interview, essays/personal statement.

COSTS AND AID

In-state tuition	$9,256
Out-of-state tuition	$17,920
Room and board	$1,400
Cost of books	$1,600
Fees	$213

Financial Aid

% students receiving aid	80
Average grant	$8,695
Average loan	$15,700
Average debt	$63,000

UNIVERSITY OF TEXAS
MEDICAL BRANCH AT GALVESTON SCHOOL OF MEDICINE

OFFICE OF ADMISSIONS, G-210, ASHBEL SMITH BUILDING, GALVESTON, TX 77555-1317 • ADMISSION: 409-772-3517 • FAX: 409-772-5753 • E-MAIL: PWYLIE@MSPO4.MED.EDU • WEBSITE: WWW.UTMB.EDU

STUDENT BODY

Type	Public
Enrollment	821
% male/female	59/41
% underrepresented minorities	15
# applied (total/out)	2,772/485
# accepted (total/out)	37/15
# enrolled (out)	12

ADMISSIONS

Application Information

Regular application	10/15
Regular notification	1/15 until filled
Are transfers accepted?	No
Admissions may be deferred?	Yes
Interview required?	No
Application fee	$45

Academics

In addition to the standard four-year MD curriculum, UTMB offers a combined MS/PhD program for students who are interested in training for a career in biomedical research. Generally, about five students enter this program each year and receive full funding for the duration of their studies. Summer and yearlong research projects are also open to medical students. As an alternative to the primarily lecture-based basic science curriculum, twenty-four incoming students each year enter an interactive learning track, which relies on small group instruction.

BASIC SCIENCES: First-year courses are the following: gross anatomy and developmental anatomy, microanatomy, biochemistry, cells and genes, physiology and biophysics, neuroscience, medical ethics, community continuity experience, and introduction to patient evaluation. Second-year courses are endocrinology, microbiology, pharmacology and toxicology, pathology, introduction to patient evaluation, immunology, introduction to clinical medicine, and community continuity experience. During the first and second years, students are in class or other scheduled sessions for about thirty hours per week. In addition to teaching basic science principles, the preclinical curriculum involves practical problem solving experiences and case studies that demonstrate the interrelationship between the basic and clinical sciences. The community continuity experience gives first- and second-year students the opportunity to work with primary care physicians, interact with patients, and apply and expand knowledge and skills that are gained in the classroom. Educational support services include academic counseling, peer tutorials, study skills workshops, and stress management workshops. An Educational Support Center provides medical students with computer-assisted educational support. For research purposes and as a place to study, students use the Moody Medical Library, which is the oldest medical library in Texas and one of the largest medical research centers in the Southwest. Collections include nearly 250,000 volumes in addition to computerized informational services.

CLINICAL TRAINING

Third-year required clerkships are internal medicine (eight weeks), surgery (eight weeks), pediatrics (four weeks), obstetrics/gynecology (six weeks), psychiatry (six weeks), family medicine (six weeks), and a multidisciplinary ambulatory clerkship (twelve weeks). Lectures in anesthesiology, medical jurisprudence, ophthalmology, and otolaryngology are also part of the third-year curriculum. Fourth-year required clerkships are neurology (four weeks), surgery (four weeks), emergency medicine (four weeks), radiology (two weeks), dermatology (two weeks), and an acting internship selective (four weeks). At least twenty weeks are reserved for elective study. Clinical training takes place primarily at UTMB hospitals and clinics. Some electives may be taken at other institutions.

Students

At least 90 percent of students are Texas residents. Typically, about 10 percent of entering students are a bit older and have taken significant time off after college. Approximately 15 percent of students are underrepresented minorities. Class size is 200.

STUDENT LIFE

Students benefit from the resources and facilities of a large, modernized campus. The Lee Hage Jamail Student Center serves as a meeting place for medical students. It has a cafeteria, meeting rooms, study areas, and recreational facilities. Coed medical fraternities located close to campus offer housing, meals, and social opportunities to medical students. The UTMB Alumni Fields House features a variety of indoor and outdoor facilities, including tennis courts, baseball diamonds, volleyball courts, an outdoor basketball court, racquetball courts, fitness centers, spa facilities, an outdoor track, and an Olympic size pool. UTMB has more than fifty student organizations that range from support groups for minority students, to community service oriented groups, to professional organizations. The university operates both dormitories and apartments for single students.

GRADUATES

Graduates are successful in securing residencies at top institutions throughout the United States.

Admissions

REQUIREMENTS

A grade of at least a C must be earned in all of the prerequisite courses. These are English (one year), biology (two years), math (one semester of college-level), physics (one year), chemistry (one year), and organic chemistry (one year). All science courses must include laboratory work. The MCAT is required, and scores should be from within the past year. For applicants who have retaken the exam, the most recent set of scores is considered.

SUGGESTIONS

As a state-supported institution, UTMB gives preference to Texas residents. Applicants are encouraged to take the spring MCAT because late receipt of scores from the fall cycle may delay application processing. Medical experience, volunteer activities, and research are all helpful.

PROCESS

The University of Texas does not participate in the AMCAS system. Applications may be obtained from The University of Texas System, Medical/Dental Application Center, Suite 6400, 702 Colorado Street, Austin, TX, 78701, Telephone: 512-499-4785. Applications must be submitted between May 15 and October 15. About 1,000 applicants are invited to interview during November and December. Candidates receive two interviews, each with a faculty member. On interview day, there are also orientation sessions, a campus tour, and several opportunities to informally meet with current medical students. About 20 percent of interviewed candidates are accepted. Other candidates are rejected or placed on a wait-list and possibly accepted later in the year.

Admissions Requirements (Required)

MCAT scores, science GPA, non-science GPA, letters of recommendation, state residency, extracurricular activities, exposure to medical profession.

Admissions Requirements (Optional)

interview, essays/personal statement.

COSTS AND AID

Tuition	$1,000
Cost of books	$2,000
Fees	$1,000

Financial Aid

Average loan	$125,141

University of Texas Health Science Center at Houston
The University of Texas Medical School at Houston

Office of Admissions, MSB 1.126, Houston, TX 77030 • Admission: 713-500-5116 • Fax: 713-500-0604 •
E-mail: msadmissions@uth.tmc.edu • Website: www.med.uth.tmc.edu

STUDENT BODY

Type	Private
Enrollment	814
% male/female	58/42
% underrepresented minorities	16
# applied (total/out)	2,795/525
# accepted (total/out)	37/24
# enrolled (out)	8
Average age	24

FACULTY

Total faculty (number)	678
% female	28
% part-time	5

ADMISSIONS

Application Information

Regular application	10/1
Regular notification	1/15 until filled
Are transfers accepted?	Yes
Admissions may be deferred?	No
Interview required?	No
Application fee	$45

Academics

Although most medical students complete studies in four years, some follow an alternate pathway curriculum, which extends first-year courses over a two-year period and leads to the MD degree in five years. Others follow a seven-year program that leads to both the MD and the PhD degrees, while others earn a master's in public health, along with the MD in five years. Summer research opportunities are available, most of which are paid. Medical students are evaluated with grades of honors, high pass, pass, marginal performance, and fail. All students must take the USMLE Steps 1 and 2.

BASIC SCIENCES: First-year courses are biochemistry, gross anatomy, developmental anatomy, histology, immunology, introduction to clinical medicine (ICM), microbiology, neuroscience, and physiology. The ICM course introduces students to interviewing, history-taking, and physical-examination skills. Instructional methods used during the first year include lectures, small group sessions, tutorials, and labs. A problem-based learning curriculum links basic and clinical sciences and allows second-year students to begin addressing complex medical problems. Problem-based learning is an important part of the second-year curriculum, serving to integrate the various courses and provide clinical skills. Second-year courses are behavioral science, genetics, fundamentals of clinical medicine, pathology, pharmacology, physical diagnosis, and reproductive biology. During the first two years, students are in class or other scheduled sessions for about twenty-two hours per week. The Learning Resource Center has textbooks, audiovisuals, anatomical models, audiotapes and videotapes of lectures, computers, files of past exams, USMLE review materials, and other instructional aids. Networked computers with free access to computer-based services and instructional materials are also provided.

CLINICAL TRAINING

Third-year required rotations are radiology (one week), medicine (twelve weeks), surgery (eight weeks), obstetrics/gynecology (eight weeks), pediatrics (eight weeks), psychiatry (eight weeks), and family medicine (four weeks). During the fourth year, required rotations are family practice (one month), medicine (one month), neurology (one month), and surgery (one month). Third and fourth-year students receive advanced technical skills training. Clinical training takes place primarily at the numerous hospitals, clinics, and care centers associated with the Texas Medical Center in Houston and in a city/county hospital in northeast Houston. There is flexibility in terms of where elective credits may be earned, and some students opt to study elsewhere in the country or at one of several international programs.

Students

At least 90 percent of students are Texas residents. Most students are recent college graduates, although there is typically a wide age range among incoming students. In terms of ethnic backgrounds, students represent the diverse population of the state.

STUDENT LIFE

There are numerous student organizations that focus on areas such as public service projects, professional interests, religious and ethnic interests, athletics, and recreation. Medical students serve on important committees, such as the Admissions Committee, the Faculty-Student Relations Committee, and the Curriculum Committee. Houston is an exciting city for students, with a wide variety of entertainment, recreational attractions, restaurants, shopping areas, and facilities for outdoor activities. The university offers apartments a short distance from school and a free shuttle runs throughout the week.

GRADUATES

Of approximately 4,200 UT Houston Medical School graduates, about 59 percent go on to practice in Texas. Among the 2001 graduates, the most popular fields for residencies were internal medicine (15 percent), anesthesiology (12 percent), family practice (9 percent), pediatrics (9 percent), surgery (7 percent), obstetrics/gynecology (6 percent), orthopedics 6 percent, emergency medicine (5.5 percent), internal medicine/pediatrics (5 percent), and psychiatry (4 percent).

Admissions

REQUIREMENTS

Prerequisites are one year of English, one semester of college-level calculus, one year of physics with lab, two years of biology with lab, one year of general chemistry with lab, and one year of organic chemistry with lab. The MCAT is required, and scores should be from within the past five years. For applicants who have retaken the exam, the last three scores will be reviewed.

SUGGESTIONS

No more than 10 percent of students may be nonresidents; thus, admission is very competitive for nonresidents. A liberal arts background is important and, as long as science requirements are fulfilled, students are encouraged to pursue a major in their area of interest while they are in college. Technological, vocational engineering, or business courses of study are not viewed as favorably as those providing a broad educational background. Important traits include intellectual capacity, interpersonal and communication skills, breadth and depth of pre-medical educational experience, potential for service to the State of Texas, motivation, and integrity.

PROCESS

The University of Texas does not participate in the AMCAS system. Applications may only be made online at the Texas Medical and Dental Schools Application Service website at www.utsystem.edu/tmdsas Applications must be submitted between May 1 and November 1. Additional information about the admissions process may be obtained from Texas Medical and Dental Schools Application Service, 702 Colorado Street, Suite 6400, Austin, TX 78701, Telephone: 512-499-4785. About 1,250 applicants are interviewed at UT Houston between August and January. Applicants generally receive two one-on-one interviews, each with a faculty member. On interview day, candidates also have lunch with medical students, tour the campus, and attend group orientation sessions. About one-fifth of interviewees are accepted and are notified via the TMDSAS website on February 1. A few wait-listed candidates are accepted later in the spring and summer.

Admissions Requirements (Required)

MCAT scores, state residency, essays/personal statement, extracurricular activities.

Admissions Requirements (Optional)

science GPA, nonscience GPA, letters of recommendation, interview, exposure to medical profession.

University of Texas Health Science Center at San Antonio
University of Texas Medical School at San Antonio

Medical School Admissions Office, 7703 Floyd Curl Drive, San Antonio, TX 78284 • Admission: 210-567-2665 • Fax: 210-567-2685 • E-mail: eliker@uthscsa.edu • Website: www.uthscsa.edu

STUDENT BODY

Type	Private
Enrollment	814
% male/female	58/42
% underrepresented minorities	16
# applied (total/out)	2,795/525
# accepted (total/out)	37/24
# enrolled (out)	8
Average age	24

Academics

Almost all medical students follow a four-year curriculum that leads to the MD. A few students enter combined MS/PhD programs after their first year of medical school. Grades of A through F are used to evaluate students in most of their courses. All students must pass Step 1 of the USMLE for promotion to year three.

BASIC SCIENCES: Basic sciences are primarily covered during the first two years, although introductory clinical training also begins in year one. San Antonio operates on a semester system, with a break scheduled around Christmas. First-year, first-semester courses are the clinical integration course, biochemistry, gross anatomy and embryology, microscopic anatomy, and microbiology. Second-semester courses are neuroscience and physiology. Other first-year courses use a combination of lectures, labs, and small group sessions. Students are in class or other scheduled sessions for about twenty-one hours per week during year one. During the second year, the curriculum is increasingly clinically oriented. First semester courses are behavioral sciences, pathology, and pharmacology. Second-semester courses are pathology and psychopathology. During year two, students are in class for about nineteen hours per week, providing ample study time. An important resource for students, faculty, and the community is the Dolph Briscoe Library, which houses more than 200,000 books and journals.

CLINICAL TRAINING

The clinical integration course is an interdisciplinary program that starts with the first month of medical school and extends through the second year. Students learn basic clinical skills in the initial month of the program, spend time with community physicians, rotate with third-year students, and assume patient responsibilities to gain experience in continuity of care. The third and fourth years are devoted primarily to clinical clerkships. However, didactic instruction is also an important part of the curriculum. Topics covered are clinical orientation, basic cardiac life support, emergency medicine, radiology, patient rehabilitation, clinical pathology, medical jurisprudence, advanced cardiopulmonary resuscitation, medial humanities, infectious disease, genetics, and epidemiology. Third-year required rotations are obstetrics/gynecology (six weeks), medicine (twelve weeks), pediatrics (six weeks), psychiatry (six weeks), surgery (twelve weeks), and family practice (six weeks). Fourth-year requirements are medicine (eight weeks), surgery (four weeks), a choice of pediatrics, obstetrics/gynecology, psychiatry, or family practice (four weeks), and other selectives (sixteen weeks). An additional eight weeks are reserved for electives. The primary teaching hospital is the University Hospital, which has 547 beds. Training also takes place at the facilities of the South Texas Veterans Health Care System and at other affiliates. University-affiliated patient care covers a geographical area from San Antonio to the Rio Grande Valley and is delivered in clinics, hospitals, traveling vans, as well as in sites in schools and churches. The Health Science Center serves the entire South Texas/Border region.

Students

At least 90 percent of students are Texas residents. Underrepresented minorities account for 16 percent of the student population. Mexican Americans are particularly well represented. The student body is slightly older than at many other medical schools. The average age of incoming students is usually about twenty-four, and about 15 percent of students in each class are in their thirties or older.

STUDENT LIFE

Medical students enjoy a collegial environment and appreciate the diversity within the student body. Mentoring and peer support programs help incoming students with the transition to medical school, and special programs are available to assist underrepresented minority students. Students are very active in community service programs and events. Activities range from volunteering at clinics to participating in health education programs in schools. All students live off campus. San Antonio offers affordable housing accessible to the medical center by public transportation.

GRADUATES

More than half of graduates enter primary care fields, and a significant number of them go on to practice in Texas.

Admissions

REQUIREMENTS

Required courses are one semester of calculus, one year each of English and physics, two years of biology (one of which may be biochemistry), and two years of chemistry (which should include both organic and inorganic chemistry). The MCAT is required, and scores must be from 1997 or later. For applicants who have retaken the exam, the best set of scores is weighed most heavily. Therefore, there is no advantage in withholding scores.

SUGGESTIONS

In addition to academic requirements, personal traits and background are considered. Some type of medically related experience or research is required.

PROCESS

The University of Texas medical schools do not participate in AMCAS. Rather, applications may be obtained from The Texas Medical and Dental Application Service, 702 Colorado, Suite 6400, Austin, Texas 78701. Applications must be completed by October 15. About one-third of applicants are interviewed between August and December. Interviews consist of two thirty-minute sessions with Admissions Committee members who may be faculty or senior students. On interview day, candidates also have lunch with students, attend group orientation sessions, and tour the campus. The initial group of accepted candidates are notified in January. Others are notified later in the spring. An alternate pool of applicants is established and candidates are admitted as positions become available.

ADMISSIONS

Application Information

Regular application	10/1
Regular notification	1/15 until filled
Are transfers accepted?	Yes
Admissions may be deferred?	No
Interview required?	No
Application fee (in/out)	$45/$80

University of Texas Southwestern Medical Center
Medical Center at Dallas

5323 Harry Hines Boulevard, Dallas, TX 75390-9162 • Admission: 214-648-5617 • Fax: 214-648-3289 • E-mail: admissions@utsouthwestern.edu • Website: www.utsouthwestern.edu

STUDENT BODY

Type	Public
Enrollment	869
% male/female	56/44
% underrepresented minorities	47
# applied (total/out)	2,630/399
# accepted (total/out)	391/44
# enrolled (total/out)	218/23
Average age	24

FACULTY

Total faculty (number)	1,459
% female	25
% minority	16
% part-time	15
# student/faculty ratio	1:1

ADMISSIONS

Average GPA and MCAT Scores

Overall GPA	3.8
MCAT Bio	11
MCAT Phys	10.8
MCAT Verbal	10.1
MCAT Essay	P

Application Information

Regular application	11/1
Regular notification	2/1
Are transfers accepted?	Yes
Admissions may be deferred?	Yes
Interview required?	Yes
Application fee	$65

Academics

The vast majority of students follow a four-year path that leads to the MD degree. A small number of students each year enter a joint MS/PhD program in conjunction with the Southwestern Graduate School of Biomedical Sciences. For the most part, students are evaluated with grades of A through F; a C is required to pass. Fourth-year courses are graded pass/fail.

BASIC SCIENCES: During the first two years, a variety of teaching/learning formats are used, including lectures, small group, problem-based learning, computerized curriculum, and standardized patient interviews. First-year courses include biology of cells and tissues, human anatomy and embryology, integrative human biology, medical biochemistry, human behavior, and endocrinology and human reproduction. In addition, clinical ethics in medicine exposes first-year students to the ethical, behavioral, and clinical perspectives of medicine in a problem-based learning format. During the ten-week period between the first and second years, numerous clinical and research opportunities are available for students who wish to participate. Clinical exposure continues in the second year through clinical medicine: principles and practice; students learn about the physical examination and experience direct, one-on-one, patient contact. Second-year courses also include immunology and medical microbiology, anatomic and clinical pathology, medical pharmacology, and psychopathology. On average, students are in scheduled sessions for twenty-five to thirty hours per week. The campus where preclinical instruction takes place is also part of a large medical complex that includes several hospitals, research centers, and the medical school library, which holds more than 229,000 volumes and currently subscribes to almost 2,000 journals. Passing the USMLE Step 1 is required to progress to the fourth year.

CLINICAL TRAINING

Building upon the clinical experiences in the first two years, the third and fourth years offer intense clinical experiences involving medical students in direct patient care. Third-year required clinical rotations are surgery (eight weeks), pediatrics (eight weeks), obstetrics and gynecology (six weeks), internal medicine (twelve weeks), psychiatry (six weeks), and family practice (four weeks). The fourth year is organized into four-week periods filled with electives, selectives, and a few remaining required rotations. Requirements include neurology (four weeks), internal medicine (four weeks of a subinternship and four weeks of ambulatory care), and women's health care (four weeks). Four four-week periods remain, two of which are for selectives and two of which are reserved for electives. Clinical training takes place at university sites and affiliated institutions, including Parkland Memorial Hospital, the James Aston Ambulatory Care Center, Zale Lipshy University Hospital, Children's Medical Center, Dallas Veterans' Affairs Medical Center, Southwestern Institute of Forensic Sciences, Baylor University Medical Center, Presbyterian Hospital of Dallas, Methodist Hospitals of Dallas, St. Paul Medical Center, Texas Scottish Rite Hospital for Children, and John Peter Smith Hospital in Fort Worth. Students may fulfill many of their senior rotations at academic or medical institutions in other parts of the state, the country, or the world.

Students

At least 90 percent of the student body are Texas residents. Underrepresented minorities account for about 10 percent of the population. The average age of incoming students is usually twenty-four; the range of ages is typically twenty to forty-five. Incoming class size at UT Southwestern is 200 students.

STUDENT LIFE

The Bryan Williams, MD Student Center has exercise and recreational facilities and offers students a convenient place to relax and socialize. Dynamic campus activity programming includes intramural sports, special interest organizations, recreational and cultural events, and parties. Students also join groups based on professional and academic interests or participate in community service projects. Dallas is an exciting city with a diverse population and many kinds of cultural, recreational, and entertainment activities. All students live off campus, and most students own cars.

GRADUATES

Graduates are successful in securing residencies at prestigious institutions all over the United States. The majority of graduates go on to become practicing physicians, typically with a large percentage choosing primary care specialties. Some of them go into academic medicine or research.

Admissions

REQUIREMENTS

Prerequisite courses include one semester of calculus or statistics, two semesters of English, two semesters of physics (with lab), four semesters of biology (two of which should be with lab and one of which may be biochemistry), and four semesters of chemistry (with lab), which should be equally divided between organic and inorganic chemistry. The MCAT is required, and scores must be no more than five years old. For applicants who have retaken the exam, the best set of scores is used.

SUGGESTIONS

Admission for out-of-state applicants is highly competitive, as Texas law requires that no more than 10 percent of each class be nonresidents. In addition to academic credentials (GPA, MCAT score, relative rigor of the undergraduate curriculum, letters of recommendation), the Admissions Committee considers extracurricular activities, socioeconomic background, any time spent in outside employment, personal integrity and compassion for others, the ability to communicate in English, motivation for a career in medicine, and other personal qualities and individual factors such as leadership, insightful self appraisal, determination, social/family support, and maturity/coping capabilities. Applicants are also evaluated for the demonstration of significant interest and experiences that parallel the mission of UT Southwestern.

PROCESS

UT Southwestern does not participate in the AMCAS system. A common application is available for the University of Texas System medical schools (Southwestern at Dallas, Galveston, Houston, and San Antonio), Texas A&M University College of Medicine, and Texas Tech University School of Medicine. An online application is available at http: //dpweb1.dp.utexas.edu/mdac/homepage.htm. Applications must be submitted between May 1 and November 1. About one-quarter of the applicants are invited to interview between September and December. Interviews consist of two sessions with individual faculty members. About 40 percent of interviewed candidates are accepted and are notified beginning on February 1.

Admissions Requirements (Required)

MCAT scores, science GPA, non-science GPA, letters of recommendation, interview, essays/personal statement, extracurricular activities, exposure to medical profession.

Admissions Requirements (Optional)

state residency.

Overlap Schools

Baylor College of Medicine, Duke University, South Texas College of Law, Texas Tech University, The University of Texas HSC at Houston, University of Texas Health Science Center at San Antonio, Vanderbilt University.

COSTS AND AID

In-state tuition	$6,920
Out-of-state tuition	$20,020
Cost of books	$1,800
Fees	$846

Financial Aid

% students receiving aid	85
Average grant	$2,500
Average loan	$18,500
Average debt	$63,000

UNIVERSITY OF TORONTO

315 BLOOR STREET WEST, TORONTO, ON, M5S1A3 • ADMISSION: 416-978-2190 • FAX: 416-978-7022 •
WEBSITE: WWW.UTORONTO.CA/

STUDENT BODY

Type	Public
# applied (total)	1,731

ADMISSIONS

Application Information

Regular application	10/15
Regular notification	5/31
Transfers accepted?	No
Admissions may be deferred?	Yes
Interview required?	Yes
Application fee	$75

Academics

The curriculum is based on four guidelines: patient-centered learning, integrated and multidisciplinary content, student-motivated learning, and structured problem-based learning. In addition to the four-year program that leads to an MD, a six-year MS/PhD program is offered jointly by the Faculty of Medicine and the School of Graduate Studies.

BASIC SCIENCES: The initial phase of the undergraduate medical program spans approximately eighty-two weeks. The curriculum consists of the following sequential blocks or units, which focus on principles of medicine: art and science of clinical medicine, brain and behavior, metabolism and nutrition, determination of community health, structure and function, pathobiology of disease, and foundations of medical practice. Students meet actual as well as simulated patients and are introduced to clinical medicine by faculty members in teaching hospitals. The emphasis is on student-centered, self directed work, and small group tutorials. Students are in scheduled sessions for approximately thirty-five hours per week. Most learning takes place in small group settings. Independent study is also important.

CLINICAL TRAINING

The third and fourth academic periods consist of mainly six-week clinical clerkships. These are medicine, surgery, obstetrics/gynecology, pediatrics, family and community medicine, psychiatry, specialty medicine, specialty surgery, emergency medicine and anesthesia, ambulatory and community experience, and three electives. Training takes place at a network of teaching hospitals and community-based health agencies. Affiliated hospitals include Baycrest Centre for Geriatric Care, Centre for Addiction and Mental Health (formerly Addition Research Foundation and the Clarke Institute of Psychiatry), The Hospital for Sick Children, Mount Sinai Hospital, St. Michael's Hospital, Toronto Rehabilitation Institute (formerly Hillcrest Hospital and Queen Elizabeth Hospital), Sunnybrook and Women's College Health Science Centre, The Toronto Hospital (formerly the Toronto Hospital and the Ontario Cancer Institute/Princess Margaret Hospital. Students are also able to learn in the community through participation in settings such as teaching health units and physicians' offices.

Students

About 15 percent of students are from outside of the province. Approximately 40 percent of students are women. Class size is 177.

STUDENT LIFE

One of the advantages of attending medical school at the University of Toronto is the city itself. The university campus is located within easy walking distance of the attractions and facilities of Toronto. Students enjoy clubs, concerts, museums, major league sporting events, and shopping. Just outside of the city, skiing and other outdoor sports are readily accessible. On- campus activities include pubs, concerts, special lectures, theaters, intramural sports, student government, special interest clubs, and the Medical Journal. Medical students benefit from the large campus of 55,000 students and its resources. Student support includes health services and a housing office that coordinates both on- and off-campus housing. Residence halls with meal plans are one of many housing options.

GRADUATES

A key aspect of the program is that it exposes students to all medical career options. Graduates enter primary care fields, specialties, academic medicine, research, and leadership positions.

Admissions

REQUIREMENTS

Academic achievement is measured by grades and MCAT results. Prerequisite courses are at least two full course equivalents in life sciences and at least one full course equivalent in humanities, social sciences, or languages. These courses should provide applicants with an understanding of the basic principles and vocabulary of physics, chemistry, and biology, a working knowledge of statistics, and the ability to gather, interpret, and present information from complex texts both in writing and orally. Students must be in their third year or higher of university to be considered for admission.

SUGGESTIONS

Students from social sciences, humanities, and physical and life sciences are encouraged to apply. Demonstrated high-level proficiency in oral and written English is considered essential for success in the curriculum and in practice, and applicants are encouraged to have completed at least two full equivalents in course that require expository writing. Generally, minimum requirements are an average grade point average of 3.6 and a minimum of 8 on each section of the MCAT. Desired personal characteristics include a perceptive nature, strong commitment, high personal standards, and a history of academic and personal achievement.

PROCESS

Applications for admission to the medical school must be submitted by October 15 to OMSAS, Ontario Universities Application Center, PO Box 1328, Guelph, Ontario N1H 7P4. The faculty will invite selected applicants for an interview. Notices of acceptance are sent to students in the spring or summer prior to the proposed date of enrollment.

COSTS AND AID

Tuition & Fees

Tuition (in/out)	$14,000/$23,750
Fees (in/out)	$919/$1,498

UNIVERSITY OF UTAH
SCHOOL OF MEDICINE

OFFICE OF ADMISSIONS, 30 NORTH 1900 EAST #1C116, SALT LAKE CITY, UT 84132-2101 • ADMISSION: 801-581-7498 • FAX: 801-581-2931 • E-MAIL: DEANS.ADMISSIONS@HSC.UTAH.EDU • WEBSITE: WWW.MED.UTAH.EDU/SOM

STUDENT BODY

Type	Public
Enrollment	407
% male/female	68/32
% underrepresented minorities	12
# applied (total/out)	1,325/859
# accepted (total/out)	34/18
# enrolled (out)	15
Average age	26

ADMISSIONS

Average GPA and MCAT Scores

Overall GPA	3.5
MCAT Bio	9.6
MCAT Phys	9.3
MCAT Verbal	8.9

Application Information

Regular application	10/15
Regular notification	rolling
Early application	6/1-8/1
Early notification	10/1
Are transfers accepted?	Yes
Admissions may be deferred?	No
Interview required?	No
Application fee	$60

Academics

The University of Utah School of Medicine implemented a new curriculum during the 1997—1998 academic year that emphasized active learning approaches, critical thinking skills, and information management techniques. The new curriculum builds upon the strengths of the traditional one and, in addition, explores areas of study opened up by the explosion of biomedical knowledge and the transformation of the U.S.'s health care delivery system. The goal of the curriculum is to produce highly skilled physicians who are technically proficient, caring and compassionate, and flexible enough to adapt to the changing demands they will face in the twenty-first century medical environment. In the first two years of medical school, students will receive a solid foundation in the sciences basic to medicine, including gross anatomy, embryology, histology, psychiatry, biochemistry, pharmacology, immunology, microbiology, genetics, physiology, pathology, and organ system pathophysiology. Courses cover such topics as health care financing and delivery, community and public health, research methodology and medical literature analysis, biostatistics, and epidemiology. The critical skills of communicating with, examining, and diagnosing patients are also covered in depth. The third year of the curriculum centers on clinical clerkships in internal medicine, surgery, obstetrics and gynecology, pediatrics, family practice, psychiatry, and neurology. During the fourth year a preceptorship in primary care medicine gives students a broader perspective on the health care issues facing medically underserved rural and urban areas; students generally live in the underserved area during the six-week preceptorship. Ample elective time is available for students to pursue areas of particular interest. Finally, a required subinternship will serve as a transition to residency. Students, with the help of faculty advisers, will apply to various post-graduate residency training programs through the National Resident Matching Program.

Students

Almost all students are from Utah or neighboring states. About 9 percent of entering students are typically from underrepresented ethnic groups. The age range of entering students is typically from nineteen to forty. A significant number of medical students at Utah are married by the fourth year. Class size is 100.

STUDENT LIFE

Medical students take advantage of the campus and the surrounding areas. The University of Utah is situated on a 1,500-acre campus that offers indoor and outdoor recreational activities. Salt Lake City is at the base of spectacular mountains and is only short drive from excellent skiing or hiking, depending on the season. Several national parks are accessible to the city. The city is relatively safe and student-friendly, with cultural activities as well as the basic amenities, such as malls, movie theaters, and restaurants. On-campus housing is available for married couples and single parents in the University Village, for all students in the Medical Plaza Towers (apartments and town houses), and for single students in university residence halls. There are organizations that unite medical students around common interests or that promote interaction with students from medical schools in neighboring states.

GRADUATES

Graduates are usually successful at obtaining their first choice of residencies. Typically, more than half of graduates enter primary care fields.

Admissions

REQUIREMENTS

The MCAT is required and must be taken within three years of application. The Admissions Committee is eager to admit students with a broad perspective on life. The school believes that a true physician who is not only skilled in medicine and the allied sciences but also who is a person of culture and broad intelligence. In addition to a bachelor's degree, the applicant must have subject matter competence in the following course work: two years of chemistry, the general chemistry series that include quantitative and qualitative analysis (AP credit accepted if at a level 4 or 5) and the organic series (AP credit not accepted), both with a laboratory; one year of physics with a laboratory (AP credit not accepted); one year of English writing/speech courses that must fulfill the institution writing/composition classification (AP credit not accepted; two college courses of biology, one of which should be in cellular biology or biochemistry (no substitutions, AP credit not accepted); one college course in social science (AP credit not accepted); and one college course in humanities (AP credit not accepted). With the exception of Advanced Placement credit for general chemistry at a level of 4 or 5, CLEP, Advanced Placement, and home study credit will not be accepted for completion of required course work. All pre-medical courses must be completed at an accredited college or university in the United States or Canada. Completion of four years of college work and a bachelor's degree are required before entering the School of Medicine. Only those students who have completed most of their undergraduate training in a U.S. or Canadian school will be considered.

SUGGESTIONS

Taking on independent research projects while in college is encouraged. Demonstration of writing skills and computer literacy is also important. Applicants should have participated in both health related and volunteer work. Applicants who have taken time off after college are advised to demonstrate recent course work.

PROCESS

Many Utah residents are asked to submit secondary applications, and 50 percent of those who submit them are invited to interview. Approximately one-third of Utah interviewees are accepted. About one-third of out-of-state applicants are sent secondary applications, and of those who submit them, 30 percent are invited to interview. Fifteen percent of out-of-state interviewees are accepted. Interviews take place from September through February and consist of two one-hour sessions with members of the faculty or administration or with students. Candidates are notified about their status on a rolling basis after they interview. A ranked wait-list is created.

Admissions Requirements (Required)

MCAT scores, science GPA, non-science GPA, letters of recommendation, state residency, extracurricular activities, exposure to medical profession.

Admissions Requirements (Optional)

interview, essays/personal statement.

COSTS AND AID

In-state tuition	$13,297
Out-of-state tuition	$25,172
Fees	$588

UNIVERSITY OF VERMONT

UNIVERSITY OF VERMONT COLLEGE OF MEDICINE

89 BEAUMONT AVENUE, E215 GIVEN BUILDING, BURLINGTON, VT 05405 • ADMISSION: 802-656-2154 • FAX: 802-656-9663 • E-MAIL: MEDADMISSIONS@UVM.EDU • WEBSITE: WWW.MED.UVM.EDU

STUDENT BODY

Type	Public
Enrollment	400
% male/female	41/59
% underrepresented minorities	20
# applied (total/out)	4,868/4,759
# accepted (total/out)	214/164
# enrolled (total/out)	101/65
Average age	24

FACULTY

Total faculty (number)	1,806
% female	30
% minority	10
% part-time	10

ADMISSIONS

Average GPA and MCAT Scores

Overall GPA	3.4
MCAT Bio	9.5
MCAT Phys	9
MCAT Verbal	9.2
MCAT Essay	Q

Application Information

Regular application	11/1
Regular notification	10/15
Early application	8/1
Early notification	10/1
Are transfers accepted?	Yes
Admissions may be deferred?	Yes
Interview required?	Yes
Application fee	$80

Academics

The curriculum progresses through three levels of increasing competency. Block courses in Level I/foundations provide students with a fundamental understanding of the basic biology of health and illness within systems that include genes, organs, individuals, populations. A comprehensive assessment of integrated knowledge and skills is planned for the end of the first year and again at the completion of the level midway through the second year of school. Level II/clinical clerkships focuses on students' development of clinical skills, decision-making skills, and their application of foundational sciences. It consists of seven clerkships with a longitudinal bridge curriculum of advanced sciences and clinical skills over a period of thirteen months. Clinical training takes place primarily at Fletcher Allen Health Care, an integrated health care delivery system formed in 1995 of the former Fanny Allen Hospital, the Medical Center Hospital of Vermont, and the University Health Center, a specialty service provider. Fletcher Allen serves the State of Vermont and beyond, attracting patients from New York and around New England. The merging of these institutions improved economic efficiency and suggests financial stability for the future.

Students advance to Level III/advanced integration after successful achievement on a clinical competency exam. During the final fifteen months of advanced integration, the student gains an understanding of the impact of economic, social, and political systems on the health care environment. This level includes acting internships, an emergency medicine rotation, a teaching practicum, and a scholarly project. During this section, there is flexibility in how students may earn elective credit. Many rotate to hospitals outside of the state, some work on Indian reservations, and others head overseas. Throughout the college's curriculum, complementary curricular themes aim to teach the student to take an integrated approach to patient care and responsibility for their own professional development. Student leadership groups provide students with opportunities to collaborate with classmates, a faculty facilitator, and various family faculty members from the community.

The MD/PhD program is designed to train future physician-scientists through a curriculum that integrates clinical care with basic research. The MD/PhD degree is awarded by the joint efforts of The College of Medicine and the Graduate College. Award of the MD degree requires completion of the entire medical curriculum. Award of the PhD degree requires fulfillment of the requirements of any of the basic science graduate programs, which include anatomy and neurobiology, biochemistry, microbiology and molecular genetics, molecular physiology and biophysics and pharmacology, or those of the multidisciplinary program in cell and molecular biology. It is anticipated that a period of seven years will be necessary to complete the combined program. Four students are chosen yearly for this program. Students who are enrolled in the program will receive financial support that includes full medical and graduate school tuition remission, as well as a stipend consistent with National Institutes of Health guidelines. Medical students use Dana Medical Library to study and to conduct research. Students use a Web-based, UVM-designed computer assisted teaching system to aid their learning. UVM is known for health information systems that it has developed, such as the Vermont Oxford Neonatal Network Database, which is in operation nationwide. The Academic Medical Center opened a new state-of-the-art facility for learning and assessment of clinical skills in January 2002. In the spring of 2005, a new educational center, library, and ambulatory center will open. The Academic Medical Center, along with the rest of the University of Vermont campus, is located in picturesque Burlington. The city is safe, affordable, and comfortable.

Students

Approximately 40 percent of students are residents of Vermont, 10 percent are from Maine, and the remainder come from out of area. In the class entering in 2002, the average age was twenty-four. Students came from fifty-nine different universities, six countries and a variety of academic backgrounds. Class size is ninety-seven.

STUDENT LIFE

Students have access to all of the university's athletic facilities. In addition, Burlington and the surrounding area offer excellent skiing, hiking, and mountain biking. On-campus choices include UVM's married student housing—about four miles from campus—and nearby apartments and residence halls. Group houses or shared apartments in walking or biking distance from school are popular off-campus choices. Student organizations are numerous and include Cyberdocs, a medical computer interest group, and The Diversity in Medicine Committee, a group that works to promote awareness of many types of diversity (ethnic, religious, age, gender, sexual orientation) in student life, medical education, and patient care.

GRADUATES

Graduates are successful in obtaining residencies at strong programs throughout the United States. In 2002, about half of the graduates entered primary care residencies. This year favored specialties were: internal medicine (23 percent), emergency medicine (12 percent), pediatrics (16 percent), and anesthesiology (10 percent).

Admissions

REQUIREMENTS

One year each of biology, chemistry, organic chemistry and physics, all with associated labs are required. Students who have taken time off after college must present some recent course work. The MCAT is required, and all sets of scores are considered.

SUGGESTIONS

We recommend that students take one course in biochemistry or molecular genetics. The MCAT should be taken no later than April of the application year to facilitate timely review of the entire application file. We encourage students who have a broad and balanced educational background during their undergraduate years. In addition to prerequisite courses in the sciences, recommended areas of study include literature, mathematics, behavioral sciences, history, philosophy, and the arts. College work must demonstrate intellectual drive, independent thinking, curiosity, and self-discipline. A career in medicine calls for excellent oral and written communication skills. Applicants should seek out opportunities to develop such skills during their college years. Successful applicants often have a history of service to community.

PROCESS

All AMCAS applicants receive a supplemental application. All well-qualified residents who apply are interviewed. Approximately 10 percent of out-of-state applicants are interviewed. Interviews take place from September through March and consist of an hour-long session with a faculty member and a third- or fourth-year medical student, if possible. Decisions are made on a rolling basis, and applicants are notified of their status—accept, reject, or wait-list—shortly after the interview. Wait-listed candidates should indicate if UVM is their first choice.

Admissions Requirements (Required)

MCAT scores, science GPA, non-science GPA, letters of recommendation, interview, essays/personal statement, extracurricular activities, exposure to medical profession.

Admissions Requirements (Optional)

state residency.

Overlap Schools

Albany Law School, Dartmouth College, Tufts University, University of Rochester.

COSTS AND AID

In-state tuition	$22,300
Out-of-state tuition	$39,020
Room and board	$10,280
Cost of books	$8,000
Fees	$981

Financial Aid

% students receiving aid	91
Average grant	$16,700
Average loan	$37,500
Average debt	$129,170

University of Virginia
School of Medicine

Box 800725, Charlottesville, VA 22908 • Admission: 804-924-5571 • Fax: 804-982-2586 •
E-mail: bab7g@virginia.edu • Website: www.med.virginia.edu/home.html

STUDENT BODY

Type	Public
Enrollment	556
% male/female	50/50
% underrepresented minorities	7
# applied (total/out)	3,577/2,866
# accepted (total)	140
# enrolled (total/out)	140/48
Average age	24

FACULTY

Total faculty (number)	800
# student/faculty ratio	1:1

ADMISSIONS

Average GPA and MCAT Scores

Overall GPA	3.7
MCAT Bio	10.83
MCAT Phys	10.94
MCAT Verbal	10.31
MCAT Essay	P

Application Information

Regular application	11/1
Regular notification	10/15
Are transfers accepted?	Yes
Admissions may be deferred?	Yes
Interview required?	Yes
Application fee	$75

Academics

Most medical students follow a four-year, highly integrated curriculum that leads to the MD. Each year six students enter a combined MS/PhD curriculum. Training for the PhD degree is usually in one of the biomedical science programs, which include anatomy, biochemistry, microbiology, pharmacology, physiology, biophysics, and neuroscience. A generalist scholars program supplements the medical education of students with special opportunities in the area of primary care. Students who participate in this program work closely with a faculty mentor and complete a thesis as part of their graduation requirements. Medical students are evaluated in a variety of ways, including both pass/fail and letter grades.

BASIC SCIENCES: First-year courses are biochemistry, cell and tissue structure, gross anatomy, physiology, human behavior, neuroscience, genetics, physical diagnosis, medical ethics, and the practice of medicine, in which topics such as human behavior and medical ethics are discussed. Basic clinical skills such as the patient interview are also introduced. Second-year courses are microbiology, pathology, pharmacology, psychiatric medicine, psychopathology, clinical epidemiology, community preceptorship, and introduction to clinical Medicine (ICM). Basic science concepts are coordinated with the ICM course, which involves discussion of clinical cases in small group tutorials. In the spring of the second year, each student completes a one-month community medicine preceptorship that provides hands-on primary care experience and serves as a transition to third-year clinical rotations. Instruction takes place at the Harvey E. Jordan Hall, a seven-story structure that houses lecture halls and laboratories. First- and second-year students also use the School of Medicine Learning Center, which contains conference rooms, tutorial rooms, and a student lounge. The Claude Moore Health Sciences Library is a modern, fully computerized facility with almost 79,000 books, 3,000 periodicals, and 4,000 audiovisual titles.

CLINICAL TRAINING

Third-year required rotations are medicine (twelve weeks), surgery (twelve weeks), psychiatry (six weeks), family medicine (four weeks), pediatrics (eight weeks), and obstetrics (six weeks). During the fourth year, a four-week neurology clerkship is required as are twenty-eight weeks of electives. Clinical training takes place primarily at the University of Virginia Medical Center University Hospital (552 beds), Kluge Children's Rehabilitation Center, and at forty outpatient clinics associated with the medical center. Students also train at affiliated hospitals, which include The Community Hospital of Roanoke Valley (400 beds), Roanoke Memorial Hospital (677 beds), and the Veterans' Affairs Medical Center (750 beds). Electives may be taken at other academic or clinical institutions in other parts of the country or abroad.

Students

About ninety of the 139 students in each class are Virginia residents. Underrepresented minorities account for approximately 10 percent of the student body. There is typically a wide age range among incoming students, with at least a few students in their thirties.

STUDENT LIFE

Students are highly active in on-campus activities and events. Many are involved in community activities such as Service, Humanity, Action, Responsibility, Education (SHARE), which initiates health education projects and other service oriented activities. Support groups for minority students are available, as are clubs that focus on professional interests and recreational pursuits such as singing. UVA also has local chapters of national medical student organizations. Medical students enjoy Charlottesville, a thriving tourist and cultural center located at the foot of the Blue Ridge Mountains and close to the Shenandoah Valley. The city of Richmond, Virginia, is an hour away by car, and Washington, DC is just two hours away.

GRADUATES

Graduates are successful in securing top residency positions in all regions of the country. A significant number stay on to do post-graduate training at UVA-affiliated hospitals.

Admissions

REQUIREMENTS

Prerequisites are one year each of biology, general chemistry, organic chemistry, and physics, all with associated labs. The MCAT is required, and scores must be no more than three years old at the time of matriculation. For applicants who have retaken the exam, the best scores are considered. Therefore, there is no advantage to withholding scores.

SUGGESTIONS

State residency is a factor in admissions decisions as about 65 percent of positions in a class are reserved for Virginia resident applicants. The Admissions Committee looks for students who will make significant contributions to society as members of the medical profession. Factors such as depth of motivation and commitment to medicine are evaluated. Some medically related experience that involves patient contact is considered important.

PROCESS

AMCAS applicants are sent secondary applications. About 25 to 30 percent of Virginia resident applicants are interviewed, while only about 10 percent of nonresidents make it to the interview stage. On interview day, applicants have two interviews, each with a member of the Admissions Committee. Candidates also attend a group orientation session and have the opportunity to tour the campus and eat lunch with current medical students. Notification begins after October 15 and continues on a rolling basis until the class is filled. Wait-listed candidates may send additional information to update their files.

Admissions Requirements (Required)

MCAT scores, science GPA, non-science GPA, letters of recommendation, interview, essays/personal statement, extracurricular activities, exposure to medical profession.

Admissions Requirements (Optional)

state residency.

Overlap Schools

Duke University, Johns Hopkins University, Vanderbilt University.

COSTS AND AID

In-state tuition	$22,486
Out-of-state tuition	$34,546
Cost of books	$1,000

Financial Aid

% students receiving aid	85
Average grant	$10,265
Average loan	$17,803
Average debt	$72,000

UNIVERSITY OF WASHINGTON
SCHOOL OF MEDICINE

A-300 HEALTH SCIENCES, BOX 356340, SEATTLE, WA 98195 • ADMISSION: 206-543-7212 • FAX: 206-616-3341 • E-MAIL: ASKUWSOM@U.WASHINGTON.EDU • WEBSITE: WWW.WASHINGTON.EDU/MEDICINE/SOM/

STUDENT BODY

Type	Public
Enrollment	734
% male/female	52/48
% underrepresented minorities	10
# applied (total/out)	3,124/2,203
# accepted (total/out)	229/39
# enrolled (total/out)	176/12

ADMISSIONS

Average GPA and MCAT Scores

Overall GPA	3.7
MCAT Bio	11.2
MCAT Phys	10.7
MCAT Verbal	10.3
MCAT Essay	Q

Application Information

Regular application	11/1
Regular notification	11/1
Are transfers accepted?	Yes
Admissions may be deferred?	Yes
Interview required?	Yes
Application fee	$35

Academics

Students who enter UW as residents of Wyoming, Alaska, Montana, and Idaho spend their first year at the university site in their home state. Twenty Washington students begin medical studies at Washington State University in Pullman and then transfer to the UW campus after completing their first year. Other students complete a four-year program based in Seattle. From eight to ten students each year enter the MSTP MS/PhD program. The doctoral degree may be earned in biochemistry, bioengineering, biomathematics/biostatistics, biological structure, epidemiology, environmental health, genetics, immunology, microbiology, molecular biotechnology, pathology, pharmacology, physiology, biophysics, and zoology. Medical students are evaluated with grades of honors, satisfactory, and not satisfactory. Passing Step 1 of the USMLE is a requirement for promotion to year three, and passing Step 2 is a requirement for graduation.

BASIC SCIENCES: First-year courses at the UW campus are microscopic anatomy; gross anatomy and embryology; mechanisms in cell physiology; biochemistry; cell and tissue response to injury; natural history of infectious diseases and chemotherapy; introduction to immunology; systems of human behavior; epidemiology; head, neck, ear, nose and throat; and nervous system. Most second-year topics are organized around body/organ systems, which are cardiovascular; complementary medicine; respiratory; pharmacology; endocrine; systemic pathology; gastrointestinal; hematology; musculoskeletal; genetics; urinary; reproduction; skin; and nutrition. Other courses are introduction to clinical medicine and medicine, health, and society. The rural/underserved opportunities program enables first-year medical students to work with practicing physicians in small towns or inner-city neighborhoods and to learn firsthand about working with underserved communities.

CLINICAL TRAINING

The clinical curriculum covers the third and fourth years and includes clerkships in medicine (twelve weeks), obstetrics/gynecology (six weeks), pediatrics (six weeks), psychiatry (six weeks), surgery (six weeks), family medicine (six weeks), emergency medicine (four weeks), and rehabilitation (two weeks). An additional twenty-four weeks of electives are required. Selected third-year students participate in an alternate, rural training program, which involves six months in a rural, primary care practice. In its teaching, patient care, and research programs, the School of Medicine is affiliated with Children's Hospital, Harborview Hospital (411 beds), UW Medical Center (450 beds), Seattle Veterans' Affairs Hospital, Fred Hutchinson Cancer Research Center, Boise Veterans' Affairs Hospital, Providence Hospital, Swedish Hospital, Madigan Hospital, and the Group Health Cooperative. Additional affiliations across the Pacific Northwest enable medical students to train in more than seventy-five communities in Washington, Alaska, Montana, and Idaho. The International Medical Education Office organizes a range of activities including exchange programs that allow UW medical students to participate in clinical electives overseas.

Students

About 93 percent of the 176 students in each class are residents of Washington, Alaska, Montana, Wyoming, or Idaho. Out-of-region students make up a total of about 10 percent of the student body and include MS/PhD students. There is a wide age range among medical students, with significant numbers of them in their late twenties and thirties.

STUDENT LIFE

UW offers countless extracurricular opportunities and attractions, including cultural programs, student groups, intercollegiate sporting events, and social functions. Medical students take advantage of these opportunities and the tremendous resources afforded by UW and its student community. Seattle is an ideal city for students, offering outstanding daytime and outdoor activities and an excellent nightlife. Around the city are beautiful areas suitable for hiking, camping, mountain climbing, running, biking, swimming, and skiing. Most students live off campus.

GRADUATES

Of the roughly 5,000 UW School of Medicine alumni, about 50 percent are practicing or training in fields designated as physician-shortage specialties, which include family physicians, general internists, general pediatricians, psychiatrists, general surgeons, and general practitioners. Among students in the 1996 graduating class, 62 percent entered residency programs in primary care fields, which encompass family medicine, internal medicine, and pediatrics.

Admissions

REQUIREMENTS

Prerequisites are biology (eight semester hours), chemistry (twelve semester hours, which can be satisfied by any combination of inorganic, organic, biochemistry, or molecular biology courses), and physics (four semester hours). In addition the understanding of basic biochemistry, an understanding molecular biology concepts is required. An additional eight semester hours of unspecified science course work is required. This requirement can be met by taking other courses in any of the above three categories. The MCAT is required, and scores must be from within three years of application.

SUGGESTIONS

Preference is given to legal residents of Washington, Wyoming, Alaska, Montana, and Idaho. Applicants from disadvantaged backgrounds or who are willing to serve the underserved are also considered. Candidates should be proficient in the use of the English language and in basic mathematics and are expected to have an understanding of personal computing and information technologies. Some biochemistry or molecular biology is also recommended.

PROCESS

All Washington residents and a limited number of highly qualified, nonresidents are sent secondary applications and invited to interview. Interviews take place between October and April and consist of one session with a panel of interviewers. Also on interview day, candidates have the opportunity to meet with current students and to tour the campus. About 30 percent of interviewed candidates are accepted. Others are rejected or put in a hold category.

Admissions Requirements (Required)

MCAT scores, letters of recommendation, interview, state residency, essays/personal statement.

Admissions Requirements (Optional)

science GPA, nonscience GPA, extracurricular activities, exposure to medical profession.

COSTS AND AID

In-state tuition	$12,450
Out-of-state tuition	$29,391

Financial Aid

% students receiving aid	83

UNIVERSITY OF WESTERN ONTARIO

ADMISSIONS/STUDENT & EQUITY AFFAIRS

MEDICAL SCIENCES BUILDING, LONDON, ON N6A 5C1 • ADMISSION: 519-661-3744 • FAX: 519-661-3797 • E-MAIL: ADMISSIONS@FMD.UWO.CA • WEBSITE: WWW.FMD.UWO.CA

STUDENT BODY

Type	Public
Enrollment	500
% male/female	55/45
# applied (total)	1,690
# accepted (total)	133
# enrolled (total)	133
Average age	23

ADMISSIONS

Average GPA and MCAT Scores

Overall GPA	3.6
MCAT Bio	9
MCAT Phys	9
MCAT Verbal	9
MCAT Essay	P

Application Information

Regular application	10/15
Regular notification	5/31
Are transfers accepted?	No
Admissions may be deferred?	No
Interview required?	Yes
Application fee	$175

Academics

The Faculty of Medicine and Dentistry and the Faculty of Graduate Studies has established a combined MD/PhD program in which the research curriculum of the graduate program is integrated into the MD program. Applicants must be accepted to the medical school as MD candidates before entering the combined program.

BASIC SCIENCES: During the third year integrated clerkship, the student will become an active member of clinical care teams in the following medical disciplines: family medicine, medicine, obstetrics and gynecology, pediatrics, psychiatry, and surgery. Under the supervision of faculty and more senior house staff, clerks will be given graded responsibility in the investigation, diagnosis, and management of patients in hospital and outpatient settings. The clerkship year incorporates rural experiences throughout Southwestern Ontario. Some students will be placed outside London for the entire clerkshiip year. Beginning in the fourth year, clinical electives will be arranged by the student in any area of medicine at UWO or other approved centers. For students who wish to arrange electives in developing countries, we have a medical electives overseas officer who advises and assists students with making their arrangements. After completion of the clinical electives, students will return to the UWO in February for the transition period which includes advanced basic sciences (surgical anatomy and medical physiology), advanced communication skills, general review, health care systems, and so on. This will permit students to further integrate the basic and clinical aspects of medicine in light of their clinical experience.

CLINICAL TRAINING

The first two years of the new curriculum will provide students with a solid grounding in the basic and clinical sciences. These two years are each divided into a series of six blocks. Within each block various subject areas are presented that integrate the basic and clinical sciences. The blocks are introduction to medicine, heart and circulation, digestive systems and nutrition, endocrine and metabolism, genito-urinary system, immunology and skin, life cycle, musculoskeletal, neurosciences, eye and ear, psychiatry and behavioural sciences, reproduction, and respiration and airways.

During each week or block, the case of a single patient will be discussed. A facilitator will help students to determine the biological, behavioral, and population issues that are pertinent to the patient; the objectives for the week's instruction will be described. Students will then receive instruction throughout the week relevant to the patient's case using a variety of teaching methods such as lectures, small group sessions, and labs. Students will also be expected to obtain information pertinent to the case objectives. The faculty has excellent library and resource facilities to support self study. In the middle of the week, students will meet to review the instruction to date and relate it to the patient case. At the end of the week, the students will meet in a plenary session to discuss the case of the week.

A particular strength of our program will be the opportunity for early patient contact. Patient-centered care recognizes the need to see the health concerns of a patient through the patient's eyes. The illness experience markedly differs from the traditional teaching in medical schools where the emphasis has been on teaching about only the disease and not on the experiences of the patient with that disease. In the patient-centered approach, the emphasis is on defining the unique illness experience of patients and their relation to family and community in economic, social, and environmental dimensions. The first two years of the program provide a variety of opportunities for students to better understand the relationship between health care and the community.

Students

Class size is 133.

STUDENT LIFE

The University of Western Ontario offers students a rich lifestyle. School-sponsored events and countless clubs and organizations are offered on campus. London is a small city of about 300,000 with a range of cultural and recreational activities. Both on- and off-campus housing is available.

GRADUATES

The curriculum is designed to allow graduates to enter any clinical or medical research field. A significant portion of graduates enter residency programs at hospitals affiliated with the University of Western Ontario.

Admissions

REQUIREMENTS

Enrollment is limited to Canadian citizens and permanent residents of Canada. Candidates who are in the third year or have successfully completed three full years of study in any degree program at a recognized university are eligible to apply. A minimum of five full or equivalent courses must be included in the final undergraduate year (September to April year only). Science prerequisites are one full course in biology, one full course in organic chemistry, and one additional full science course. Nonscience prerequisites are two full nonscience courses from different disciplines and one senior-level course in one of these two subjects. Interested applicants should contact the faculty for more detailed course requirements. The MCAT is required. The latest date that applicants should take the exam is August in the year of application. Only applicants who have achieved a certain grade point average and MCAT scores will be considered for admission. Typically, the minimum GPA is 3.5 and minimum MCAT scores are a 9 on Biological Sciences, an 8 on Physical Sciences, a 9 on Verbal Reasoning, and a Q on the Writing Sample. English proficiency is a requirement.

SUGGESTIONS

For entrance in fall 2002, there were 1,690 applicants for 133 positions. Thus, admission is competitive. Apart from science prerequisites, there is no prescribed pre-med program. Students at Western Ontario come from a variety of undergraduate programs and a wide variety of disciplines. For those who have retaken the MCAT, only the most recent scores is used.

PROCESS

The deadline for application is October 15 for the following September. Applicants now apply online at www.ouac.on.ca/omsas/. Applicants who satisfy the course load, GPA, and MCAT requirements will generally be invited for an interview. Letters indicating admissions decisions are sent to applicants beginning in the end of May until the class is full.

Admissions Requirements (Required)

MCAT scores, science GPA, non-science GPA, letters of recommendation, interview, state residency.

Admissions Requirements (Optional)

essays/personal statement, extracurricular activities, exposure to medical profession.

COSTS AND AID

Tuition	$14,280
Cost of books	$2,200
Fees	$808

University of Wisconsin

Medical School

Medical Sciences Center, Room 1140, 1300 University Avenue, Madison, WI 53706-1532 • Admission: 608-263-4925 • Fax: 608-262-2327 • E-mail: lwall@wisc.edu • Website: www.med.wisc.edu

STUDENT BODY

Type	Public
Enrollment	619
% male/female	47/53
% underrepresented minorities	8
# applied (total/out)	652/218
# accepted (total/out)	230/53
# enrolled (total/out)	150/19
Average age	24

ADMISSIONS

Average GPA and MCAT Scores

Overall GPA	3
MCAT Bio	10.6
MCAT Phys	10.2
MCAT Verbal	10
MCAT Essay	P

Application Information

Regular application	11/1
Regular notification	rolling
Early application	8/1 and 9/1
Early notification	10/1
Are transfers accepted?	Yes
Admissions may be deferred?	Yes
Interview required?	Yes
Application fee	$45

Academics

The UW Medical School offers an MD degree and a dual MD/PhD degree option. In addition, students can combine training for the MD degree with earning a master's degree in population health. Medical students are evaluated with letter grades. Students must pass Step 1 of the USMLE for promotion to year three and must take Steps 2 and 3 to graduate.

BASIC SCIENCES: The revised curriculum features fewer lectures and more small group discussions, practical laboratories, multimedia computer programs and videos, and significant opportunities to learn through real life clinical examples. An important component of the new curriculum is the generalist partners program (GPP) which matches first-year medical students with primary care physicians who practice in the community and who serve as teachers and mentors to students. Through GPP, students learn firsthand about generalist medicine, and enjoy early patient care opportunities. Also during the first and second years, students take an interdisciplinary course that addresses practicing medicine in a variety of modern day environments. Other first-year courses are gross anatomy, biomolecular chemistry, genetics, histology, neuroscience, pathology, and physiology. The second-year pathophysiology courses are organized around body/organ systems, including hematology, cardiovascular, renal, respiratory, neoplastic disease, endocrine, gastrointestinal, and hepatic. Other courses are infection and immunity, pharmacology, psychiatry, and nutrition. The William S. Middleton Medical Library is used by students for research and for studying. It houses 150,000 volumes and 2,000 publications.

CLINICAL TRAINING

The third- and fourth-year clerkships expose students to a wide variety of clinical settings (outpatient, inpatient, community based, rural, and inner city). Training takes place at university hospitals in Madison as well as in affiliated sites in Milwaukee, La Crosse, and Marshfield. Third-year required clerkships are medicine (eight weeks), primary care (eight weeks), surgery (eight weeks), pediatrics (six weeks), obstetrics/gynecology (six weeks), anesthesia (two weeks), neuroscience (six weeks), psychiatry (four weeks), and ophthalmology (one week). During the fourth year, students complete an acting internship in medicine (four weeks), an advanced surgery clerkship (four weeks), a preceptorship (six weeks), and eighteen weeks of electives. A portion of electives may be taken at other academic and clinical institutions, both in the United States and overseas. The UW International Health Exchange is an affiliated nonprofit foundation that increases awareness of international health issues through a range of activities that include promoting overseas clinical experiences for students.

Students

Each class consists of 150 students. Approximately 80 percent of students are Wisconsin residents. During the past four years, about 50 percent of all students attended UW for their undergraduate education. About 14 percent of students are underrepresented minorities. About 10 students in each class are in their late twenties or thirties.

STUDENT LIFE

The medical school benefits from the resources of one of the top public universities in the U.S. Medical students have access to the facilities of the large campus and enjoy the lively environment of a popular college city. Students are active in community service projects such as volunteering at homeless shelters and clinics and organizing AIDS or other education projects. On-campus housing is available for all students, including students who are married. Most students prefer to live in shared apartments off campus. Madison is a midsized city located around three lakes.

GRADUATES

Graduates are successful in securing residency positions at prestigious institutions throughout the United States.

Admissions

REQUIREMENTS

Minimum science requirements are general biology with lab (one semester), advanced biology/zoology with lab (one semester) or biochemistry, general chemistry with lab (one year), organic chemistry with lab (one year), general physics with lab (one year), and mathematics (two semesters). The MCAT is required; for the 2005 entering class, scores must be from 2001 or later. For candidates who have retaken the exam, the higher values of the two most recent scores are used.

SUGGESTIONS

UW gives preference to residents of Wisconsin; however, about 15 to 20 percent of each incoming class consists of nonresidents. A sound liberal arts education, including both humanities and social sciences, is considered important. While specific courses are not required, the applicant's preparation should include courses in areas that prepare them for the social, psychological, and economic aspects of medical practice. The Admissions Committee members rely heavily on applicant essays, letters of recommendation, and the personal interviews to assess motivation and personal character.

PROCESS

Upon receipt of the AMCAS application, the UW Secondary Application is sent to Wisconsin residents who meet the minimal academic thresholds (GPA greater than 2.8 and MCAT scores greater than 7, 7, and 8) and to highly qualified nonresidents. All applicants who receive a secondary application are invited to interview. Interviews take place between August and March and consist of one session with a faculty member and one with a medical student. Interview-day activities include group informational sessions, a tour, and lunch with medical students.

Admissions Requirements (Required)

MCAT scores, science GPA, non-science GPA, letters of recommendation, interview, essays/personal statement, extracurricular activities, exposure to medical profession.

Admissions Requirements (Optional)

state residency.

COSTS AND AID

In-state tuition	$21,153
Out-of-state tuition	$32,277
Cost of books	$2,000
Fees	$584

Financial Aid

% students receiving aid	85
Average grant	$15,000
Average loan	$37,000
Average debt	$115,000

Vanderbilt University

Vanderbilt University School of Medicine

215 Light Hall, Nashville, TN 37232-0685 • Admission: 615-322-2145 • Fax: 615-343-8397 • E-mail: hal.helderman@vanderbilt.edu • Website: www.mc.vanderbilt.edu/medschool/admissions/index.php

STUDENT BODY

Type	Private
Enrollment	415
% male/female	53/47
% underrepresented minorities	4
# applied (total/out)	3,507/3,267
# accepted (total/out)	270/248
# enrolled (total/out)	104/88
Average age	23

FACULTY

Total faculty (number)	1,444
% female	30
% minority	5
% part-time	2
# student/faculty ratio	2:1

ADMISSIONS

Average GPA and MCAT Scores

Overall GPA	3.8
MCAT Bio	11.13
MCAT Phys	10.97
MCAT Verbal	10.19
MCAT Essay	Q

Application Information

Regular application	11/15
Regular notification	Rolling
Early application	6/1-8/1
Early notification	10/1
Are transfers accepted?	Yes
Admissions may be deferred?	Yes
Interview required?	Yes
Application fee	$50

Academics

Most students complete a four-year curriculum that leads to an MD degree. Some students opt to take an additional year to work on research or independent projects. A few students each year enter a combined MS/PhD program that leads to the doctoral degree in cell biology, biochemistry, biomedical engineering, microbiology and immunology, molecular biology, pathology, pharmacology, or molecular physiology and biophysics. Many joint degree candidates are sponsored and supported by the medical scientist training program. Medical students are evaluated with grades of A, B, C, and F, with the exception of first- and second-year electives, which are pass/fail.

BASIC SCIENCES: During the first year, students focus on the basic sciences, which are primarily taught through lectures and labs. courses are biochemistry, gross anatomy, microbiology, cell and tissue biology, introduction to biomedical research, physiology, and behavioral science. Several afternoons each week are reserved for electives, many of which are problem-based. During the second year, introductory clinical training is integrated into basic science instruction, and small group discussions complement the lecture/lab format. Second-year courses are pathology, neurobiology, laboratory diagnosis, radiology, pharmacology, preventive medicine, psychiatry, and physical diagnosis. During the first two years, students are in class or other scheduled sessions for about thirty-four hours per week. Most instruction takes place in Light Hall, which is connected by tunnels to clinical and research facilities. For research and study purposes, students and faculty use the Eskind Biomedical Library, which houses more than 200,000 volumes and 2,000 periodicals, in addition to computer-based informational resources. The Vanderbilt University Computer Center provides a full range of computing services and resources to faculty, staff, and students.

CLINICAL TRAINING

Required third-year clerkships are medicine (ten weeks), surgery (ten weeks), pediatrics (eight weeks), psychiatry-neurology (eight weeks), and obstetrics/gynecology (eight weeks). During their fourth year, students must also complete advanced clerkships selected from medical, surgical, primary care, and emergency medicine fields. Sixteen weeks of electives are also required. Most clinical training takes place at the Vanderbilt University Hospital (660 beds), at other VUMC institutions, and at clinical affiliates such as Veterans' Administration Medical Center (439 beds), Howard Hughes Medical Institute, Saint Thomas Hospital, Baptist Hospital, and Middle Tennessee Mental Health Institute. With permission, some elective requirements may be fulfilled at other academic or clinical institutions.

Students

The 2002 entering class came from thirty-three states and five foreign countries. Fifty-seven undergraduate institutions were represented. The age range was twenty to fifty, 5 percent of students were underrepresented minorities, and 46 percent were females.

STUDENT LIFE

Vanderbilt's attractive campus provides a focal point for student life and promotes cohesiveness within the student body. Students interact in common areas such as dining halls, cafés, study areas, and the student center. Athletic facilities include fitness centers, indoor and outdoor tracks, a tennis center, playing fields, a swimming pool, basketball, racquetball and squash courts, and a rock climbing wall. Medical students participate alongside other graduate and professional students in intramural sports, fitness classes, and recreational clubs. In addition to being a world renowned hub for live music, Nashville offers many attractions that include a historic riverfront district, many restaurants, brew pubs, coffeehouses, nightclubs, bookstores, seasonal street fairs, farmers' markets, museums, and a large performing arts center. Nashville is also an academic center and is home to more than a dozen colleges and universities. Conveniently located, university-owned apartments are available to single and married students and to students with larger families. In addition, off-campus housing is readily available.

GRADUATES

Students perform exceptionally well on the USMLE, which contributes to their success in securing residency positions at prestigious institutions nationwide.

Admissions

REQUIREMENTS

Prerequisites are eight semester hours each of biology, chemistry, organic chemistry, and physics. Six semester hours of English are also required. The MCAT is required, and scores should be from within the past three years. For applicants who have retaken the exam, the most recent set of scores is weighed most heavily. Thus, there is no real advantage in withholding scores. No AP credit nor pass/fail credit is accepted for required courses.

SUGGESTIONS

The school seeks students who have strong backgrounds in both the sciences and liberal arts. The April MCAT is preferred over the August one. Extracurricular activities, particularly activities that involve hospital and medical exposure, are important.

PROCESS

For 2004 secondary applications will be sent only to candidates who are granted an interview. Interviews are conducted between September and March and consist of one session with a faculty member or administrator. On interview day, applicants also take part in a group orientation session, lunch with students, and a tour of the campus. About 30 percent of interviewees are accepted and are notified on a rolling basis. Wait-listed candidates may send supplementary information to update their files.

Admissions Requirements (Required)

MCAT scores, science GPA, non-science GPA, letters of recommendation, interview, essays/personal statement.

Admissions Requirements (Optional)

state residency, extracurricular activities, exposure to medical profession.

Overlap Schools

Duke University, Harvard University, Johns Hopkins University, University of Pennsylvania, Washington University.

COSTS AND AID

Tuition	$30,100
Room and board	$8,280
Cost of books	$4,993
Fees	$2,057

Financial Aid

% students receiving aid	87
Average grant	$22,400
Average loan	$30,300
Average debt	$110,500

Virginia Commonwealth University
School of Medicine

Box 980565, Richmond, VA 23298 • Admission: 804-828-9629 • Fax: 804-828-1246 • E-mail: somume@hsc.vcu.edu • Website: www.medschool.vcu.edu

STUDENT BODY

Type	Public
Enrollment	698
% male/female	51/49
% underrepresented minorities	7
# applied (total/out)	3,471/2,750
# accepted (total/out)	394/201
# enrolled (total/out)	184/69
Average age	23

FACULTY

Total faculty (number)	982
% female	33
% minority	4
% part-time	26
# student/faculty ratio	1:1

ADMISSIONS

Average GPA and MCAT Scores

Overall GPA	3.5
MCAT Bio	9.9
MCAT Phys	9.6
MCAT Verbal	9.3
MCAT Essay	0

Application Information

Regular application	11/15
Regular notification	10/15
Early application	6/1-8/1
Early notification	10/1
Are transfers accepted?	Yes
Admissions may be deferred?	Yes
Interview required?	Yes
Application fee	$80

Academics

The MD Degree program is four years long. A combined MS/PhD program is also offered and generally takes seven years to complete. Medical students who are interested in public health can earn an MPH concurrently with the MD degree. A fellowship program gives medical students the opportunity to participate in research projects, either during summers or throughout the school year. Medical students are evaluated with grades of honors, high pass, pass, marginal, and fail.

BASIC SCIENCES: Although the emphasis is on the basic sciences, the following are also taught during the first two years: behavioral science, preventive medicine, epidemiology, and public health. Laboratory and classroom time is supplemented by a longitudinal experience designed to give students early clinical exposure. First-year courses are cell biology; biochemistry; anatomical sciences; physiology; behavioral sciences; human genetics; population medicine/biostatistics; neuroscience; pathogenesis; immunology; ethics; and foundations of clinical medicine, which meets two half-days per week, uses community physicians as mentors, and teaches the basics of patient interviewing and physical diagnosis. The second-year curriculum is organized largely by body/organ systems. Courses are autonomic pharmacology, microbiology/infectious diseases, preventive medicine, hematology/oncology, central nervous system, gastroenterology, behavioral science, respiratory, cardiovascular, musculoskeletal/dermatology, renal, endocrine, reproduction, and continuation of foundations of clinical medicine. Two libraries—the University Library and the Tompkins-McCaw Library—support the research needs of students and faculty. Another important educational resource is the computer-based instructional laboratory, which features computer workstations and audiovisual equipment.

CLINICAL TRAINING

Third-year required clerkships are the following: medicine (twelve weeks), surgery (eight weeks), psychiatry (six weeks), obstetrics/gynecology (six weeks), pediatrics (eight weeks), family practice (four weeks), and neurology (four weeks). An additional requirement is one week of a workshop that covers topics such as nutrition, ethics, legal medicine, health economics, and clinical pharmacology. Fourth-year requirements are an acting internship, a board review course, a clinical update course, and twenty-four weeks of electives. For training purposes, medical students have access to over 1,050 beds at MCV hospitals. A Level I trauma center, a transplant center, and one of the nation's most prominent head injury centers are among MCV's clinical facilities. Students also have contact with outpatients at McGuire Veterans' Administration Medical Center.

Students

Approximately 70 percent of students are Virginia residents. The average age of incoming students is usually twenty-three, and each year about thirty students are in their late twenties and thirties. Underrepresented minorities account for about 10 percent of the student body. Class size is 184.

STUDENT LIFE

VCU has at least twenty student organizations. These include groups that are focused on professional pursuits, community service, and religious interests. A variety of facilities, services, and programs designed to meet the leisure and health needs of students are coordinated by the recreational sports staff. The Cary Street Recreation complex and the main VCU gym offer fitness facilities, including a pool, weight rooms, areas for fitness classes, and squash, tennis, and basketball courts. Students have the opportunity to interact outside of class in the new student lounge and in other common areas. Richmond offers many recreational attractions such as parks, museums, historical centers, and shopping areas. While some medical students live in campus residence halls, most live in nearby restored neighborhoods or in surrounding suburban areas.

GRADUATES

MCV students score above the national average on the USMLE, which contributes to their success in obtaining post-graduate positions. About 25 percent of each graduating class enters residency programs administered by MCV hospitals, while others are successful at securing positions in other parts of the state and country. VCU alumni sponsor a unique bed-and-breakfast program, whereby members of the alumni host medical students who are traveling for residency interviews.

Admissions

REQUIREMENTS

Prerequisites are eight semester hours each of biology, chemistry, organic chemistry, and physics, all with associated labs. Two semesters of English and two semesters of college-level math are also required. The MCAT is required and must have been taken within three years of application. For applicants who have taken the exam more than once, the best set of scores is considered.

SUGGESTIONS

Students are encouraged to pursue their own intellectual interests in college. VCU recognizes that studying medicine requires commitment, strong analytical abilities, good judgment, and sound communication skills. In addition to academic abilities, the Admissions Committee looks for important attributes of character and personality.

PROCESS

About 75 percent of AMCAS applicants who are Virginia residents and about 40 percent of nonresidents are sent secondary applications. Applicants returning secondary applications are further screened, and some of them are invited to interview on campus. Interviews take place between August and March, and consist of one session with a faculty member, medical student, or administrator. On interview day, students also attend group informational sessions, have lunch with current medical students, and tour the campus. Notification occurs on October 15, in mid-December, and in mid-March.

Admissions Requirements (Required)

MCAT scores, science GPA, non-science GPA, letters of recommendation, interview, essays/personal statement, extracurricular activities, exposure to medical profession.

Admissions Requirements (Optional)

state residency.

Overlap Schools

Duke University, Eastern Virginia Medical School, Emory University, Georgetown University, Johns Hopkins University, The George Washington University, University of Virginia.

COSTS AND AID

In-state tuition	$12,025
Out-of-state tuition	$30,350
Room and board	$8,630
Cost of books	$1,480
Fees	$1,306

Financial Aid

Average grant	$4,069
Average loan	$27,338
Average debt	$94,681

WAKE FOREST UNIVERSITY
WAKE FOREST UNIVERSITY SCHOOL OF MEDICINE

OFFICE OF ADMISSIONS, MEDICAL CENTER BOULEVARD, WINSTON-SALEM, NC 27157-1090 • ADMISSION: 336-716-4264 • FAX: 910-716-9593 • E-MAIL: MEDADMIT@WFUBMC.EDU • WEBSITE: WWW.WFUBMC.EDU

STUDENT BODY

Type	Private
Enrollment	438
% male/female	60/40
% underrepresented minorities	15
# applied (total/out)	5,152/4,572
# accepted (total/out)	297/201
# enrolled (total/out)	108/68
Average age	23

FACULTY

Total faculty (number)	1,362
% female	21
% minority	13
% part-time	40
# student/faculty ratio	1:1

ADMISSIONS

Average GPA and MCAT Scores

Overall GPA	3.6
MCAT Bio	10
MCAT Phys	10
MCAT Verbal	10
MCAT Essay	P

Application Information

Regular application	11/1
Regular notification	rolling
Early application	6/1-8/1
Early notification	10/1
Are transfers accepted?	Yes
Admissions may be deferred?	Yes
Interview required?	Yes
Application fee	$55

Academics

The curriculum which combines features of traditional and problem-based learning methodologies was implemented in 1998. For details about the curriculum, contact the admissions office. Joint-degree programs include the MD/MBA in conjunction with The Babcock Graduate School of Management, the MD/MS (epidemiology), the MB/MA intercultural studies, and the MS/PhD. The PhD degree is offered in the following fields: anatomy, biochemistry, genetics, immunology, microbiology, molecular biology, neuroscience, pathology, pharmacology, and physiology. Students are evaluated with grades of 0 to 3, and both steps of the USMLE are required for graduation.

BASIC SCIENCES: The preclinical curriculum emphasizes self directed and lifelong learning skills, core biomedical science knowledge, problem solving/reasoning, interviewing and communication skills, information management, and professional attitudes and behavior. The course foundations of clinical medicine is taken throughout year one and two and provide students with instruction in interviewing and physical examination skills. First-year courses focus on helping students to build a foundation in the core biomedical sciences, and second-year courses are organized around body/organ systems. The course medicine as a profession is an interdisiplinary course that touches on a range of issues related to the practice of medicine. Most preclinical instruction takes place in the Hanes Research Building. The James A Gray Building houses the library, which contains more than 120,000 volumes and 3,800 medical and scientific journals, in addition to audiovisual and computer-based educational aids.

CLINICAL TRAINING

Third-year required rotations are inpatient medicine (eight weeks), surgery (eight weeks), obstetrics/gynecology (six weeks), pediatrics (eight weeks), neurology/rehibilitation medicine (four weeks), anesthesiology (one week), and radiology (one week). Required Outpatient clerkships are internal medicine (four weeks), obstetrics/gynecology and women's health (six weeks), and family medicine (four weeks). During the fourth year, students fullfill the remaining requirements, which are emergency medicine (four weeks), intensive care (four weeks), eight weeks of required advancement patient management clerkships, and electives (twenty-four weeks). Training takes place at North Carolina Baptist Hospital (806 beds), which includes a children's hospital and a rehibilitation unit, among other specialty facilities. Other sites used for instruction that are located in both rural and urban areas include Forsyth Memorial Hospital and the Downtown Health Plaza.

Students

Approximately 30 to 40 percent of each class is made up of North Carolina residents, and about 10 percent are from Wake Forest's undergraduate program. The remainder represent up to 100 different colleges. About 14 percent of students are underrepresented minorities, most of whom are African American. Class size is 108.

STUDENT LIFE

A student life and fitness center gives students the opportunity to work out, study, gather, or simply relax. The fitness center includes Nautilus equipment, free weights, showers, and a steam room. Other features are a quiet, twenty-four-hour study area, vending machines, a TV lounge, and rooms suitable for small group discussions. The School of Medicine is located on the Bowman Gray campus, about four miles from the Reynolds campus of Wake Forest, where many academic and cultural events take place. Two state parks are within an hour's drive of Wake Forest, and the Carolina beaches are about four hours away. There is no on-campus housing, but apartments and rooms are readily available in the surrounding areas.

GRADUATES

Wake Forest's reputation, coupled with its students above-average scores on national boards, allows graduates to enter competitive residency programs all over the country.

Admissions

REQUIREMENTS

Requirements are eight semester hours in biology, chemistry, organic chemistry, and physics. The MCAT is required, and scores must be no more than three years old. For applicants who have retaken the exam, the best set of scores is considered.

SUGGESTIONS

A well-rounded academic experience, including courses in the humanities, is strongly advised. For students who have taken significant time off after college, recent course work is suggested. The April MCAT is recommended over the August one, as it allows applicants to retake the exam if necessary. Medically related or community-service experiences are considered valuable.

PROCESS

Approximately half of AMCAS applicants are sent secondary application materials. About 10 percent of those returning secondary applications are invited to interview sometime between September and March. Interviews are one-on-one and consist of three fifteen- to twenty-minute sessions with faculty and/or Admissions Committee members. On interview day, candidates also receive a tour and a group orientation. Candidates are notified on a rolling basis whether they are accepted, rejected, or wait-listed. Wait-listed candidates are generally not encouraged to submit supplemental materials. An alternate path to admissions is through an early assurance program that accepts competitive college juniors even though they have not taken the MCAT. If successful, these students complete their senior year knowing that they have been admitted to medical school for the year following college graduation.

Admissions Requirements (Required)

MCAT scores, science GPA, non-science GPA, letters of recommendation, interview, essays/personal statement, extracurricular activities, exposure to medical profession.

Overlap Schools

Duke University, Emory University, University of North Carolina at Chapel Hill, Vanderbilt University, Virginia Commonwealth University.

COSTS AND AID

Tuition	$32,056
Cost of books	$1,460

Financial Aid

% students receiving aid	85
Average grant	$6,000
Average loan	$27,900
Average debt	$126,000

Washington University in St. Louis

Washington University School of Medicine

Campus Box 8107, 660 South Euclid Avenue, St. Louis, MO 63110 • Admission: 314-362-6848 • Fax: 314-362-4658 • E-mail: wumscoa@msnotes.wustl.edu • Website: http://medschool.wustl.edu/admissions

STUDENT BODY

Type	Private
Enrollment	578
% male/female	55/45
% underrepresented minorities	40
# applied (total)	3,733
# accepted (total)	337
# enrolled (total)	122
Average age	23

FACULTY

Total faculty (number)	2,787
% female	26
% minority	10
% part-time	41
# student/faculty ratio	2:1

ADMISSIONS

Average GPA and MCAT Scores

Overall GPA	3.8
MCAT Bio	12.5
MCAT Phys	12.6
MCAT Verbal	11.3
MCAT Essay	Q

Application Information

Regular application	12/1
Regular notification	rolling
Are transfers accepted?	Yes
Admissions may be deferred?	Yes
Interview required?	Yes
Application fee	$50

Academics

In addition to the four-year MD program, students may apply for a five-year combined MA/MD program, which involves a year of funded research and the completion of a thesis. The MSTP-sponsored MS/PhD program is one of the largest in the country, with up to twenty-three positions available each year. During the first year, students are evaluated with grades of pass and fail, but grades of honors, high pass, pass, and fail are used from the second year onward.

BASIC SCIENCES: During the first two years, students are in class for about twenty hours per week. Scheduled sessions are divided among lectures, labs, and problem-based sessions conducted in small groups. Topics covered in lectures are documented by a transcript service, to which most students subscribe. Most first-year courses address normal human structure and function. They are anatomy, the molecular foundations of medicine, cell and organ systems biology, immunology, genetics, and neuroscience. The course physicians, patients, and society offers first-year students a multidisciplinary perspective on practicing medicine and continues into the second year. Patient contact begins in the first year, in introduction to clinical medicine. Second-year courses focus on the effects of disease and are organized into blocks, most of which are defined by body systems or physiological concepts. these are cardiovascular, clinical epidemiology, dermatology, nervous system, ENT, endocrinology and metabolism, gastrointestinal and liver disease/nutrition, hematology and oncology, infectious disease, obstetrics/gynecology, ophthalmology, pathology, pediatrics, nervous system, pulmonary, renal and genitourinary, and rheumatology. Clinical experience is expanded and integrated into pathology, pathophysiology, and pharmacology. Students have significant input in curriculum development and revision. The library is extensive, housing about 300,000 volumes and equipped with computer and Internet facilities. The gross anatomy lab is particularly renowned.

CLINICAL TRAINING

The third year is reserved for core, required clerkships, which are medicine (twelve weeks); surgery (twelve weeks); neurology (four weeks); psychiatry (four weeks); combined obstetrics/gynecology and pediatrics (twelve weeks); and ambulatory care, which involves emergency medicine, family practice, and psychiatric consultation (twelve weeks). The fourth year (twenty-four weeks) is entirely reserved for electives, which may be in clinical and/or basic science departments. Students are permitted to fulfill up to twelve weeks of clinical clerkships at nonaffiliated institutions. While many other academic health care institutions are struggling, Washington University's Medical Center and their other Barnes-Jewish associated hospitals and clinics are thriving and expanding. Children's Hospital ranks as one of the premier pediatric hospitals in the United States. In total, affiliated hospitals provide over 2,000 patient beds. Students are exposed to a local population in need of basic care and to patients who have come from around the world for the most advanced treatments. The School of Medicine expects students to play important roles in the provision of patient care.

Students

The current student body represents forty-three states and twenty-one foreign countries. Although most of the students are recent college graduates with degrees in one of the hard sciences, there is tremendous diversity in terms of age and undergraduate background. Class size is 120.

STUDENT LIFE

Since most students come from out-of-state (and from overseas), they are eager to get to know each other and tend to form a cohesive group quickly. An extensive orientation session at the beginning of the year aids in this process. Student groups are extremely active, and include groups that focus on community service projects such as operating a free clinic on weekends, intramural sports clubs, and Hot Docs (a musical group). On-campus facilities include the Hilltop Campus Athletic Facility, which is a comprehensive gym and sports center. Social life often centers on the restaurants and bars of the Central West End and the tree-lined paths of Forest Park. Campus housing is available adjacent to the medical school, but many students prefer to live in the surrounding areas since housing is affordable and attractive.

GRADUATES

Graduates gain acceptance to the nation's most competitive residency programs. About half of them enter a primary care field.

Admissions

REQUIREMENTS

Washington University expects applicants to have completed one year of biology, general chemistry, organic chemistry, and physics, in addition to math through the calculus level. The MCAT is required, and scores must be no more than three years old.

SUGGESTIONS

The Admissions Committee looks favorably on candidates who have pursued in-depth study of a particular subject, whether in the natural sciences, social sciences, or humanities. Successful applicants also demonstrate commitment and leadership through their extracurricular activities. Since the medical school offers rolling admissions beginning October 15, applicants should make every attempt to complete materials early.

PROCESS

About 20 percent of AMCAS applicants are interviewed between September and March. Interviews consist of one session with a member of the school's faculty or administration. Notification occurs on a rolling basis, and about one-third of interviewees are accepted. Wait-listed candidates are not ranked and are generally not encouraged to send supplementary material.

Admissions Requirements (Required)

MCAT scores, science GPA, non-science GPA, letters of recommendation, interview, essays/personal statement.

Admissions Requirements (Optional)

state residency, extracurricular activities, exposure to medical profession.

COSTS AND AID

Tuition	$37,032
Cost of books	$1,613

Financial Aid

% students receiving aid	72
Average grant	$27,192
Average loan	$25,264
Average debt	$49,905

Wayne State University

Wayne State University School of Medicine

1310 Scott Hall, 540 E. Canfield, Detroit, MI 48201 • Admission: 313-577-1466 • Fax: 313-577-9420 •
E-mail: admissions@med.wayne.edu • Website: www.med.wayne.edu/admissions

STUDENT BODY

Type	Public
% male/female	100/0
# applied (total/out)	2,722/1,640
# accepted (total/out)	504/102
# enrolled (total/out)	257/30
Average age	24

ADMISSIONS

Average GPA and MCAT Scores

Overall GPA	3.5
MCAT Bio	9.8
MCAT Phys	9.5
MCAT Verbal	8.8
MCAT Essay	0

Application Information

Regular application	12/15
Regular notification	10/15
Early application	6/1-8/1
Early notification	10/1
Are transfers accepted?	Yes
Admissions may be deferred?	Yes
Interview required?	Yes
Application fee	$50

Academics

The School of Medicine administers academic programs that lead to the MD, MS, and PhD. Some medical students pursue a combined MS/PhD that leads to the doctoral degree in anatomy and cell biology, cellular and clinical neurobiology, immunology/microbiology, medical physics, molecular biology and genetics, pathology, pharmacology, and physiology. Other students earn an MS in biomedical or behavioral sciences along with the MD. The standard medical curriculum consists of two years of basic sciences, a year of clinical clerkships, and a year of clinical electives. Evaluation of medical student performance uses grades of honors, pass, and fail. Students must pass Step 1 of the USMLE to receive promotion to year three and must record a score on Step 2 of the USMLE to graduate.

BASIC SCIENCES: Basic science courses are taught primarily in a lecture/lab format, with some use of small group sessions. Students are in class for about twenty hours per week. This schedule gives students the time they need to study, pursue independent projects, and take part in community service or other extracurricular activities. During year one, students learn about the normal functions of the human body. Courses are anatomy, histology, embryology, evidence based medicine, physiology, biochemistry, genetics, neuroscience, clinical nutrition, introduction to the patient, human sexuality, and behavioral medicine. Second-year courses focus on the effects of disease and the principles of drug action and therapy. The pathophysiology course is organized by body/organ systems, which are connective tissue, cardiovascular, hematology, pulmonary, renal, endocrine, gastrointestinal, and neuroscience. Other courses are pathology, microbiology, psychiatry, pharmacology, public health and preventive medicine, physical diagnosis/interviewing, introduction to the patient, medical ethics, and human sexuality. The majority of first- and second-year classes are conducted in Scott Hall, a modern building that houses laboratories, lecture halls, and faculty offices. The Shiffman Medical Library has more than 150,000 volumes, computer facilities, and ample space for studying. Students can view recorded lectures and take advantage of other audiovisual study aids in the self-instruction center.

CLINICAL TRAINING

During the third year, students complete eight-week, required clerkships in internal medicine, surgery, pediatrics, and obstetrics/gynecology. There are also four-week clerkships in family medicine, neurology, and psychiatry. During the fourth year, selectives in ambulatory medicine (four weeks) and emergency medicine (four weeks), in addition to a subinternship (four weeks), are required. Five months of electives are also required, a significant portion of which may be taken at other institutions. Clinical training takes place at the Detroit Medical Center (DMC), which consists of numerous hospitals, institutes, and care centers and has over 2,400 beds. DMC includes Harper Hospital, Grace Hospital, Hutzel Hospital, Children's Hospital of Michigan, Rehabilitation Institute of Michigan, Detroit Receiving Hospital/University Health Center, Gershenson Radiation Oncology Center, Kresge Eye Institute, and Huron Valley Hospital. Medical students also rotate to affiliated hospitals in suburban areas.

Students

About 90 percent of the 256 students in each class are Michigan residents. Approximately 12 percent of students are underrepresented minorities, most of whom are African American. Although a few students are older or nontraditional, most entering students are in their early twenties.

STUDENT LIFE

Medical students are involved in chapters of national organizations such as the American Medical Student Association, professionally oriented groups such as the Family Medicine Interest Group, production of a student newspaper, and numerous community service projects. Volunteer activities involve working with the city's youth, elderly, underinsured and noninsured populations. Medical students also enjoy the extensive extracurricular offerings of Wayne State University, as well as the diverse culture of Detroit. Students live off campus, usually in apartments in the Detroit metropolitan area or in surrounding suburbs. Parking is available on campus, and most students own cars.

GRADUATES

About 65 percent of graduates chose residency programs in Michigan hospitals, and more than 50 percent stay in the Detroit area. In recent years, more than half of all graduates entered primary care fields.

Admissions

REQUIREMENTS

One year each of biology, chemistry, organic chemistry, and physics, all with associated labs, is required. The MCAT is required, and scores should be from the spring or fall of the year prior to entrance. For applicants who have retaken the exam, the most recent set of scores is weighed most heavily; therefore, it is not advantageous to withhold scores.

SUGGESTIONS

Although most positions are reserved for Michigan residents, well-qualified, nonresidents are also considered. In addition to academic credentials, the Admissions Committee is interested in extracurricular activities and work. Health-related volunteer work and research are valuable.

PROCESS

About 50 percent of AMCAS applicants are sent secondary applications, of which about 20 percent are interviewed between September and April. The interview consists of one session with a member of the Admissions Committee. Candidates also receive a tour and have the opportunity to meet with current students. About one-third of interviewed candidates are accepted and are notified shortly after the interview. Wait-listed candidates are generally not encouraged to send additional information.

Admissions Requirements (Required)

MCAT scores, science GPA, non-science GPA, letters of recommendation, interview, essays/personal statement, extracurricular activities, exposure to medical profession.

Admissions Requirements (Optional)

state residency.

Overlap Schools

Michigan State University, University of Michigan.

COSTS AND AID

In-state tuition	$14,204
Out-of-state tuition	$29,556
Cost of books	$1,000

Financial Aid

% students receiving aid	83
Average grant	$5,452
Average loan	$22,649
Average debt	$62,468

West Virginia University

West Virginia University School of Medicine

PO Box 9111, Morgantown, WV 26506 • Admission: 304-293-2408 • Fax: 304-293-7814 •
E-mail: medadmissions@hsc.wvu.edu • Website: www.hsc.wvu.edu

STUDENT BODY

Type	Public
Enrollment	391
% male/female	60/40
% underrepresented minorities	2
# applied (total/out)	845/617
# accepted (total/out)	151/49
# enrolled (total/out)	107/27
Average age	22

FACULTY

Total faculty (number)	611
% female	32
% minority	17
% part-time	16

ADMISSIONS

Average GPA and MCAT Scores

Overall GPA	3.7
MCAT Bio	9.4
MCAT Phys	8.7
MCAT Verbal	9.1
MCAT Essay	0

Application Information

Regular application	12/1
Regular notification	rolling
Early application	8/1
Early notification	10/1
Are transfers accepted?	Yes
Admissions may be deferred?	Yes
Interview required?	Yes
Application fee	$100

Academics

While most medical students follow a four-year curriculum and earn the MD degree, about two medical students each year pursue joint MS/PhD degrees that lead to the doctorate in anatomy, biochemistry, medical technology, microbiology, pathology, pharmacology and toxicology, and physiology. Medical students are evaluated with grades of honors, satisfactory, or unsatisfactory for all courses and clerkships. All students must pass Step 1 of the USMLE to be promoted to year three. Passing Step 2 is a graduation requirement.

BASIC SCIENCES: First-year courses are physiology, gross anatomy, biochemistry, genetics, histology, embryology, microanatomy, and problem based learning (which integrates clinical correlation to the basic sciences). Second-year courses are pathology, microbiology, behavioral medicine and psychiatry, pharmacology and toxicology, genetics, community medicine, and introduction to clinical medicine (ICM). The ICM courses use faculty mentors as teachers and train students in basic clinical techniques such as the physical examination and patient interview. Instructional aids include computer-assisted learning programs. For research purposes and for studying, students use the Health Sciences Library, which has a collection of more than 205,000 volumes and an extensive amount audiovisual equipment.

CLINICAL TRAINING

Third-year, required clerkships are eight weeks each of medicine, surgery, behavioral medicine and psychiatry, obstetrics/gynecology, pediatrics, and family medicine (which includes a rural rotation). Fourth-year requirements include one month of a subinternship in internal medicine, pediatrics, or family medicine, a one-month critical care clerkship, an additional one-month surgery clerkship, and two months of a rural primary care experience. Half of the fourth year is reserved for electives. Five months of fourth-year clerkships must be taken at WVU sites, leaving ample opportunity for students to rotate to other academic and clinical institutions. Clinical training takes place primarily at the Ruby Memorial Hospital (376 beds), which is part of the West Virginia University Robert C. Byrd Health Sciences Center Complex. The complex also includes the Physicians Office Center, the Mary Babb Randolph Cancer Center, Chestnut Ridge Psychiatric Hospital (seventy beds), Southview Regional Rehabilitation Hospital (sixty beds), and the National Institute of Occupational Safety and Health (NIOSH). About one-third of third year students enter a clinical training program at university-affiliated hospitals in Charleston. All students also have the opportunity to rotate to facilities that are part of a large network of hospitals and physicians in rural areas of the state.

Students

At least 95 percent of students are West Virginia residents, and more than one-third attended WVU for undergraduate studies. About forty other undergraduate institutions are represented in a typical class. Approximately 68 percent of students were biology or chemistry majors in college. In a recently admitted class of eighty-eight students, twenty-five of them were twenty or twenty-one years of age, fifty-six were twenty-two or twenty-three, and seven were twenty-four or older.

STUDENT LIFE

With more than 1,700 students enrolled in programs at the Health Sciences Center, a camaraderie exists among WVU students. Small class sizes promote class cohesion and cooperation. Student organizations include local chapters of national medical student organizations, community service-based groups, and clubs that focus on professional interests. University-owned housing is available to medical and graduate students.

GRADUATES

About one-third of the practicing physicians in the state of West Virginia are graduates of WVU. At least half of all graduates enter the primary care fields of family medicine, internal medicine, pediatrics, and obstetrics/gynecology.

Admissions

REQUIREMENTS

Prerequisites are one year each of English, social sciences, biology, general chemistry, organic chemistry, and physics. All science courses should include lab work. The MCAT is required and is used, along with undergraduate transcripts, to assess academic achievement. For applicants who have retaken the exam, all scores are considered.

SUGGESTIONS

State residents are given strong preference in admission. However, a limited number of highly qualified nonresidents may also be admitted. Beyond required course work, recommended courses are biochemistry, cell and molecular biology, and calculus. The Committee on Admissions expects strength in the sciences but gives no preference to any particular major. Demonstration of an understanding of the medical profession is considered important.

PROCESS

All qualified West Virginia resident applicants and highly qualified nonresidents are sent secondary applications. Of those returning secondaries, about 50 percent of residents and 10 percent of nonresidents are interviewed between September and February. Interviews generally consist of one two-on-one session, usually with medical school faculty, fourth-year students, or administrators. On interview day, students also have the opportunity to tour the campus and meet current students. Approximately one-third of interviewed candidates are accepted on a rolling basis. Others are either rejected or wait-listed. West Virginia residents on the wait-list have a reasonable chance of being accepted later in the spring.

Admissions Requirements (Required)

MCAT scores, science GPA, non-science GPA, letters of recommendation, interview, essays/personal statement, extracurricular activities, exposure to medical profession, computer literacy.

Admissions Requirements (Optional)

state residency.

Overlap Schools

Marshall University, University of Pennsylvania, West Virginia School of Osteopathic Medicine.

COSTS AND AID

In-state tuition	$1,640
Out-of-state tuition	$4,550
Room and board	$10,005
Cost of books	$4,950
In-state fees	$11,800
Out-of-state fees	$26,630

Financial Aid

% students receiving aid	92
Average grant	$8,348
Average loan	$26,225
Average debt	$90,403

Wright State University
School of Medicine

Office of Student Affairs/Admissions, PO Box 1751, Dayton, OH 45401-1751 • Admission: 937-775-2934 • Fax: 937-775-3322 • E-mail: som_saa@desire.wright.edu • Website: www.med.wright.edu

STUDENT BODY

Type	Public
Enrollment	364
% male/female	45/55
% underrepresented minorities	24
# applied (total/out)	2,774/1,888
# accepted (total/out)	232/44
# enrolled (total/out)	91/11
Average age	23

FACULTY

Total faculty (number)	1,500
% female	25
# student/faculty ratio	4:1

ADMISSIONS

Average GPA and MCAT Scores

Overall GPA	3.6
MCAT Bio	9.04
MCAT Phys	8.51
MCAT Verbal	8.64
MCAT Essay	0

Application Information

Regular application	11/15
Regular notification	10/15
Early application	6/1-8/1
Early notification	10/1
Are transfers accepted?	Yes
Admissions may be deferred?	Yes
Interview required?	Yes
Application fee	$45

Academics

Although most students complete the MD curriculum in four years, a few enter the MS/PhD program, which requires additional course work. Graduate degrees are offered in most biomedical sciences including anatomy, physiology, biochemistry, pathology, and pharmacology. Medical students are evaluated with percentile scores and grades of pass and fail. Students take the USMLE Step 1 after completion of year two and Step 2 after completion of year three.

BASIC SCIENCES: Basic science instruction includes use of small groups, clinical case studies, problem-based learning, and computer-aided instruction. First-year courses are human structure, human development, introduction to clinical medicine I (ICM I), molecular, cellular, and tissue biology, social and ethical issues in medicine, principles of disease, and evidence-based medicine. The second year is organized around organ/body systems. These are pathobiology and therapeutics blood, cardiology, endocrine, GI, integument, musculoskeletal, neuroscience, renal, reproductive, and respiratory. Students also learn about infectious diseases and continue clinical training in ICM II. The ICM course provides clinical contact from the very first week of class. In this series, students learn to take medical histories, conduct physical exams, and identify common diseases. Three two-week elective periods during the first two years give students the opportunity to pursue intensive research or clinical projects. Students are also encouraged to participate in faculty-guided research during the summer in between the first and second years. The Fordham Health Sciences Library is fully computerized and provides 106,000 volumes, in addition to journals and special collections. Students also study in the student lounge and the main university's libraries. The Interdisciplinary Teaching Laboratory enhances learning through the use of audiovisual equipment, hardwired labs, and medical software.

CLINICAL TRAINING

Third-year required rotations are family medicine (six weeks), internal medicine (twelve weeks), women's health (eight weeks), pediatrics (eight weeks), psychiatry (six weeks), and surgery (eight weeks). Fourth-year requirements are emergency medicine (four weeks), neurology (four weeks), surgical specialties (four weeks), and a variety of electives (five months). Students also participate in a senior seminar program. Training takes place at Children's Medical Center (155 beds), Dayton Veterans' Affairs Medical Center, Good Samaritan Hospital and Health Center (560 beds), Green Memorial Hospital (210 beds), Kettering Medical Center (486 beds), Miami Valley Hospital (811 beds), and Wright-Patterson Air Force Base Medical Center (301 beds). Some students rotate overseas as part of individually designed or faculty-led experiences.

Students

About 90 percent of entering students are Ohio residents. In the class that will graduate in 2002, 19 percent of students are underrepresented minorities. Typically, about 10 percent of entering students took significant time off between college and medical school. Class size is ninety.

STUDENT LIFE

Medical students have active extracurricular lives and take advantage of the offerings of the medical school, the main university, and the greater community. Students are involved in community service organizations and projects such as the Center for Healthy Communities, which provides health education services to the Dayton community. Other student organizations are chapters of state and national medical organizations, honor societies, support groups and clubs that are focused on professional or recreational interests. Athletic facilities on campus include racquetball, squash, basketball and tennis courts, indoor and outdoor tracks, and several fitness centers. The university's 200 acres of woods are used for walking and jogging. The university is located twelve miles Northeast of Dayton, a city of nearly one million residents. Students live in privately owned apartments and houses, which are generally affordable and conveniently located.

GRADUATES

Among students who graduated in 2001, 61 percent entered primary care residencies, which are defined as family medicine, internal medicine, and pediatrics. About 50 percent choose residency programs in Ohio.

Admissions

REQUIREMENTS

Prerequisites are one year each of biology, chemistry, organic chemistry, and physics, all with associated labs. In addition, one year each of English and mathematics are required. The MCAT is required, and scores should be from within the past three years. For applicants who have retaken the exam, all scores are considered.

SUGGESTIONS

Ohio residents are given strong preference, which makes admission for nonresidents very competitive. The April MCAT is preferred over the August one. In addition to academic strength, selection is based on a student's dedication to human concerns, communication skills, maturity, and motivation. Some hospital or other medically related experience is recommended.

PROCESS

All AMCAS applicants receive secondary applications, of which about 10 percent are invited to interview between September and March. Interviews consist of two sessions, each with a member of the admissions committee. On interview day, students also attend group information presentations, have lunch with faculty and students, and tour the campus. About 45 percent of interviewed candidates are accepted on a rolling basis. Others are rejected or put on a wait-list. Wait-listed candidates are not encouraged to send additional information.

Admissions Requirements (Required)

MCAT scores, science GPA, non-science GPA, letters of recommendation, interview, essays/personal statement, extracurricular activities, exposure to medical profession.

Admissions Requirements (Optional)

state residency.

COSTS AND AID

In-state tuition	$16,602
Out-of-state tuition	$23,496
Cost of books	$1,757
Fees	$980

Financial Aid

Average grant	$5,483
Average loan	$21,500

YALE UNIVERSITY
SCHOOL OF MEDICINE

367 CEDAR STREET, NEW HAVEN, CT 06510 • ADMISSION: 203-785-2643 • FAX: 203-785-3234 • E-MAIL: MEDICAL SCHOOL.ADMISSIONS@QUICKMAIL.YALE.EDU • WEBSITE: HTTP://INFO.MED.YALE.EDU/EDUCATION/ADMISSIONS/INDEX.
HTML

STUDENT BODY

Type	Private
Enrollment	479
% male/female	51/49
% underrepresented minorities	18
# applied (total/out)	3,093/3,472
Average age	24

ADMISSIONS

Application Information

Regular application	10/15
Regular notification	3/15 until filled
Early application	6/1-8/1
Early notification	10/1
Are transfers accepted?	Yes
Admissions may be deferred?	Yes
Interview required?	No
Application fee	$60

Academics

Although most students complete courses, clerkships, and a thesis in four years, about 30 to 50 percent of students extend their studies over a five-year period at no extra cost. Some students take an extra year to earn an MPH along with the MD. Other combined degree programs offered are the MD/JD, MD/MDiv, and MS/PhD. Entering students are assigned a clinical tutor who serves as a mentor during all four years. Also throughout all four years, students take a series of lectures, workshops, and clinical discussion under the broad topic of medicine, society and public health. Evaluation of students uses grades of strictly pass and fail. Students must pass Steps 1 and 2 of the USMLE to graduate.

BASIC SCIENCES: The first two years are spent building a foundation in the basic sciences as well as learning skills and techniques for training in clinical responsibilities. Year one is devoted to understanding normal relevant biological form and function. Year two concentrates on the study of disease. Formats include lecture, small group discussion, laboratories, demonstrations, and individual tutorials; many of these involve patients, both at the bedside and in the classroom. First year students must pass the following courses: cellular and physiologic basis of medicine (physiology and cell biology), human genetics, human anatomy and development, molecular foundations of medicine (biochemistry), neurobiology, psychological basis of medical practice, biological basis of behavior, and aspects of child and adolescent development. In addition there is an umbrella course called medicine, society and public health that includes the following related but distinct subcourses: biostatistics, history of medicine, professional responsibility, and health policy. preclinical training is included in the course the doctor/patient encounter. The major, second-year course is called mechanisms of disease and is organized into two segments. The initial offering, called basic principles, includes immunobiology, pathology, pharmacology, microbiology, and basics of diagnostic radiology, and laboratory medicine. The second segment is called mechanisms of disease: organs/systems. Each integrated module, organized around body systems or organs, includes pathology, pharmacology, pathophysiology, diagnostic radiology, laboratory medicine, and prevention. the modules are blood/hematology; neoplasias/oncology; cardiovascular system; respiratory system; digestive system; musculoskeletal system; renal, urinary tract and male reproductive system; female reproductive system; endocrine systems; skin; clinical neuroscience; and psychiatry. Medicine, society and public health continues, and offers epidemiology and public health in the first semester, and relevant prevention during the modules. The doctor/patient encounter course also continues, building as it progresses.

CLINICAL TRAINING

There are seven required clerkships in the third year, one of which may be completed early in the fourth year. These are internal medicine (twelve weeks), general surgery/surgical subspecialties (twelve weeks), pediatrics (eight weeks), psychiatry (six weeks), obstetrics/gynecology (six weeks), and clinical neuroscience (four weeks). During the fourth year, an integrated clinical medicine clerkship (three weeks) and a primary care clerkship (four weeks) are required. The primary care clerkship takes place in a variety of community- and practice-based sites. Most clinical rotations are completed at the Yale New Haven Hospital and the West Haven Veterans' Administration Hospital. Other affiliated hospitals are Bridgeport Hospital, Danbury Hospital, Greenwich Hospital, Griffin Hospital in Derby, Hospital of Saint Raphael, Lawrence and Memorial Hospital, Norwalk Hospital, Saint Mary's Hospital in Waterbury, Saint Vincent's Medical Center in Bridgeport, and Waterbury Hospital. Several clinics and mental health centers are also used for training. Although some students begin working on their theses early in medical school, the majority of research and writing takes from four to seven months and is completed in the fourth year. Some students publish their work, while others continue developing their research after graduation.

Students

Yale attracts students from all regions of the country. Approximately 15 to 20 percent of entering students are underrepresented minorities. Among students in the 1997 entering class, the average age was twenty-four, with a considerable age range. Class size is 100.

STUDENT LIFE

The School of Medicine is a short walk from the university's main campus. This gives medical students access to athletic facilities, student meeting areas, libraries, and university-sponsored events. Medical students participate in intramural sports, competing against other graduate and professional school teams. About three-quarters of medical students are involved in community service activities such as STATS (Students Teaching AIDS to Students), the Prenatal Care Project, and ASAP (the Adolescent Substance Abuse Prevention Project). The Office for Women in Medicine is the oldest of its kind in the nation and provides support, guidance, and special programs of interest for women medical students. The Office for Multicultural Affairs recruits and supports minority students, serves as a link between the school and its surrounding community, and sponsors various cultural events and centers. The Edward S. Harkness Memorial Hall is a residence hall for medical, physician associate, nursing, public health, and other graduate students. Both dormitory-style rooms and apartments are available.

GRADUATES

Among 1998 graduates, the most popular areas for residency training were internal medicine (40 percent), pediatrics (12 percent), surgery (5 percent), diagnostic radiology (1 percent), orthopedics (8 percent), plastic surgery (4 percent), dermatology (3 percent), and otolaryngology (5 percent).

Admissions

REQUIREMENTS

Prerequisites are one year each of general biology or zoology, general chemistry, organic chemistry, and general physics, all of which should be taken with associated labs. The MCAT is required, and scores should be from within the past four years. For applicants who have retaken the exam, the best set of scores is considered.

SUGGESTIONS

In addition to academic credentials, the Committee on Admissions looks for intelligent, mature, and highly motivated students who possess integrity, common sense, personal stability, dedication to service, and the ability to inspire and maintain confidence.

PROCESS

Yale does not participate in AMCAS. Applications should be requested from the address above or downloaded from http://info.med.yale.edu/medadmit. About 25 percent of applicants are interviewed between October and February. Interviews consist of two sessions, each with a faculty member or medical student committee member. Candidates attend group information sessions and have the opportunity to eat lunch and tour the campus with current medical students. About 15 percent of interviewed candidates are accepted and are notified in mid-March.

Admissions Requirements (Required)

MCAT scores, state residency, essays/personal statement, extracurricular activities, exposure to medical profession.

Admissions Requirements (Optional)

science GPA, nonscience GPA, letters of recommendation, interview.

COSTS AND AID

Tuition	$33,800
Room and board	$9,650
Cost of books	$1,700
Fees	$300

Financial Aid

% students receiving aid	2

Yeshiva University

Albert Einstein College of Medicine

Jack and Pearl Resnick Campus, 1300 Morris Park Avenue, Bronx, NY 10461 • Admission: 718-430-2106 • Fax: 718-430-8825 • E-mail: admissions@aecom.yu.edu • Website: www.aecom.yu.edu

STUDENT BODY

Type	Private
Enrollment	724
% male/female	51/49
% underrepresented minorities	7
# applied (total/out)	5,943/4,522
# accepted (total/out)	521/336
# enrolled (total/out)	180/92
Average age	23

FACULTY

Total faculty (number)	3,510
% female	35
% part-time	42
# student/faculty ratio	1:1

ADMISSIONS

Average GPA and MCAT Scores

Overall GPA	3.6
MCAT Bio	10.6
MCAT Phys	10.5
MCAT Verbal	9.4
MCAT Essay	P

Application Information

Regular application	12/31
Regular notification	1/15
Early application	8/1
Early notification	10/1
Are transfers accepted?	No
Admissions may be deferred?	Yes
Interview required?	Yes
Application fee	$90

Academics

In addition to the requirements described below, all students conduct research projects through the independent scholars program. Such research often leads to publication or to distinction at the time of graduation. Projects involve a faculty mentor and can be in traditional or nontraditional medical science fields. Students may apply for joint PhD/MD programs when they initially apply or while they are enrolled in the MD program. Candidates who are accepted into this program receive stipends, either through the MSTP program or from institutional sources. The PhD may be earned in the following fields: anatomy, biochemistry, biophysics, cell biology, genetics, immunology, microbiology, molecular biology, neuroscience, pathology, pharmacology, and physiology. Evaluation of student performance uses grades of honors, pass, and fail. Passing the USMLE Steps 1 and 2 are requirements for graduation.

BASIC SCIENCES: Throughout the first and second years, introduction to clinical medicine complements the basic science curriculum by addressing practical and personal issues related to the patient interview and examination. About forty entering students participate in a generalist mentorship program, which involves shadowing a primary care physician. First-year courses, taught primarily with lectures and labs, are histology, anatomy, cardiovascular physiology, principles of pharmacology, and disease mechanisms. The course molecular and cellular foundations of medicine uses both lectures and small group sessions. During the second part of year one, and throughout all of year two, instruction is organ-based, is carried out in small groups, and uses a case-based approach. Courses are renal physiology and pathobiology, nervous system and behavior, endocrine system, reproductive system and human sexuality, cardiovascular system, respiratory system, gastrointestinal system and liver, hematology, and rheumatologic and orthopedic disease. Other second-year courses are microbiology and infectious disease and parasitology. On average, students spend about twenty hours per week in class. A cognitive skills program offers reviews for the USMLE and tutoring for students who will benefit from it. Basic science instruction takes place in the Arthur B. and Diane Belfer Educational Center for Sciences, which is open twenty-four hours a day and contains classrooms, laboratories, study areas, a student bookstore, and computer rooms. The D. Samuel Gottesman Library has 250,000 volumes, 2,400 journal subscriptions, computer databases, and other informational technology. Electronic search mechanisms allow easy access to several large collections in the New York area.

CLINICAL TRAINING

Third-year required clerkships are medicine (eleven weeks), pediatrics (seven weeks), psychiatry (six weeks), obstetrics/gynecology (six weeks), surgery (eight weeks), family medicine (six weeks), geriatrics (two weeks), and neurology (two weeks). During the fourth year, two months of a subinternship in either medicine or pediatrics is required, as are two months in an ambulatory care program. For clinical training, Einstein students have access to six prominent hospitals in New York, all of which have a total of 6,988 beds. These are Jacobi Medical Center (537 beds), Montefiore Medical Center (745 beds), Long Island Jewish Medical Center (829 beds), Beth Israel Medical Center (212 beds), and the Bronx-Lebanon Medical Center (two centers, 540 beds). Training also takes place at mental health facilities and long-term care centers for primarily older populations. Several nationally recognized research institutes are part of Einstein's resources and provide further opportunities for students. Fellowships are available for up to twenty fourth-year students, which enables them to fulfill elective requirements overseas. Numerous organized exchange programs also exist with countries such as Germany, Sweden, Israel, France, Japan, and Cuba.

Students

Students come from around the country. Undergraduate institutions that are particularly well represented are Yeshiva, State Universities of New York, private Northeastern colleges and universities, and public universities in California. In a typical entering class, about 9 percent of students are minorities, most of whom are African American. Students who have taken time off after college account for about one-third of entering classes, and those over thirty years old account for about 5 to 10 percent. Class size is 180.

STUDENT LIFE

Central meeting areas such as the Lubin Student Lounge and the Max and Sadie Friedman Lounge feature music, food, television, and an opportunity for interaction outside of the academic environment. There are full athletic facilities for student use. School-sponsored activities include class parties, clubs focused on films or the outdoors, and organizations based on cultural, religious, or ethnic affiliations. Einstein has its own symphony orchestra. The beaches of Long Island and the culture, entertainment, and excitement of Manhattan are easily accessible by car or public transportation. Most students live on campus, in the Eastchester Road or Rhinelander residences, where studios and one- and two-bedroom apartments are available.

GRADUATES

Among the 1999 graduates, the predominant residency choices were internal medicine (45 percent), pediatrics (12 percent), surgery or general surgery (10 percent), obstetrics/gynecology (6 percent), emergency medicine (6 percent), psychiatry (5 percent), family practice (4 percent), and ophthalmology (3 percent). Einstein has the largest postgraduate training program in the country and is the destination of about 40 percent of Einstein School of Medicine graduates. Programs at other New York institutions, in the Philadelphia area, and in California are also popular choices.

Admissions

REQUIREMENTS

Requirements are biology (eight semester hours), chemistry (eight hours), organic chemistry (eight hours), physics (eight hours), college math (six hours), and English (eight hours). The MCAT is required and should be no more than three years old. For those who have retaken the MCAT, the best score is counted. Thus, there is no advantage to withholding scores.

SUGGESTIONS

College students should pursue studies in their areas of interest, as no particular major is considered more appropriate than the next. Course work in the humanities and social sciences is important. Statistics is useful, and computer literacy is necessary. Einstein looks closely at the personal interaction skills of its applicants and at their ability to work with people from diverse backgrounds.

PROCESS

All AMCAS applicants are sent secondary applications, of which about 20 percent are invited to interview. Interviews are about one hour long and take place between August and May; applicants meet with faculty members. On interview day, applicants tour the campus and have a lunch period with current Einstein students. Candidates are notified about whether they are accepted, wait-listed, or rejected begining in January. Wait-listed candidates may submit additional material.

Admissions Requirements (Required)

MCAT scores, science GPA, non-science GPA, letters of recommendation, interview, essays/personal statement, extracurricular activities, exposure to medical profession.

Admissions Requirements (Optional)

state residency.

Overlap Schools

New York University, SUNY at Stony Brook, UMDNJ.

COSTS AND AID

Tuition	$35,925
Room and board	$4,000
Cost of books	$1,600
Fees	$1,600

Financial Aid

% students receiving aid	75
Average grant	$8,500
Average loan	$20,000
Average debt	$65,000

8 Osteopathic Profiles

A. T. Still University of Health Sciences

Kirksville College of Osteopathic Medicine

800 West Jefferson, Kirksville, MO 63501 • Admission: 660-626-2237 • Fax: 660-626-2969 •
E-mail: admissions@atsu.edu • Website: www.atsu.edu

Academics

The Kirksville College of Osteopathic Medicine is the founding school of osteopathic medicine and offers an education firmly based on holistic care, wellness, and academic excellence. Kirksville has a reputation for training physicians in primary care areas, as well as providing a strong clinical and basic science education for specialization. Although the first two years are reserved for basic science instruction, a clerkship with a primary care physician is included in the first-year curriculum. Traditional tenets of osteopathic medicine are coupled with the use of all modern technology, thus providing a well-rounded, comprehensive education. Problem solving and critical thinking are emphasized in both the basic science courses and clinical training. Clinical rotations take place in one of the following areas: Arizona, Michigan, Missouri, Ohio, and Utah. Additional fourth-year rotations take place in Georgia, New York, and Texas. Kirksville is a community of approximately 20,000 residents. With a 2002 class size of 158, the average age is twenty-five, the composite MCAT is 26, and the overall GPA is 3.5.

Admissions

REQUIREMENTS

Since this is a private institution, no preference is given to Missouri residents, and almost all states are represented in the student body. Course requirements are biology (eight semester hours), chemistry (eight hours), organic chemistry (eight hours), physics (eight hours), and English (six hours). To be considered for admission, applicants should have a minimum GPA of 2.5 in both the sciences and overall. The MCAT is required, and scores must be no more than three years old. About 10 percent of AACOMAS applicants are interviewed; interviews consist of two sessions with faculty or administrators. Financial aid, both merit- and need-based, is available in the form of grants and loans.

STUDENT BODY

Type	Private
Enrollment	629
% male/female	65/35
% underrepresented minorities	2
# applied (total)	2,441
# accepted (total)	445
# enrolled (total/out)	168/136
Average age	25

FACULTY

Total faculty (number)	92
# student/faculty ratio	3:1

ADMISSIONS

Average GPA and MCAT Scores

Overall GPA	3.4
MCAT Bio	8.5
MCAT Phys	8.5
MCAT Verbal	7.5
MCAT Essay	0

Application Information

Regular application	2/1
Regular notification	rolling
Early application	8/1
Early notification	10/15
Are transfers accepted?	Yes
Admissions may be deferred?	Yes
Interview required?	Yes
Application fee	$60

Admissions Requirements (Required)

MCAT scores, science GPA, non-science GPA, letters of recommendation, interview, essays/personal statement, extracurricular activities, exposure to medical profession.

Admissions Requirements (Optional)

exposure to osteopathic medicine.

COSTS AND AID

Tuition	$28,456
Cost of books	$1,575
Fees	$495

Financial Aid

% students receiving aid	94
Average grant	$1,425
Average loan	$39,675
Average debt	$139,340

BASTYR UNIVERSITY

SCHOOL OF NATUROPATHIC MEDICINE

14500 JUANITA DRIVE NE, KENMORE, WA 98028 • ADMISSION: 425-602-3330 • FAX: 425-602-3090 •
E-MAIL: ADMISS@BASTYR.EDU • WEBSITE: WWW.BASTYR.EDU/ACADEMIC/PROFILES/

Academics

Bastyr's naturopathic medicine (ND) department educates future physicians in the tradition of medical science and the art of natural healing. The school does this by providing students with a comprehensive understanding of the basic medical sciences, accurate diagnostic skills, and the ability to apply the natural and minimally invasive methods of whole person health care, which is characteristic of naturopathic medicine. Bastyr University will be the world's leading academic center for advancing knowledge in the natural health sciences. We educate future leaders in the natural health sciences that integrate mind, body, spirit, and nature. Through natural health education, research, and clinical services, we improve the health and well-being of the human community. Original research is conducted regularly and a research fellowship has been funded. The university has established an AIDS Research Center with funding from the NIH Office of Complementary and Alternative Medicine. Students are engaged in primary clinical research at the Natural Health Clinic. The university maintains a library with current journals; special collections in alternative medicine, acupuncture, nutrition, midwifery, and naturopathic medicine; and audio-visual aids. Students also have access to the nearby University of Washington Health Sciences libraries.

Admissions

SUGGESTIONS

For priority consideration, applications should be received by February 1 for admission the following fall, although late applications are considered on a space-available basis. When requesting an application or program information, please be sure to indicate the specific program of interest and what materials you would like sent.

PROCESS

Admission baed on academic achievement, personal and social development, relevant experience, financial planning, and demonstrated humanistic qualities.

STUDENT BODY

Type	Private
Enrollment	539
% male/female	29/71
% underrepresented minorities	6
# applied (total/out)	241/190
# accepted (total/out)	169/125
# enrolled (total/out)	115/90
Average age	28

FACULTY

Total faculty (number)	28
% female	60
% part-time	64

ADMISSIONS

Average GPA and MCAT Scores

Overall GPA	3.3
MCAT Bio	1
MCAT Phys	1

Admissions (continued)

MCAT Verbal	1
MCAT Essay	J

Application Information

Regular application	2/1
Regular notification	4/15
Early application	11/1
Early notification	2/1
Are transfers accepted?	Yes
Admissions may be deferred?	Yes
Interview required?	Yes
Application fee	$75

Admissions Requirements (Required)

science GPA, nonscience GPA, letters of recommendation, interview, essays/personal statement, exposure to medical profession.

Admissions Requirements (Optional)

MCAT scores, state residency, extracurricular activities.

COSTS AND AID

Tuition	$18,000
Cost of books	$1,560
Fees	$1,200

Financial Aid

% students receiving aid	80
Average grant	$800
Average loan	$18,500
Average debt	$100,000

DES MOINES UNIVERSITY
COLLEGE OF OSTEOPATHIC MEDICINE AND SURGERY

3200 GRAND AVENUE, DES MOINES, IA 50312-4198 • ADMISSION: 515-271-1499 • FAX: 515-271-7085 •
E-MAIL: DOADMIT@DMU.EDU • WEBSITE: WWW.DMU.EDU

Academics

At the Des Moines University College of Osteopathic Medicine, students learn in a supportive environment. This includes a solid basic sciences education, extensive practical experience in the clinical setting, and one-on-one interaction with seasoned educators and clinicians. The curriculum emphasizes state-of-the-art standardized patient assessment laboratories and problem-based learning opportunities that emphasize critical thinking and problem solving. The college is the second oldest osteopathic school. Located in a safe metropolitan setting, the campus offers proximity to affordable housing. A new 143,000-square-foot student education center will provide students with modern facilities and a location where they can exercise, relax, and learn. Other distinguishing features of DMU include a wireless campus, laptop and hand-held computers for incoming students, and a dual master's degree program in health care administration or public health. The College of Osteopathic Medicine provides a flexible program that allows students to explore a range of professional goals. Students learn to consider the overall needs of the patient rather than an isolated medical problem.

Admissions

REQUIREMENTS

Eight semester hours each in biology, chemistry, organic chemistry, and physics (all with labs) are required. In addition, applicants must have taken six semester hours of English. We accept students without regard to legal state of residence. Usually 75 percent of students are from states other than Iowa. You can apply while you are working on your undergraduate degree, but you should have plans to receive the degree by the time you register with the college. The MCAT (taken within the last two years) is required. Those AACOMAS applicants who meet the minimum requirements for GPA and MCAT are sent secondary applications. About half of those who return secondary applications are invited for an interview. Notification occurs on a rolling basis.

STUDENT BODY

Type	Private
Enrollment	795
% male/female	56/44
% underrepresented minorities	9
# applied (total/out)	2,161/2,048
# accepted (total/out)	541/487
# enrolled (total/out)	201/161
Average age	25

FACULTY

Total faculty (number)	62
% female	32
% minority	1
% part-time	35
# student/faculty ratio	13:1

ADMISSIONS

Average GPA and MCAT Scores

Overall GPA	3.5
MCAT Bio	8.7
MCAT Phys	8.2
MCAT Verbal	8.2
MCAT Essay	0

Application Information

Regular application	2/1
Regular notification	rolling
Early application	rolling
Early notification	3/1
Are transfers accepted?	Yes
Admissions may be deferred?	Yes
Interview required?	Yes
Application fee	$50

Admissions Requirements (Required)

MCAT scores, science GPA, non-science GPA, letters of recommendation, interview, essays/personal statement, extracurricular activities, exposure to medical profession.

Admissions Requirements (Optional)

state residency.

COSTS AND AID

Tuition	$26,350
Cost of books	$3,890
Fees	$1,050

Financial Aid

% students receiving aid	96
Average grant	$22,287
Average loan	$37,426
Average debt	$138,000

Edward Via Virginia College of Osteopathic Medicine

Office of Admissions, VCOM, 2265 Kraft Drive, Blacksburg, VA 24060 • Admission: 540-231-6138 •
E-mail: admissions@vcom.vt.edu • Website: www.vcom.vt.edu

Academics

The curriculum for students who are enrolled in VCOM is modern and innovative. The basic science and clinical content are interwoven throughout the four years. In the first two years, students learn about the normal state of homeostasis of the human body, the propensity for health and ability of the human body to heal, the clinical conditions that most often affect the human body, and the presentations of those conditions. The curriculum is patient centered and integrates patient cases throughout the four years that focus on physical health (the body), mental health (the mind), and spiritual health. The curriculum also emphasizes the community centered approach to health care. The curriculum is based upon a learner centered approach. Students are given the opportunity to learn relevant material through a clinical systems organized approach. Students attend lectures and labs that are interwoven with small group conferences, self directed learning computer tutorials, and clinical experiences. Students are given patient centered cases to integrate biomedical and clinical curriculum. Students must employ problem solving through third year clinical based modules that require literature searches, group analysis, and collaboration. Assessment of knowledge occurs often to assure students are meeting the educational objectives. The clinical and basic science integration throughout the four years provides an opportunity for a continuous curriculum. The same clinical faculty physicians who provide instruction in the classroom will be the faculty who plan and provide instruction in the clinical setting. The principles of primary care clinical course in the first year emphasizes patient communication, the patient-doctor relationship, physical exam skills, professionalism and ethics, preventive medicine, community health, diversity issues, social issues, and clinical problem solving. Each month the principles learned in this course are reinforced and assessed by primary care physicians in the ambulatory office setting, public health and community settings, and the hospital. VCOM has a predominance of primary care physician faculty who accept the responsibility to teach, mentor, and assess students.

STUDENT BODY

Type	Public
Enrollment	155
% male/female	52/48
% underrepresented minorities	10
# applied (total/out)	657/558
# accepted (total/out)	155/110
# enrolled (total/out)	155/110
Average age	25

ADMISSIONS

Average GPA and MCAT Scores

Overall GPA	3.4
MCAT Bio	8
MCAT Phys	8
MCAT Verbal	8
MCAT Essay	P

Admissions (continued)

Application Information

Regular application	2/5
Regular notification	2/4
Are transfers accepted?	No
Admissions may be deferred?	Yes
Interview required?	Yes
Application fee	$75

Admissions Requirements (Required)

MCAT scores, science GPA, non-science GPA, letters of recommendation, interview, essays/personal statement, extracurricular activities, exposure to medical profession, Letter of recommendation from an osteopathic physician.

Admissions Requirements (Optional)

state residency.

Overlap Schools

Lake Erie College of Osteopathic Medicine, Nova Southeastern University, University of Virginia, West Virginia School of Osteopathic Medicine.

COSTS AND AID

Tuition	$29,500
Cost of books	$2,500

Financial Aid

% students receiving aid	90
Average grant	$1,000
Average loan	$50,000

MICHIGAN STATE UNIVERSITY

COLLEGE OF OSTEOPATHIC MEDICINE

C110 EAST FEE HALL, MSUCOM, EAST LANSING, MI 48824-1316 • ADMISSION: 517-353-7740 • FAX: 517-355-3296 • E-MAIL: COMADM@COM.MSU.EDU • WEBSITE: WWW.COM.MSU.EDU

Academics

The Michigan State University College of Osteopathic Medicine (MSUCOM) was created by the Michigan legislature in 1971 to provide osteopathic physicians with the necessary means to meet the health care needs of the state's population. Educating primary care and specialty care osteopathic physicians occurs in a spectrum that includes pre-medical programs, an osteopathic medical college, internships, residencies, and fellowships. The college has partnerships for clinical education with twenty osteopathic hospitals in Michigan in its statewide campus system; clinical education also occurs in private clinics and other environments. Medical research is a high priority of the college, and MSUCOM provides educational opportunities for physician/scientists, especially in its joint DO/PhD curriculum, the medical scientist training program. The curriculum, based on a study of the body's organ systems, emphasizes osteopathic principles and practices, early patient care, behavioral and diversity aspects of medicine, lifelong learning, and use of technology. The smallest college in a university with nearly 45,000 students, MSUCOM is a close-knit community known for compassionate care and its volunteer work in the communities.For further information, see www.com.msu.edu.

Admissions

REQUIREMENTS

Requirements are eight semester hours of biology, chemistry, organic chemistry, and physics, in addition to six hours of English and behavioral science. Grades in these courses must be a 2.0 or better, and the combined science and overall GPAs must be a 2.5 or better. The MCAT is required, and scores must not be more than three years old. For those who have retaken the exam, all results are considered. All in-state residents and about one-quarter of out-of-state residents who submit preliminary applications through AACOMAS receive secondary applications. About 10 percent of returning secondaries are interviewed, of which about 25 percent of those interviewed are accepted. Interviews take place from October through March and consist of two sessions with faculty members or administrators. About 80 percent of the 125 positions are reserved for Michigan residents.

STUDENT BODY

Type	Public
Enrollment	527
% male/female	54/46
% underrepresented minorities	6
# applied (total/out)	1,621/1,224
# accepted (total/out)	194/24
# enrolled (total/out)	124/5
Average age	25

FACULTY

Total faculty (number)	177
% female	37
% minority	19
% part-time	11
# student/faculty ratio	3:1

ADMISSIONS

Average GPA and MCAT Scores

Overall GPA	3.5

Admissions (continued)

MCAT Bio	8.7
MCAT Phys	8
MCAT Verbal	8.2
MCAT Essay	0

Application Information

Regular application	12/1
Regular notification	rolling
Early application	8/15
Early notification	10/15
Are transfers accepted?	Yes
Admissions may be deferred?	Yes
Interview required?	Yes
Application fee	$75

Admissions Requirements (Required)

MCAT scores, science GPA, non-science GPA, letters of recommendation, interview, essays/personal statement, extracurricular activities, exposure to medical profession.

Admissions Requirements (Optional)

state residency.

COSTS AND AID

In-state tuition	$17,838
Out-of-state tuition	$39,438
Room and board	$10,656
Cost of books	$2,605
Fees	$1,112

Financial Aid

% students receiving aid	93
Average grant	$2,720
Average loan	$25,455
Average debt	$117,220

Midwestern University
Arizona College of Osteopathic Medicine

Office of Admissions, 19555 North 59th Avenue, Glendale, AZ 85308 • Admission: 623-572-3275 •
Fax: 623-572-3229 • E-mail: admissaz@arizona.midwestern.edu • Website: www.midwestern.edu

Academics

The Arizona College of Osteopathic Medicine (AZCOM) was founded in 1995. The college, along with its sister college, the Chicago College of Osteopathic Medicine (CCOM), is part of Midwestern University. In addition to the Colleges of Osteopathic Medicine, Midwestern University also includes a college of pharmacy and a college of health sciences. The school is located on a 124-acre site in scenic Glendale, Arizona, a suburb of Phoenix. Facilities include three main academic centers that house lecture halls, conference rooms, a student services facility and numerous lecture and laboratory classrooms that boast the finest in educational equipment, cadavers for anatomy laboratories rather than plastic models, on-campus housing that features one- and two-bedroom student apartments and a heated pool, a comprehensive library with computer resources and study rooms, a researcy facility, a clinic, and a student clubhouse. The mission of Arizona College of Osteopathic Medicine of Midwestern University responds to the contemporary societal need for physicians by emphasizing primary care and education experiences needed to serve in rural and underserved urban communities.

Admissions

REQUIREMENTS

As a private institution, the college attracts a national applicant pool, and out-of-state residents account for over 80 percent of the group. Only 125 positions are available in each class, and in recent years there have been over 3,000 applicants. The average GPA of successful applicants is about 3.4 in both sciences and overall. Minimum course work includes six semester hours in English and eight semester hours in each of the following: biology, inorganic chemistry, organic chemistry, and physics. The MCAT is required and must be no more than three years old. In addition to the AACOMAS application, applicants must submit a supplemental application (provided by the college after the AACOMAS application has been received).

STUDENT BODY

Type	Private
Enrollment	664
% male/female	52/48
% underrepresented minorities	22
# applied (total/out)	2,747/2,423
# accepted (total/out)	410/304
# enrolled (total/out)	177/114
Average age	24

FACULTY

Total faculty (number)	294
% female	23
% minority	11
% part-time	50
# student/faculty ratio	2:1

ADMISSIONS

Average GPA and MCAT Scores

Overall GPA	3.5
MCAT Bio	8.8
MCAT Phys	8.3
MCAT Verbal	8.4

Application Information

Regular application	1/1
Regular notification	rolling
Are transfers accepted?	Yes
Admissions may be deferred?	Yes
Interview required?	Yes
Application fee	$50

Admissions Requirements (Required)

MCAT scores, science GPA, non-science GPA, letters of recommendation, interview, essays/personal statement, extracurricular activities, exposure to medical profession, oral and written communication skills.

Admissions Requirements (Optional)

state residency.

COSTS AND AID

Tuition	$28,142
Room and board	$8,730
Cost of books	$1,900
Fees	$335

Financial Aid

% students receiving aid	85
Average grant	$12,121
Average loan	$40,542
Average debt	$150,000

Midwestern University

Chicago College of Osteopathic Medicine

Office of Admissions, 555 31st Street, Downers Grove, IL 60515 • Admission: 800-458-6253 • Fax: 630-971-6086 • E-mail: admissil@midwestern.edu • Website: www.midwestern.edu

Academics

Midwestern University administers the Chicago College of Osteopathic Medicine (CCOM), the Chicago College of Pharmacy, and the College of Health Sciences, in addition to related programs in Glendale, Arizona. The MWU campus is located in a western suburb of Chicago, Illinois. Clinical training takes place at various sites around the city and throughout the Midwest region. Students enjoy early clinical exposure through volunteering, preceptor programs, and formal patient contact in the second semester of year one. Research is also important at CCOM, which offers a combined DO/PhD program and has summer research awards for medical students. The Downers Grove campus offers modern academic and recreational facilities, in addition to on-campus housing. The male/female ratio is 40:60 and average age of incoming students is about twenty-seven. In fall 2002, the Downers Grove campus enrolled 1,590 students while the Glendale, Arizona, campus enrolled 1,154 students.

Admissions

REQUIREMENTS

Residents of Illinois account for 65 percent of the student body of the Downers Grove campus. Residents of Arizona account for 42 percent of the student body on the Glendale, Arizona, campus. See www.midwestern.edu for specific admissions requirements.

STUDENT BODY

Type	Private
Enrollment	507
% male/female	64/36
% underrepresented minorities	23
# applied (total)	2,200
# accepted (total)	280
# enrolled (total/out)	134/102
Average age	26

ADMISSIONS

Average GPA and MCAT Scores

Overall GPA	3.4
MCAT Bio	8.72
MCAT Phys	8.21
MCAT Verbal	7.86
MCAT Essay	Q

Admissions (continued)

Application Information

Regular application	1/2
Regular notification	3/1
Are transfers accepted?	Yes
Admissions may be deferred?	Yes
Interview required?	Yes
Application fee	$50

Admissions Requirements (Required)

MCAT scores, science GPA, non-science GPA, letters of recommendation, interview, essays/personal statement, extracurricular activities, exposure to medical profession.

Admissions Requirements (Optional)

state residency.

Overlap Schools

Midwestern University.

COSTS AND AID

Cost of books	$2,060

Financial Aid

% students receiving aid	90
Average grant	$1,910
Average loan	$23,500

NEW YORK INSTITUTE OF TECHNOLOGY

NEW YORK COLLEGE OF OSTEOPATHIC MEDICINE

DIRECTOR OF ADMISSIONS, NYCOM/NYIT, OLD WESTBURY, NY 11568 • ADMISSION: 516-626-6947 • FAX: 516-626-6946 • WEBSITE: WWW.NYIT/NYCOM/NYCOM

Academics

The New York College of Osteopathic Medicine is part of the New York Institute of Technology, an independent institution that encompasses numerous academic and professional programs at the undergraduate and graduate level. In conjunction with some of these programs, medical students may pursue joint degrees such as a DO/MBA or DO/MS. The College of Medicine is located twenty-two miles east of New York City and uses more than twenty clinical facilities in and around Manhattan, on Long Island, in upstate New York, and in northern New Jersey. With such a diverse patient population, students learn to be excellent clinicians in both primary and specialty fields. The medical student population itself is diverse, largely as a result of special efforts at recruiting immigrants who were trained as physicians in other countries, women, and minorities. Women account for 48 percent of the student body, and underrepresented minorities account for about 13 percent.

Admissions

REQUIREMENTS

Course requirements are eight semester hours of biology, chemistry, organic chemistry, and physics in addition to six semester hours of English. A minimum grade of 2.75 is expected in all of the required courses; applicants' combined science and cumulative GPAs must be higher than 2.75 for serious consideration. The MCAT is required as well as a baccalaureate degree. About 20 percent of AACOMAS applicants are interviewed between November and May. The supplementary application is given to candidates at the time of interview. Interviews are conducted with basic science faculty and/or osteopathic physicians from the community. About two-thirds of interviewed candidates are accepted. Preference is given to New York residents and to residents of states in the northeastern United States.

STUDENT BODY

Type	Private
% male/female	60/40
% underrepresented minorities	16

ADMISSIONS

Application Information

Regular application	2/1
Are transfers accepted?	No
Admissions may be deferred?	No
Interview required?	Yes

Admissions Requirements (Required)

science GPA, nonscience GPA, letters of recommendation, interview, state residency, extracurricular activities, exposure to medical profession.

Admissions Requirements (Optional)

MCAT scores, essays/personal statement.

COSTS AND AID

Tuition	$21,000

Nova Southeastern University
College of Osteopathic Medicine

3200 South University Drive, Fort Lauderdale, FL 33328 • Admission: 954-262-1101 • Fax: 954-262-2282 •
E-mail: com@nova.edu • Website: www.nova.edu

Academics

The Colleges of Osteopathic Medicine, Optometry, Allied Health, Pharmacy, and Biomedical Science are among the many schools featured at Nova Southeastern University, which is situated on a 232-acre campus in Fort Lauderdale. The curriculum includes two years of basic science instruction followed by two years of clinical training. One of the required clinical rotations is a three month clerkship in a rural, underserved area. Some students are admitted to a special seven-year primary medicine track that ensures residency placement. Other students jointly pursue an MPH along with the DO. Seventy percent of graduates enter primary care fields. The male/female ratio is 70:30, and the average age of incoming students is approximately twenty-six.

Admissions

REQUIREMENTS

Nova Southeastern University receives over 3,000 application each year to fill a class of 180 students. All AACOMAS applicants receive a secondary application, but not everyone who applies is granted an interview. Interviews begin in October and consist of a session with a panel of health professionals including a DO. Science prerequisites must include eight hours of each in biology, chemistry, organic chemistry, and physics (all with labs). In addition, three semester hours of English literature and three hours of English composition are required. The MCAT is required and should be no more than three years old. The best set of scores will be used.

SUGGESTIONS

Applicants are advised to send materials early because of the time it takes for AACOMAS to provide all of the student information and because of NSU's rolling admissions policy.

STUDENT BODY

Type	Private
Enrollment	760
% male/female	55/45
% underrepresented minorities	32
# applied (total/out)	1,218/914
# accepted (total/out)	324/185
# enrolled (total/out)	202/91
Average age	25

FACULTY

Total faculty (number)	604
% female	88
% minority	20
% part-time	2

ADMISSIONS

Average GPA and MCAT Scores

Overall GPA	3.5
MCAT Bio	8.26

Admissions (continued)

MCAT Phys	7.76
MCAT Verbal	7.87
MCAT Essay	N

Application Information

Regular application	1/15
Regular notification	rolling
Are transfers accepted?	Yes
Admissions may be deferred?	Yes
Interview required?	Yes
Application fee	$50

Admissions Requirements (Required)

MCAT scores, science GPA, non-science GPA, letters of recommendation, interview, state residency, essays/personal statement, extracurricular activities, exposure to medical profession.

Overlap Schools

Des Moines University, New York Medical College, Philadelphia College of Osteopathic Medicine.

COSTS AND AID

Tuition	$25,130
Room and board	$9,448
Cost of books	$6,300
Fees	$160

Financial Aid

% students receiving aid	96
Average grant	$13,417
Average loan	$34,724
Average debt	$162,000

Ohio University

Ohio University College of Osteopathic Medicine

102 Grosvenor Hall, Athens, OH 45701 • Admission: 800-345-1560 • Fax: 740-593-2256 • E-mail: admissions@exchange.oucom.ohiou.edu • Website: www.oucom.ohiou.edu

Academics

The Ohio University College of Osteopathic Medicine (OU-COM) is dedicated to preparing well-rounded primary care and specialty physicians for service to the state of Ohio as well as the nation. Students begin their first two years of training in Athens and spend the final two years at one of twelve hospitals in our Centers for Osteopathic Research and Education (CORE). The learning environment at OU-COM and the CORE is constructed based on the principles of adult learning that include student empowerment and clinical relevance. Students will enroll in one of two tracks: the Patient-Centered Continuum (PCC) curriculum or the Clinical Presentation Continuum (CPC) curriculum. Both curricula view medical education as an organized building process that extends from the first day of medical school through residency training and beyond. Students in both curricula begin interacting with real patients in the first weeks of their medical education.

Admissions

REQUIREMENTS

Eight semester hours each in biology, chemistry, organic chemistry, and physics are required. In addition, applicants must have taken six semester hours of English and social science. As a state-affiliated institution, the college gives preference to Ohio residents, who make up about 80 percent of the student body. About 80 percent of AACOMAS applicants are sent supplemental applications. About 16 percent of those who submit supplemental applications are invited to interview from October to April. Interviews consist of three thirty-minute sessions with members of the faculty and administration. Approximately half of interviewees are accepted and are notified on a rolling basis. In the past, successful candidates have had a mean GPA of 3.5 and an average of at least 8 on each section of the MCAT.

STUDENT BODY

Type	Public
Enrollment	433
% male/female	44/56
% underrepresented minorities	24
# applied (total/out)	2,041/1,581
# accepted (total/out)	191/33
# enrolled (total/out)	107/18
Average age	24

FACULTY

Total faculty (number)	106
% female	30
% minority	8
% part-time	22
# student/faculty ratio	4:1

ADMISSIONS

Average GPA and MCAT Scores

Overall GPA	3.5
MCAT Bio	8.46
MCAT Phys	7.8
MCAT Verbal	7.76
MCAT Essay	P

Application Information

Regular application	2/4
Regular notification	rolling
Are transfers accepted?	Yes
Admissions may be deferred?	Yes
Interview required?	Yes
Application fee	$155

Admissions Requirements (Required)

MCAT scores, science GPA, non-science GPA, letters of recommendation, interview, essays/personal statement, extracurricular activities, exposure to medical profession.

Admissions Requirements (Optional)

state residency.

Overlap Schools

A. T. Still University of Health Sciences, Lake Erie College of Osteopathic Medicine, Medical College of Ohio, Philadelphia College of Osteopathic Medicine, The Ohio State University, University of Cincinnati, Wright State University.

COSTS AND AID

In-state tuition	$18,015
Out-of-state tuition	$26,253
Cost of books	$4,175
Fees	$2,046

Financial Aid

% students receiving aid	92
Average grant	$2,500
Average loan	$24,909
Average debt	$108,000

Oklahoma State University

Oklahoma State University College of Osteopathic Medicine

Student Affairs Office, 1111 West 17th Street, Tulsa, OK 74107 • Admission: 800-677-1972 • Fax: 918-561-8243 • E-mail: bblaster@chs.okstate.edu • Website: www.healthsciences.okstate.edu

Academics

The curriculum at the College of Osteopathic Medicine includes hands-on clinical experiences, student-centered, and problem-based methods of instruction, as well as frequent consultation with faculty and community-based physicians. The first year focuses on biomedical sciences, and the second year emphasizes case-based learning and problem solving as it relates to conditions seen in primary care environments. The third and fourth years are composed of clinical rotations, most of which take place at Tulsa Regional Medical Center, the country's largest osteopathic hospital (521 beds). Students also rotate to adjacent rural areas, and they may fulfill requirements at various medical institutions across the country. Although 64 percent of graduates enter primary care, they are prepared to enter residencies in all medical specialty fields. The medical school, a college of Oklahoma State University, is located in Tulsa, a very livable city with a population of 500,000.

Admissions

REQUIREMENTS

Of the eighty-eight positions in a class, sixty-eight are reserved for Oklahoma residents. Prerequisites for application are eight to ten semester hours of biology, physics, chemistry, and organic chemistry (all with labs), in addition to six to eight hours of English, and one upper-level science course. The minimum undergraduate GPA is 3.0, and an average of 7.0 on the MCAT is required. All AACOMAS applicants meeting these requirements receive a secondary application, but only about 10 percent of those secondary applicants are interviewed. Interviews begin in August and continue until early March. Applicants will interview simultaneously with two faculty members for thirty-five to forty minutes. Notification occurs on a rolling basis, and about 35 to 40 percent of interviewees are accepted.

STUDENT BODY

Type	Public
Enrollment	349
% male/female	56/44
% underrepresented minorities	19
# applied (total/out)	410/208
# accepted (total/out)	151/32
# enrolled (total/out)	88/8
Average age	25

FACULTY

Total faculty (number)	367
% female	25
% minority	5
% part-time	80
# student/faculty ratio	6:1

ADMISSIONS

Average GPA and MCAT Scores

Overall GPA	3.6
MCAT Bio	9
MCAT Phys	8
MCAT Verbal	9
MCAT Essay	0

Application Information

Regular application	2/15
Regular notification	rolling
Are transfers accepted?	Yes
Admissions may be deferred?	No
Interview required?	Yes
Application fee	$25

Admissions Requirements (Required)

MCAT scores, science GPA, non-science GPA, letters of recommendation, interview, essays/personal statement, extracurricular activities, exposure to medical profession, familiar with osteopathic physician.

Admissions Requirements (Optional)

state residency.

Overlap Schools

University of Oklahoma.

COSTS AND AID

In-state tuition	$13,774
Out-of-state tuition	$30,144
Cost of books	$4,100
Fees	$776

Financial Aid

% students receiving aid	90
Average grant	$5,500
Average loan	$26,000
Average debt	$91,000

Philadelphia College of Osteopathic Medicine

Office of Admissions, 4170 City Avenue, Philadelphia, PA 19131 • Admission: 800-999-6998 • Fax: 215-871-6719 • E-mail: admissions@pcom.edu • Website: www.pcom.edu

Academics

Philadelphia College of Osteopathic Medicine (PCOM) is among the five largest medical schools in the country, with 250 students per class. Early clinical exposure through community service activities and formal course work complement basic science instruction. The curriculum is interdisciplinary, includes topics such as medical ethic and medical law, and emphasizes primary care and prevention. Clinical training takes place at thirty-three affiliated institutions in and around Philadelphia. In addition, students may arrange to fulfill elective requirements in other states or in other countries. Joint-degree programs lead to the DO/MBA or DO/MPH. The entering class of 1999 included students from twenty states. The male/female ratio was 55:45, and the average age was twenty-five.

Admissions

REQUIREMENTS

As a private institution, PCOM accepts applicants from all over the country and does show preference for Pennsylvania residents. Science preparation must include eight semester hours each in biology, inorganic chemistry, organic chemistry, and physics. In addition, six hours of English literature/composition are required. The MCAT is required and the best set of scores is used for applicants who have retaken the exam. All AACOMAS applicants receive secondary applications. About 18 percent of the approximately 4,000 returning secondaries are invited to interview on campus beginning in September. The interview consists of one session with a panel that could include faculty, students, and administrators. Notification of committee decision occurs on a rolling basis. In a recently accepted class, the average GPA was 3.36 overall, and the average combined MCAT score was 26.

STUDENT BODY

Type	Private
Enrollment	1,011
% male/female	56/44
% underrepresented minorities	19
# applied (total/out)	3,154/2,678
# accepted (total/out)	410/209
# enrolled (total/out)	256/88
Average age	24

FACULTY

Total faculty (number)	969
% female	11
% part-time	5
# student/faculty ratio	5:1

ADMISSIONS

Average GPA and MCAT Scores

Overall GPA	3.4
MCAT Bio	8.31
MCAT Phys	8.04
MCAT Verbal	8.2
MCAT Essay	P

Application Information

Regular application	2/1
Regular notification	rolling
Are transfers accepted?	No
Admissions may be deferred?	No
Interview required?	Yes
Application fee	$50

Admissions Requirements (Required)

MCAT scores, science GPA, non-science GPA, letters of recommendation, interview, essays/personal statement.

Admissions Requirements (Optional)

state residency, extracurricular activities, exposure to medical profession.

Overlap Schools

Temple University, University of Medicine and Dentistry of New Jersey.

COSTS AND AID

Tuition	$28,500
Room and board	$13,190
Cost of books	$1,950
Fees	$525

Financial Aid

% students receiving aid	93
Average grant	$2,500
Average loan	$42,250
Average debt	$149,800

PIKEVILLE COLLEGE

PIKEVILLE COLLEGE SCHOOL OF OSTEOPATHIC MEDICINE

147 SYCAMORE STREET, PIKEVILLE, KY 41501 • ADMISSION: 606-218-5406 • FAX: 606-218-5442 •
E-MAIL: JTHOMAS@PC.EDU • WEBSITE: WWW.PCSOM.EDU

Academics

PCSOM uses a new curriculum that features increased hours in behavior and community medicine, physical diagnosis, and OP&P. Traditional subjects are covered using case-based learning, tradition lectures, labs, and computer simulation. All the medical school facilities have been completed in the last five years. The physical plant features new classrooms, new labs, and the state-of-the-art telemedicine center/medical library. The medical school's computer system is wireless and available campus wide. Pikeville College's Board of Trustees has decided that no student should be organizationally or academically disadvantaged in an osteopathic medical school because of a lack of adequate personal funding. To this end PCSOM supplies each student with the following: a state-of-the-art Pentium laptop computer, Windows NT, Office 2002, a modem, all required CD ROMs, free Internet access, all required texts and workbooks (to be provided each year), all necessary anatomy dissection equipment, a new portable OP&P table, stethoscope, ophthalmoscope, otoscope, lab coats, scrub suits, outside board review, and the cost of taking Part I and Part II of NBOME once.

Admissions

REQUIREMENTS

There is a supplemental application.

PROCESS

Pikeville participates in the AACOMAS application process. Requirements for admission include twelve hours of biology, four hours of chemistry, eight hours of physics, and eight hours of organic chemistry. The MCAT exam is required.

STUDENT BODY

Type	Private
Enrollment	253
% male/female	62/38
% underrepresented minorities	8
# applied (total/out)	1,334/1,236
# accepted (total/out)	102/62
# enrolled (total/out)	75/42
Average age	27

FACULTY

Total faculty (number)	22
% female	29
# student/faculty ratio	6:1

ADMISSIONS

Average GPA and MCAT Scores

Overall GPA	3.3
MCAT Bio	7.64
MCAT Phys	7.08
MCAT Verbal	7.78
MCAT Essay	0

Application Information

Regular application	2/5
Regular notification	rolling
Are transfers accepted?	Yes
Admissions may be deferred?	No
Interview required?	Yes
Application fee	$75

Admissions Requirements (Required)

MCAT scores, science GPA, non-science GPA, letters of recommendation, interview, essays/personal statement, extracurricular activities, exposure to medical profession.

Admissions Requirements (Optional)

state residency.

Overlap Schools

Marshall University, Ohio University, University of Kentucky, University of Louisville, West Virginia School of Osteopathic Medicine.

COSTS AND AID

Tuition	$26,000

Financial Aid

% students receiving aid	96
Average grant	$12,110
Average loan	$25,000
Average debt	$96,000

TOURO UNIVERSITY—CALIFORNIA

TOURO UNIVERSITY COLLEGE OF OSTEOPATHIC MEDICINE

OFFICE OF ADMISSIONS, 1310 JOHNSON LANE, VALLEJO, CA 94592 • ADMISSION: 707-638-5270 • FAX: 707-638-5250 • E-MAIL: SDAVIS@TOURO.EDU • WEBSITE: WWW.TUMI.EDU

Academics

The Touro University College of Osteopathic Medicine, San Francisco, is located in the northeast part of San Francisco Bay, on Mare Island. Touro University is an international institution based in New York that has branches in Israel and the Russian Federation. The mission of the TUCOM is to train osteopathic, family practice physicians to help meet the need for primary care practitioners in California and throughout the country. Although preventative medicine and primary care are emphasized, graduates are also prepared to enter residency programs that train osteopathic specialists. Patient contact begins in the first year, and clinical training takes place at sites throughout the greater Bay Area, including hospitals, clinics, and physicians' offices. Students have the opportunity to experience both urban and rural patient populations.

Admissions

REQUIREMENTS

TUCOM requires eight semester units each of biology/zoology, inorganic chemistry, organic chemistry, and physics. Six semester units each of English, humanities, and behavioral science courses are also required. Computers are an integral part of the educational process, and candidates are strongly encouraged to be computer literate. TUOCOM participates in AACOMAS. The MCAT is required, and scores must be no more than three years old. Successful candidates typically have minimum science and cumulative GPAs of 3.0 and minimum cumulative MCAT scores of 23 or higher.

STUDENT BODY

Type	Private
Enrollment	500
% male/female	53/47
% underrepresented minorities	2
# applied (total)	3,250
# accepted (total)	131
# enrolled (total)	131
Average age	27

ADMISSIONS

Average GPA and MCAT Scores

Overall GPA	3.5
MCAT Bio	9.6
MCAT Phys	9.27
MCAT Verbal	8.13

Application Information

Regular application	2/15
Regular notification	rolling
Early application	8/1
Early notification	9/1
Are transfers accepted?	Yes
Admissions may be deferred?	Yes
Interview required?	Yes
Application fee	$100

Admissions Requirements (Required)

MCAT scores, science GPA, non-science GPA, letters of recommendation, interview, essays/personal statement, extracurricular activities, exposure to medical profession.

Admissions Requirements (Optional)

state residency.

COSTS AND AID

Tuition	$29,650
Cost of books	$1,615

Financial Aid

% students receiving aid	93

The University of Health Sciences
College of Osteopathic Medicine

1750 Independence Avenue, Kansas City, MO 64106-1453 • Admission: 800-234-4847 • Fax: 816-283-2484 • E-mail: admissions@uhs.edu • Website: www.uhs.edu

Academics

UHS-COM is the largest medical school in the state of Missouri and the oldest in Kansas City, Missouri. Affordable and friendly, Kansas City's metropolitan area encompasses counties in both Kansas and Missouri. The college's goal, as stated in its mission statement is to "... prepare men and women to be exceptionally competent osteopathic physicians." In 2000, 38 percent of the entering class was female, the average age was twenty-six, the age range was twenty-forty-four, and class size was 220. For its exemplary curriculum devoted to understanding the relationship between healing and patients' spiritual beliefs, the university recieved the coveted Spirituality and Medicine Award from the John Templeton Foundation.

Admissions

REQUIREMENTS

As a private school, no preference is given to Missouri residents. Course requirements are fifteen semester hours of biology, three of which must be in genetics; sixteen semester hours of chemistry, three of which must be in biochemistry; eight semester hours of physics; and six semester hours of English and/or literature. Science courses must have labs. The MCAT is required and must be no more than three years old. For those who have retaken the exam, the best set of scores is considered. AACOMAS applicants who meet minimum requirements are sent secondary applications. About 25 percent of applicants are interviewed between September and May. The interview consists of one session with a group of faculty members, including osteopathic physicians on staff. Applicants are advised to not only know the history and tenets of osteopathic medicine but also to be able to articulate their personal motivation for wanting to practice osteopathic medicine. About 85 percent of interviewees are accepted and are notificatied on a rolling basis. The average GPA of successful applicants is about 3.4, and the average MCAT is 8.4.

STUDENT BODY

Type	Private
Enrollment	887
% male/female	40/60
% underrepresented minorities	40
# applied (total/out)	2,040/1,926
# accepted (total/out)	487/433
# enrolled (total/out)	227/199
Average age	25

FACULTY

Total faculty (number)	983
% female	19
% minority	6
% part-time	1
# student/faculty ratio	1:1

ADMISSIONS

Average GPA and MCAT Scores

Overall GPA	3.4
MCAT Bio	8.64
MCAT Phys	7.76
MCAT Verbal	8.09
MCAT Essay	Q

Application Information

Regular application	2/1
Regular notification	rolling
Are transfers accepted?	No
Admissions may be deferred?	Yes
Interview required?	Yes
Application fee	$50

Admissions Requirements (Required)

MCAT scores, science GPA, non-science GPA, letters of recommendation, interview, essays/personal statement, extracurricular activities, exposure to medical profession, community service/volunteer work.

Admissions Requirements (Optional)

state residency.

Overlap Schools

A. T. Still University of Health Sciences, University of Osteopathic Medicine and Health Sciences.

COSTS AND AID

Tuition	$31,200
Cost of books	$1,483
Fees	$60

Financial Aid

% students receiving aid	96
Average grant	$1,500
Average loan	$40,000
Average debt	$154,000

UNIVERSITY OF NEW ENGLAND
COLLEGE OF OSTEOPATHIC MEDICINE

ADMISSIONS OFFICE, UNECOM, HILLS BEACH ROAD, BIDDEFORD, ME 04005 • ADMISSION: 207-283-0171 • FAX: 207-294-5900 • E-MAIL: ADMISSIONS@MAILBOX.UNE.EDU • WEBSITE: WWW.UNE.EDU

Academics

The UNE College of Osteopathic medicine is a private, nonprofit institution, largely focused on training physicians for family practice and other primary health care fields. Rural medicine is also emphasized in keeping with the school's goal of graduating health practitioners who will help meet the health care needs of underserved populations in the New England region. A portion of the basic science curriculum at UNE uses a body systems approach and incorporates osteopathc principles and topics such as human behavior, community health, health maintenence, and ethics. Clinical rotations begin early in the third year and take place in over twenty community hospitals and medical centers throughout the country. The UNE campus offers a health science library, computer resources, a fitness center, and university-owned-apartments. Biddeford is a small city situated on the water, with a population just under 20,000. The male/female ratio is about 55:45, and the average age of entering students in a recent class was twenty-eight. Underrepresented minorities account for about 9 percent of the student body. Class size is 115.

Admissions

REQUIREMENTS

Residents of New England are given some preference in admissions, although qualified applicants from other regions are considered. The minimum course requirements are one year each of biology, physics, chemistry, and organic chemistry, all with associated labs. Applicants should have at least a 2.7 GPA in both sciences and overall, as the average overall GPA of successful applicants is about 3.3. The MCAT is required and must be no more than two years old. The average MCAT of successful applicants is in the eight to nine range. Most of the 2,700 ACOMAS applicants receive secondary applications. Of those returning secondaries, approximately 10 percent are interviewed between August and April. The interview consists of one session, usually with a team of interviewers. About 80 percent of interviewed candidates are accepted on a rolling basis. Wait-listed candidates may send supplemental information to update their files.

STUDENT BODY

Type	Private
Enrollment	458
% male/female	54/46
% underrepresented minorities	9
# applied (total)	602
# accepted (total)	162
# enrolled (total)	115
Average age	27

ADMISSIONS

Average GPA and MCAT Scores

Overall GPA	3.4
MCAT Bio	8.5
MCAT Phys	8.1
MCAT Verbal	8.4
MCAT Essay	Q

Admissions (continued)

Application Information

Regular application	1/2
Regular notification	rolling
Are transfers accepted?	Yes
Admissions may be deferred?	No
Interview required?	Yes
Application fee	$55

Admissions Requirements (Required)

MCAT scores, science GPA, non-science GPA, letters of recommendation, interview, essays/personal statement, extracurricular activities, exposure to medical profession.

Admissions Requirements (Optional)

state residency.

COSTS AND AID

Tuition	$27,690
Cost of books	$1,000
Fees	$260

Financial Aid

% students receiving aid	91
Average grant	$1,000

UNIVERSITY OF NORTH TEXAS HEALTH SCIENCE CENTER

TEXAS COLLEGE OF OSTEOPATHIC MEDICINE

EAD-248, 3500 CAMP BOWIE BOULEVARD, FORT WORTH, TX 76107-2699 • ADMISSION: 817-735-2204 • FAX: 817-735-2225 • E-MAIL: TCOMADMISSIONS@HSC.UNT.EDU • WEBSITE: WWW.HSC.UNT.EDU/EDUCATION/TCOM/ADMISSIONS.CFM

Academics

The University of North Texas Health Science Center at Fort Worth trains osteopathic physicians, physician assistants, biomedical scientists, and public health professionals. Its academic components are the Texas College of Osteopathic Medicine, the Graduate School of Biomedical Sciences, and the School of Public Health. Dual-degree programs combine medical training with research and public health. U.S. News & World Report and the Texas Academy of Family Physicians have both recognized TCOM's commitment to primary care.

BASIC SCIENCES: The first portion of the curriculum is designed to help students integrate the basic and clinical sciences, further develop their ability to diagnose illness, and increase their understanding of the context within which medicine is practiced. The integrated systems approach is built on the same strong foundation of scientific and clinical knowledge that has long characterized TCOM's outstanding academic program.

Admissions

REQUIREMENTS

At least 90 percent of the positions in each class of 125 are reserved for Texas residents. One year of traditional pre-medical sciences is required, in addition to one year of English composition. The MCAT is required, and scores must be from within the past three years. Applications are accepted through the Texas Medical and Dental Schools Application Service (TMDSAS). Selected applicants are invited to interview between August and December. Initial offers of acceptance are sent on February 1 and continue until the incoming class is full.

STUDENT BODY

Type	Public
Enrollment	492
% male/female	48/52
% underrepresented minorities	9
# applied (total/out)	1,350/97
# accepted (total/out)	155/16
# enrolled (total/out)	127/7
Average age	25

FACULTY

Total faculty (number)	198
% female	22
% minority	8

ADMISSIONS

Average GPA and MCAT Scores

Overall GPA	3.6
MCAT Bio	9.2
MCAT Phys	8.72
MCAT Verbal	8.49
MCAT Essay	0

Admissions (continued)

Application Information

Regular application	11/1
Regular notification	2/1
Early application	8/1
Early notification	10/1
Are transfers accepted?	Yes
Admissions may be deferred?	Yes
Interview required?	Yes

Admissions Requirements (Required)

MCAT scores, science GPA, non-science GPA, letters of recommendation, interview, essays/personal statement, exposure to medical profession, secondary application.

Admissions Requirements (Optional)

state residency, extracurricular activities.

Overlap Schools

Baylor College of Medicine, South Texas College of Law, Texas Tech University, The University of Texas HSC at Houston, University of Texas, University of Texas Health Science Center at San Antonio, University of Texas Southwestern Medical Center.

COSTS AND AID

In-state tuition	$6,550
Out-of-state tuition	$19,650
Cost of books	$2,426
Fees	$2,480

Financial Aid

% students receiving aid	91
Average grant	$5,000
Average loan	$24,418
Average debt	$86,000

West Virginia School of Osteopathic Medicine

West Virginia School of Osteopathic Medicine

Director of Admissions, 400 North Lee Street, Lewisburg, WV 24901 • Admission: 800-356-7836 •
Fax: 304-645-4859 • E-mail: admissions@wvsom.edu • Website: www.wvsom.edu

Academics

West Virginia School of Osteopathic Medicine is part of the West Virginia state system of higher education. As a state school located in rural Appalachia, it is geared toward meeting the primary care needs of West Virginia's significantly rural population. Nine other states have loose affiliations with the school and are also served by its programs. This curriculum includes a system-based and problem-based approach to learning basic sciences, and clinical training at community sites. Among all students the average age is twenty-seven, and the male/female ratio is 54:49.

Admissions

REQUIREMENTS

Residents of West Virginia account for 50 percent of the student body and are given priority in admissions. The minimum course requirements are eight semesters of biology, physics, general chemistry, and organic chemistry, all with associated labs, and six semester hours of English. The MCAT is required and the test must be taken no later than the fall prior to the entering class year. The average MCAT of successful applicants is in the seven to eight range. About 26 percent of approximately 1,400 applicants are interviewed between August and April.

STUDENT BODY

Type	Public
Enrollment	336
% male/female	51/49
% underrepresented minorities	8
# applied (total/out)	1,432/1,276
# accepted (total/out)	265/188
# enrolled (total/out)	103/53
Average age	27

FACULTY

Total faculty (number)	40
% female	30
% minority	1
% part-time	0
# student/faculty ratio	5:1

ADMISSIONS

Average GPA and MCAT Scores

Overall GPA	3.4
MCAT Bio	7.5
MCAT Phys	7
MCAT Verbal	7.8
MCAT Essay	N

Application Information

Regular application	2/15
Regular notification	rolling
Are transfers accepted?	Yes
Admissions may be deferred?	No
Interview required?	Yes
Application fee	$155

Admissions Requirements (Required)

MCAT scores, science GPA, letters of recommendation, interview, essays/personal statement, expo

Admissions Reuirements (Required/continued)

sure to medical profession, minimum 90 semester hours.

Admissions Requirements (Optional)

nonscience GPA, state residency, extracurricular activities.

COSTS AND AID

In-state tuition	$15,272
Out-of-state tuition	$37,794
Cost of books	$4,704

Financial Aid

% students receiving aid	95
Average grant	$1,000
Average loan	$36,000
Average debt	$141,742

WESTERN UNIVERSITY OF HEALTH SCIENCES

COLLEGE OF OSTEOPATHIC MEDICINE OF THE PACIFIC

OFFICE OF ADMISSIONS, POMONA, CA 91766-1854 • ADMISSION: 909-469-5335 • FAX: 909-469-5570 •
E-MAIL: ADMISSIONS@WESTERNU.EDU • WEBSITE: WWW.WESTERNU.EDU

Academics

The Western University of Health Sciences (Western U.) is made up of five colleges: College of Osteopathic Medicine of the Pacific (COMP), College of Allied Health Professions, College of Graduate Nursing, College of Pharmacy, and College of Veterinary Medicine. The College of Veterinary Medicine welcomed its first students in the fall of 2003. Western U. is a leader in training primary care practitioners, including nurses, osteopathic physicians, physician assistants, physical therapists, pharmacists, and family practitioners. Clinical training facilities include the Arrowhead Regional Medical Center and many affiliated ambulatory sites. The university is located thirty-five miles east of Los Angeles.

Admissions

REQUIREMENTS

Eight semester hours each in biology, chemistry, organic chemistry, and physics (with labs) are required. In addition, applicants must have taken six semester hours of behavioral science and English. We accept students without regard to legal state of residence. Usually 85 percent of students are from California. You can apply while working on your undergraduate degree, but you should have plans to receive it by the time you register with the college. The MCAT (taken within the last three years) is required. Those AACOMAS applicants who are academically competitive are sent secondary applications, and about half of those who return secondary applications are invited for an interview. Notification occurs on a rolling basis.

STUDENT BODY

Type	Private
Enrollment	700
% male/female	55/45
% underrepresented minorities	55
# applied (total/out)	1,994/1,300
# accepted (total/out)	371/25
# enrolled (total/out)	181/60
Average age	27

FACULTY

Total faculty (number)	28
% female	11
% minority	11
% part-time	11
# student/faculty ratio	4:1

ADMISSIONS

Average GPA and MCAT Scores

Overall GPA	3.4
MCAT Bio	9.2
MCAT Phys	8.8
MCAT Verbal	8.3
MCAT Essay	P

Application Information

Regular application	2/1
Regular notification	rolling
Early application	5/30
Early notification	9/1
Are transfers accepted?	Yes
Admissions may be deferred?	Yes
Interview required?	Yes
Application fee	$60

Admissions Requirements (Required)

MCAT scores, science GPA, non-science GPA, letters of recommendation, interview, essays/personal statement, extracurricular activities, exposure to medical profession.

Admissions Requirements (Optional)

state residency.

Overlap Schools

Touro College, University of California at Irvine.

COSTS AND AID

Tuition	$31,115
Cost of books	$2,000
Fees	$30

Financial Aid

% students receiving aid	90
Average grant	$19,376
Average loan	$38,928
Average debt	$145,608

SCHOOL SAYS

In this section you'll find schools with extended listings describing admissions, curriculum, internships, and much more. This is your chance to get in-depth information on programs that interest you. The Princeton Review charges each school a small fee to be listed, and the editorial responsibility is solely that of the university.

NATIONAL UNIVERSITY OF HEALTH SCIENCES

National University of Health Sciences has been the leader in educating chiropractic physicians since its founding in 1906. Formerly called the National College of Chiropractic, the institution's name was changed to reflect its expanded offerings in alternative and complementary methods of health care beginning with the establishment of a massage therapy certification program in 1999. The education of chiropractic physicians, however, continues to be National University's main focus.

CHIROPRACTIC

Chiropractic medicine is one of the three branches of healing along with osteopathic and allopathic medicine. As a school of healing, chiropractic may be defined as the diagnosis and treatment of human ailments without the use of drugs, prescriptive medicines, or invasive surgery. The consistently steady increase in the public's use of complementary and alternative medicine has escalated the chiropractic profession to the second largest primary health care profession in the United States.

GENERAL INFORMATION

National University of Health Sciences (NUHS) offers a broad scope, comprehensive program that leads to the doctor of chiropractic (DC) degree and also allows the student the option of earning a bachelor of science degree with a major in human biology (BS).

National University takes the designation of doctor most seriously and believes the chiropractic physician must undertake the same rigorous learning processes as all other doctors. Our students are educated as primary health care providers—able to diagnose, treat, and manage a wide range of conditions. They refer patients to other health care providers when their conditions are beyond the scope of chiropractic care.

LOCATION

National University is located on a 32-acre campus in Lombard, Illinois, in a family-oriented suburban community of 42,000, just 20 miles from downtown Chicago.

FACILITIES

National University is proud of its comprehensive facilities for educating students in the basic sciences, chiropractic therapeutics, and massage therapy. Our main building consists of fully equipped physiology, biochemistry, and microbiology laboratories, as well as a gross anatomy laboratory where students learn and perform a full cadaver dissection. Our on-campus clinic includes treatment rooms as well as research and X-ray laboratories.

National students can also take advantage of a fully equipped fitness center, on-campus health services, on-campus student housing, and the Learning Resource Center, the largest health-oriented library in DuPage County.

The university has one of the most prestigious research facilities among chiropractic colleges with laboratories dedicated to spinal biomechanics, interdisciplinary research, and biological resources. The NUHS Department of Research promotes the advancement of knowledge pertaining to the practice of chiropractic and other aspects of complementary and alternative medicine by performing and encouraging high quality, efficiently conducted ethical research.

National is the only chiropractic college to be equipped with a Magnetic Resonance Imaging (MRI) facility for student, patient and research situations, and a Training and Assessment Center (TAC). The TAC is utilized for remote observation and recording of student/patient interactions with standardized patients, small group discussion using the problem-based learning process, review of videotaped patient encounters, training in interpersonal skills, faculty development, and performance-based clinical competence assessment.

PROGRAM

National's program consists of ten trimesters of study, including one year of uninterrupted internship. New classes are admitted each January, May, and September. By enrolling for ten consecutive trimesters, the program can be completed in three years and four months. If students take a break each summer, they can graduate in five years.

At the conclusion of the fourth trimester, students are eligible to receive the bachelor of science degree in human biology. After completion of all academic requirements, the doctor of chiropractic degree is conferred.

CURRICULUM

National students undergo a thorough grounding in the basic and clinical sciences, which enhances further instruction in our unique Guided Discovery Curriculum. The format incorporates, lectures, small groups, case-based learning, and self-directed study. Students' education concludes with an intensive one-year clinical internship in one of the health care facilities operated by or affiliated with the university or with a community-based chiropractic physician. We also have an exclusive practice management program, which gives students the necessary business skills necessary to manage a successful, ethical chiropractic practice.

National's curriculum fully qualifies students for licensure in all 50 states, Canada, and several foreign countries and results in consistently top-ranking pass rates on national board examinations.

ADMISSION REQUIREMENTS

Because we believe a good solid foundation is necessary to be successful in our program, our admissions requirements have always been the highest in the profession. We are the only chiropractic college that requires a bachelor's degree for entrance along with a minimum cumulative GPA of 2.5 on a 4.0 scale and the completion of specific science course requirements.

For students who lack certain science courses, an accelerated prerequisite program has been developed to address these needs.

FINANCIAL AID

The university offers Federal Stafford Loans, Federal Perkins Loan, Veterans Educational Benefits, federal work-study, institutional grants and loans, scholarships, and student employment. National's Office of Financial Aid will work with you to determine the loan or grant program for which you may qualify.

ACCREDITATION

National University's doctor of chiropractic degree program is accredited by the Higher Learning Commission of the North Central Association of Colleges and Schools and the Commission on Accreditation of the Council on Chiropractic Education.

APPLICATION

To request an application packet, e-mail us at issions@nuhs.edu" admissions@nuhs.edu or visit our website at www.nuhs.edu to apply online or download an application. Then, submit your application with transcripts, $55 application fee, and two character references. The Admissions Committee will evaluate your file for acceptance.

CAMPUS VISIT

National University holds official Campus Visit Days during the year but tours may be arranged Monday to Friday on an individual basis. For information on the next visit day or to arrange a personal tour, call 800-826-6285 or e-mail us at admissions@nuhs.edu.

ROSS UNIVERSITY

Ross University promises to challenge and empower students to achieve their full professional and personal potential as a physician.

The Medical School was founded in 1978 and offers a doctor of medicine (MD) degree. The educational program is fully comparable to those offered by medical schools in the United States and is designed to prepare students for general medical practice and to provide the foundation for post-graduate specialty training in the United States. The first four semesters (16 months) are taught in Dominica and consist of basic science and preclinical courses. Students spend the fifth semester in clinical studies in Miami, Florida, and the remaining five semesters in clinical clerkships at affiliated hospitals located throughout the United States.

Ross University School of Medicine maintains a technologically advanced campus in Dominica. Academic facilities include classrooms and auditoriums equipped with the latest audiovisual instructional technology, modern laboratories, two simulation facilities housing patient simulators, medical education computer room, a medical library, and learning resource centers that are equipped with over 100 computers for student use. Student support services include a food court and an outdoor café, athletic playing fields, a fitness facility, and a U.S.-modeled day care and preparatory school (K-8).

The basic science courses are taught by experienced full-time faculty members who have been selected for their teaching ability and their devotion to students. Members of the faculty hold an MD, a PhD, or both. Many faculty members are board certified in their specialties in the United States or are members of the Royal Colleges of the United Kingdom. The school's Academic Curriculum Committee meets on a routine basis to review and revise the educational program to respond to changes in medical training in the United States.

Ross University School of Medicine operates a ten semester program of instruction that offers three academic semesters per year and enrolls a new class of students in January, May, and September.

Over the first four semesters, students focus primarily on basic science disciplines such as gross anatomy, biochemistry, and microbiology. Courses are presented employing both traditional didactic and lab based methodologies (75 percent) and problem-based learning (PBL) techniques (25 percent). During their fourth semester, students are introduced to clinical medicine at the Princess Margaret Hospital on Dominica and affiliated clinics. Each semester is fifteen weeks long with two- or three-week breaks between semesters. Each course is concluded with a subject based Comprehensive Shelf Exam prepared by the Educational Commission for Foreign Medical Graduates (ECFMG), which serves as the final exam. Students receive traditional letter grades with corresponding grade points for each course.

Upon completing the four basic science semesters, any student with a 2.9 grade point average or higher is promoted to the Advanced Introduction to Clinical Medicine (AICM) course conducted at Area Health Education Training Centers in Miami, Florida, and certified by the university to sit for the Step 1 of the United States Medical Licensing Examination (USMLE).

Students who complete the basic science with less than a 2.9 GPA will sit for the National Board of Medical Examiners comprehensive examination (NBME), and if they receive a passing score on the exam they will be promoted to fifth semester. Students who do not pass the exam must remain in Dominica and complete the ten-week basic medical sciences integration (BMSI) course (conducted in affiliation with Princeton Review). Upon passage of BMSI, students are promoted to AICM and certified for USMLE Step 1.

The AICM/fifth semester serves as a vital transition from the basic sciences to clinical medicine. Students refine their physical diagnosis skills; through supervised patient encounters, they develop skills in evaluating and assessing medical problems.

Before beginning their clinical rotations, students must take and pass USMLE Step 1. The exam tests the student's ability to integrate and apply basic science knowledge to solving problems presented in the form of clinical vignettes. Over the past ten years, 97 percent of Ross medical students have passed the USMLE Step 1.

Upon successful completion of USMLE Step 1, the students rotate through mandatory and elective medical specialty areas in clinical programs with affiliated hospitals located in the United States. Students are placed for 81 weeks of "clinical clerkships" in which they gain practical experience alongside their peers from U.S. medical schools.

These clerkships consist of 48 weeks of required (core) rotations and 33 weeks of elective rotations, encompassing the sixth through the tenth semesters of the program. The educational objectives of the clinical program are: (1) to train students in the clinical aspects of the basic areas of medical practice; (2) to prepare students to function effectively in subsequent graduate residency programs; (3) to provide students with an overview of different levels of medical practice; and (4) to provide students with an opportunity to assess areas of medical practice in which they might wish to continue in a residency program.

The core clinical clerkships consist of medicine, family medicine, obstetrics/gynecology, surgery, pediatrics, and psychiatry. The remaining 33 weeks are spent in elective clerkships, which include, but are not limited to, general medicine or medical subspecialties and general surgery or surgical subspecialties. Rotations are conducted at more than 40 teaching hospitals that have ACGME-approved residency programs. Students can elect to participate in clinical training in affiliated teaching hospital located in California; Connecticut; Florida; Illinois; Maryland; Massachusetts; Nevada; New Jersey; New York; Ohio; Washington, DC; and the Commonwealth of Dominica, West Indies.

Upon completion of core rotations, students must complete and pass USMLE Step 2 Clinical Skills (Step 2 CS) and USMLE Step 2 Clinical Knowledge (Step 2 CK) in addition to completing elective rotations to graduate. Unlike many U.S. schools of medicine, the Medical School requires passage of USMLE Step 2 for graduation. Over the past ten years, 99 percent of Ross medical students have passed the USMLE Step 2.

Concurrently, graduates enlist in the National Residency Match Program, which is a paired choice system for matching applicants to available residencies that takes place every March. Typically, 96 percent of eligible Ross University graduates obtain ACGME-accredited residency positions following graduation. Students train in a residency program for two to three years during which they sit for the USMLE Step 3.

Upon completion of their residency and passage of USMLE Step 3, candidate physicians are prepared for licensure.

The Medical School has graduated over 4,000 physicians since 1978 who have gone into virtually every specialty of medicine; however, the majority of graduates select residencies in primary care (internal medicine, family medicine, pediatrics, obstetrics or gynecology). A number of Ross alumni are now practitioners in specialties such as transplant nephrology, invasive cardiology, plastic surgery, pulmonary medicine, cardiovascular, anesthesiology, neonatology, endocrinology, rheumatology, geriatric medicine, infectious diseases, and hematology/oncology. Over 1,250 Ross alumni have obtained Board Certification in one or more specialties. Some Ross alumni hold faculty appointments at United States medical schools across the country.

SPARTAN UNIVERSITY

STUDENT SERVICES

Periodicals, books, and audiovisual materials are important supplements to a medical education. Therefore, students are encouraged to take advantage of the available facilities. Microscopes, microscopic slides, and skeletons are available for student use. However, all equipment must remain in the laboratory. Student housing is available off-campus. The university approves the facilities. For further information, contact the Director of Housing, Vieux Fort, St.Lucia, at 758-454-6128. Student Government Association (SGA): The SGA represents collective interests of students with regard to the proper administration and improvement of the university. Individual student grievances will be channeled through the SGA president to appropriate committees.

FINANCIAL AID

The university offers financial aid in the form of The Education Resources Institute (TERI) loans. TERI, in partnership with International Education Finance Corporation (IEFC), has developed the affordable solution called ISLP to help students finance their international education.

The ISLP Graduate Loan is available to U.S. or foreign students who are enrolled at least half-time at approved colleges and universities. ISLP Loans are guaranteed by TERI, a national not-for-profit guarantor of educational loans. Funding is made possible with private capital from Bank of Boston.

IEFC Telephone: 781-843-5334

TERI Telephone: 800-837-4326

Facsimile: 888-329-8374

Address: PO Box 312

Boston, MA 02117

CANADIAN LOANS

Financial assistance may be available through the Canadian Student Loan Program for eligible Canadian citizens. Their address and telephone number is as follows:

Ministry of Education and Training

PO Box 4500

189 RED RIVER ROAD, 4th Floor

Thunder Bay, Ontario P7B 6G9

Canada

Telephone 807-343-7260

The Veterans' Administration approved benefits may also be available for Veterans.

ACADEMICS

Spartan Health Sciences University, School of Medicine, offers a four academic year (36 calendar months) program leading to the doctor of medicine degree (MD) and is taught on a trimester (four-month) schedule. The curriculum of the university's doctor of medicine degree program encompasses a comprehensive course of basic sciences (BS), preclinical and clinical sciences (CS) that lasts for four (4) academic years. The trimester periods start in January, May, and September of each year. A student may elect to enter in any one of the three trimesters. All students are required to demonstrate competency in the basic medical sciences before being permitted to begin clinical rotations.

BASIC SCIENCES

The initial four trimesters of the program represent an integrated course presentation of the basic sciences (BS), which include anatomy, physiology, pharmacology, biochemistry, immunology, pathology, microbiology, behavioral sciences, neuroanatomy, general introduction to medicine, including physical diagnosis. Didactic lectures in internal medicine, pediatrics, psychiatry, obstetrics/gynecology, and surgery are offered. Clinical correlated conferences are conducted for related basic sciences to clinical medicine.

CLINICAL SCIENCES

The final five trimesters are committed to broad clinical exposure in the major clinical disciplines of internal medicine (12 weeks), surgery and its subspecialties (20 weeks), pediatrics (6 weeks), obstetrics and gynecology (8 weeks), psychiatry (6 weeks), family medicine (6 weeks), radiology (4 weeks), pathology (4 weeks), and clinical electives (14 weeks).

ADMISSIONS

The minimum requirement for admission is ninety (90) semester credit hours of college level work. Prerequisites are one year each of general chemistry, organic chemistry, biology, physics, English and mathematics. The MCAT is not required. Applicants from the United Kingdom, British Commonwealth of Nations, and other countries with similar educational standards must possess a baccalaureate degree and have completed courses in biology, chemistry, mathematics, and physics. However, applicants with high grades in the general certificate of education (GCE) advanced level with courses in the sciences may be considered. Prospective students from other countries with educational systems different from the British or U.S. will be evaluated on their merits.

ADMISSIONS PROCESS

In evaluating individual applicant's credentials, the Admissions Committee looks for the applicant's capacity to do academic work for absorption of the material needed for sound foundation in the basic medical sciences. Evaluation is also carried out on grade point average (GPA) from individual colleges and universities and letters of recommendation. However, academic background is not the main criterion for selection; an individual's character and motivation to become a physician are essential determinants for admission.

MISSION & OBJECTIVES

The mission of Spartan Health Sciences University, School of Medicine is to train doctors of all races and from all nations of the world rather than to indulge in parochialism of medical education. The primary objective of the university is to provide qualified students an opportunity to fulfill their lifelong ambition of serving humanity with medical education, prolongation of human life through medical care and research. The university strives hard to attain a high standard of education with affordable tuition fees ever since its inception. This does not in anyway compromise the standard of medical education offered by this institution.

STUDENT LIFE

The university's student body is made up of multiracial backgrounds. Some of the students were professionals in their fields before they were admitted; some were pharmacists, biochemists, and researchers with post-graduate degrees. The university is a microcosm of the United Nations in the pursuit of eradication of diseases that plague the human race.

9 Post-baccalaureate Pre-medical Programs

Colleges and universities offer organized post-baccalaureate pre-medical programs. Although this list is quite comprehensive, it is likely to be incomplete because many schools have just recently adopted post-bacc programs. In addition, many undergraduate institutions that do not offer formal programs have flexible enrollment policies that facilitate post-bacc studies.

For further listings of post-bacc programs, Syracuse University Health Professions Advisory Program (315-443-2321) has an online compilation at: http://services.aamc.org/postbac/.

AGNES SCOTT COLLEGE: POST-BACCALAUREATE PRE-MEDICAL PROGRAM

Dr. Lerita Coleman Brown
Program Director
141 E. College Avenue
Decatur, GA 30030
Contact: Amy Whitworth
404-471-6361
E-mail: awhitworth@agnesscott.edu

ALBRIGHT COLLEGE: POST-BACCALAUREATE PRE-MEDICAL PROGRAM

Dr. Karen A. Campbell
Program Director
Biology Department
Albright College
Reading, PA 19612-5234
610-921-7720
Fax: 610-921-7728
E-mail: kcampbell@alb.edu

AMERICAN UNIVERSITY

Post-baccalaureate Pre-medical Certificate Program
Dr. Frederick W. Carson, Pre-medical Programs Coordinator
Department of Chemistry
American University
4400 Massachusetts Avenue NW
Washington, DC 20016-8014
202-885-1770
Fax: 202-885-1752
E-mail: fcarson@american.edu

ARMSTRONG ATLANTIC STATE UNIVERSITY: POST-BACCALAUREATE PRE-MEDICAL PROGRAM

Dr. W. C. Zipperer
11935 Abercorn Street
Savannah, GA 31419
912- 921-5660
Fax: 912-961-3226
E-mail: zipperwc@mail.armstrong.edu

ASSUMPTION COLLEGE

Steven Theroux, PhD
Biology Department, Assumption College
500 Salisbury Street
Worcester, MA 01615-0005
508-767-7545
E-mail: stheroux@assumption.edu

AVILA COLLEGE: POST-BACCALAUREATE PRE-MEDICAL PROGRAM

Dr. C. Larry Sullivan, Pre-medical Advisor
11901 Wornall Road
Kansas City, MO 64145
816-501-3655
Fax: 816-501-2457
E-mail: sullivancl@mail.avila.edu

BARRY UNIVERSITY: BIOMEDICAL SCIENCES

Dr. Ralph Lauden, Associate Dean and Director
School of Natural & Health Sciences
11300 NE Second Avenue
Miami Shores, FL 33161-6695
305-899-3227 or 800-756-6000, Ext. 3541
Fax: 305-899-3232
Program Contact: Ms. Jocelyn Goulet
E-mail: healthsciences@mail.barry.edu

BENNINGTON COLLEGE: POST-BACCALAUREATE PRE-MEDICAL PROGRAM
Dr. Janet Foley
Office of Admissions
Bennington College
1 College Drive
Bennington, VT 05201
800-833-6845
Fax: 802-440-4320
Program Contact: Rachel Emmons-Bradley
E-mail: rachel@bennington.edu

BOSTON UNIVERSITY
Post-baccalaureate Certificate in Pre-medical Studies
PMC Program Coordinator
725 Commonwealth Avenue, Room 102
Boston, MA 02215
617-353-2980
617-353-4190

BOSTON UNIVERSITY SCHOOL OF MEDICINE
Susan Wilcox
GMS, Boston University School of Medicine
715 Albany Street, Suite L-317
Boston, MA 02446
617-638-5120
Fax: 617-638-4842
E-mail: wilcox@bu.edu

BRANDEIS UNIVERSITY
Post-baccalaureate Certificate Program
Jennifer Lewis
Office of Undergraduate Academic Affairs
Kutz 108/MS 001
Waltham, MA 02254-9110
781-736-3470
E-mail: jlewis@brandeis.edu

BRYN MAWR COLLEGE
Post-baccalaureate Pre-medical Program
Bryn Mawr College Canwyll House
101 North Merion Ave.
Bryn Mawr, PA 19010-2899
610-526-7350
E-mail: 610-526-7350

CARSON-NEWMAN COLLEGE
Dr. Frank Pinkerton
Program Director
Carson-Newman College
Box 71992
Jefferson City, TN 37760
865-471-3257
Fax: 865-471-3578
E-mail: fpinkerton@cn.edu

CHAPMAN UNIVERSITY
Dr. Virginia Carson,
Post-baccalaureate Pre-professional Program
One University Drive
Orange, CA 92866
714-997-6696
Fax: 714-532-6048
E-mail: carson@chapman.edu

CUNY—CITY COLLEGE
Dr. Robert Goode
J-529 Program in Pre-medical Studies
138th Street at Convent Avenue
New York, NY 10031
212-650-7843
Fax: 212-650-7816
Program Contact: L. Wood-Hill
E-mail: woodhill@sci.ccny.cuny.edu

CLEVELAND STATE UNIVERSITY
Post-baccalaureate Program
Dr. Madeline M. Hall
BGES Department 2121 Euclid, SI 219
Cleveland, OH 44115
216-687-2418
Fax: 216-687-6972
E-mail: m.hall@csuohio.edu

COLUMBIA UNIVERSITY
Post-baccalaureate Program
Mail Code 4101
2970 Broadway
New York, NY 10027
212-854-2772
E-mail: postbacc@columbia.edu

COLUMBIA UNIVERSITY
Post-baccalaureate Pre-medical Program
Dr. Mary McGee
2970 Broadway
404 Lewissohn Hall, MC 4109
New York, NY 10027
212-854-0467
Fax: 212-854-7257
E-mail: gspostbacc@columbia.edu

DARTMOUTH MEDICAL SCHOOL: CENTER FOR THE EVALUATIVE CLINICAL SCIENCES
Hinman Box 7252
Karen A. Tombs, MEd
14 MML Building
Hanover, NH 03755
603-650-1782
Fax: 603-650-1900
E-mail: karen.a.tombs@dartmouth.edu

DOMINICAN UNIVERSITY
Post-baccalaureate Pre-medical Program
7900 West Division Street
River Forest, IL 60305-1066
708-366-2490
Program Contact: Mary Woods
E-mail: woodssrm@email.dom.edu

DOWLING COLLEGE
Certificate Program in the Pre-health Professions
Dr. Richard Wilkens
Department of Biology
Oakdale, NY 11769
631-244-3491
Fax: 631-244-1033
E-mail: wilkensr@dowling.edu

DREXEL UNIVERSITY
Laura Mangano
Medical Science Preparatory Program
Drexel University College of Medicine
245 M 15th Street, MS 344, Room 4122 NCB
Philadelphia, PA 19102
215-762-4692
Fax: 215-762-7434
E-mail: imsinfo@drexel.edu

DUQUESNE UNIVERSITY
Post-baccalaureate Pre-medical Program
Dr. Kyle Selcer
B101 Bayer Learning Center
Pittsburgh, PA 15282
412-396-6335
Fax: 412-396-5587
Program Contact: Cathy Dvorak
MSW/LSW, Associate Director
E-mail: dvorak@dug.edu

EAST TENNESSEE STATE UNVERSITY
FasTrack Program
Dr. Lattie Collins
PO Box 70592—ETSU
East Tennessee State University
Johnson City, TN 37614
423-439-6903
Fax: 423-439-4840
E-mail: collinsl@mail.etsu.edu

EASTERN VIRGINIA MEDICAL SCHOOL
Medical Master's Program
Toni Dorn, Administrator
700 West Olney Road
Norfolk, VA 23507
757-446-8424
Fax: 757-446-8449
dornma@evms.edu

FISK UNIVERSITY
Mary Welsh, PhD
UNCF Pre-medical Summer Institute
1000 17th Avenue, North
Nashville, TN 37208-3051
615-329-8796
Fax: 615-329-8636
mckelvey@fisk.edu

GEORGETOWN UNIVERSITY
Adam Myers, Program Director
Special Master's Program, Department of Physiology
Georgetown University, Box 571460
Washington, DC 20057-1460
Program Contact: Ms. Aureller Cabiness
202-687-1179
Fax: 202-687-7407
E-mail: physio@georgetown

GOUCHER COLLEGE
Liza Thompson, Program Director
Post-baccalaureate Pre-medical Program
1201 Dulaney Valley Road
Baltimore, MD 21204-2794
800-414-3437
Fax: 410-337-6461
E-mail: pbpm@goucher.edu

IMMACULATA COLLEGE
Post-baccalaureate Pre-professional Program
Susan Cronin
Box 650
Immaculata, PA 19345-0650
610-647-4400, Ext. 3273
E-mail: scronin@immaculata.edu

INDIANA UNIVERSITY SCHOOL OF MEDICINE
Master of Science in Medical Science Program
Indiana University School of Medicine
Dr. William Agbor Baiyee
Medical Science Building 207
635 Barnhill Drive
Indianapolis, IN 46202
317-278-1724
317-278-5211
E-mail: msms@iupui.edu

INDIANA UNIVERSITY SCHOOL OF MEDICINE
Dr. Stephen Kempson
MS in Health Sciences
635 Barnhill Drive
Physiology—MS 309
Indianapolis, IN 46202-5120
317-274-7772
E-mail: msphysio@iupui.edu

IOWA STATE UNIVERSITY
102 Carrie Chapman Catt Hall
Ames, IA 50011
515-294-4831
Fax: 515-294-7446
E-mail: jowens@iastate.edu

JOHNS HOPKINS UNIVERSITY
Post-baccalaureate Pre-medical Program
David Trabilsy
3003 N. Charles Street
Wyman Park Building, Suite G1
Baltimore, MD 21218
410-516-7748
Fax: 410-516-6017
Program Contact: Candy Kidwell, Coordinator
E-mail: postbacc@jhu.edu

LA SALLE UNIVERSITY
Post-baccalaureate Pre-medical Certificate Program
Dr. Geri Seitchik
1900 West Olney
Philadelphia, PA 19141-1199
215-951-1248
E-mail: seichik@lasalle.edu

LAKE ERIE COLLEGE OF OSTEOPATHIC MEDICINE (LECOM)
Dr. R. Nassiri
LECOM
1858 West Grandview Boulevard
Erie, PA 16509
814-866-8146
Fax: 814-886-8411
E-mail: rnassiri@lecom.edu

LAMAR UNIVERSITY
Dr. James Westgate
College of Arts and Sciences
PO Box 10058
Beaumont, TX 77710
409-880-7972
Fax: 409-880-8007
E-mail: westgatejw@hal.lamar.edu

LOMA LINDA UNIVERSITY
Biomedical Sciences Certificate
Dr. Ramon Gonzalez, Jr.
School of Graduate Studies
West Hall, Room 1301
Loma Linda, CA 92350
909-558-4564
Fax: 909-558-0119
E-mail: rgonzalez@som.llu.edu

LOYOLA MARYMOUNT UNIVERSITY
1 LMU Drive
MS 8140
Los Angeles, CA 90045-2659
310-338-2823
Fax: 310-338-7339
E-mail: sscheck@lmu.edu

LOYOLA UNIVERSITY OF CHICAGO
Post-baccalaureate Pre-health Program
Loyola University Chicago Grad. & Prof. Enrollment
820 North Michigan Avenue, LT 800
Chicago, IL 60611-2196
773-508-3636 or 312-915-8900

LOYOLA UNIVERSITY OF CHICAGO
Master of Arts in Medical Sciences
Dr. Diane Suter, Graduate Program Director
Department of Biology
6525 North Sheridan Road
Chicago, IL 60626
773-508-3285
E-mail: dsuter@luc.edu

MANHATTANVILLE COLLEGE
Post-baccalaureate Pre-health Professions Program
Academic Advising Office
2900 Purchase Street
Purchase, NY 10577
914-798-2755
Fax: 914-323-5338
Program Contact: Andrew Bodenrader
E-mail: bodenradera@mville.edu

MIDWESTERN UNIVERSITY
Fred D. Romano, PhD
555 31st Street
Downers Grove, IL 60515
630-515-6392
Fax: 630-971-6414
E-mail: froman@midwestern.edu

MILLS COLLEGE
Post-baccalaureate Program
5000 MacArthur Boulevard
Oakland, CA 94613
510-430-2317
Fax: 510-430-3314
Program Contact: Nancy Hutcheon
E-mail: nhutcheo@mills.edu

MOUNT HOLYOKE
Frances Perkins Post-baccalaureate Studies Program
Kay Althoff
6 Safford Hall
50 College Street
South Hadley, MA 01075
413-538-2077
Fax: 413-538-3013
E-mail: frances-perkins@mtholyoke.edu

NATIONAL INSTITUTES OF HEALTH
NIH Post-baccalaureate Training Program
Building 2, Room 2E6
2 Center Drive MSC 0240
Bethesda, MA 20892-0240
301-402-1917
Fax: 301-402-8975
Program Contact: Debbie Cohen
E-mail: cohend@od.nih.gov

NEW YORK MEDICAL COLLEGE
Graduate School of Basic Medical Sciences
Basic Sciences Building, Room A-41
Valhalla, NY 10595
Program Contact: Marge Riley
914-594-4110
Fax: 914-594-4944
E-mail: marge_riley@nymc.edu

NEW YORK UNIVERSITY
Pre-health Advisor
College of Arts and Science
Main Building
100 Washington Square East
Room 904
New York, NY 10003
212-998-8160

NEW YORK UNIVERSITY
Post-baccalaureate/Pre-health Studies
Ms. Charlene Visconti
Silver Professional Center
100 Washington Square East, #901
New York, NY 10003-6699
212-998-8160
Fax: 212-995-4549
E-mail: prehealth@nyu.edu

NORTHWESTERN UNIVERSITY SCHOOL OF CONTINUING STUDIES
Pre-medical Professional Health Careers Program
Admissions Coordinator
Annenberg Hall, Suite 162
2120 Campus Drive
Evanston, IL 60208-2650
847-491-0990
Fax: 491-3660
E-mail: a-simmons@northwestern.edu

OLD DOMINION UNIVERSITY
Pre-health Advisory Committee
Ms. Sharon Melone-Orme
College of Sciences
OCNPS 131
Norfolk, VA 23529-0163
757-683-5200
Fax: 757-683-3034
E-mail: smelone@odu.edu

PENNSYLVANIA STATE UNIVERSITY
Post-baccalaureate Pre-medical Certificate Program
Dr. Rodriguez
213 Whitmore Lab
University Park, PA 16802
814-865-7620
Fax: 814-865-7214
E-mail: mxr22@psu.edu

PHILADELPHIA COLLEGE OF OSTEOPATHIC MEDICINE
Biomedical Sciences Program
Office of Admissions
4170 City Avenue
Philadelphia, PA 19131
800-999-6998
Fax: 215-871-6719
admissions@pcom.edu

RICHARD STOCKTON COLLEGE OF NEW JERSEY
Post-baccalaureate Certificate Program in Health Professions
Dr. Ralph Werner
Jim Leeds Road
Pomona, NJ 08240
609-652-4462
E-mail: ralph.werner@stockton.edu

RIDER UNIVERSITY
Department of Biology
Dr. Julie Drawbridge
2083 Lawrenceville Road
Lawrenceville, NJ 08648
609-895-5428
Fax: 609-895-5782
E-mail: drawbridge@rider.edu

ROCKHURST UNIVERSITY
Post-baccalaureate Pre-medical Program
Dr. James Wheeler
Department of Chemistry
1100 Rockhurst Road
Kansas City, MO 64110
816-501-4068
Fax: 816-501-4169
E-mail: james.wheeler@rockhurst.edu

RUTGERS UNIVERSITY—NEWARK
Post-baccalaureate Pre-medical Program
Dr. John M. Maiello
306 Hill Hall
Newark, NJ 07102-1801
973-353-5705
Fax: 973-353-1419
E-mail: jmaiello@andromeda.rutgers.edu

SAN DIEGO STATE UNIVERSITY
Pre-professional Health Advising Office
Barbara Huntington
5500 Campanile Drive
MC-1017
San Diego, CA 92182-1017
619-594-6638
Fax: 619-594-0244
E-mail: healthpr@sciences.sdsu.edu

SAN FRANCISCO STATE UNIVERSITY
Health Professions Prep and Re-applicant Program
Dr. Barry Rothman
1600 Holloway Avenue
San Francisco, CA 94132
415-338-2410
Fax: 415-338-2295
E-mail: hpac@sfsu.edu

SAN JOSE STATE UNIVERSITY
Post-baccalaureate Pre-medical Program
Dr. Robert Fowler
Department of Biological Sciences
San Jose, CA 95192
408-924-4900 or 408-924-4843
Fax: 408-924-4840
E-mail: rfowler@email.sjsu.edu

SCRIPPS COLLEGE
Post-baccalaureate Pre-medical Program
Ms. Jodi Olson
W. M. Keck Science Center
925 North Mills Avenue
Claremont, CA 91711
909-621-8764
Fax: 909-8588
E-mail: Jolson@scrippscollege.edu

SEATTLE UNIVERSITY
Post-baccalaureate Pre-medical Program
Dr. Margaret Hudson
Biology Department Seattle University
Seattle, WA 98122
206-296-5486
E-mail: mhudson@seattleu.edu

SOUTHERN ILLINOIS UNIVERSITY SCHOOL OF MEDICINE
Medical/Dental Education Preparatory Program (MEDPREP)
Dr. Harold Bardo, Program Director
Wheeler Hall
Carbondale, IL 62901-4323
618-453-1554
Fax: 618-453-1919
Program Contact: Vera Felts
E-mail: vfelts@siumed.edu

SPRING HILL COLLEGE
Post-baccalaureate Pre-medical Studies
Dr. David Dean
4000 Dauphin Street
Mobile, AL 36608
215-380-3067
Fax: 215-460-2190
Program Contact: Nick Saacks
E-mail: nsaacks@shc.edu

SUNY AT BUFFALO
Roswell Park Cancer Institute
Interdisciplinary Biomed/Oncology MS Program
Mr. Craig Johnson
408 Research Studies Center
Buffalo, NY 14263-0001
716-845-2339
Fax: 716-845-8178
E-mail: gradapp@roswellpark.org

SUNY AT STONY BROOK
Post-baccalaureate Pre-medical Program
James Montren
Room E2360
Stony Brook, NY 11704-3353
631-632-7093
E-mail: prehealth@notes.cc.sunysb.edu

TEXAS CHRISTIAN UNIVERSITY
Ruth Eakin
Box 298800
Fort Worth, TX 76129
817-257-5337
Fax: 817-257-6177
E-mail: r.eakin@tcu.edu

TUFTS UNIVERSITY
Post-baccalaureate Pre-medical Program
Carol Baffi-Dugan
419 Boston Avenue
Dowling Hall
Medford, MA 02155
Program Contact: Liz Regan
617-627-2321
Fax: 617-627-3907
E-mail: liz.regan@tufts.edu

TULANE UNIVERSITY
Hayward Genetics Center One-year Master's Degree Program
Gayle Pullen
1430 Tulane Avenue
New Orleans, LA 70112
504-584-1981
Fax: 504-584-3684
E-mail: hgcedprg@tulane.edu

UNIVERSITY OF CALIFORNIA DAVIS SCHOOL OF MEDICINE
Post-baccalaureate Re-applicant Program
Edward Dagang
One Shields Avenue
Davis, CA 95616
Program Contact: Alan Blakely
503-754-6033
Fax: 503-754-6252
E-mail: awblakely@ucdavis.edu

UNIVERSITY OF CALIFORNIA IRVINE COLLEGE OF MEDICINE
Pre-medical Post-baccalaureate Enhancement Program
Emma Ledesma
Office of Admissions and Outreach
College of Medicine
Medical Education Building 802
Irvine, CA 92697-4089
800-824-5388
Fax: 949-824-2485
E-mail: ppep@uci.edu

UNIVERSITY OF CALIFORNIA IRVINE COLLEGE OF MEDICINE
Post-baccalaureate Re-applicant Program
Ms. Ellen Munoz
Medical Education Building 802
PO Box 4089
Irvine, CA 92697-4089
949-824-8930
E-mail: pbreapp@uci.edu

UNIVERSITY OF CALIFORNIA LOS ANGELES, DAVID GEFFEN SCHOOL OF MEDICINE
13-154 CHS Office of Academic Enrichment and Outreach
10833 Le Conte Avenue
Los Angeles, CA 90095
310-825-3575
Fax: 310-206-7180
E-mail: aeotemp2@mednet.ucla.edu

UNIVERSITY OF CALIFORNIA SAN DIEGO SCHOOL OF MEDICINE
Re-applicant Post-baccalaureate Program
Saundra Kirk
Student Outreach Services
Date Building, Room 105
La Jolla, CA 92093-0655
858-534-4171
Fax: 858-534-5293
E-mail: sjkirk@ucsd.edu

UNIVERSITY OF CALIFORNIA SAN FRANCISCO
UCSF Post-baccalaureate Programs
Valerie Margol
1855 Folsom Street
MCB: Room 566H
San Francisco, CA 94143-0409
Program Contact: Gabrielle Fisher
415-514-1390
Fax: 415-502-1680
E-mail: fisherg@medsch.ucsf.edu

UNIVERSITY OF CONNECTICUT SCHOOL OF MEDICINE
Post-baccalaureate Program
Keat Sanford
Admissions Center
263 Farmington Avenue
Farmington, CT 06030-3906
Program Contact: Tricia Avolt
860-679-4306
Fax: 860-679-1899
E-mail: robertson@nso2.uchc.edu

UNIVERSITY OF MARYLAND—COLLEGE PARK
Science in the Evening
Dr. Joelle Presson
1322 Symons Hall
University of Maryland
College Park, MD 20742
301-405-6892
E-mail: jpresson@umd.edu

UNIVERSITY OF MASSACHUSETTS—BOSTON
Post-baccalaureate Pre-medical Program
Grace McSorley
University Career Services
100 Morrissey Boulevard
Boston, MA 02125
617-287-5519
Fax: 617-287-5525
E-mail: grace.mcsorley@umb.edu

UMDNJ, GRADUATE SCHOOL OF BIOMEDICAL SCIENCES
Master's in Biomedical Sciences
Dr. Nicholas Ingoglia
ADMC 1, Suite 110
Newark, NJ 07103
973-972-4776 or 973-972-4511
Fax: 973-972-5656
E-mail: ingoglia@umdnj.edu

UNIVERSITY OF MIAMI
Pre-medical Post-baccalaureate Program
Deborah Paris
205 Ashe Building
Coral Gables, FL 33124-4622
Program Contact: Kathleen Kelly
305-284-5176
Fax: 305-284-4686
E-mail: kkelly@miami.edu

UNIVERSITY OF NORTH CAROLINA—GREENSBORO
Pre-medical Program
Post-Baccalaureate Premed Program, UNC—Greensboro
Robert E. Cannon, PhD
Department of Biology, PO Box 26170
Greensboro, NC 27402-6170
336-256-0071
Fax: 336-334-5839
E-mail: Robert_Cannon@uncg.edu

UNIVERSITY OF NORTH FLORIDA
Post-baccalaureate Pre-medical Program
Dr. Ray Bowman
4567 St. Johns Bluff Road South
Jacksonville, FL 32224
904-620-2608
E-mail: rbowman@unf.edu

UNIVERSITY OF OREGON
Post-baccalaureate Pre-medical Program
Office of Academic Advising 5217
University of Oregon
Eugene, OR 97403-5217
541-346-3211
Fax: 541-346-6048
E-mail: karenc@darkwing.uoregon.edu

UNIVERSITY OF PENNSYLVANIA
Pre-health Program
Dr. Lynne Hunter
3440 Market Street, Suite 100
College of General Studies
Philadelphia, PA 19104-3335
215-898-3110
Fax: 215-573-2053
E-mail: lynneh@sas.upenn.edu

UNIVERSITY OF PITTSBURGH
CAS Post-baccalaureate Program
Donna Walker
252 Thackeray Hall
Pittsburgh, PA 15260
412-624-6444
Fax: 412-624-3707
E-mail: dlw5@pitt.edu

UNIVERSITY OF PITTSBURGH
Arts and Sciences Post-baccalaureate Program
Donna Walker
252 Thackeray Hall
Pittsburgh, PA 15260
412-624-6444
Fax: 412-624-3707
E-mail: dlw5@pitt.edu

UNIVERSITY OF SOUTH FLORIDA
Biomedical Sciences
4202 E. Fowler Ave.
SCA 400
Tampa, FL 33620
813-974-2144
Fax: 813-974-5314
E-mail: chemadvising@cas.usf.edu

UNIVERSITY OF SOUTHERN CALIFORNIA
Post-baccalaureate Pre-medical Program
Admissions Coordinator
CAS 120, USC College
Los Angeles, CA 90089-0151
213-821-2354
Fax: 213-740-3664
E-mail: CAS@usc.edu

UNIVERSITY OF UTAH SCHOOL OF MEDICINE
Summer MCAP Preparation & Research/Clinical Training Program
Ms. Sunshine Nakae-Gibson
30 North 1900 East
Room 1C117
Salt Lake City, UT 84132-2101
801-585-2430
Fax: 801-585-3300
E-mail: sunny.gibson@hsc.utah.edu

UNIVERSITY OF VERMONT
Post-baccalaureate Pre-medical Program
Beth Taylor-Nolan
1322 South Prospect Street
Burlington, VT 05401
802-656-2085
Fax: 802-656-0306
E-mail: Beth.Taylor-Nolan@uvm.edu

VIRGINIA COMMONWEALTH UNIVERSITY
Pre-medical Basic Sciences
Dr. Jan Chlebowski
Office of Graduate Education VCU School of Medicine
1101 E. Marshall Street Box 980565
Richmond, VA 23298-9565
804-828-8366
Fax: 804-828-6011
E-mail: jfchlebo@vcu.edu

WAKE FOREST UNIVERSITY SCHOOL OF MEDICINE
Brenda Latham-Sadler
Medical Center Boulevard
Office of Student Services
Winston-Salem, NC 27157
Program Contact: Shirley Dockery
336-716-4271
Fax: 336-716-4271
E-mail: sdockery@wfubmc.edu

WEST CHESTER UNIVERSITY
Pre-medical Program
Dr. Melissa Cichowicz
117 Schmucker Science Center South
West Chester, PA 19383
610-436-2978
Fax: 610-436-3277
E-mail: pmed@wcupa.edu

WORCESTER STATE COLLEGE
Dr. Allan Cooper
Pre-medical Advisor
486 Chandler Street
Worcester, MA 01602
508-929-8600
E-mail: acooper@worcester.edu

ALPHABETICAL INDEX

INDEX BY LOCATION

USA

ALABAMA

ARIZONA

ARKANSAS

CALIFORNIA

COLORADO

CONNECTICUT

DISTRICT OF COLUMBIA

FLORIDA

GEORGIA

HAWAII

ILLINOIS

INDIANA

IOWA

KANSAS

KENTUCKY

LOUISIANA

MAINE

MARYLAND

ABOUT THE AUTHOR

Malaika Stoll is a recent graduate of Stanford Medical School. She grew up in Berkeley, California, and graduated from Dartmouth College. After college she worked for two years as a Health Educator with the Peace Corps in Zaire. She earned a master's degree in public affairs from Princeton University, and went on to work in international health and development for the World Bank and the United States Agency for International Development. She completed her science requirements at Goucher College's Post-bacc Pre-medical Program. She is about to begin her family practice residency at Lehigh Valley Hospital in Pennsylvania.

More expert advice from **The Princeton Review**

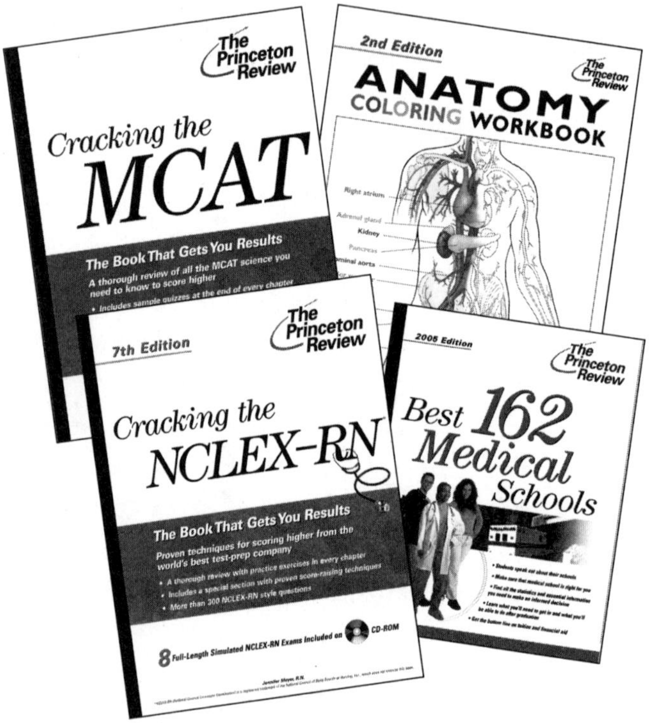

CRACKING THE MCAT WITH PRACTICE QUESTIONS ON CD-ROM
0-375-76352-X • $59.95

PRACTICE MCATs
0-375-76456-9 • $22.95

CRACKING THE NCLEX-RN
7TH EDITION
0-375-76316-3 • $25.00

CRACKING THE NCLEX-RN WITH SAMPLE TESTS ON CD-ROM
7TH EDITION
0-375-76302-3 • $34.95
WIN/MAC COMPATIBLE

ANATOMY COLORING WORKBOOK
2ND EDITION
0-375-76342-2 • $19.00

BIOLOGY COLORING WORKBOOK
0-679-77884-5 • $18.00

HUMAN BRAIN COLORING WORKBOOK
0-679-77885-3 • $17.00

PHYSIOLOGY COLORING WORKBOOK
0-679-77850-0 • $18.00

BEST 162 MEDICAL SCHOOLS
0-375-76420-8 • $22.95

GUIDE TO CAREERS IN THE HEALTH PROFESSIONS
0-375-76158-6 • $24.95

If you want to give yourself the best chance for getting into the medical school of your choice, we can help you get the highest test scores, make the most informed choices, and make the most of your experience once you get there. Whether you want to be an M.D., a nurse, or any other kind of health care professional, we can even help you ace the tests and make a career move that will let you use your skills and education to their best advantage.

The Princeton Review

Available at Bookstores Everywhere.
www.PrincetonReview.com